EXPRESSION OF DIFFERENTIATED FUNCTIONS IN CANCER CELLS

Expression of Differentiated Functions in Cancer Cells

Editors

Roberto P. Revoltella
Laboratory of Cell Biology
National Research Council
Rome, Italy

Giuseppe M. Pontieri
Institute of General Pathology
University of Rome
Rome, Italy

Claudio Basilico
Department of Pathology
New York University Medical Center
New York, New York

Giovanni Rovera
The Wistar Institute of Anatomy and
Biology
Philadelphia, Pennsylvania

Robert C. Gallo
Laboratory of Tumor Cell Biology
National Cancer Institute
National Institutes of Health
Bethesda, Maryland

John H. Subak-Sharpe
Department of Virology
Institute of Virology
Glasgow, United Kingdom

Raven Press ■ New York

Raven Press, 1140 Avenue of the Americas, New York, New York 10036

Made in the United States of America

Library of Congress Cataloging in Publication Data
Main entry under title:

Expression of differentiated functions in cancer cells.

"Proceedings of the first Workshop on Cell Differenti-
ation and Neoplastic Transformation...held in Venice, Italy, April 6–10, 1981."—
Pref.
"Sponsored by the Italian National Council of Research
...[et al.]."—Acknowl.
Includes bibliographical references and index.
1. Cancer cells—Congresses.   2. Cell differentiation
—Congresses.   3. Cell proliferation—Congresses.
4. Host-virus relationships—Congresses.   I. Revoltella,
Roberto P.   II. Workshop on Cell Differentiation and
Neoplastic Transformation (1st : 1981 : Venice, Italy)
III. Consiglio nazionale delle ricerche (Italy) [DNLM:
1. Cell differentiation—Congresses.   2. Cell transforma-
tion, Neoplastic—Congresses. QZ 202 E96 1981]
RC267.E94   616.99'407   81–23483
ISBN 0–89004–693–X   AACR2

Preface

This volume presents an up-to-date comprehensive review of cell differentiation and neoplastic transformation. The complexity and the ever-increasing variety of pertinent data point to the need for such a review in order to provide a coherent picture and a dialogue with members of this vast community of scientists.

A large number of outstanding experts with a wide range of perspectives have contributed to this volume. The authors were invited to report new experimental data and provide recent references in their field of expertise. The topics covered include determination and segregation of cell lineages during development and differentiation, immunologic and genetic markers during development and differentiation of different cell lineages, control of growth and normal differentiation in malignant cells, and interaction of virus and host cells. Many new, interesting data are presented, resulting in a volume that provides a precious source of up-to-date accumulated information and delineates the needs, opportunities, and stimuli for new approaches and prospects for this exciting and rapidly developing research field.

This volume will be of interest to research oncologists and to cellular and molecular biologists.

Roberto P. Revoltella
Giuseppe M. Pontieri

Acknowledgments

This volume results from the proceedings of the first Workshop on Cell Differentiation and Neoplastic Transformation, entitled "Expression Of Differentiated Functions In Cancer Cells," held in Venice, Italy, April 6–10, 1981. This is the first of a series of workshops that will be held every two years.

The Workshop was officially sponsored by the Italian National Council of Research, the State Departments of Public Education and Foreign Affairs, the European Molecular Biology Organization, and the City Council of Venice. Grants were also obtained from the Fondazione Giovanni Lorenzini, Milan, several national and local banks, private institutions such as Farmitalia, Lepetit, Fidia, Lagitre, scientific laboratory product companies, and other local sources that we wish to thank for their generous support which made this workshop possible.

In particular, we wish to express our thanks to Dr. Mario Rigo, the Mayor of Venice, Dr. Nereo Laroni, Head of the Health Department Planning of the City of Venice, and to all of their collaborators for the gracious hospitality and for helping us to enjoy both the meeting and the beauty of the city. We are deeply grateful to the Advisory Scientific Committee (Drs. C. Basilico, G. Rovera, R. C. Gallo, L. Diamond, C. Friend, J. Subak-Sharpe), to the session chairpersons for many helpful suggestions and critical surveys of the topics of their sessions and for regulating the presentations, and to all of the speakers for coming to Venice and sharing their most recent findings and thoughts with us. We also wish to thank Drs. Luisa Lenti, Giuliana Boera, and Oliviero Vernier for their invaluable assistance in organizing the meeting and gratefully acknowledge the help of Dr. Emanuela Folco of the Fondazione Lorenzini and the editorial office of Raven Press, New York, in chasing late-coming manuscripts and handling the editorial process as well.

Opening Address

The Community Administration is pleased to welcome all the guests, on behalf of the City of Venice, gathered together for this important workshop.

The topics which have been dealt with by you in these past few days, remind me of some general considerations that I would like to pass on to you. The first refers to the relationship between the verification of certain pathologies and the presence of environmental conditions that can affect to some degree, the same pathological processes. As you know, the problem of environmental pollution is not unique to Venice. Our greatest hope is to save the city, and above all, the inhabitants, by means of comprehensive methods of cleaning up environmental conditions, so as to guarantee the equilibrium of the lagunal ecosystem. The necessity to promote scientific research aimed at different problems converges on that of the defense of the environment and of the citizen. Here, then, our enthusiasm rests on all those initiatives of the present workshop that are aimed directly or indirectly towards this end of civilized progress. It will also be remembered that the City of Venice, characterized as a place promoting and valuing culture, wishes to make a contribution to the improvement of the living conditions of man. For this reason, Venice is extremely happy and honoured to give space, time, and hospitality, now and in the future, to initiatives such as this. Great prestige will be derived from hosting this workshop.

Some ten years ago, an international team of researchers at Massachusetts Institute of Technology began a study of the implications of continued worldwide growth. They launched the appeal towards "global equilibrium," through the auspices of the "Club di Roma." Today, you scientists with this "Venice Workshop" could launch a message of hope to man. The effort in the field of cancer research over these last ten years has been enormous and many contributions have been achieved, particularly regarding the relationship of cell-differentiation and neoplastic transformation. This research field will probably contribute significantly to a better understanding of the mechanisms that regulate the deviation from normality. This approach may be a truly useful one for studying cancer. It is true that great progress has been made in the finer diagnostic processes, technology, and treatment of the disease. It is true that suitable therapies have been found, at least for some types of tumors (in surgery, and also in chemotherapy and radiotherapy). However, it is also true that the level of positive results after therapeutic treatment, in time, if compared with the rate of mortality, has changed little or not at all, in the majority of types of tumors, in the last 45 years. Moreover, if one looks at the explosive growth in the production of chemical substances, and the consequent deterioration of the environment from the 1960s, an increase in the incidence of tumors in the 1980s is understandable.

It is therefore the general conviction at the moment that it would be worthwhile to define a new strategy and new avenues of research in the fight against cancer. If prevention of tumors is perhaps now of primary importance, in order to obtain valid results, it is necessary to be more aware of the etiopathogenesis of the neoplastic disease, the mechanism of onset, and the regulation of the tumor cells. It is for this reason that we believe it has been a suitable and productive moment to organise a workshop that is aimed at focusing on the problem of cellular differentiation and its relationship to cancer.

The title of the workshop has underlined this objective. You, who represent highly qualified world experts in the field of cellular differentiation and of tumor cells, in particular, who have, in the recent past, produced much significant and original work, you know that the city of Venice is with you in the effort aimed at reducing this spreading illness.

Congratulations on the excellent work carried out in your research laboratories. We sincerely hope that we shall have the opportunity to meet again soon.

Dr. Mario Rigo
City Council of Venice

Contents

ix

Interaction of Virus and Host Cell

Effects of Virus Expression on Normal Cell Differentiation

Short Communications

Contributors

L. Adorini
CNEN-Euratom Immunogenetics Group
Laboratory of Radiopathology
CSN Casaccia
00060 Rome, Italy

N. Affara
Beatson Institute for Cancer Research
Glasgow G61 1BD, Scotland

André van Agthoven
Sidney Farber Cancer Institute and Department
of Pathology
Harvard Medical School
Boston, Massachusetts 02115

S. Alemà
Laboratory of Cell Biology
C.N.R.
00196 Rome, Italy

F. Ameglio
Laboratorio di Biologia Cellulare
National Research Council
Rome, Italy

Leif C. Andersson
Transplantation Laboratory and Department of
Pathology
University of Helsinki
SF-00290 Helsinki 29, Finland

J. T. August
Department of Pharmacology and Experimental
Therapeutics
The Johns Hopkins University School of
Medicine
Baltimore, Maryland 21205

Judy Banks
Memorial Sloan-Kettering Cancer Center
New York, New York 10021

E. Barbanti
CNR Center of Cytopharmacology
Department of Pharmacology
University of Milan
20129 Milan, Italy

Claudio Basilico
Department of Pathology
New York University School of Medicine
New York, New York 10016

Thomas L. Benjamin
Department of Pathology
Harvard Medical School
Boston, Massachusetts 02115

G. Bennett
Department of Anatomy
School of Medicine
University of Pennsylvania
Philadelphia, Pennsylvania 19104

J. Bilello
Institute of Physiological Chemistry
University of Hamburg
2000 Hamburg 13, West Germany

K. Bister
Department of Molecular Biology
University of California
Berkeley, California 94720

C. Blat
Institut de Recherches
Scientifiques sur le Cancer
Laboratoire de Dynamique Cellulaire
B.P. No. 8
94082 Villejuif, France

Jannie Borst
Sidney Farber Cancer Institute and Department
of Pathology
Harvard Medical School
Boston, Massachusetts 02115

Theodore R. Breitman
Laboratory of Tumor Cell Biology
National Cancer Institute
Bethesda, Maryland 20205

Samuel Broder
Metabolism Branch
National Cancer Institute
National Institutes of Health
Bethesda, Maryland 20205

R. H. Butler
Laboratorio di Biologia Cellulare
National Research Council
Rome, Italy

Franco Calabi
Gruppo di Microbiologia e Patologia Generale
Facoltà di Scienze
University of Rome
00185 Rome, Italy

M. R. Capobianchi
Instituto di Virologia
University of Rome
Rome, Italy

M. D. Cappellini
Terza Cattedra di Clinica Medica
Università degli Studi di Milano
Milan, Italy

Graham Carpenter
Department of Biochemistry and Division of
    Dermatology
Department of Medicine
Vanderbilt University
School of Medicine
Nashville, Tennessee 37232

C. Casimir
Beatson Institute for Cancer Research
Glasgow G61 1BD, Scotland

Zi-xing Chen
Memorial Sloan-Kettering Cancer Center
New York, New York 10021

R. Ciccariello
Istituto Patologia Medica
University of Naples
Naples, Italy

Livia Cioé
The Wistar Institute
Philadelphia, Pennsylvania 19104

J. B. Clements
Institute of Virology
University of Glasgow
Glasgow G11 5JR, Scotland

John M. Coffin
Department of Molecular Biology and
    Microbiology
Tufts University School of Medicine
Boston, Massachusetts 02111

Stanley Cohen
Department of Biochemistry and Division of
    Dermatology
Vanderbilt University School of Medicine
Nashville, Tennessee 37232

G. Colletta
Centro di Endocrinologia e Oncologia
    Sperimentale del C.N.R.
Istituto di Patologia Generale
II Facoltà di Medicina e Chirurgia
Università di Napoli
80131 Naples, Italy

P. Comi
Centro per lo Studio della Patologia Cellulare
Istituto Patologia Generale
Università di Milano
Milan, Italy

Kathleen F. Conklin
Department of Molecular Biology and
    Microbiology
Tufts University School of Medicine
Boston, Massachusetts 02111

Giorgio Corte
Istituto di Chimica Biologica
University of Genoa
16132 Genoa, Italy

G. Cosu
Istituto di Istologia
University of Rome
Rome, Italy

A. Covelli
Istituto Patologia Medica
University of Naples
Naples, Italy

A. Cowie
Transcription Laboratory
Imperial Cancer Research Fund
London WC2A 3PX, England

Carlo M. Croce
The Wistar Institute of Anatomy and Biology
Philadelphia, Pennsylvania 19104

H. H. M. Dahl
Laboratory of Gene Structure and Expression
National Institute for Medical Research
London NW7 1AA, United Kingdom

E. de Boer
Laboratory of Gene Structure and Expression
National Institute for Medical Research
London NW7 1AA, United Kingdom

Giuliano Della Valle
Department of Pathology
New York University
School of Medicine
New York, New York 10016

Joseph E. De Larco
Laboratory of Viral Carcinogenesis
National Cancer Institute
Frederick Cancer Research Facility
Frederick, Maryland 21701

Leila Diamond
The Wistar Institute
Philadelphia, Pennsylvania 19104

F. Dieterlen-Lièvre
Institut d'Embryologie du CNRS et du Collège
  de France
49 bis
Avenue de la Belle Gabrielle
94130 Nogent-sur-Marne, France

P. P. Di Fiore
Centro di Endocrinologia e Oncologia
  Sperimentale del C.N.R.
Istituto di Patologia Generale
II Facoltà di Medicina e Chirurgia
Università di Napoli
80131 Naples, Italy

Dino Dina
Department of Genetics
Albert Einstein College of Medicine
Bronx, New York 10461

A. Dlugosz
Department of Anatomy
School of Medicine
University of Pennsylvania
Philadelphia, Pennsylvania 19104

A. Dolei
Cattedra di Patologia Generale
University of Camerino
Camerino, Italy

G. Doria
CNEN-Euratom Immunogenetics Group
  Laboratory of Radiopathology
CSN Casaccia
00060 Rome, Italy

P. Duesberg
Department of Molecular Biology
University of California
Berkeley, California 94720

R. P. Eglin
Institute of Virology
University of Glasgow
Glasgow G11 5JR, Scotland

Elliot Epner
Memorial Sloan-Kettering Cancer Center
New York, New York 10021

Eleanor Erikson
Department of Pathology
University of Colorado
School of Medicine
Denver, Colorado 80262

R. L. Erikson
Department of Pathology
University of Colorado
School of Medicine
Denver, Colorado 80262

Jeffrey Faust
The Wistar Institute of Anatomy and Biology
Philadelphia, Pennsylvania 19104

J. Favaloro
Transcription Laboratory
Imperial Cancer Research Fund
London WC2A 3PX, England

Robert G. Fenton
Department of Pathology
New York University School of Medicine
New York, New York 10016

M. Ferrentino
Centro di Endocrinologia e Oncologia
  Sperimentale del C.N.R.
Istituto di Patologia Generale
II Facoltà di Medicina e Chirurgia
Università di Napoli
80131 Naples, Italy

R. A. Flavell
Laboratory of Gene Structure and Expression
National Institute for Medical Research
London NW7 1AA, United Kingdom

M. Freshney
The Beatson Institute for Cancer Research
Bearsden, Glasgow G61 1BD, Scotland

C. Friend
Center for Experimental Cell Biology
Mollie B. Roth Laboratory
Mount Sinai School of Medicine
Cit University of New York
New York, New York 10029

D. K. Fujii
Cancer Research Institute
University of California Medical Center
San Francisco, California 94143

A. Fusco
Centro di Endocrinologia e Oncologia
Sperimentale del C.N.R.
Istituto di Patologia Generale
II Facoltà di Medicina e Chirurgia
Università di Napoli
80131 Naples, Italy

Carl G. Gahmberg
Department of Biochemistry
University of Helsinki
SF-00290 Helsinki 29, Finland

Robert C. Gallo
Laboratory of Tumor Cell Biology
National Cancer Institute
National Institutes of Health
Bethesda, Maryland 20205

Roberto Gambari
Memorial Sloan-Kettering Cancer Center
New York, New York 10021

C. Garon
Tumor Virus Genetics Laboratory
National Cancer Institute
National Institutes of Health
Bethesda, Maryland 20205

A. M. Gianni
Clinica Medica I
Università di Milano
Milan, Italy

B. Giglioni
Centro per lo Studio della Patologia Cellulare
Istituto Patologia Generale
Università di Milano
Milan, Italy

D. W. Golde
Division of Hematology-Oncology
Department of Medicine
UCLA School of Medicine
Los Angeles, California 90024

P. Goldfarb
Beatson Institute for Cancer Research
Glasgow G61 1BD, Scotland

D. Gospodarowicz
Cancer Research Institute
University of California Medical Center
San Francisco, California 94143

E. Gresick
Laboratorio di Biologia Cellulare
C.N.R.
Rome, Italy

M. Grieco
Centro di Endocrinologia e Oncologia
Sperimentale del C.N.R.
Istituto di Patologia Generale
II Facoltà di Medicina e Chirurgia
Università di Napoli
80131 Naples, Italy

J. E. Groopman
Division of Hematology-Oncology
Department of Medicine
UCLA School of Medicine
Los Angeles, California 90024
and Veterans Administration Hospital
Sepulveda, California 91343

F. G. Grosveld
Laboratory of Gene Structure and Expression
National Institute for Medical Research
London NW7 1AA, United Kingdom

G. C. Grosveld
Laboratory of Gene Structure and Expression
National Institute for Medical Research
London NW7 1AA, United Kingdom

L. Harel
Institut de Recherches
Scientifiques sur le Cancer
Laboratoire de Dynamique Cellulaire
B.P. No. 8
94082 Villejuif, France

P. R. Harrison
Beatson Institute for Cancer Research
Glasgow G61 1BD, Scotland

John K. Heath
University of Oxford
Department of Zoology
Oxford OX1 3PS, England

H. Holtzer
Department of Anatomy
School of Medicine
University of Pennsylvania
Philadelphia, Pennsylvania 19104

Kay Huebner
The Wistar Institute of
Anatomy and Biology
Philadelphia, Pennsylvania 19104

D. Hughes
The Beatson Institute for Cancer Research
Bearsden, Glasgow G61 1BD, Scotland

E. N. Hughes
Department of Pharmacology and Experimental
*   Therapeutics*
The Johns Hopkins University
School of Medicine
Baltimore, Maryland 21205

T. Huyn
Mollie B. Roth Laboratory
Center for Experimental Cell Biology
Mount Sinai School of Medicine
City University of New York
New York, New York 10029

Rudolf Jaenisch
Heinrich-Pette Institut für Experimentelle
*   Virologie und Immunologie an der*
*   Universität Hamburg*
200 Hamburg 20, Federal Republic of Germany

C. Jasmin
ICIG
Department of Virology
94800 Villejuif, France

G. R. Johnson
Cancer Research Unit
Walter and Eliza Hall
Institute of Medical Research
P.O. Royal Melbourne Hospital
3050 Victoria, Australia

V. S. Kalyanaraman
Laboratory of Tumor Cell Biology
National Cancer Institute
National Institutes of Health
Bethesda, Maryland 20205

R. Kamen
Transcription Laboratory
Imperial Cancer Research Fund
London WC2A 3PX, England

H. C. Kitchener
Institute of Virology
University of Glasgow
Glasgow G11 5JR, Scotland

B. Klein
Laboratoire d'Immunopharmacologie des
*   Tumeurs*
Centre Paul Lamarque
Hôpital St.-Eloi
34033 Montpellier, France

F. Lacour
Institut Gustave Roussy
C.N.R.S.
Laboratoire d'Immunologie
94800 Villejuif, France

G. Lambertenghi-Deliliers
Prima Cattedra di Clinica Medica
Università degli Studi di Milano
Milan, Italy

Beverly Lange
The Division of Oncology
Children's Hospital of Philadelphia
Philadelphia, Pennsylvania 19104

Debra Laskin
The Wistar Institute of Anatomy and Biology
Philadelphia, Pennsylvania 19104

Deborah Lebman
The Wistar Institute of Anatomy and Biology
Philadelphia, Pennsylvania 19104

Kenneth LeClair
Sidney Farber Cancer Institute and Department
*   of Pathology*
Harvard Medical School
Boston, Massachusetts 02115

W.-H. Lee
Department of Molecular Biology
University of California
Berkeley, California 94720

Eero Lehtonen
Department of Pathology
University of Helsinki
SF-00290 Helsinki 29, Finland

JoAnn Leong
Department of Microbiology
Oregon State University
Corvallis, Oregon 97441

F. Lettieri
Clinica Medica I
Università di Milano
Milan, Italy

Jay A. Levy
Department of Medicine
University of California
San Francisco, California 94143

Alban Linnenbach
The Wistar Institute of
Anatomy and Biology
Philadelphia, Pennsylvania 19104

A. J. Lusis
Division of Hematology-Oncology
Department of Medicine
UCLA School of Medicine
Los Angeles, California 90024
and Veterans Administration Hospital
Sepulveda, California 91343

A. Lyons
Beatson Institute for Cancer Research
Glasgow G61 1BD, Scotland

J. C. M. Macnab
Institute of Virology
University of Glasgow
Glasgow G11 5JR, Scotland

Paul A. Marks
Memorial Sloan-Kettering Cancer Center
New York, New York 10021

G. Mengod
Department of Pharmacology and Experimental
* Therapeutics*
The Johns Hopkins University
School of Medicine
Baltimore, Maryland 21205

A. R. Migliaccio
Istituto di Patologica Medica II
Università di Napoli
Naples, Italy

G. Migliaccio
Istituto di Patologica Medica II
Università di Napoli
Naples, Italy

G. Monaco
Istituto di Anatomia Comparata
Università degli Studi di Roma
Rome, Italy

M. A. S. Moore
Department of Developmental Hematopoiesis
Sloan Kettering Institute for Cancer Research
New York, New York 10021

Carlo Moscovici
Department of Pathology
College of Medicine
University of Florida and Tumor Virology
* Laboratory Research Service*
Veterans Administration Medical Center
Gainesville, Florida 32602

M. G. Moscovici
Department of Pathology
College of Medicine
University of Florida and Tumor Virology
* Laboratory Research Service*
Veterans Administration Medical Center
Gainesville, Florida 32602

P. Musiani
Istituto di Anatomia Patologica dell'Università
* Cattolica del Sacro Cuore*
Rome, Italy

I. Nathan
Division of Hematology-Oncology
Department of Medicine
UCLA School of Medicine
Los Angeles, California 90024
and Veterans Administration Hospital
Sepulveda, California 91343

U. Novak
Transcription Laboratory
Imperial Cancer Research Fund
London WC2A 3PX, England

Thomas G. O'Brien
The Wistar Institute of Anatomy and Biology
Philadelphia, Pennsylvania 19104

Hermann Oppermann
Department of Microbiology and Cancer
* Research Institute*
University of California
San Francisco, California 94143

W. Ostertag
The Beatson Institute for Cancer Research
Bearsden, Glasgow G61 1BD, Scotland

S. Ottolenghi
Centro per lo Studio della Patologia Cellulare
Istituto Patologia Generale
Università di Milano
Milan, Italy

M. Pacifici
Department of Anatomy
School of Medicine
University of Pennsylvania
Philadelphia, Pennsylvania 19104

T. Papas
Tumor Virus Genetics Laboratory
National Cancer Institute
National Institutes of Health
Bethesda, Maryland 20205

R. Payette
Department of Anatomy
School of Medicine
University of Pennsylvania
Philadelphia, Pennsylvania 19104

Bice Perussia
The Wistar Institute of Anatomy and Biology
Philadelphia, Pennsylvania 19104

C. Peschle
Istituto di Patologia Medica II
Università di Napoli and Istituto Superiore di
Sanità
Rome, Italy

M. Piantelli
Istituto di Anatomia Patologica dell'Università
Cattolica del Sacro Cuore
Rome, Italy

A. Pinto
Centro di Endocrinologia e Oncologia
Sperimentale del C.N.R.
Istituto di Patologia Generale
II Facoltà di Medicina e Chirurgia
Università di Napoli
80131 Naples, Italy

Mikulas Popovic
Laboratory of Tumor Cell Biology
National Cancer Institute
National Institutes of Health
Bethesda, Maryland 20205

I. B. Pragnell
The Beatson Institute for Cancer Research
Bearsden, Glasgow G61 1BD, Scotland

Marvin S. Reitz, Jr.
Laboratory of Tumor Cell Biology
National Cancer Institute
National Institutes of Health
Bethesda, Maryland 20205

R. P. Revoltella
Laboratorio di Biologia Cellulare
National Research Council
Rome, Italy

P. Ricciardi-Castagnoli
CNR Center of Cytopharmacology
Department of Pharmacology
University of Milan
20129 Milan, Italy

Richard A. Rifkind
Memorial Sloan-Kettering Cancer Center
New York, New York 10021

F. Robbiati
CNR Center of Cytopharmacology
Department of Pharmacology
University of Milan
20129 Milan, Italy

Marjorie Robert-Guroff
Laboratory of Tumor Cell Biology
National Cancer Institute
National Institutes of Health
Bethesda, Maryland 20205

T. Robins
Department of Molecular Biology
University of California
Berkeley, California 94720

Harriet L. Robinson
Worcester Foundation for Experimental Biology
Shrewsbury, Massachusetts 01545

G. B. Rossi
Istituto Superiore di Sanità
Rome, Italy

Giovanni Rovera
The Wistar Institute of Anatomy and Biology
Philadelphia, Pennsylvania 19104

Ugo Rovigatti
Istituto Fisiologia Generale
Università degli Studi di Roma
00100 Rome, Italy

Janice Rowe
Imperial Cancer Research Fund
Lincoln's Inn Fields
London WC2A 3PX, England

Ivor Royston
Department of Medicine
Division of Hematology/Oncology
University of California
San Diego, California 92093

Francis W. Ruscetti
Laboratory of Tumor Cell Biology
National Cancer Institute
National Institutes of Health
Bethesda, Maryland 20205

David J. Shealy
Department of Pathology
University of Colorado
School of Medicine
Denver, Colorado 80262

C. K. Shewmaker
Laboratory of Gene Structure and Expression
National Institute for Medical Research
London NW7 1AA, United Kingdom

Martti A. Siimes
Department of Pediatrics
University of Helsinki
SF-00290 Helsinki 29, Finland

Peter Snow
Sidney Farber Cancer Institute and Department
of Pathology
Harvard Medical School
Boston, Massachusetts 02115

Rosa Sorrentino
Gruppo di Microbiologia e Patologia Generale
Facoltà di Scienze
University of Rome and Laboratory of Cell
Biology
C.N.R.
Rome, Italy

Christa Stoscheck
Department of Biochemistry and Division of
Dermatology
Department of Medicine

Vanderbilt University School of Medicine
Nashville, Tennessee 37232

E. A. Stringer
Center for Experimental Cell Biology
Mollie B. Roth Laboratory
Mount Sinai School of Medicine
CUNY
New York, New York 10029

J. H. Subak-Sharpe
Institute of Virology
University of Glasgow
Glasgow G11 5JR, Scotland

Nobuyunki Tanigaki
Roswell Park Memorial Institute
Buffalo, New York 14263

S. Tapscott
Department of Anatomy
School of Medicine
University of Pennsylvania
Philadelphia, Pennsylvania 19104

F. Tato
Gruppo di Microbiologia e Patologia Generale
Facoltà di Scienze
University of Rome
Rome, Italy

Natalie M. Teich
Imperial Cancer Research Fund
Lincoln's Inn Fields
London WC2A 3PX, England

Cox Terhorst
Sidney Farber Cancer Institute and Department
of Pathology
Harvard Medical School
Boston, Massachusetts 02115

George J. Todaro
Laboratory of Viral Carcinogenesis
National Cancer Institute
Frederick Cancer Research Facility
Frederick, Maryland 21701

Roberto Tosi
Laboratory of Cell Biology
C.N.R.
00196 Rome, Italy

R. H. Treisman
Transcription Laboratory
Imperial Cancer Research Fund
London WC2A 3PX, England

Giorgio Trinchieri
The Wistar Institute of Anatomy and Biology
Philadelphia, Pennsylvania 19104

Philip N. Tsichlis
Department of Molecular Biology and
*   Microbiology*
Tufts University School of Medicine
Boston, Massachusetts 02111

N. Tsuchida
The Wistar Institute
Philadelphia, Pennsylvania 19104

G. Vecchio
Centro di Endocrinologia e Oncologia
*   Sperimentale del C.N.R.*
Istituto di Patologia Generale
II Facoltà di Medicine e Chirurgia
Università di Napoli
80131 Naples, Italy

K. Vehmeyer
Department of Hematology
School of Medicine
University of Goettingen
3400 Goettingen, West Germany

E. Vigneti
Laboratorio di Biologia Cellulare
C.N.R.
Rome, Italy

I. Vlodavsky
Cancer Research Institute
University of California Medical Center
San Francisco, California 94143

Paul Volberding
Department of Medicine
University of California
San Francisco, California 94143

G. Warnecke
Institute of Physiological Chemistry
University of Hamburg
2000 Hamburg 13, West Germany

R. H. Weisbart
Division of Hematology-Oncology
Department of Medicine
UCLA School of Medicine
Los Angeles, California 90024
and Veterans Administration Hospital
Sepulveda, California 91343

N. M. Wilkie
Institute of Virology
University of Glasgow
Glasgow G11 5JR, Scotland

Y. P. Yung
Department of Developmental Hematopoiesis
Sloan Kettering Institute for Cancer Research
New York, New York 10021

Nancy Zeller
Department of Pathology
College of Medicine
University of Florida and Tumor Virology
*   Laboratory Research Service*
Veterans Administration Medical Center
Gainesville, Florida 32602

Expression of Differentiated Functions in Cancer Cells, edited by R. F. Revoltella et al., Raven Press, New York © 1982.

The Segregation of Intraembryonic Blood Stem Cells During Avian Development

F. Dieterlen-Lièvre

Institut d'Embryologie du CNRS et du Collège de France, 94130 Nogent-sur-Marne, France

The ontogeny of the hemopoietic system implies precise mechanisms of recognition between stem cells (SC), and the endomesodermal or mesodermal frame of organ rudiments which become colonized according to patterns specific for each of them. Recently it could be shown that the thymus receives successive waves of colonizing SC (Le Douarin and Jotereau, 1980). Short influx period (24 hours) are separated by longer phases (around 5 days) during which the thymus is incapable of attracting or retaining new SC. By contrast the bursa of Fabricius becomes colonized during a continuous period lasting most or all of incubation (Le Douarin et al., 1981) ; after that time the SC pool of the chicken appears to contain no precursors capable of entering the bursal follicles and differentiating there (Toivanen et al., 1972). Finally the spleen begins receiving SC at a very early date (Dieterlen-Lièvre, 1973), while the bone marrow is seeded from a later date than any other hemopoietic organ (Jotereau and Le Douarin, 1978).

Thus it appears that, during a long period of development, SC are available for the establishment of hemopoiesis in the definitive organ rudiments. It is not known whether they all originate from a common pool, where this pool is located at different times of ontogeny or whether this original pool may give off sub-populations of committed precursors. It was held for some years that the yolk sac was the progenitor of all SC (Moore and Owen, 1967). We could show that in fact yolk sac stem cells are relayed by intraembryonic SC (Dieterlen-Lièvre, 1975 ; Dieterlen-Lièvre et al., 1976). This paper will report our current knowledge about intraembryonic SC and how they become segregated, an event which only begins to be understood.

Abbreviations :
MHC : Major Histocompatibility Complex
SC   : Stem Cells
YS   : Yolk sac.

1. Intraembryonic SC are the only founders of definitive hemopoiesis.

Long held as sole seeders of the hemopoietic system,the YS-SC are indeed capable of entering the thymus and becoming lymphoid (Jotereau and Houssaint, 1977), and of giving rise to the first definitive ery- throcytes (Hagopian and Ingram, 1971 ; Beaupain et al., 1979). However when unfolding of hemopoiesis was followed in chimeras composed of a quail embryo and a chick yolk sac (fig. 1a) (YS chimeras), it could be concluded that, despite considerable pliability, the YS-SC do not usually participate in the establishment of definitive hemopoiesis. The thymus, bursa and bone marrow always contained quail lymphoid or hemo- poietic cells ; the spleen showed minimal chimerism in a few cases. The data about blood evolution were rather dispersed, showing that some 13-day chimeras derived a major proportion of their erythrocytes from intraembryonic SC, while in others most red cells still descended from YS-SC. It could be surmised that interspecies differences, such as YS sizes, rhythm of development, etc...., were responsible for the discre- pancy (it should be noted that it was not attempted to obtain hatching of these interspecific chimeras and that the reverse combination - chick embryo on quail YS - is technically difficult to realize).

For all these reasons, it seemed interesting to study homospecific chick◄──►chick chimeras built with several markers (fig. 1b, c, d). These were purposefully raised past hatching as far as adulthood, when the immune system is mature and erythropoiesis has reached a steady state. With all the marker systems, the results confirmed quail/ chick data. First it should be emphasized that the adult chimeras exhi- bited normal immune responses to various antigenic stimuli (Martin et al., 1979). Second, cells in the lymphoid organs and bone marrow were always derived from the embryonic component of the chimera, never from the YS (Martin et al., 1979). But the most specific contribution from chick◄──►chick chimeras concerns erythropoiesis (Lassila et al., submitted for publication). Chimeras were made from components differing by MHC alleles expressed on the surface of red cells, so that the pro- portion of intraembryonic SC-derived to YS-SC-derived erythrocytes could be established at different points of development (Table 1). It can be presumed that this evolution is very similar, if not identical, to normal since all other parameters are normal in these chimeras. Table 1 shows that YS-SC derived erythrocytes are rapidly and consis- tently diluted by intraembryonic SC and disappear completely around hatching. The graph is in fact strikingly similar to that picturing the replacement pattern of primitive by definitive erythrocytes (fig. 2). Thus the YS-SC contribution to definitive erythropoiesis must be very small, if it exists at all.

Establishing precisely this last point will require more data in the 5-10 day period of incubation, as well as a study of the hemoglobin patterns of each population. In quail◄──►chick chimeras such a study showed that the type of erythrocytes formed depended entirely on the time of development and not on the site of origin of the SC (Beaupain et al., 1979, 1980).

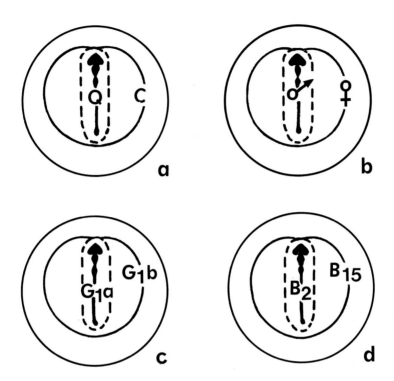

Figure 1 : YS chimeras are constructed surgically at 2 days of incubation by suturing an embryo on a foreign YS (Martin, 1972). Here are
schematized the associations realized with different types of markers,
used to follow the movements and fates of hemopoietic cells.
a. Quail embryo (Q) on a chick YS (C). Cells are identified by the
   quail/chick nuclear marker (Le Douarin, 1969). Erythrocytes in the
   blood are separated according to species by an immune hemolysis technique (Dieterlen-Lièvre et al., 1976).
b. Chick⟷chick association relying on the chance combination of the
   two sexes in 50% of the cases. The reciprocal combination is also
   obtained.
c. Chick⟷chick combination of two lines differing by presumptive Ig
   allotypes. Each is homozygous g1a/g1a or g1b/g1b and the two reciprocal grafts were made.
d. Chick⟷chick association between two lines differing by histocompatibility alleles. The reciprocal combination was not made.

TABLE 1 : <u>Origin of erythroid cells in blood of chick↔chick yolk sac chimeras.</u>
(B_2 embryos were grafted on B_{15} YS).

Number of chimeras	Age	anti-B_2 % *	anti-B_{15} %	NCS
	Embryo			
4	7-d	7.7	80.5	0.0
3	10-d	75.5	21.3	0.0
4	17-18-d	93.2	3.7	0.0
	Post-hatch.			
1	2 wks	98.5	0.0	0.0
2	4 wks	99.2	0.0	0.0

* % immunofluorescent cells after antiserum + FITC antichicken IgG.
NCS : normal chicken serum.

2. Origin of intraembryonic SC :

Both chick and quail embryos exhibit diffuse hemopoiesis in the me-senchyme, outside individualized organs (Miller, 1913 ; Dieterlen-Lièvre and Martin, 1981). This process is particularly intense in the dorsal mesentery between 6 and 9 days of incubation. Highly basophilic cells build up "para-aortic foci" (fig. 3) which eventually disappear, cells having undergone <u>in situ</u> granulopoiesis or erythropoiesis. Some of the basophilic cells enter neighbouring veins or more frequently large lacunae which are the rudiments of lymph channels. They are also seen to approach and enter the thymus rudiment (fig. 4a and b).

The foci are preceded at earlier stages by basophilic cells scattered in the dorsal mesentery. In quail↔chick YS chimeras, the foci are always quail, i.e. intraembryonic in origin. The basophilic cells, which may be either stem cells or committed precursors, are seen to travel in the aorta and liver sinusoids from 3 to 7 days of incubation, usually isolated, or sometimes in groups as illustrated in figure 5 ; in this particular group it can be seen, after Feulgen staining, that cells are

Figure 2

Comparison between replacements of :

and { primitive (P) by definitive (D) erythrocytes

vitelline stem cell-derived by intraembryonic stem cell derived erythrocytes.

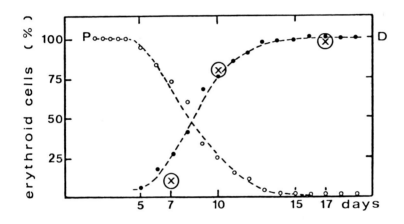

o--o--o % primitive erythrocytes } in normal chick embryos (data
●--●--● % definitive erythrocytes } from Bruns & Ingram, 1973).

Ⓧ % erythrocytes bearing the B_2 antigen in chimeras (B_2 embryos were grafted on B_{15} YS)

Figure 3

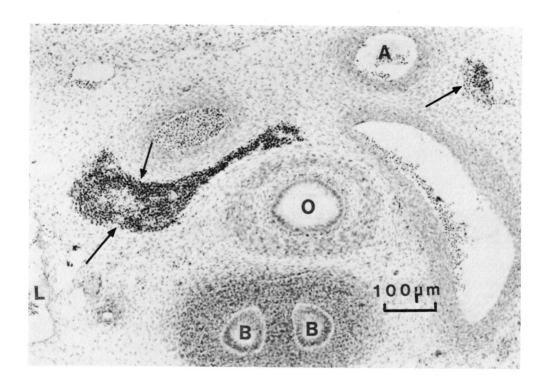

Para-aortic foci in the dorsal mesentery of the 7-day chick embryo
(arrows). Feulgen-Rossenbeck staining. A = systemic artery ; B = Bronchi
O = oesophagus ; L = anlage of lymph channel.

Figure 4 a and b

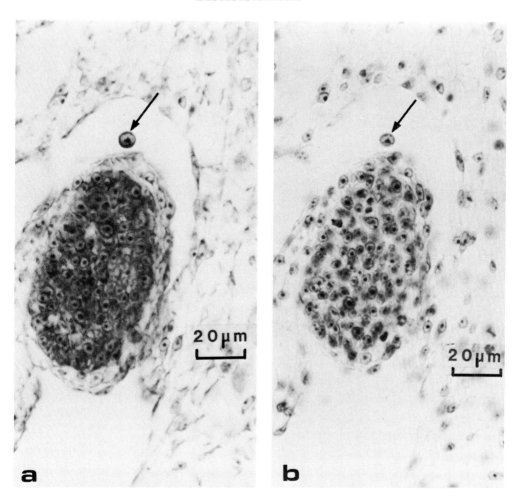

Thymus of a 6-day quail⟷chick YS chimera. The same section was stained by the methylgreen-pyronine technique (a) and poststained by the Feulgen reaction (b). A basophilic cell (arrow) is sitting in a vessel near the thymus (a). The nucleus of the same cell displays the nucleolus-associated heterochromatin typical of the quail (b) ; it is a colonizing lymphoid precursor whose intraembryonic origin is attested.

Figure 5 a and b

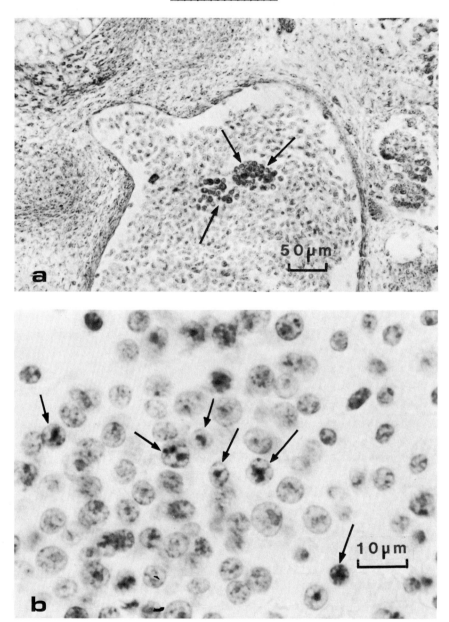

a. Aorta of a 5-day quail⟷chick YS chimera. Methylgreen pyronine
   staining. A group of basophilic cells is circulating among erythrocytes (arrow).
b. In a neighbouring section, this same group of cells has been stained
   by the Feulgen reaction. A few quail nuclei (arrows) can be identified among chick.

mixed quail and chick ; thus the "blood-borne" traffic between the
embryo and the yolk sac is visualized here as a double way exchange.
Indeed , in these chimeras, from 7 days onwards, the YS blood islands
appear colonized to different degrees by quail erythroid cells (Martin
et al., 1978). The proportions of quail and chick basophilic cells in
vessels have been quantified and appear to shift very rapidly from chick
to quail around 5 days (fig. 6) (Dieterlen-Lièvre and Martin, 1981).

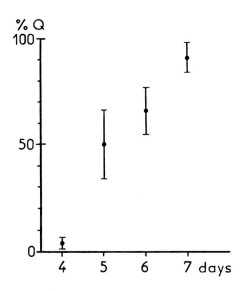

Figure 6 : Evolution of the percentage of quail cells among hemopoietic cells in the circulation of quail←—→chick YS chimeras. For each
day, a total of 200 cells was counted from 3 to 6 chimeras (Feulgen
preparations). At 4 and 5 days cells were counted in the aorta, at 6
and 7 days in the aorta and liver sinusoids.

The presence of hemopoietic cells in the mesenchyme of 7-day chick
embryos was further investigated by functional tests. In a first set
of experiments, the cells were obtained by mechanically dissociating
chick embryos, which had been beheaded and eviscerated. This obviously
rather crude preparation did contain precursors capable of homing to
hemopoietic organs of irradiated 14-day embryos (table 2) as shown with
sex chromosomal markers (Lassila et al., 1980, 1981). The 7-day cell
suspension was also capable of reconstituting the bursa of cyclophospha-
mide-treated-embryos (table 3) (Lassila et al., 1979, 1981).
In another set of experiments, the region where the para-aortic foci
are located was taken out and a cell suspension was prepared using dissociating agents (table 4). Finally the para-aortic foci were dissected
and dissociated mechanically. These two types of preparations generated
numerous colory-forming-cells in agar (granulocyte-macrophage lineage) ;
the highest yield was obtained by the dissection of the foci themselves
(Dieterlen-Lièvre, Moscovici and Moscovici, in preparation) (table 4).

TABLE 2 : <u>Homing of cells present in 7-day intraembryonic mesenchyme (sex chromosome tracing) to hemopoietic organs of syngeneic chickens.</u>

Organ	Mitogen	Number of chickens	No. of cells analysed ♂	No. of cells analysed ♀	% donor cells
Bursa	None	10	47	211	36.4
Thymus	Anti-Ig	5	13	50	41.3
	Con A	8	44	206	35.2
Spleen	Anti-Ig	8	20	107	31.5
	Con A	8	60	205	45.3
Bone marrow	Anti-Ig	8	22	71	47.3
	Con A	10	55	177	47.4

10^7 cells from pooled ♂ and ♀ embryos were injected into 14 day X-irradiated embryos. Six weeks after hatching, organs from ♀ were scanned for ♂ metaphases.

TABLE 3 : Restoration of cyclophosphamide-treated chickens by cells present in 7-day intraembryonic mesenchyme.

CY	Cell transpl.	N° of chickens	Body weight(g)	Bursa weight	Thymus weight	Spleen weight
+	-	9	257 + 38	73 + 35	323 + 82	185 + 58
+	+	12	318 + 33**	287 + 163***	411 + 101**	203 + 42
-	-	15	361 + 51***	417 + 177***	446 + 94**	211 + 45

Mean values + SD
*p < 0.01   when compared to cyclophosphamide-treated
**p < 0.001   chickens ; Student's *t*-test.
Embryos were injected I.V. with 1.50 mg Cy on days 15, 16 and 17
and with 10⁷ mesenchyme cells on day 18.

TABLE 4 : <u>Development of chicken CFC in agar from several embryonic origins.</u>

Organ or rudiment	Stage when taken	Number of colonies developed from	
		10^5 cells	10^4 cells
Bone marrow	hatching	Too many to count	16
Spleen	13-d. embryo	"	214
Area of heart vessels (trypsinized)	8-d. embryo	80	0
Area of heart vessels (Trypsin + EDTA)	8-d. embryo	40	0
Para-aortic foci (mechanical dissection and dissociation)	8-d. embryo	Too many to count	31

Each figure was determined from 3 or 4 culture dishes.

Thus in the 7-day embryo it is possible to correlate the presence of the para-aortic foci with that of SC which appear pluripotent in several functional tests. However nothing indicates that these foci are the primordial site where these SC arise. To investigate this point, younger embryos were studied and a special test of hematogenic potentialities had to be devised in order to recover and identify a small number of cells differentiated from early rudiments.

3. <u>The hemopoietic cells present in the para-aortic foci arise at an earlier stage from the wall of the aorta.</u>

In the 4-5-day embryo, scarce basophilic cells are present, dispersed in the dorsal mesentery. They are absent from the 3-day embryo. At that stage, aggregated basophilic cells built two symmetrical, ventrolateral, thickenings to the wall of the aorta. It was thought that these might represent the earliest process in the segregation of the SC. The dorsal mesentery, found to be an excellent microenvironment for the multiplication of hemopoietic cells, was used as a grafting site.(When quail bone marrow from a newly hatched quail was grafted into the chick, hemopoietic cells left the transplant and invaded the mesentery, precisely in the sites where hemopoietic cells are normally found; if the embryo was left to develop long enough, these cells reached the thymus, bursa or spleen, and gave rise to an erythrocytic progeny in the host's blood). Grafted in the chick mesentery, fragments of the 3-day quail aorta, dissected surgically,and in some cases treated with trypsin to remove outer cells, yielded such foci. Finally aortas, dissociated into a cell suspension, gave rise to CFC in agar.

As a conclusion to these data, I wish to propose an interpretation about the events through which intraembryonic SC segregate during onto-geny. Their arisal from the aorta is not surprising, since it is a similar process to what occurs in the yolk sac.

In this site, it is known that a common precursor, the hemangioblast, gives rise to either blood cells or endothelial cells, depending whether the hemangioblasts are located centrally or peripherally in the blood islands.

As to the aorta, the morphological aspects suggest that some cells in the ventrolateral thickenings are emitted towards the lumen and some towards the external aspect of the wall. According to the hypothesis considered, the cells emitted into the lumen undergo erythropoiesis, and circulating basophilic cells (whether from the embryo or the YS in fact) become committed at short term. On the other hand, cells emit-ted towards the mesentery meet a cellular environment which promotes their multiplication and maintains them in an uncommitted state until the hemopoietic organ rudiments become attractive. Indeed the para-aortic foci are at the height of their activity at the time when the thymus and bursa enter their receptive period. Evidently the correct unfolding of these events hinges on the simultaneous availability of totipotent SC and attractivity of the organ rudiments. It is likely that the latter parameter determines which SC go where.

REFERENCES :

1. Beaupain, D., Martin, C., and Dieterlen-Lièvre, F. (1979): Blood, 53:212-225.

2. Beaupain, D., Martin, C., and Dieterlen-Lièvre, F. (1980).In "In vivo and in vitro erythropoiesis : the friend system" edited by J.B.Rossi, Elsevier, Biomedical Press, pp. 21-32.

3. Bruns, G.A.P. and Ingram, V.M. (1973):Phil.Trans.Roy.Soc.B 266:225-305

4. Dieterlen-Lièvre, F. (1973):Année Biologique 12:481-490.

5. Dieterlen-Lièvre, F. (1975). J. Embryol. exp. Morph. 33, 607-619.

6. Dieterlen-Lièvre, F., Beaupain. D and Martin, C. (1976) : Ann. Immu-nol. (Inst. Pasteur) 127c : 857-863.

7. Dieterlen-Lièvre, F.,and Martin, C. (1981):Submitted for publication.

8. Hagopian, H.K. and Ingram, V.M. (1971):J.Cell. Biol. 51:440-551.

9. Jotereau, F.V. and Houssaint, E. (1977): In : Developmental Biology, edited by J.B. Solomon and J.D. Horton, pp. 123-130, Elsevier/North Holland, Amsterdam.

10.Jotereau, F.V. and Le Douarin, N.M. (1978): Dev. Biol. 63:253-265.

11. Lassila, O., Eskola, J. and Toivanen, P. (1979): J. Immunol. 123: 2091-2094.

12. Lassila, O., Eskola, J., Toivanen, P. and Dieterlen-Lièvre, F. (1980): Scand. J. Immunol. 11:445-448.

13. Lassila, O., Eskola, J., Dieterlen-Lièvre, F. and Toivanen, P. (1980) in Aspects of Developmental and Comparative Immunology - I, pp. 211-215. Solomon, ed. Pergamon Press, Oxford and New-York

14. Lassila, O., Martin, C., Toivanen, P. and Dieterlen-Lièvre, F. (1981): submitted for publication.

15. Le Douarin, N. (1969):Bull. biol. Fr. Belg. 103:435-442.

16. Le Douarin, N. and Jotereau, F. (1980). In : Immunology 80, edited by M. Fougereau and J. Dausset, Academic Press, pp. 285-302.

17. Le Douarin, N., Jotereau, F., Houssaint, E., Martin, C. and Dieterlen-Lièvre, F. (1981). In : The reticulo-endothelial system edited by N. Cohen and M. Sigel, Plenum publ. Corp. New York, in press.

18. Martin, C. (1972): C.R. Séanc. Soc. Biol. (Paris). 166:283-285.

19. Martin, C., Beaupain, D. and Dieterlen-Lièvre, F. (1978): Cell Diff. 7:115-130.

20. Martin, C., Lassila, O., NUrmi, T., Eskola, J., Dieterlen-Lièvre, F. and Toivanen, P. (1979): Scand. J. Immunol. 10:333-338.

21. Miller, A.M. (1913): Amer. J. Anat. 15:131-198.

22. Moore, M.A.S. and Owen, J.J.T. (1967): Lancet, 2:658-659.

23. Toivanen, P., Toivanen, A., Linna, T.J. and Good, R.A. (1972): J. Immunol. 109:1071-1080.

Expression of Differentiated Functions in Cancer Cells, edited by R. F. Revoltella et al., Raven Press, New York © 1982.

Lineage and Mechanism in the Early Mouse Embryo

John K. Heath

University of Oxford, Department of Zoology, Oxford OX1 3PS, England

In most organisms there is often observed a regularity in the division and deployment of cells such that specific cell types of the adult arise as the mitotic progeny of particular cells of the early embryo. A cell lineage is a description of such a pattern of division and deployment leading to the formation of a certain tissue type. In order to study the molecular and cellular mechanisms involved in the generation of cell types it is clearly valuable to know their respective lineages.

Cell lines are best described from direct observation of living material, since their pattern may well depend upon the integrated behaviour of the whole embryo. This approach has been successfully applied in a few invertebrate species (29, 23). The mouse is an organism which is unfortunately poorly suited to this approach: the embryo has a complex tissue architecture and most of its development occurs attached to the wall of the maternal uterus. These problems can be partially resolved by tracing the progeny of genetically marked cells introduced into particular locations in the preimplantation embryo at a time when it is amenable to experimental manipulation. This approach relies on the assumption that the behaviour of orthotopically transplanted cells closely resembles the behaviour of their unmanipulated normal counterparts. The level of resolution which can be achieved with transplantation techniques is presently limited by the genetic markers available in mouse stocks. There is unfortunately no general genetic marker which allows the resolution of progeny cells at the single cell level (see Dewey (4), however). Transplanted cells generally differ from their host at isoenzymic loci; the progeny cells can be traced by measuring the relative isoenzymic contributions to dissected tissues in the later embryo.

Preimplantation Development

The development of the mouse prior to implantation occupies approximately four days. First cleavage occurs 24-30 hours after fertilization. The following five cleavages occur asynchronously over the next 48 hours (21). The most striking event during this time is the phenomenon of compaction, whereby the cleavage blastomeres change from focal contacts with their neighbours to a more tightly associated

configuration in which individual cell outlines are hard to see. This
phenomenon is associated with the appearance of tight junctions between
adjacent cells (6). At $3\frac{1}{2}$ days after fertilization the embryo forms the
blastocyst, a structure which is composed of two distinct tissue types;
an outer hollow sphere of some 45 flattened polygonal cells, the trophectoderm, and a small group of some 15 cells apposed to the inside
surface of the trophectoderm, the inner cell mass (I.C.M.). These two
cell types are the earliest to be formed in the embryo. They are biochemically distinct (30), presumably as the result of differential gene
activity. The trophectoderm and the I.C.M. further represent founder
members of different lineages. If microsurgically isolated I.C.M.s are
injected into genetically marked vesicles of trophectoderm which are
allowed to implant and develop it is found that the progeny of the
I.C.M. cells have colonised the foetus, whereas the trophectoderm cells
have formed some of the specialized tissues required for implantation;
the ectoplacental cone, extraembryonic ectoderm and trophoblast (12).

The trophectoderm is formed from cells located on the outside of the
embryo during cleavage. The I.C.M. is formed from cells located inside
the cleaving embryo. This has been demonstrated by introducing oil
droplets into the outside cells of the embryo at the 16-cell stage. The
injected cells are located in the trophectoderm of the blastocyst (32).

Normal spatial relationships within the cleavage embryo can be
simulated by completely enclosing an embryo of one genotype with
cleavage embryos of another. These structures will develop normally to
the blastocyst stage and beyond. In these cases, the enclosed embryo
gives rise to I.C.M. cells, whereas the enclosing embryos predominantly
form trophectoderm (16). Thus the allocation of cells to these two
lineages occurs during cleavage, and is not the direct result of the
segregation of intrinsic cellular factors.

An isolated 8-cell blastomere can continue cleavage and cytodifferentiation will occur before there is an opportunity for 'inside' cells
to be formed. The embryo that develops is composed solely of trophectodermal tissue (26). Similarly, if a cleavage embryo is prevented
from compacting by prolonged incubation in certain antibody preparations
(20) cell division and cytodifferentiation will occur in the loose
aggregate of cells that are formed. The decompacted embryo forms an
abnormal blastocyst with little or no recognisable I.C.M. cells. Thus
it would seem that cytodifferentiation of trophectoderm is independent
of normal cell interactions that occur during cleavage. However, the
formation of the I.C.M. lineage, and the resulting differential gene
expression is dependent upon the microenvironment created inside the
cleaving embryo as a result of compaction, or upon a certain sequence of
cellular interactions resulting from an inside location during cleavage.
These are not, of course, mutually exclusive possibilities. How microenvironment and/or cell interaction may control gene expression in this
instance is unknown. These observations have, however, naturally
focussed attention upon the normal sequence of events leading to the
generation of inside cells during cleavage, and the cell interactions
which are unique to an inside location.

The process of cleavage has been followed in intact embryos, or
isolated blastomere groups by semi-continuous observation (21, 14). It
was first observed that, although cleavage divisions are usually
asynchronous, the first cell to divide to the 4-cell stage (second
cleavage division) tended to produce progeny which divided ahead of
other cells in the embryo (21). Thus the order of cell division was

preserved through cleavage. Cells which divided first in a given cleavage cycle tended to lie deeper in the embryo by virtue of their more extensive cell contacts (14). The position of later dividing cells tended to be more peripheral. At the 4-8 cell division an asymmetry in the positioning of daughter cells was noted, in that one daughter would retain the cell contacts of the parent, whereas the other assumed a more peripheral location. Thus the allocation of cells to the inside of the morula could be envisaged as a consequence of retaining a greater number of cell contacts through cleavage; this is affected by the order in which the cells divide, and the positioning of the parent cell in successive cleavage divisions.

A second property of cleavage blastomeres which may be valuable in understanding the forces that govern the formation of inside cells during cleavage is the ability of some cells to form polarized areas of microvilli when placed in contact with other cells (33). This pheno-menon was first described as a distinguishing feature of outside cells and thus gives the embryo a radial organisation (15). The polarised regions can be inherited through cell division (19). The polarised phenotype is therefore a characteristic of cells that are destined to form trophectoderm (19). It is possible that a polarised microvillar cell surface would lead to a smaller number of possible cell contacts, and hence to an outer location and trophectodermal form of differen-tiation.

The cytodifferentiation of the first two tissues in the mouse embryo can therefore be seen as a consequence of differing cell contacts and microenvironment which can be generated by very simple properties of cleavage blastomeres.

The Formation of Primitive Endoderm

Less than 24 hours after the blastocyst is formed, a third layer of cells appears in the embryo. This is the primitive endoderm, which is a layer of cells which delaminate from the inner cell mass, facing the inside of the trophectoderm. These cells proliferate and eventually spread over the inside surface of the trophectoderm, and invest the developing extraembryonic regions of the embryo.

The primitive endoderm is almost certainly formed from the I.C.M., since microsurgically isolated inner cell masses will form primitive endoderm (but not trophectoderm) over the exposed surface when cultured in the oviduct or in vitro (25, 27). Furthermore, if dissociated I.C.M.s from $4\frac{1}{2}$ d.p.c. embryos are dissociated and single cells are transplanted into genetically marked host blastocysts two distinct patterns of colonisation are evident. One form is manifested as the colonisation of foetal tissues (including representatives of all three germ layers) and the second type is purely colonisation of the primitive endoderm overlying the embryo, extraembryonic regions and yolk sac (11). The primitive endoderm is therefore the third distinct lineage to be formed in the mouse embryo.

The observation that primitive endoderm cells form on the outside of isolated I.C.M. has led to the suggestion that position effects may be important in the differentiation of primitive endoderm and primitive ectoderm (the presumptive foetal tissues). Supporting evidence for this view comes from three types of experiment. First, it is possible to perform xenografts in the early mouse embryo by injecting I.C.M.

cells from synchronous rat embryos. One can trace the fate of individual rat cells by the use of species-specific antisera (9). It is observed that in some of these transplants the rat cells lie on the outside surface of the inner cell mass, and in these cases they tend to form primitive endoderm structures (10). Secondly, if the blastocyst is surgically bisected the I.C.M.s are reduced in number and tend to form primitive endoderm at the expense of primitive ectoderm (8). This is perhaps because all the cells in a reduced sized I.C.M. are exposed to the blastocoele. Thirdly, it is possible to clone single I.C.M. cells. Daughter cell pairs can then be transferred to different locations within the I.C.M. It is observed that daughters transferred to an outside location show a primitive endoderm pattern of colonisation upon development, whereas the homologous daughter transplanted inside the inner cell mass gives rise exclusively to foetal tissues (R.L. Gardner, personal communication). Taken together, these observations suggest a role for position and/or contact effects in the formation of trophectoderm and I.C.M.

The primitive endoderm lineage further divides into two related cell types: the visceral endoderm overlying the developing egg cylinder, and the parietal endoderm overlying the trophectoderm. These tissues are biochemically distinct; visceral endoderm cells produce alpha foetoprotein whereas parietal endoderm cells produce type IV procollagen (1) and laminin (17).

The synthesis of AFP by the visceral endoderm is furthermore under the control of tissue interactions. In situ AFP is only found in those regions of the visceral endoderm which overlie the presumptive foetal regions (the primitive ectoderm). The visceral endoderm overlying the extraembryonic regions can synthesise AFP is isolated and cultured free of the underlying tissue (7). The phenotype of primitive endoderm derivatives in the embryo is therefore partly determined by location rather than history.

The colonisation of host blastocysts by visceral and parietal endoderm cells has been recently investigated by Gardner (personal communication). Parietal endoderm did not colonise host embryos with high frequency. A single visceral endoderm cell could give rise to both parietal and visceral endoderm cells. Further evidence for the formation of parietal endoderm from visceral endoderm has been provided by in vitro culture experiments (18). If the extraembryonic regions of the 6.5 day embryo are dissected free of the embryo and cultured as fragments, it is observed that the visceral extraembryonic endoderm cells undergo marked morphological changes and start to synthesise laminin and type IV procollagen. Secondly, if visceral extraembryonic endoderm layer is removed from an isolated embryo, the visceral embryonic endoderm cells recolonise the extraembryonic regions. The recolonising cells assume a parietal endoderm morphology, and again secrete significant amounts of laminin and type IV procollagen (18).

Parietal endoderm in vivo is formed from those cells which have migrated farthest from the site of origin at the I.C.M., and so have presumably undergone more cell divisions than the more proximal visceral endoderm. Little DNA synthetic activity is observed in parietal endoderm cells in vivo (J. Warshaw, personal communication). It is plausible that the derivatives of the primitive endoderm have a defined proliferative capacity. The cytodifferentiation of primitive endoderm cells is therefore a function of age (cell divisions) and positioning within the embryo. The progeny of primitive endoderm cells

all have the capacity to go through a defined sequence of differentiative steps to the end-point of the lineage, parietal endoderm. In
the living embryo, only those cells which have migrated farthest (and
thus formed earliest) reach the terminal stage. Other derivatives of
the primitive endoderm are constrained from further development by their
position within the embryo. A second possibility is that parietal and
visceral endoderm phenotypes are interchangeable, and that the pattern
of gene expression in the primitive endoderm derivatives is modulated
by the tissue environment, particularly the derivation of the underlying tissue. Confirmation of this view, however, awaits a demonstration
of the formation of visceral endoderm cells from parietal endoderm.

Prospects and Conclusions

The lineages that are best understood in the mouse are those which
are destined to form structures which are only needed for the life of
the embryo in utero. It would be most valuable to be able to follow
lineages in those tissues destined to form adult structures, the
descendants of the primitive ectoderm. Some success in this direction
has been made in analysing haemopoietic lineages, derived from the
mesoderm of the yolk sac, by transplantation of cells to adult (22) or
foetal mice in utero (31). Primitive ectoderm cells do not seem to be
capable of colonising the embryo following transfer to the blastocyst
with any reliability. There are three potential avenues by which this
problem may be overcome. First, teratocarcinoma are malignant tumours
which form from the primitive ectoderm (5). They are capable of undergoing differentiation in vitro (13) and, more dramatically, giving rise
to functional adult tissue following injection into the blastocyst (24)
or aggregation with the cleavage embryo (28). An analysis of the
in vitro differentiation of teratocarcinoma cells may give clues as to
mechanisms and events in the real embryo. Secondly, valuable advances
have been made in the techniques for culturing whole post-implantation
embryos in vitro. It is possible to perform similar kinds of grafting
experiments on cultured embryos as those performed with preimplantation
embryos (3). These cultured embryos are not, however, as yet capable of
developing through to the stage of the newborn mouse. The third
possibility is the development of techniques for culturing clonal
populations of primitive ectoderm cells in vitro. These expanded
populations may then be transferred back to the embryo, or allowed to
differentiate in vitro. The development of these techniques is greatly
aided by the study of the hormonal requirements for proliferation of
differing tissues in the mouse embryo (2).

Acknowledgments

I would like to thank Christopher Graham and Richard Gardner for
valuable discussions and permission to quote unpublished observations.
The author is a Beit Memorial Fellow.

References

1. Adamson, E., and Ayers, S. (1979): Cell, 16: 953-965.
2. Adamson, E., Deller, M., and Warshaw, J. (1981): Nature, in press.
3. Beddington, R. (1981): J.E.E.M., in press.

4. Dewey, M., and Mintz, B. (1978): Dev. Biol., 66: 550-559.
5. Diwan, S., and Stevans, L. (1976): J. Natn. Cancer Inst., 57: 937-942.
6. Ducibella, T., Ukena, T., Karnovsky, M., and Anderson, E. (1977): J. Cell. Biol., 74: 153-167.
7. Dziadek, M. (1978): J. Embryol. exp. Morph., 46: 135-146.
8. Gardner, R. (1975): In : The Developmental Biology of Reproduction, edited by C. Markert, pp. 207-238. Academic Press, New York.
9. Gardner, R., and Johnson, M. (1973): Nature (new biology), 246: 86-89.
10. Gardner, R., and Johnson, M. (1975): In: Cell Patterning. Ciba Symp. 29, edited by G. Wolstenholme, pp. 183-195. Elsevier Excerpta Medica Amsterdam.
11. Gardner, R., and Rossant, J. (1979): J. Embryol. exp. Morph., 52: 141-152.
12. Gardner, R., Papaioannou, V., and Barton, S. (1973): J. Embryol. exp. Morph., 30: 561-572.
13. Graham, C. (1979): In: Concepts in Mammalian Embryogenesis, edited by M. Sherman, pp. 315-394. MIT Press, London.
14. Graham, C., and Deussen, Z. (1978): J. Embryol. exp. Morph., 48: 53-72.
15. Handyside, A. (1980): J. Embryol. exp. Morph., 60: 99-116.
16. Hillman, N., Sherman, M., and Graham, C. (1972): J. Embryol. exp. Morph., 28: 263-278.
17. Hogan, B., Cooper, A., and Kurkinen, M. (1980): Dev. Biol., 80: 289-300.
18. Hogan, B., and Tilly, R. (1981): J.E.E.M.: 62: 379-394.
19. Johnson, M., and Ziomek, C. (1981): Cell: 24: 71-80.
20. Johnson, M., Chakraborty, J., Handyside, A., Willison, K., and Stern, P. (1979): J. Embryol. exp. Morph., 54: 241-261.
21. Kelly, S., Mulnard, J., and Graham, C. (1978): J. Embryol. exp. Morph., 48: 37-51.
22. Metcalf, D., and Moore, M. (1971): Haematopoietic cells, North Holland, Amsterdam.
23. Ortolani, G. (1964): Acta. Embryol. Morph. Expt., 7: 191-200.
24. Papaioannou, V., McBurney, M., Gardner, R., and Evans, M. (1975): Nature, 258: 70-73.
25. Rossant, J. (1975): J. Embryol. exp. Morph., 33: 991-1001.
26. Rossant, J. (1976): J. Embryol. exp. Morph., 36: 283-290.
27. Solter, D., and Knowles, B. (1975): Proc. Natn. Acad. Sci. (U.S.A.), 72: 5099-5102.
28. Stewart, C. (1981): J.E.E.M., in press.
29. Sulston, J., and Horvitz, H. (1977): Dev. Biol., 56: 110-156.
30. Van Blerkom, J., Barton, S., and Johnson, M. (1976): Nature, 259: 319-321.
31. Weissman, I., Baird, S., Gardner, R., Papaioannou, V., and Raschke, W. (1976): Cold Spring Harbour Symp. Q. Biol., 41: 9-21.
32. Wilson, I., Bolton, E., and Cutler, R. (1972): J. Embryol. exp. Morph., 27: 467-479.
33. Ziomek, C., and Johnson, M. (1980): Cell, 21: 935-942.

Expression of Differentiated Functions in Cancer Cells, edited by R. F. Revoltella et al., Raven Press, New York © 1982.

Insertion of Leukemia Virus Genomes into the Germ Line of Mice: A Model System to Study Gene Expression During Development and Differentiation

Rudolf Jaenisch

Heinrich-Pette-Institut für Experimentelle Virologie und Immunologie an der Universität Hamburg, 2000 Hamburg 20, Federal Republic of Germany

SUMMARY

The exogenous Moloney leukemia virus (= M-MuLV) was inserted into the germ line of mice by exposing embryos to virus at different stages of embryogenesis. Mice derived from exposed embryos were mosaics with respect to integrated virus. Thirteen substrains, designated Mov-1 to Mov-13, were derived which carry each a single M-MuLV genome at a different chromosomal position in their germ line. Restriction enzyme analyses demonstrated that with the exception of Mov-4 and Mov-6 mice no major rearrangements or deletions have occurred in the integrated proviral genomes.

Infectious virus is not activated in the majority of substrains (Mov-4 to Mov-8 and Mov-10 to Mov-12), whereas the other mice develop viremia. A detailed comparison between Mov-1 and Mov-13 mice demonstrated that the time of virus activation is different. Whereas Mov-13 mice activate infectious virus during embryogenesis leading to a distinct pattern of virus expression in all tissues of the adult, the viral genome in Mov-1 mice is activated only during the first two weeks after birth leading to virus expression predominantly in lymphatic organs. The available data distinguish at least four different phenotypes of virus expression among the thirteen substrains: early virus activation during embryogenesis in Mov-13 mice, virus activation after birth in Mov-1 mice, virus activation late in life in Mov-2 mice and no expression of infectious virus at all in the majority of the substrains. Our results suggest that the chromosomal region at which a viral genome is integrated influences its expression during development and differentiation. This is of relevance for attempts to correct a genetic defect by inserting a functional gene into the germ line of an individual (= gene therapy).

INTRODUCTION

Gene regulation at the transcriptional level appears to be a fundamental process underlying differentiation and development (3). This view is supported by recent evidence measuring the specific transcription of selected genes in differentiated tissues of animals (6,20). The mechanisms responsible for tissue-specific gene activation, however, are not known.

Our approach to study gene regulation involved in development has been to introduce retrovirus genomes into the germ line, thus deriving substrains of mice which transmit the viral information as new Mendelian genes. Endogenous retroviruses are stable genetic elements and they can serve as models to study the regulation of normal cellular genes.

In the first successful attempts along these lines, the BALB/Mo strain was derived which transmits the exogenous Moloney leukemia virus (= M-MuLV) as a Mendelian gene (8). The viral genome was shown to be integrated on chromosome No. 6 and this new genetic locus was named Mov-1 (1). Expression of the M-MuLV-specific sequences in BALB/Mo mice occurs in the lymphatic "target tissues" spleen and thymus, and little or no viral specific RNA is found in the other "non-target" organs (9). In more recent experiments, twelve new substrains of mice, designated as Mov-2 to Mov-13, were derived, each carrying the M-MuLV genome at different chromosomal positions (7,14). Four dissimilar phenotypes, i.e., patterns of virus activation, can be distinguished among the mouse strains derived so far. Our results support the hypothesis that the chromosomal position of a gene is of importance for its activation during development.

RESULTS AND DISCUSSION

Derivation of Substrains of Mice Transmitting M-MuLV Genetically

The derivation of mouse sublines transmitting M-MuLV as a Mendelian gene was achieved by exposing mouse embryos to virus at different stages of development. Fig. 1 is a summary of the experimental approach and the techniques involved in characterizing the integrated viral genes (= Mov loci). Three different protocols to infect mouse embryos were used: (i) 4-16 cell stage mouse embryos were exposed to virus in vitro, (ii) mouse blastocysts were microinjected with a Cl 1-1a fibroblast cell producing virus, and (iii) mouse embryos were microinjected with virus in utero at day 8 or 9 of gestation. Preimplantation embryos were transplanted to foster mothers to assure further development and viremic animals were selected and tested for germ line integration of virus by two approaches: (i) by segregation analysis to define genetically a virus locus (designated as Mov-1 to Mov-13) and (ii) by restriction enzyme analysis using DNA from liver biopsies (see Fig. 1). The

GERM LINE INTEGRATION OF LEUKEMIA VIRUS

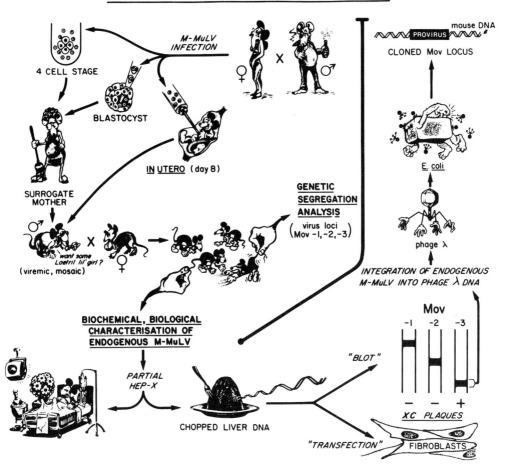

FIG. 1. The figure illustrates on the left side the derivation and characterization of Mov substrains and on the right side the experimental approach to molecularly clone integrated provirus (= Mov locus).

experimental details of deriving the mouse sublines have
been described previously (7,8,14).

So far, thirteen mouse sublines have been derived carrying M-MuLV at a different genetic locus in their germ line.
Table 1 is a summary of the substrains designated as Mov-1
to Mov-13. The size of the EcoRI fragment carrying the
M-MuLV genome is different for each mouse substrain, indicating a different integration site (for details, see 7,14).

TABLE 1. <u>Mouse strains with germ line integrated Moloney
leukemia virus</u>

Strain	M-MuLV sequences		Expression of virus		Other charac-teristics
	Genetic locus	Size of EcoRI fragm. (Kbp)	Viremia	Time of activation	
BALB/c	Mov-1	28	+	after birth	virus on chromo-some 6
ICR	Mov-2	21	+	in 20% as adults	
	Mov-3	18	+		
	Mov-4	9	−		del. env.
129	Mov-5	21	−		
	Mov-6	15.5	−		del. env.
	Mov-7	14.5	−		
	Mov-8	17	−		
	Mov-9	14.7	+		
	Mov-10	17.5	−		
	Mov-11	30	−		
	Mov-12	18	−		
C57BL	Mov-13	24	+	during em-bryogenesis	"gray hair"

<u>Activation of the Mov Locus During Development and Differentiation</u>

The expression of the M-MuLV genome in the different
mouse substrains was monitored by testing the mice (i) for
viremia using an RIA, (ii) for the presence of M-MuLV-specific RNA in different organs using molecular hybridization,
(iii) for appearance of infectious virus using an infectious
center assay, and (iv) by in situ hybridization of organ
sections to ^{3}H-labeled M-MuLV cDNA. The results have been

described (7,8,9,14) and are summarized in Table 1. The majority of the Mov substrains do not activate their endogenous M-MuLV genome and therefore do not develop viremia. Some substrains, i.e., Mov-1, Mov-2, Mov-3, Mov-9 and Mov-13, develop viremia. The time of activation of the viral genome, however, is different in these strains (Table 1). Mov-13 mice activate the virus already at the embryo stage (day 16 of gestation) leading to a distinct pattern of virus expression in the adult. Mov-1 mice activate infectious virus one week after birth leading to a "lymphotropic" virus expression. Virus activation occurs even later and only in 20% of animals carrying the Mov-2 gene.

CONCLUSIONS

Exposure of Embryos to Virus: Frequency of Germ Line Integration

Exposure of early embryos to viral genetic information has been used to insert new genes into the germ line of mice. In our first experiments, SV40 DNA was microinjected into mouse blastocysts. A high percentage of animals derived from the embryos carried SV40-specific DNA sequences in some of their tissues (12). Genetic transmission or virus expression was not observed in these animals. Exposure of preimplantation embryos to M-MuLV, however, led to the derivation of substrains of mice transmitting the virus as a Mendelian gene (Table 1). These substrains are congenic with the parental mouse strain. Most substrains of mice transmitting M-MuLV genetically were derived from 4 to 16 cell embryos exposed to virus or from a blastocyst microinjected with a virus-producing fibroblast. The efficiency of integration of new genetic information into the germ line appears to change markedly during development. Thus, every viremic animal derived from a preimplantation embryo exposed to virus carried one or more viral copies integrated into germ line cells (for details, see 7,14). As these animals were mosaics in their germ cell population, as well as in somatic tissues, genetically defined substrains of mice were only derived after segregating the genes in the N-1 generations. Integration of virus into germ cells of animals which were exposed to virus at midgestation, however, was detected in less than 0.5%, although virus-specific DNA sequences are found in cells of every organ (10). Animals infected as newborns with virus never transmit the viral gene to the next generation (5,8, 15). It thus appears that the probability of inserting new genetic information into an animal's germ cells decreases during the process of embryonal development.

Activation of Endogenous M-MuLV Sequences During Differentiation

The appearance of infectious virus in the serum of all substrains of mice transmitting M-MuLV was monitored and

used as criterium for virus expression. Viremia develops as
a consequence of superinfection of susceptible cells with
virus. Table 1 is a summary of the phenotypes observed among
the different substrains transmitting M-MuLV. The majority
of mice carrying M-MuLV in their germ line do not develop
viremia (Mov-4 to Mov-8, Mov-10 to Mov-12). This indicates
that the endogenous M-MuLV copy is not activated as an infectious agent during the life of the respective animals.
The remaining substrains activate infectious virus and develop viremia. The age at which virus activation occurs,
however, is different in the respective substrains. The appearance of infectious centers during the development of
Mov-1 and Mov-13 mice was compared in detail. Whereas infectious centers in livers of Mov-13 mice are observed as
early as the 16th gestation day, in Mov-1 mice the first appearance of infectious centers in the spleen is not observed
earlier than 6 days after birth. In situ hybridization data
revealed a high concentration of viral specific RNA in cells
of all organs of Mov-13 mice, contrasting Mov-1 mice where
viral specific RNA was seen in lymphoid organs only (for
experimental details, see 14). An even later activation of
virus than in Mov-1 mice occurs in Mov-2 mice. These animals are non-viremic at 3 weeks of age, but the Mov-2 gene
becomes activated in 20% of the animals between 2 and 4
months of age leading to virus expression in lymphatic organs and to viremia (7). Thus, at least four different phenotypes can be distinguished (Table 1): early virus activation during embryogenesis in Mov-13 mice, virus activation
during the first weeks of life in Mov-1 mice, occasional
appearance of virus late in life in Mov-2 mice, and no virus
activation in the negative Mov substrains. The time of virus
activation in Mov-3 and Mov-9 mice has not been determined.

It should be emphasized here that the different genetic
background of the mice used in these experiments will not
influence the efficiency or likelihood of replication or
the spread of NB tropic M-MuLV once infectious virus has
appeared. This is indicated by infecting mice of different
genotype as midgestation embryos or as newborns (10). In
all cases the development of viremia was not influenced by
the genetic background of the infected mouse.

Restriction enzyme analysis with EcoRI has shown that
integration of virus into the germ line occurred at a different chromosomal position in all substrains of mice
(Table 1). The use of enzymes with multiple recognition
sites within the viral genome demonstrated that the proviral DNAs carried in eleven substrains were indistinguishable. The proviral genomes in Mov-4 and Mov-6 mice, however,
showed an identical deletion or rearrangement at the 3' end
(14). Our results therefore suggest that the different patterns of virus activation in the different substrains are
due to the chromosomal position at which virus integration
took place rather than a major change in the viral genome
itself. The present data do not exclude mutations in proviral DNA not detected by the methods employed.

The mechanisms by which chromosomal regions flanking an inserted gene influence its expression are not known. Evidence, however, is accumulating that chromosomal regions distant of the structural gene which is expressed in a given tissue are in an "active" conformation as well as the structural gene itself. Thus, the chromatin structure regions surrounding the chicken globin genes are in a DNase I sensitive conformation in erythroid cells but not in other tissues (19). Similarly, non-coding genetic regions surrounding the human β genes are undermethylated in tissues that express globin sequences (17). These observations suggested that a cis acting mechanism may be involved in gene regulation affecting development and differentiation. The effect of deletions on regulation of distant genes (4,18) or the differential infectivity of DNA of integrated retroviral genomes (2,16) has also been explained by cis acting control mechanisms. Thus, a viral gene integrated into a given chromosomal region may come under the control of adjacent regulatory elements as has been discussed previously (11). One approach to study the conformation of host sequences flanking the integrated provirus is to molecularly clone the respective Mov locus (see Fig. 1). First experiments along these lines support the hypothesis that cis acting control elements influence the expression of adjacent genes.

The results obtained in our system are relevant for experiments involving the manipulation of the genetic composition of animals. The most efficient way to insert new genetic information into the germ line appears to be introduction of genes into preimplantation embryos. Virus replication or virus spread is not a prerequisite for integrating genes into the germ line because preimplantation embryos are non-permissive for virus expression (13). Our results emphasize the difficulty of attempts to correct genetic defects by inserting a functional gene into the germ line of an individual. Selection for tissue-specific expression on the germ line level appears not to be possible. To derive animals which express an inserted gene in the correct tissues, one may have to insert this gene into a specific chromosomal region of the animal's genome.

ACKNOWLEDGMENTS

The work summarized in this article was supported by research grants from the National Cancer Institute, the Deutsche Forschungsgemeinschaft and the Volkswagen Foundation. The Heinrich-Pette-Institut is supported by Freie und Hansestadt Hamburg and Bundesministerium für Jugend, Familie und Gesundheit.

REFERENCES

1. Breindl, M., Doehmer, J., Willecke, K., Dausman, J., and Jaenisch, R. (1979): <u>Proc. Nat. Acad. Sci. USA</u>, 76: 1938-1942.

2. Cooper, G., and Silverman, L. (1978): <u>Cell</u>, 15:573-577.

3. Davidson, E. (1976): <u>Gene Activity in Early Development</u>. Academic Press, New York, San Francisco, London.

4. Fritsch, E., Lawn, R., and Maniatis, T. (1979): <u>Nature</u>, 279:598-603.

5. Gross, L. (1961): <u>Proc. Soc. Exp. Biol. Med.</u>, 107:90-93.

6. Groudine, M., Holtzer, H., Scherrer, K., and Therwath, K. (1974): <u>Cell</u>, 3:243-250.

7. Jähner, D., and Jaenisch, R. (1980): <u>Nature</u>, 287:456-458.

8. Jaenisch, R. (1976): <u>Proc. Nat. Acad. Sci. USA</u>, 73:1260-1264.

9. Jaenisch, R. (1979): <u>Virology</u>, 93:80-90.

10. Jaenisch, R. (1980): <u>Cell</u>, 19:181-188.

11. Jaenisch, R. (1980): In: <u>The Molecular Biology of Tumor Viruses</u>, edited by J. Stephenson, pp. 131-162. Academic Press, New York.

12. Jaenisch, R., and Mintz, B. (1974): <u>Proc. Nat. Acad. Sci. USA</u>, 71:1250-1254.

13. Jaenisch, R., Fan, H., and Croker, B. (1975): <u>Proc. Nat. Acad. Sci. USA</u>, 72:4008-4012.

14. Jaenisch, R., Jähner, D., Nobis, P., Simon, I., Löhler, J., Harbers, K., and Grotkopp, D. (1981): <u>Cell</u>(May issue), in press.

15. Law, L. (1966): <u>Nat. Cancer Inst. Monogr.</u>, 22:267-282.

16. O'Rear, J., Mizutani, S., Hoffman, G., Fiandt, M., and Temin, H. (1980): <u>Cell</u>, 20:423-430.

17. Ploeg, L., and Flavell, R. (1980): <u>Cell</u>, 19:947-958.

18. Ploeg, L., Konings, A., Oort, M., Roos, D., Bernini, L., and Flavell, R. (1980): <u>Nature</u>, 283:637-642.

19. Stalder, J., Groudine, M., Dodgson, J., Engel, J., and Weintraub, H. (1980): <u>Cell</u>, 19:973-980.

20. Yamamoto, K., and Alberts, B. (1976): <u>Annu. Rev. Biochem.</u>, 45:721-746.

Expression of Differentiated Functions in Cancer Cells, edited by R. F. Revoltella et al., Raven Press, New York © 1982.

Molecular Basis of Differential Gene Expression in Murine Teratocarcinoma Derived Stem Versus Differentiated Cells

Alban Linnenbach, Kay Huebner, and Carlo M. Croce

The Wistar Institute of Anatomy and Biology, Philadelphia, Pennsylvania 19104

Murine teratocarcinoma derived stem cells seem to be equivalent to cells of the inner mass of the mouse blastocyst (5,11-12,18,20). Results of in vivo experiments of injection of teratocarcinoma derived stem cells into mouse blastocysts indicate that these cells are totipotent and can differentiate into any normal tissue of chimeric animals (5,11,20). Teratocarcinoma stem cells like early embryonal cells do not express the major H-2 histocompatibility antigens and do not express β_2 microglobulin (2,5,7,22). On the contrary all differentiated cells express H-2 antigens and β_2 microglobulin. Teratocarcinoma stem cells also restrict the expression of oncogenic viruses such as SV40, polyoma virus, and retro viruses (3,9,23,28,29,31). On the contrary, teratocarcinoma derived differentiated cells allow the expression of the viral genomes (3,9,23,28,29,31).

Recently Strickland and Mahdavi (27) have shown that nullipotent F9 teratocarcinoma derived stem cells, which are incapable of differentiating significantly in vitro and in vivo, can be induced to differentiate in the presence of retinoic acid (25,27). We have taken advantage of this finding to study the molecular basis of differential gene expression of histocompatibility antigens and oncogenic viruses in stem versus differentiated cells. In order to transfer oncogenic viral genomes into teratocarcinoma derived stem cells, we have introduced the viral DNAs into a plasmid pBR322 vector carrying a segment of the genome of herpes simplex virus type 1 containing a thymidine kinase gene (pHSV106) (10) and we have used these recombinant DNA molecules to transform thymidine kinase deficient F9 cells. Since the molecular mechanisms involved in the regulation of the expression of oncogenic viral genetic information might be similar to those involved in gene regulation during embryonal development, we intended to define the molecular basis of the suppression of oncogenic virus gene expression in teratocarcinoma derived stem cells and to determine whether the same molecular mechanisms affected the regulation of mouse endogenous genes which are also differentially regulated in stem versus differentiated cells.

29

RECOMBINANT PLASMIDS

The restriction map of the plasmid **pC6** containing the entire SV40 genome which has been used to transform F9TK⁻ cells is shown in Fig. 1. Using a similar approach we have also introduced the entire genomes of polyoma virus and Kirsten sarcoma virus in the pHSV106 vector that contains the 3.6 Kb fragment carrying the HSV-1 tk gene in pBR322(21). Polyoma virus and Kirsten sarcoma virus F9 transformants have already been obtained and are presently being characterized.

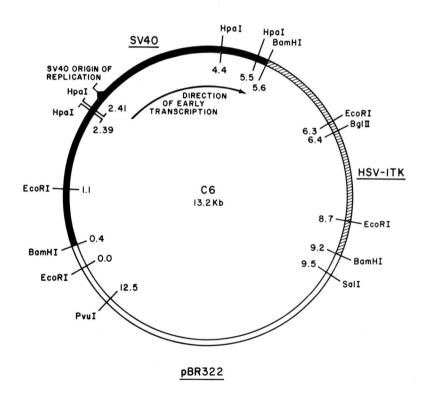

FIG. 1. Restriction map of 13.2-kb plasmid C6. One copy of Bam H1-digested SV40 DNA is inserted into the pBR322/HSV-1 tk vector, pHSV-106.

As shown in fig. 1 the pC6 plasmid is formed by three DNA segments linked at Bam H1 sites: the entire SV40 genome (5.2Kb), the HSV-1 tk genome (3.6 Kb) and the pBR322 genome (4.4 Kb) (14). By the calcium phosphate precipitation method (6) we have introduced the pC6 genome into F9-TK⁻ cells and selected the transformants in HAT medium (15, 30). Two HAT selected transformants (12-1 and 13-1) were then studied for the expression of thymidine kinase. As shown in figure 2 the transformants expressed the herpes simplex thymidine kinase activity (14).

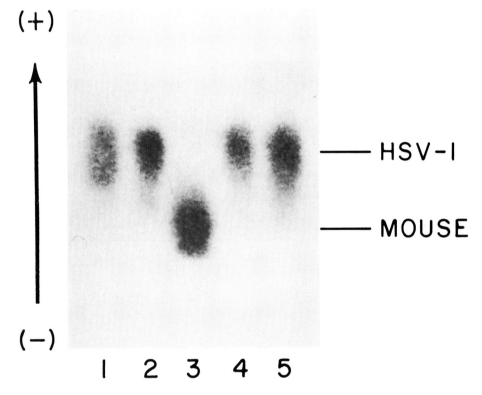

FIG.2. Starch gel electrophoretic separation of tk gene products. Enzyme migration is visualized by the binding of tritiated thymidine monophosphate product to DE-81 paper overlaid on electrophoretically separated TK enzymes. Enzymes in lanes 2 and 5 are from F9 stem cell transformants 13-1 and 12-1, respectively; lane 3, murine TK derived from MC57G cells; lane 4, HSV-1 TK derived from HSV transformed LM-TK⁻ cells. Lane 1 contains HSV-1 TK derived from an F9 stem cell transformant not described in this report.

CHARACTERIZATION OF pC6 DNA IN TRANSFORMED CELLS

We have fractionated the DNA extracted from 12-1 and 13-1 cells into a supernatant (free unintegrated DNA) and a pellet fraction (chromosomal DNA) by the Hirt procedure (8). These DNAs were then cleaved with the restriction enzymes XbaI, that does not cut the pC6 plasmid, and KpnI that cuts the SV40 genome once. The digested DNAs were fractionated through an agarose gel and blotted to a nitro-cellulose filter according to the method described by Southern (26). The filter was then hybridized with ^{32}P labeled nick translated (16) SV40 DNA. As shown in figure 3, no SV40 DNA was detectable in the Hirt supernatant DNA fraction of clones 12-1 and 13-1. On the con-trary, one single band of the size of 15 Kb was detected in the XbaI digested 12-1 P DNA (fig. 3, lane 3).

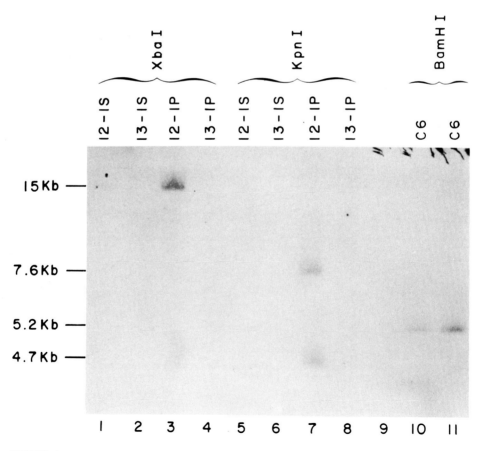

FIGURE 3

These findings indicated that a single pC6 molecule is integrated in the chromosomal DNA of clone 12-1. Since the size of the pC6 plasmid is 13.2 Kb, the 15 Kb XbaI fragments contain at least 1.8 Kb of flanking cellular DNA sequences. No SV40 was detected in clone 13-1 P DNA. Further analysis of this clone indicated that it had just retained the selectable HSV-1 DNA. Following digestion of 12-1 DNA with KpnI only two DNA fragments (7.6 Kb and 4.7 Kb respectively) hybridizing with SV40 DNA was observed. This finding is consistent with a single integration site of the pC6 genome in the chromosomal DNA of 12-1 cells. We then intended to determine whether all three components of our pC6 plasmid were part of the 15 Kb XbaI DNA fragment. Therefore, we cleaved the 12-1 DNA with XbaI, fractionated it through an agarose gel and cut the gel into three parts that were blotted to three different nitrocellulose filters. The filters were then hybridized with ^{32}P labeled pBR322 DNA, with ^{32}P labeled HSV-1 tk DNA and with ^{32}P labeled SV40 DNA respectively (fig.4). As shown in figure 4, the XbaI 15 Kb band hybridized with all three probes. These results indicate that all components of the pC6 plasmid are part of the same 15 Kb XbaI DNA fragment.

As shown in figure 4a-3, following Bam H1 digestion of the 12-1 cell DNA no 4.4 Kb pBR322 band was observed. In its place we observed a 12.5 Kb band; there should theoretically be another band in this lane, and this fragment is detected in other experiments with higher specific activity probes. This finding indicates that the pC6 plasmid is integrated through a site in the pBR322 genome. As shown in figure 4c (lane 3), an intact SV40 linear 5.2 Kb DNA molecule was detected in Bam H1 digested 12-1 DNA. We have been able, therefore, to introduce a single intact linear molecule of SV40 in the genome of teratocarcinoma stem cells by the DNA mediated gene transfer approach (14).

← ───

FIG. 3. Hybridization of ^{32}P labeled SV40 DNA to 13-1 and 12-1 cellular DNA after restriction endonuclease digestion and transfer from agarose gel. Hirt supernatant (S) and pellet (P) DNA (10 μg per lane) from 12-1 and 13-1 stem cells were cleaved with XbaI (lanes 1-4) and KpnI (lanes 5-8); electrophoresed in a 0.7% agarose slab gel; denatured; transferred to a nitrocellulose sheet; and hybridized to ^{32}P labeled SV40 DNA. BamH1-cleaved and similarly treated pC6 DNA (lane 10, lane 11) was included as a marker.

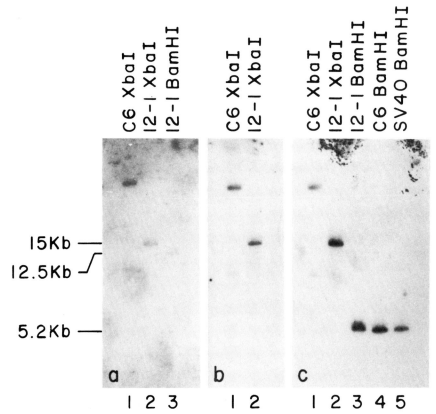

FIG. 4. Hybridization of ^{32}P labeled pBR322 DNA (a), HSV-1 tk DNA
(b), and SV40 DNA (c) to XbaI- and Bam HI- cleaved 12-1 cellular
DNA. Hirt pellet DNA (10 μg/lane) from 12-1 cells was cleaved with
XbaI and Bam HI restriction endonucleases and applied to an agarose
slab gel as indicated above each lane in this figure. After electrophoresis, the gel was cut into three parts, and the DNA in each gel
was denatured and transferred to nitrocellulose sheets. Each of the
three nitrocellulose sheets was hybridized to a different ^{32}P labeled probe: (a) hybridized to ^{32}P labeled pBR322 DNA; (b) hybridized
to ^{32}P labeled HSV-1 tk DNA; and (c) hybridized to ^{32}P labeled SV40
DNA. pC6 DNA, Bam HI-cleaved pC6 DNA, and Bam HI-cleaved SV40 DNA
are included as markers.

EXPRESSION OF SV40 T ANTIGEN IN TERATOCARCINOMA
DERIVED STEM VERSUS DIFFERENTIATED CELLS

The 12-1 cells were studied for the expression of SV40 T antigen
by indirect immunofluorescence using either mouse monoclonal antibodies against the SV40 large T antigen (19) or hamster anti T antigen antisera. As shown in figure 5a the 12-1 cells were SV40 T antigen negative. Following their exposure to retinoic acid, however,
the 12-1 cells differentiated and became SV40 T antigen positive
(figure 5b). Since the retinoic acid induced differentiated 12-1
cells are SV40 T antigen positive and phenotypically transformed it
becomes easy to obtain 12-1 derived differentiated cell lines; one
of these differentiated clones, named 12-1a, was used in experiments
described below.

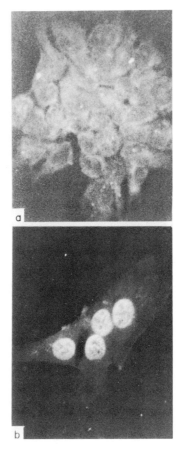

FIG.5. Indirect immunofluorescence of SV40 T antigen in transformant
12-1 cells before (a) and after (b) induction of differentiation
with 0.1 μM retinoic acid.

We have also used monoclonal antibodies specific for the SV40
large T antigen to immunoprecipitate T antigen from lysates of 12-1
and 12-1a cells. As shown in figure 6, no large T antigen (M.W. 94,000
daltons) was detected in 12-1 cells following immunoprecipitation
and SDS polyacrylamide gel electrophoresis (17). On the contrary
SV40 large T antigen was detected in lysates of 12-1a differentiated
cells (17).

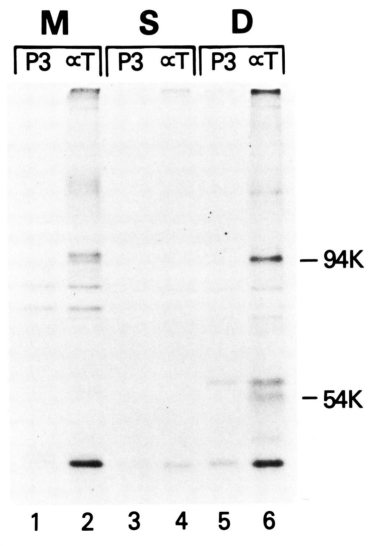

FIGURE 6

EXPRESSION OF SURFACE ANTIGENS IN TERATOCARCINOMA DERIVED STEM VERSUS DIFFERENTIATED CELLS

We have also studied the expression of the SV40 tumor specific transplantation antigen (TSTA) in stem and differentiated cells. By using a cytotoxic assay we have shown that 12-1 cells do not express TSTA (13). On the contrary retinoic acid induced 12-1 cells express this antigen (13). By using monoclonal antibodies directed against the H-2D^b private specificity 2 and immunofluorescence techniques we have shown that 12-1 cells do not express H-2,while 12-1a cells express H-2 antigens (13). Similarly we did not detect the expression of β_2 microglobulin in F9 and 12-1 cells, but we have detected it in retinoic acid induced F9 cells and 12-1a differentiated cells(fig.7)(5). We have also studied the expression of the stage specific embryonal antigen 1 (SSEA-1) that is recognized by a monoclonal antibody against teratocarcinoma stem cells (24), in 12-1 stem and 12-1a differentiated cells. The SSEA-1 was detected in F9 and 12-1 cells but not in retinoic acid induced F9 and 12-1 differentiated cells (13). A summary of these findings is reported in table 1.

TABLE 1. Surface antigen expression in teratocarcinoma derived stem and differentiated cells

Antigen	Cells		
	F9	12-1	12-1a
H-2 D (1)	−	−	+
beta-2 microglobulin (2)	−	−	+
SSEA-1 (1)	+	+	−

(1) More than 97% of the stem cells were negative for H-2 antigen and 90% were positive for SSEA-1 by indirect immunofluorescence; conversely, more than 99% of the differentiated cells were positive for H-2 antigen and all of the differentiated cells were negative for SSEA-1.

(2) More than 98% of the stem cells were negative and 99% of the differentiated cells were positive for beta-2 microglobulin by indirect immunofluorescent assay. Furthermore, detergent extracts of 12-1 stem cells did not inhibit the immunoprecipitation of radiolabeled purified mouse beta-2 microglobulin. Detergent extracts of 12-1a differentiated cells inhibited immunoprecipitation of up to 85% of radiolabeled purified mouse beta-2 microglobulin.

FIG. 6. Immunoprecipitation of SV40 T-antigen from 12-1 and 12-1a cells. (^{35}S) methionine-labeled extracts from SV40-transformed monkey kidney cells (M), 12-1 stem cells (S), and 12-1a differentiated cells (D) were reacted with monoclonal anti-SV40 T-antigen antibody (αT) or with nonimmune antibody (P3) and precipitated by addition of rabbit anti-mouse immunoglobulins. The 12% polyacrylamide gel was fluorographed, dried, and exposed for 7 days.

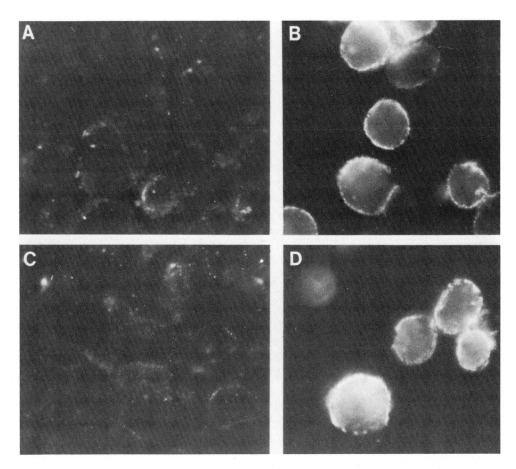

FIG. 7. Immunofluorescent assay for beta-2 microglobulin on teratocarcinoma derived cells. Single cell suspensions of teratocarcinoma
derived stem cells, F9TK⁻ and 12-1, differentiated cells, F9ACcl9 and
12-1a, and control cells, P3, Daudi, and MP, were exposed to rabbit
anti-human beta-2 microglobulin antibody. The second reagent was
anti-rabbit immunoglobulin tagged with fluorescein isothiocyanate:
A) F9TK⁻ stem cells, B) F9ACcl9 differentiated cells, C) 12-1 stem
cells, D) 12-1a differentiated cells. P3 mouse myeloma cells and
MP human lymphoblastoid cells stained positively for beta-2 microglobulin while Daudi human Burkitt lymphoma cells did not express
beta-2 microglobulin as expected (5) (data for control cells not
shown).

ORGANIZATION OF THE SV40 GENOME IN TERATOCARCINOMA
DERIVED STEM AND DIFFERENTIATED CELLS

As shown in figure 1 the pC6 plasmid was constructed by ligating Bam H1 linearized SV40 DNA into one of the two Bam H1 sites of the pHSV106 vector (14). The pHSV106 vector was formed by inserting the 3.6 Kb fragment of HSV-1 DNA carrying the TK gene into the Bam H1 site of the plasmid pBR322 (21). Therefore Bam H1 cleaves the pC6 genome into its three components. As we have shown in figures 3 and 4, XbaI cleavage of 12-1 DNA results in the appearance of a single 15 Kb band that hybridizes with all three probes and Bam H1 cleavage of 12-1 DNA results in the appearance of a single 5.2 Kb band that hybridizes with SV40 DNA. We intended to determine whether the organization of the SV40 genome within the 12-1 genome changed during the process of differentiation. As shown in figure 8, retinoic acid induced 12-1 cell DNA and 12-1a cell DNA contain the same 15 Kb XbaI DNA fragment hybridizing with ^{32}P labeled SV40 DNA. Similarly they contain a linear 5.2 Kb SV40 genome (fig.8). Therefore we can conclude that no gross rearrangement of the pC6 genome occurs in 12-1 cells during the process of differentiation.

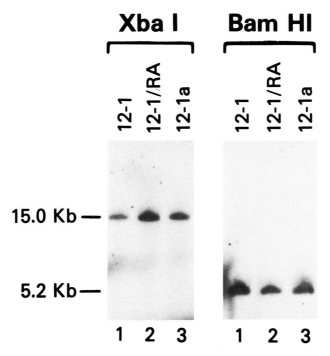

FIG. 8. Arrangement of the SV40 genome in stem and differentiated cells. Cellular DNA from 12-1 cells, 12-1 cells after 12 days of exposure to retinoic acid, and 12-1a cells, was cleaved with restriction enzymes XbaI (left panel) and Bam H1 (right panel), electrophoresed, transferred to nitrocellulose filters and filters were hybridized to ^{32}P labeled SV40 DNA.

TRANSCRIPTION OF THE SV40 GENOME IN TERATOCARCINOMA
DERIVED STEM AND DIFFERENTIATED CELLS

Total RNA was extracted from 12-1 stem and 12-1a differentiated
cells, selected by oligo (dT) cellulose chromatography, glyoxalated,
separated by agarose gel electrophoresis and transferred to nitrocellulose filters (17, 32). Hybridization with a ^{32}P labeled SV40
DNA probe detected a 2900 base and a 2600 base mRNA in the poly A$^+$
mRNA fractions of both stem and differentiated cells (fig. 9, lanes
2 and 4 respectively). The observed sizes of these two SV40 transcripts are in agreement with those found early after infection of
monkey kidney cells with SV40 DNA (4).

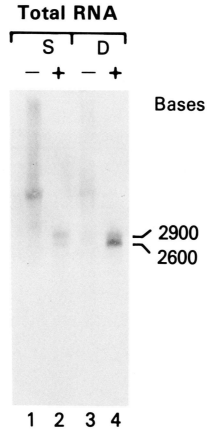

FIG. 9. SV40 RNA in 12-1 and 12-1a cells. Poly A$^+$ and non-polyaden-
ylated (poly A$^-$) fractions of total cellular RNA from 12-1 stem
cells (S) and 12-1a differentiated cells (D) were denatured, separated electrophoretically, transferred to nitrocellulose filters and
hybridized to ^{32}P labeled SV40 DNA. Lanes 1 and 2, contained 10 µg
poly A$^-$ RNA and 1 µg poly A$^+$, respectively, from 12-1 stem cells
(S); lanes 3 and 4, contained 10 µg poly A$^-$ RNA and 1 µg poly A$^+$ RNA,
respectively, from 12-1a differentiated cells (D).

When total cytoplasmic RNA from stem and differentiated cells
were analyzed, the same two SV40 RNAs were detected in the 12-1 stem
cells (Fig. 10, lane 1) and, as expected, in the 12-1a differentiated
cell (fig. 10, lane 2). Interestingly, the 2900 base RNA species,
which is the size of small t mRNA is present in stem cells in
larger amounts than the 2600 base species, which is the size of
large T mRNA, while the reverse is true for the differentiated cells.

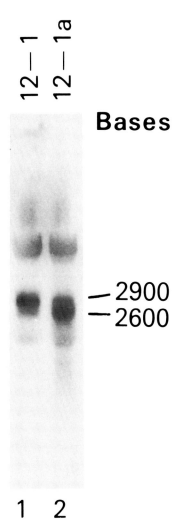

FIG. 10. SV40 RNA in cytoplasm of 12-1 and 12-1a cells. Cytoplasmic
RNA (10 μg/lane) from 12-1 stem and 12-1a differentiated cells were
electrophoresed, blotted and hybridized to ^{32}P labeled SV40 DNA.

S₁ NUCLEASE ANALYSIS OF SV40 TRANSCRIPTS

The sizes of the SV40 RNAs we have detected in the stem cells (fig. 9 and 10) were suggestive of mature SV40 transcripts. A direct demonstration of spliced mature SV40 RNAs was carried out according to the technique developed by Berk and Sharp (4) modified as outlined in figure 11.

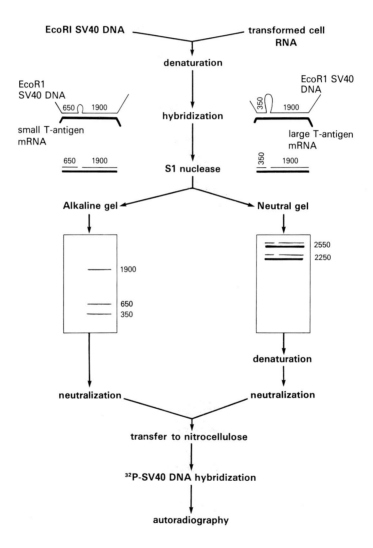

FIG. 11. Outline of method used for analysis of S₁ nuclease resistant duplexes obtained after hybridization of 12-1 and 12-1a cellular RNAs with linear SV40 DNA. The various steps in the analysis were described in detail elsewhere (17).

Alkaline agarose gel electrophoresis of S₁ resistant duplexes,
Southern transfer to nitrocellulose filters, and hybridization with
32P labeled SV40 DNA, revealed a 1900 base fragment in the 12-1 stem
cells (fig. 12a, lane 2 and 12b, lane 1) and in the 12-1a differentiated cells (fig. 12, lane 3). The 650 and 350 base leader
fragments were not detected under the experimental conditions used.
The 1900 base fragments is common to both large T- and small t-
antigen mRNAs and can occur only if the cellular RNA contained
spliced messenger RNA.

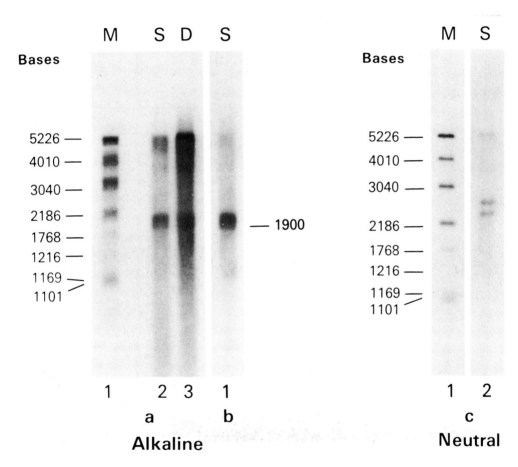

FIG. 12. Spliced SV40 mRNA in 12-1 and 12-1a cells. Total cellular
RNA from 12-1 stem (S) and 12-1a differentiated (D) cells was hybridized to EcoR1 cleaved SV40 DNA, treated with S₁ nuclease, electrophoresed on alkaline or neutral gels, blotted and hybridized with
32P labeled SV40 DNA. Results after alkaline gel electrophoresis
are shown in panels a and b and results after neutral gel electrophoresis are shown in panel c. Marker lanes (M) contained SV40 DNA
fragments prepared by digestions of SV40 DNA with Bam H1, Pst1,
Hind III and Bam H1 plus Hpa II; lanes labeled S contained duplexes
derived from 12-1 RNA and lanes marked D contained duplexes derived
from 12-1a RNA.

Splicing of the SV40 RNA in teratocarcinoma-derived stem cells
was confirmed by neutral gel electrophoresis of intact S₁ digested
DNA-RNA hybrids. The observed 2250 and 2550 base pair duplexes
(fig. 12c, lane 2) are identical to those observed for spliced
large T- and small t- antigen mRNAs in SV40-infected monkey kidney
cells (4).

The results of these experiments indicate that the integrated
SV40 genome is transcribed and the SV40 RNA spliced in teratocarcinoma stem cells. The simplest interpretation of these results is
that stem cells which carry integrated SV40 genomes, are capable of
synthesizing authentic early SV40 mRNAs and that the lack of
expression of SV40 early region genes is due to a post-transcriptional
event. In vitro translation of SV40-specific mRNAs from stem cells
will determine whether the block to SV40 T-antigen expressed in stem
cells occurs at the translational level or whether the mRNAs
produced in stem cells are defective.

TRANSCRIPTIONS OF THE GENES FOR HISTOCOMPATIBILITY ANTIGENS IN TERATOCARCINOMA DERIVED STEM AND DIFFERENTIATED CELLS

Since no H-2 antigens and β_2 microglobulin are expressed in teratocarcinoma derived stem cells, in collaboration with Drs. Ettore Appella
and Jonathan G. Seidman we attempted to determine whether the genes
coding for these surface antigens are transcribed in the stem cells(5).
By using DNA probes specific for H-2 and β_2 microglobulin we have
studied the transcription of the H-2 and the β_2 microglobulin genes in
stem and differentiated cells (5). As shown in figure 13, Northern
blotting analysis of RNA produced by stem and differentiated cells,
indicates that 12-1 cells do not contain detectable RNA that hybridizes
with the H-2 and β_2 microglobulin DNA probes. On the contrary 12-1a
cells express a 1850 bases long H-2 mRNA and two β_2 microglobulin mRNAs,
1250 and 1050 bases in length.

Similar experiments were carried out within total and polyA' cytoplasmic RNA derived from F9 cells with identical results. Therefore
we can conclude that at least two different molecular mechanisms are
involved in the regulation of gene expression in teratocarcinoma
derived stem cells: One post-transcriptional as in the case of the
expression of integrated SV40 genomes, and one transcriptional as in
the case of the expression of the H-2 and β_2 microglobulin genes (5,
17).

DEOXYRIBONUCLEASE 1 SENSITIVITY OF PLASMID GENOMES AND CELLULAR GENES IN TERATOCARCINOMA DERIVED STEM AND DIFFERENTIATED CELLS

DNase 1 sensitivity of the Simian virus 40 (SV40) genome, the pBR322
genome, the herpes simplex virus type 1 thymidine kinase (HSV-1 tk)
gene, the H-2 genes and the β_2 microglobulin genes were compared in
teratocarcinoma derived stem (12-1) and differentiated (12-1a) cell
lines which were established after transfection of TK deficient F9
cells with pC6 DNA. All five of these genomes are more sensitive to
DNase 1 digestion in stem cells than in differentiated cells, reflect-
ing the DNase 1 hypersensitivity of total stem cell chromatin (10).
The HSV-1 tk gene is the least sensitive to DNase 1 digestion in both
cell types (10).

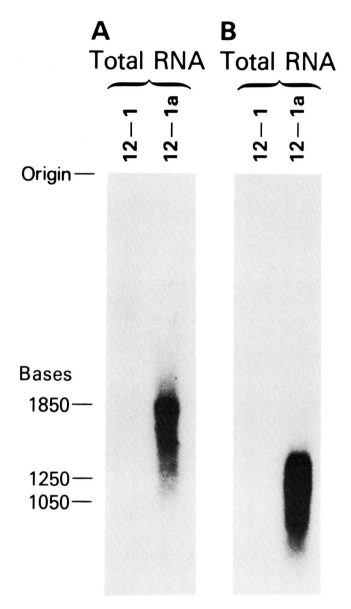

FIG. 13. Detection of H-2 and beta-2 microglobulin specific RNA in teratocarcinoma derived cells. Total RNAs were extracted from stem cells, 12-1, and differentiated cells, 12-1a. Ten μg/lane of RNA was glyoxalated, electrophoresed, and transferred to nitrocellulose filters. H-2 and beta-2 microglobulin specific transcripts were identified by hybridization to ^{32}P labeled H-2 and beta-2 microglobulin probes: a) total cellular RNA from stem (12-1) and differentiated (12-1a) cells hybridized to ^{32}P labeled H-2 DNA; and b) total cellular RNA from stem (12-1) and differentiated (12-1a) cells hybridized to ^{32}P labeled beta-2 microglobulin DNA).

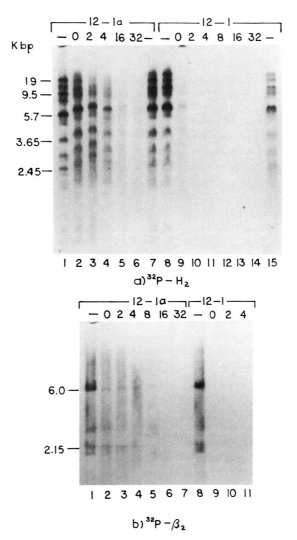

FIG.14. DNase 1 sensitivity of H-2 and beta-2-microglobulin genes in stem and differentiated cells. 12-1a and 12-1 nuclei were DNase 1 digested (10 µg DNase 1/mg DNA) for various times (0-32 minutes) as indicated above lanes (a) and (b). The minus sign (-) above lanes means that nuclei were incubated without DNase 1. DNA was prepared for each time point, cleaved with Bam H1, or EcoR1 electrophoresed, blotted and hybridized. a) Hybridization of DNase 1/Bam H1 digested DNA with ^{32}P labeled H-2 DNA probe. Lanes 1 and 8 contained 10 µg/lane of DNA extracted from 12-1a and 12-1 nuclei after incubation in RSB buffer at 37°C for 2 minutes without DNase 1. Lanes 7 and 15 contained 10 µg/ lane of 12-1a and 12-1 DNA extracted from nuclei incubated at 37°C in RSB buffer without DNase 1 for 32 minutes. b) Hybridization of DNase 1/ EcoR1 digested DNA with ^{32}P labeled beta-2 microglobulin DNA probe.

To examine the DNase 1 sensitivity of the H-2 and beta-2-microglo-
bulin genes, nuclei from 12-1 and 12-1a cells were digested with
DNase 1, then their DNA was subsequently extracted, restricted with
either Bam H1 or EcoR1, electrophoresed, blotted on to nitrocellulose
filters and hybridized to ^{32}P nick translated H-2 or beta-2-micro-
globulin probes. Results of these hybridizations are shown in
figure 14. When ^{32}P labeled H-2 DNA is hybridized with Bam H1 digested 12-1a DNA (fig. 14a, lanes 1 (-), 7(-)) and 12-1 DNA (fig.14a,
lanes 8(-), 15(-)), several major and minor bands are detected and
the pattern seems to be the same in both cell types (compare fig. 14a
lanes 7 and 8). In DNase 1/Bam H1 treated DNAs from 12-1a cells, the
hybridization pattern decreases in intensity with increase in time of
exposure to DNase 1 (fig. 14a, lanes 2-6) but hybridization is still
detectable even after 32 minutes (fig. 14a, lane 6) of DNase 1
digestion of 12-1a nuclei (when only 60% of total DNA remains, fig.
15). On the other hand, after 2 minutes of digestion of 12-1 nuclei
with DNase 1 (when 85% of total DNA remains undigested, fig. 15), no
Bam H1 fragments remain which hybridize with ^{32}P labeled H-2 DNA.

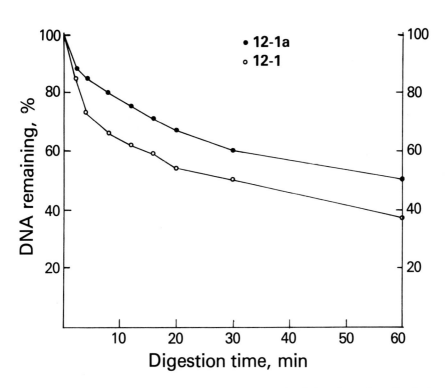

FIG. 15. Digestion of 12-1 and 12-1a nuclei with DNase 1. Nuclei
were isolated, resuspended in RSB buffer to 1 mg/ml and 10 µg/ml
DNase 1 was added. 1 ml aliquots of nuclei were removed at indicated
times and nuclei sedimented at low speed. Percentage DNA remaining
was determined by measuring the release into supernatants of material
absorbing at 260 nM.

Similar results were observed with DNase 1/EcoR1 digested DNA from the two cell types after hybridization with beta-2 microglobulin ^{32}P-labeled DNA (fig. 14b); after 8 minutes of DNase 1 digestion of 12-1a nuclei (when 80% of total DNA is undigested), the EcoR1 cleaved fragments homologous to beta-2 microglobulin cDNA are still faintly detectable; these fragments are not present after DNase 1/EcoR1 digestion of 12-1 DNA even at the first time point (fig. 14b, lane 9). We conclude that H-2 and beta-2 microglobulin genes, like total chromatin and the specific plasmid genomes are, within stem cell nuclei, in a configuration which makes them more accessible to DNase 1, than are the same genes within nuclei of differentiated cells.   Normally, transcriptionally inactive genes are DNase 1 resistant, while active genes are DNase 1 sensitive. In contrast the major histocompatibility antigen genes of teratocarcinoma stem cells, which are transcriptionally inactive, are more DNase 1 sensitive than the active genes of the differentiated cells.

CONCLUSIONS

The results of the experiments described in this paper indicate that at least two different mechanisms are involved in the differential regulation of gene expression in teratocarcinoma derived stem and differentiated cells. In the case of integrated SV40 genomes, the early SV40 DNA coding for the large T-and small t-antigens is transcribed, and SV40 spliced RNAs of the size of the mRNAs for small t-and large T-antigens are produced in stem cells. However, contrary to this, the genes for histocompatibility antigens are not transcribed in stem cells. At present we are investigating whether the SV40 RNAs detected (but not translated) in stem cells can be translated into large T- and small t- antigens in an in vitro translation system. If this is the case, this result would indicate that the block in T-antigen expression in teratocarcinoma stem cells occurs at the translational level. We are also attempting to define the factors that allow the transcription of histocompatibility antigen genes during the process of differentiation. Interestingly, we have also observed that the DNA of teratocarcinoma stem cells in toto is much more sensitive to DNase 1 digestion than the DNA of teratocarcinoma derived differentiated cells (5, 10). This finding indicates that the chromatin structure of the genome of teratocarcinoma stem cells and, by analogy, early embryonal cells makes the cellular DNA more accessible to DNase 1 digestion. At present we are investigating the differences in chromosomal proteins between stem and differentiated cells in order to understand the molecular basis of the hypersensitivity of teratocarcinoma stem cells to DNase 1 digestion.

REFERENCES

1. Artz, K., and Jacob, F. (1974): Transplantation., 17:632-634.
2. Baccara, M., and Kelly, F. (1978): Virology., 90:147-150.
3. Berk, A. J., and Sharp, P. A. (1978): Proc. Natl. Acad. Sci. USA., 75:1274-1278.
4. Brinster, R. L. (1974): J. Exp. Med., 140:1049-1056.

5. Croce, C. M., Linnenbach, A., Huebner, K., Parnes, J., Margulies, D. H., Appella, E., and Seidman, J. G. (1981) Proc. Natl. Acad. Sci. USA., Sept. 1981 in press.
6. Graham, F. L., and Van de Eb, A. J. (1973): Virology., 52: 456-467.
7. Heyner, S., Brinster, R. L., and Palm, J. (1969): Nature., 222: 783-784.
8. Hirt, B. (1967): J. Mol. Biol., 26:365-369.
9. Huebner, K., Tsuchida, N., Green, C., and Croce, C. M. (1979): J. Exp. Med., 150: 392-405.
10. Huebner, K., Linnenbach, A., Weidner, S., Glenn, G., and Croce, C. M. (1981): Proc. Natl. Acad. Sci. USA, in press.
11. Illmensee, K., and Mintz, G. (1976): Proc. Natl. Acad. Sci. USA., 73:549-553.
12. Kleinsmith, L. J., and Pierce, G. B., (1964): Cancer Res., 24: 1544-1552.
13. Knowles, B. B., Pan, S., Solter, D., Linnenbach, A., Croce, C. M., and Huebner, K. Nature., 288:615-618.
14. Linnenbach, A., Huebner, K., and Croce, C. M. (1980): Proc. Natl. Acad. Sci. USA., 77:4875-4879.
15. Littlefield, J. W., (1965): Exp. Cell. Res., 41:190-196.
16. Maniatis, T., Kee, S. G., Efstradiatis, A., and Kafatos, F. C., (1976): Cell., 8:163-182.
17. Linnenbach, A., Huebner, K., and Croce, C. M., (1981): Proc. Natl. Acad. Sci. USA., in press.
18. Martin, G., and Evans, M. J., (1975): Cell., 6:467-474.
19. Martinis, J., and Croce, C. M., (1978): Proc. Natl. Acad. Sci. USA., 75:2320-2323.
20. Mintz, B., and Illmensee, K. (1975): Proc. Natl. Acad. Sci. USA, 72:3585-3589.
21. McKnight, S. L., and Croce, C. M. (1979): Carnegie Institute Yearbook, 98:56-61.
22. Palm, J., Heyner, S., and Brinster, R. L. (1971) J. Exp. Med., 133, 1282-1293.
23. Paries, J., Alves-Cardosa, E., Carivet, M., Dehans-Guillemin, M.C., and Lasveret, J., (1977): J. Natl. Cancer Inst., 59: 463-465.
24. Solter, D., and Knowles, B. B., (1978): Proc. Natl. Acad. Sci. USA, 75:5565-5569.
25. Solter, D., Shevinsky, L., Knowles, B. B., and Strickland, S. (1979): Develop,. Biol., 70:515-521.
26. Southern, E. (1975): J. Mol. Biol., 98:503-517.
27. Strickland, S., and Mahdavi, V., (1978): Cell 15: 393-403.
28. Swartzendruber, D. E., and Lehman, J. M., (1975): J. Cell. Physiol. 93:25-30.
29. Swartzendruber, D. E., Freidrich, T. D., and Lehman, J. M., (1977): J. Cell. Physiol., 93:25-30.
30. Szybalski, W., Szybalski, E., and Ragni, G. (1962): Natl. Cancer Inst. Monograph. 7:75-88.
31. Teich, N. M., Meiss, R., Martin, G. R., and Long, D. P. (1977): Cell., 12:973-982.
32. Thomas, P. S., (1980): Proc. Natl. Acad. Sci. USA., 77:5201-5205.

Expression of Differentiated Functions in Cancer Cells, edited by R. F. Revoltella et al., Raven Press, New York © 1982.

Transcription of Globin Genes *In Vivo* and *In Vitro*

R. A. Flavell, G. C. Grosveld, C. K. Shewmaker, F. G. Grosveld, H. H. M. Dahl, and E. de Boer

Laboratory of Gene Structure and Expression, National Institute for Medical Research, London NW7 1AA, United Kingdom

INTRODUCTION

For a number of years the haemoglobin genes have proved a successful model for the study of gene expression in higher eukaryotes. The availability of recombinant DNA technology has permitted the elucidation of the structure and the linkage arrangement of numerous globin genes from diverse species. As a pre-requisite for studies on gene expression, we have studied the structure and linkage arrangement of the human and rabbit β-related globin genes. The structural data have been considered in other recent symposium articles (8, 9).

To analyse how globin genes are expressed, and how this expression is regulated, we have analysed the in vivo transcription products of the rabbit β-globin gene in rabbit bone marrow.

TRANSCRIPTION OF THE RABBIT β-GLOBIN GENE IN VIVO

The rabbit β-globin gene consists of three non-contiguous blocks of mRNA-coding sequences separated by two introns of 126 and 573 base pairs. S_1 mapping experiments using the procedure of Berk and Sharp (1) have shown (12) the structure of in vivo RNAs in Fig. 1. The largest globin pre-mRNA detectable is a colinear transcript of the gene, including the introns and exons, but lacking sequences derived from the extragenic DNA. The 5' and 3' termini of the colinear transcript have been mapped using 5' and 3' terminally labelled probes in S_1 nuclease experiments and then sizing the products on a thin polyacrylamide gel with as marker a G + A sequence lane of the fragment used as probe. In these experiments, the size of the S_1 nuclease digestion products for both the 5' and 3' ends fits with the size expected if the 5' and 3' termini of the globin mRNA are coincident with those of the colinear pre-mRNA. We conclude that, within experimental error, the 5' and 3' ends of β-globin mRNA and pre mRNA are co-terminal. A similar conclusion has been drawn for the 5' end of mouse β-globin pre mRNA (22).

In addition to the colinear RNA spliced β-globin pre-mRNAs can be detected by the same method (Fig. 1). Splices are found within both the small and large introns, together with molecules where the entire small intron has apparently been spliced out, but where the entire large intron is still present. Inspection of Fig. 1 shows that the RNAs can be

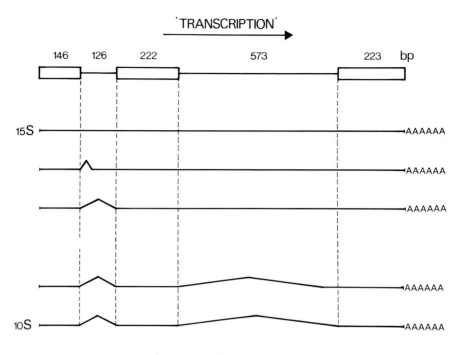

FIG. 1.

Structure of β-globin pre-mRNAs in rabbit bone marrow RNA.   The β-globin
gene is depicted as three coding blocks separated by two intervening
sequences.   The horizontal lines indicate the RNA in a given species and
indicates the region removed by splicing.   The 5' splice junction of the
intermediates, drawn here at the intron-exon boundary, has not been experimentally verified.

arranged in a scheme where sequential splicing of first the small intron,
then the large intron, each in two steps, could occur.   While this is
the most plausible explanation, two critical points should be noted.
First, it is not proven that the intermediate spliced molecules are indeed to be processed to give β-globin mRNA.   These molecules may also
be the result of splicing errors in vivo and may only be destined to be
degraded.   Second, other partially spliced molecules may be present,
but undetected in our experiments.   Thus, the pathway, suggested by
Fig. 1 may only be the way most, but not all, β-globin mRNA is produced.

TRANSCRIPTION OF THE RABBIT β-GLOBIN GENE IN VITRO

Weil et al. (23) and Manley et al.(15) have shown that the Adenovirus
2 (Ads) late genes can be transcribed in vitro in cell-free extracts to
give specific products whose 5' end is capped and coincident in position
with the 5' end of the major late Ad2 RNA.   These data suggest strongly
that RNA synthesis initiates at this site in vitro although rapid processing followed by capping of the transcript remains to be excluded.

We have used the Hela cell extract of Manley et al. (15) to characterize the in vitro transcripts of the rabbit β-globin gene and to define
the DNA sequences required to give specific RNA synthesis in vitro. By
analogy with bacterial systems we shall refer to these DNA sequences as
the rabbit β-globin promotor.

The rabbit β-globin gene is transcribed efficiently in this system.
Since the β-globin gene is presumably not expressed in Hela cells, it is
clear that positive erythroid-cell specific factors are not required for
the transcription of the β-globin gene in this type of extract. If the
rabbit β-globin DNA is cut at the intragenic Taq I site (at 308 nucleotides past the cap site; + 308) and then used as template in this system,
labelled RNAs can be detected in the in vitro product of 308 and 310
nucleotides respectively, together with larger RNAs that derive from nonspecific initiations further upstream. Similarly, if the DNA is cut at
the Bam HI site (+475) major RNA products of 471, 475 and 480 are seen;
DNA cut at the EcoRI site (+ 1120) gives two products of about 1160 NT
(Fig. 2).

Clearly, specific RNAs are synthesized with 5' ends at the same site
as in vivo globin pre-mRNA. We have also mapped the 5' ends of the in
vitro product by S_1 mapping experiments using as probe a 5' labelled
Bst NI fragment containing the 5' end of the β-globin gene. By this
criterion, the 5' end of the in vitro transcript also maps at the same
position as that of in vivo β-globin mRNA (not shown). The heterogeneity of the run off transcripts is at least partially the result of
heterogeneity of the 3' ends. The RNA polymerase apparently stutters
when it reaches the 3' end of the DNA molecule, some polymerase termin-
ate at the end of the double stranded region, while others copy the four
nucleotide sticky end (GATC in the case of Bam HI) on the non-coding
strand. This gives two transcripts which differ in length by four
nucleotides. Removal of the sticky ends by S_1 nuclease, or by DNA re-
pair using DNA polymerase I essentially eliminates this heterogeneity.

DNA SEQUENCES REQUIRED FOR THE TRANSCRIPTION OF THE RABBIT β-GLOBIN GENE: THE RABBIT β-GLOBIN GENE PROMOTOR

Sequence comparison of a number of eukaryotic genes has pointed to at
least 3 regions that have been conserved in evolution: the 'Hogness'
box (16) CATAAAAG in the case of the rabbit β-globin gene, located about
30 nucleotides upstream from the cap site; the capping box Py CATTC Pu
(4) located just after the cap site; and the so-called CCAAT box located
about 80 nucleotides upstream from the cap site (7). To determine if
any of these sequences are required for transcription in vitro we have
constructed a series of deletion mutants that lack DNA sequences in the
5' extragenic region of the rabbit β-globin gene. The map-coordinates
of some of these deletion mutants are described in Table I, together
with their ability to direct transcription. It can be seen that removal of sequences upstream of -100 has no pronounced effect on the transcription efficiency, whereas deletion of DNA between -100 and -12 eliminates transcription entirely. At least part of the rabbit β-globin
gene promotor must therefore lie between -100 and -12. We have constructed a large number of deletion mutants in the region close to the
Hogness box, and analysed their transcription in vitro (14). A mutant
lacking the sequences -20 to +7 is transcribed well in this system. A
mutant lacking -30 to -4, and therefore lacking the Hogness box, is not
transcribed at all in this system. Similarly, when the DNA sequences

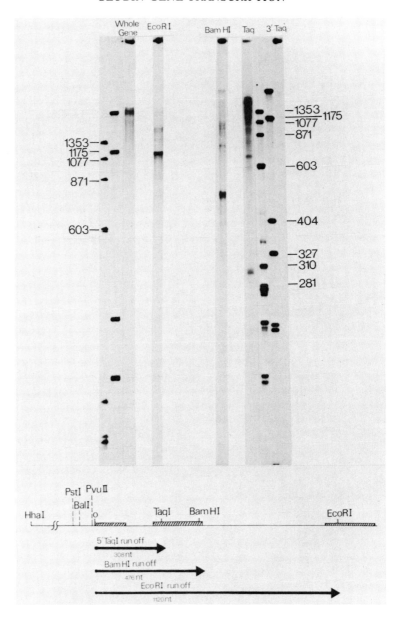

FIG. 2.

Transcription of the rabbit β-globin gene <u>in vitro</u>.   Restriction fragments of the rabbit β-globin gene truncated at the Taq I (+308), Bam HI
(+475) or Eco RI (+1120) was incubated with a Hela cell extract prepared
as in ref. 15 in a volume of 25 μl with α-^{32}P GTP (16 Ci/mmol) as labelled
substrate.   The RNA was recovered by proteinase K digestion, phenol
extraction and ethanol precipitation.   The RNA and 5' end labelled DNA
markers (ØX DNA x Taq I and ØX DNA x Hae III) were heat denatured in 98%
Formamide, 10 mM Hepes pH 6.5 0.1% SDS containing 0.02% each of Bromo-
phenol blue and Xylene cyanol FF, and analysed on a 0.3 mm thick 5% poly-
acrylamide-urea gel.

TABLE 1

Transcription of the rabbit β-globin gene <u>in vivo</u> and <u>in vitro</u>

DNA sequences deleted	Transcription	
	In vitro	In vivo
none (wild type)	+	+++
−11 to −7	+	+++
−11 to +11	+	+++
−20 to +7	+	+++
−30 to −4	−	−
upstream of −424	N.D.	+++
upstream of −100	+	+++
upstream of −58	+	+
upstream of −43	+	N.D.
upstream of −34	+	+
upstream of −15	−	−
upstream of −12	−	N.D.

The <u>in vitro</u> transcription efficiencies have been estimated from the intensities of the run off products on the polyacrylamide gels. Transcription <u>in vivo</u> was estimated by hybridization of RNA from β-globin gene-transformed Hela cells with a 5' labelled 223 NT Bst NI fragment spanning the 5' end of the rabbit β-globin gene as described in ref 11. The hybrids were treated with S_1 nuclease as described (4) and analysed by polyacrylamide gel electrophoresis. The efficiency of transcription <u>in vivo</u> is represented by the level of the 138-140 NT band, which indicates RNAs initiated at the rabbit β-globin cap site.

upstream from −58, −43 or −34 are deleted the rabbit β-globin gene is transcribed specifically in this system. Deletion of the sequences upstream from −15, and therefore removing the Hogness box, eliminates transcription entirely. Since the only conserved region between −20 and −34 is the Hogness box (−31 to −24) we consider it likely that the Hogness box is required for transcription <u>in vitro</u>. In addition, deletion of the CCAAT box does not appear to have a pronounced affect on transcription <u>in vitro</u>.

A second point comes out of the analysis of mutants lacking DNA downstream from the Hogness box. These deletions cause the 5' end of the transcripts to be displaced by approximately the same number of nucleotides as the size of the deletion (14). We believe therefore that the polymerase is (ultimately) bound to the Hogness box and then measures about 30 nucleotides downstream in the same way that is believed to occur for <u>E.coli</u> polymerase.

There is reason to believe that the <u>in vitro</u> results do not reflect perfectly the <u>in vivo</u> situation. We have linked the mutant rabbit β-globin genes discussed above to an SV40 plasmid which contains the early region. W. Schaffner (personal communication) has shown recently that plasmids containing this region of SV40 enhance the expression of a linked β-globin gene in <u>cis</u> and that neither the active production of T/t antigen nor an active replication origin is required for this transcriptional stimulation. The rabbit β-globin-SV40 recombinants were

introduced into Hela cells as a calcium phosphate co-precipitation. RNA
was isolated after 48h and β-globin gene expression assayed by S_1 nuclease mapping using as probe a 5' labelled 223 NT Bst NI fragment which
contains 138 NT of the rabbit β-globin gene.   Table I describes the
results obtained with these mutants in the in vivo system and compares
them with those obtained with the same templates in vitro.   A DNA template which contains 424 nucleotides of 5' upstream DNA sequences (∇ upstream −424) generates a large amount of β-globin mRNA with the same 5'
terminus (defined as +1) as native rabbit β-globin mRNA, together with
a minor amount of RNA with heterogeneous 5' termini at 42 to 47 nucleotides (+42 to +47) downstream from the cap site of native β-globin mRNA.
The removal of the DNA sequences upstream from −100 has no pronounced
effect on the level of β-globin mRNA with the correct 5' terminus, although the level of the aberrant RNAs (with termini at +42 to +47) is
significantly greater.   Deletion of the DNA sequences from −100 to −58,
and which include the CCAAT box, caused a dramatic drop in the level of
β-globin mRNA produced with the correct 5' termini, although the aberrant globin mRNAs discussed above are present at a similar level to that
found for the ∇ −100 mutant template.   Thus, in vivo, deletion of the
region containing the CCAAT box causes a profound drop in the level of
β-globin mRNA suggesting that this conserved DNA sequence is part of the
rabbit β-globin promotor.   A similar result to this has been obtained
by Dierks et al. (6) when the expression of mutant rabbit β-globin genes
is studied in mouse L cells.

Deletions to the 3' side of the Hogness box have the same effect as
observed in vitro (Table I)-in particular, the deletion of the Hogness
box caused the elimination of the specific β-globin mRNA transcript discussed above, although again, the aberrant RNAs are produced at the same
level as discussed above.   This result differs from that obtained by
Grosschedl and Birnstiel (11) for the sea urchin histone H_2A gene, where
a similar deletion causes the synthesis of a heterogeneous population of
RNAs with a limited number of 5' termini.   The cause of this difference
between the two gene systems must be the subject of further experimen-
tation.

DNA SEQUENCES FAR FROM GLOBIN GENES ARE PROBABLY REQUIRED FOR EXPRESSION
IN VIVO

The human globin genes have been useful in defining DNA sequences required for the expression of eukaryotic genes in vivo.   Of particular
interest is the DNA sequence requirement for the effective performance
of the γ -> δ + β globin switch around birth in man.   In δβ° thalassaemia, and in Hereditary Persistence of Foetal Haemoglobin (HPFH) this
switch apparently fails either partially or completely, respectively
(see e.g. 21).

Since these diseases appear to be the result of deletion of DNA in
the globin-gene region (but see below) we believe that the analysis of a
large number of deletion mutants which exhibit this type of phenotype,
and the comparison of these with deletion mutants where the switch is
normal should point to DNA sequences in this region that are essential
for the switch.   A large number of such deletions have been mapped with
respect to the human β-globin gene cluster using Southern blotting by
ourselves and Maniatis, Forget and their respective colleagues, and
these results are shown in Fig. 3.

These results point to two regions which may be important for the
switch.   First, removal of the 3' extragenic regions of the β-globin

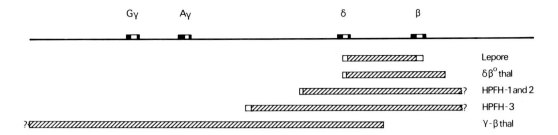

FIG. 3.

The structure of the ∈γδβ globin region in normal DNA and in a number of hereditary diseases.

The structure of the locus is considered in other articles in this volume. The DNA deleted in the hereditary diseases indicated is depicted by the horizontal line. A dashed line indicates that the precise location of the end point of the deletion in that area is not known. The deletion in Hb Kenya has not been established at the DNA level.

gene, in δβ⁰ thalassaemia appears to cause an enhancement of the γ-gene expression in adults when compared with Hb Lepore patients who retain this DNA region (2). Second, removal of the sequences 5' to the δ-globin gene appears to cause still more γ-globin gene expression in adults when two types of GγAγ HPFH cases are compared with δβ⁰ thalassaemia (3, 10, 18, 19) and when the putative deletion in Hb Kenya, which has not yet been mapped at the DNA level, is considered. The possible significance of these deletions has been discussed at length elsewhere. In short, the working hypothesis (2, 3, 10) is that these deletions remove DNA sequences that are required to organize the chromatin into an active δ + β-globin domain. Deletion of these sequences inactivates the adult β-globin gene domain and therefore forces expression of the alternative, but in adults less favoured foetal domain. In support of this idea, deletion of sequences far upstream of the β-globin gene and including the 5' extragenic regions of the δ-globin gene apparently inactivates the β-globin gene in γ-β thalassaemia (20).

A note of caution is necessary at this point. It is not established that the phenotype observed in any of these diseases is the result of the deletion observed. It is also possible that the phenotype is the result of some other mutation, perhaps even a point mutation. Indeed, at least the Greek Aγ-HPFH does not exhibit a detectable deletion in the β-globin gene cluster (3, 19).

In order to test these ideas, it is necessary to set up assay systems for developmental switching. Here the following protocol can be envisaged:

1. The isolation of the entire γδβ-globin locus as a large recombinant DNA molecule.
2. Its introduction into committed erythroid cells (either foetal, or adult) under conditions that allow developmental stage specific expression in vivo.
3. Manipulation of the recombinant DNA in vitro to delete regions suspected of being required for the switching process, reintroduction of this DNA in the cells followed by reassaying the developmental expression of the DNA.

As a first step along these lines, we have applied the cosmid technology of Collins and Hohn (5) and Kourilsky and his colleagues (17) to the cloning of the human globin genes (13). We have at present isolated several overlapping cosmid clones (Fig. 4). One of these may be a suitable candidate for 1. above since it contains the Gγ Aγ δ and β-globin genes together with the intergenic DNA regions. We are currently introducing this DNA into erythroid cells to test these ideas.

ACKNOWLEDGEMENTS

Work from this laboratory was supported by the British Medical Research Council. We are grateful to Cora O'Carroll for preparing the manuscript.

REFERENCES

1. Berk, A. J. and Sharp, P. A. (1977): Cell, 12: 721-732.
2. Bernards, R., Kooter, J. M. and Flavell, R. A. (1979): Gene, 6: 265-280.
3. Bernards, R. and Flavell, R. A. (1980): Nucl. Acids Res., 8: 1521-1534.
4. Busslinger, M., Portmann, R., Irminger, J. C. and Birnstiel, M. L. (1980): Nucl. Acids Res., 8: 957-977.
5. Collins, J. and Hohn, B. (1978): Proc. Natl. Acad. Sci. U.S.A., 75: 4242-4246.
6. Dierks, P., van Ooyen, A., Mantei, N. and Weissmann, C. (1981): Proc. Natl. Acad. Sci. U.S.A.) in press.
7. Efstratiadis, A., Posakony, J. W., Maniatis, T., Lawn, R. M., O'Connell, C., Spritz, R. A., DeRiel, J. K., Forget, B., Weissman, S. M., Slightom, J. L., Blechl, A. E., Smithies, O., Baralle, F. E., Shoulders, C. C. and Proudfoot, N. J. (1980): Cell, 21: 653-668.
8. Flavell, R. A., Bernards, R., Grosveld, G. C., Hoeijmakers-van-Dommelen, H. A. M., Kooter, J. M., de Boer, E. and Little, P. F. R. (1979): In: Eukaryotic Gene Regulation, edited by R. Axel, T. Maniatis and C. F. Fox, pp. 335-354, Academic Press, New York.
9. Flavell, R. A., Grosveld, G. C., Grosveld, F. G., Bernards, R., Kooter, J. M., de Boer, E. and Little, P. F. R. (1979): In: From Gene to Protein: Information Transfer in Normal and Abnormal Cells, edited by T. R. Russell, K. Brew, H. Faber and J. Schultz, pp. 149-164, Academic Press, New York.
10. Fritsch, E. F., Lawn, R. M. and Maniatis, T. (1979): Nature, 279: 598-603.
11. Grosschedl, R. and Birnstiel, M. L. (1980): Proc. Natl. Acad. Sci. U.S.A., 77: 1432-1436.
12. Grosveld, G. C., Koster, A. and Flavell, R. A. (1981): Cell, 23: 573-584.
13. Grosveld, F. G., Dahl, H. H. M., de Boer, E. and Flavell, R. A. (1981): Gene, in press.
14. Grosveld, G. C., Shewmaker, C. K., Jat, P. and Flavell, R. A. (1981): Cell, in press.
15. Manley, J. L., Fire, A., Cano, A., Sharp, P. A. and Gefter, M. L. (1980): Proc. Natl. Acad. Sci. U.S.A., 77: 3855-3859.
16. Proudfoot, N. J. (1979): Nature, 279: 376.

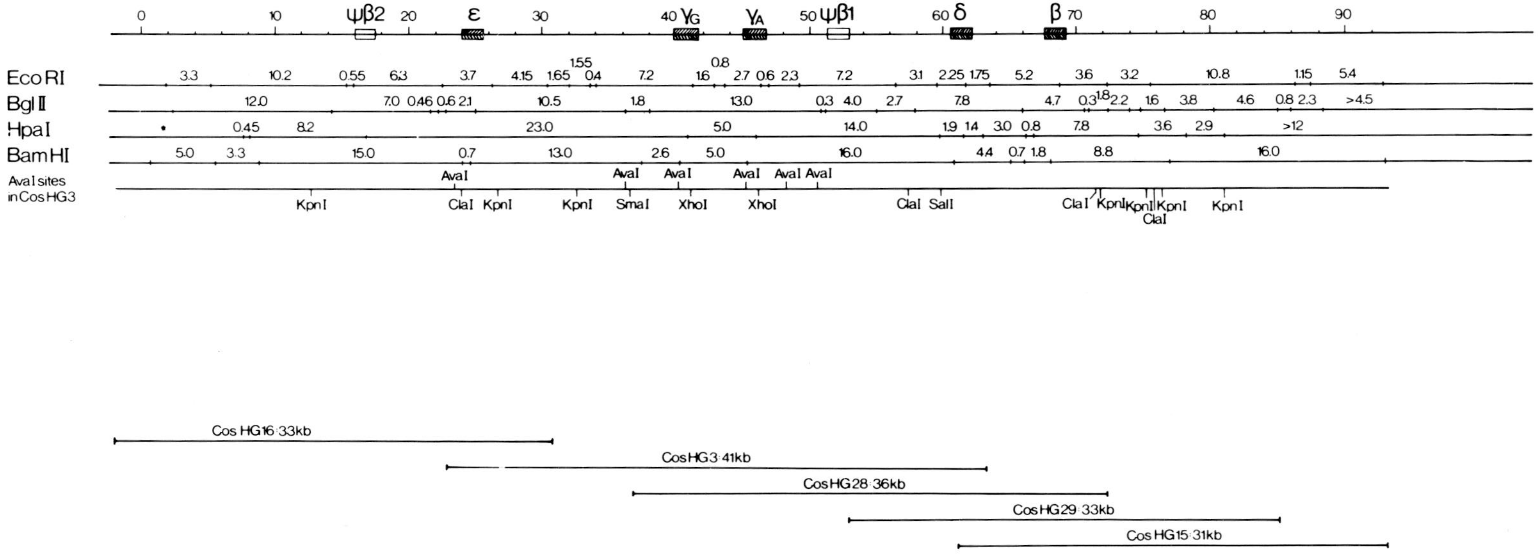

FIG. 4. The structure of a series of overlapping cosmids containing the human β-globin gene locus. The structure of the locus is shown together with maps for a series of restriction endonucleases. The map-coorinates and sizes of the cosmids are indicated (ref. 23 and F.G.G., H.H.M.D. and R.A.F, unpublished data).

17. Royal, A., Garapin, A., Cami, B., Perrin, F., Mandel, J. L., LeMeur,M., Bregegegre, F., Gannon, F., Lepennec, J. P., Chambon, P. and Kourilsky, P. (1979): Nature, 279: 125-132.

18. Tuan, D., Biro, P. A., de Riel, J. K., Lazarus, H. and Forget, B. G. (1979): Nucl. Acids Res., 6: 2519-2544.

19. Tuan, D., Murnane, M. J., de Riel, J. K. and Forget, B. G. (1980): Nature, 285: 335-337.

20. Van der Ploeg, L. H. T., Konings, A., Oort, M., Roos, D., Bernini, L. and Flavell, R. A. (1980): Nature, 283: 637-642.

21. Weatherall, D. J. and Clegg, J. B. (1979): Cell, 16: 467-479.

22. Weaver, R. F. and Weissmann, C. (1979): Nucl. Acids Res., 6: 1175-1193.

23. Weil, P. A., Luse, D. S., Segall, J. and Roeder, R. B. (1979): Cell, 18: 469-484.

Expression of Differentiated Functions in Cancer Cells, edited by R. F. Revoltella et al., Raven Press, New York © 1982.

Cellular Mechanisms for Regulation of HbF Synthesis

S. Ottolenghi, P. Comi, B. Giglioni, *A. M. Gianni, **A. R. Migliaccio, **G. Migliaccio, **F. Lettieri, and **†C. Peschle

*Centro per lo Studio della Patologia Cellulare, Istituto Patologia, Generale, Università di Milano, Milano; *Clinica Medica I, Università di Milano, Milano; **Instituto di Patologia Medica II, Università di Napoli; †Istituto Superiore di Sanità, Roma, Italy*

In humans, embryonic hemoglobins Gower 1 ($\zeta_2 \varepsilon_2$) , Gower 2 ($\alpha_2 \varepsilon_2$) and Portland ($\zeta_2 \gamma_2$) represent most of the hemoglobin during the early phases of intrauterine development (6). Rather soon, however, embryonic hemoglobins are replaced mostly by fetal ($\alpha_2 \gamma_2$) hemoglobin (HbF) and a small amount (5–10% of the total) of adult hemoglobin,(HbA,$\alpha_2 \beta_2$). At birth, a rapid transition to predominant·HbA production occurs (HbF–HbA switch), leading to the almost complete disappearance of HbF, that in normal adults represents less than 1% of total hemoglobin. Concurrently with the switch, the relative proportion of the non-allelic Gγ and Aγ globin chains of HbF changes (Gγ –Aγ. switch) from ~ 3/1 (fetal ratio) to ~ 2/3 (adult ratio) (16). An important feature of HbF production is that it is apparently confined to a low proportion (less than 8%) of cells in adults (F cells)(18). Two extreme models, not necessarily mutually exclusive, might explain these findings: (i) a single cell lineage exists, from the embryonic to the adult stage, that is modulated at different periods of development to yield erythroid cells synthesizing the appropriate type of globin chain. (ii) Two or more cell lineages exist, which are programmed with different biosynthetic properties; the predominance of either the 'fetal' or the 'adult' lineage would determine which is the prevalent Hb species at a given developmental stage.

These problems can be assessed by a simple approach, which was introduced by G.Stamatoyannopoulos ' group in 1977 (8); undifferentiated erythroid precursors (from either peripheral blood or erythropoietic organs) are plated onto semisolid substrates and stimulated to erythroid differentiation by erythropoietin addition. Under suitable dilution conditions, colonies of erythroid cells (bursts) of monoclonal origin (8) appear, which can be analyzed for Hb synthesis. In order to assess the Hb synthetic program of each erythroid undifferentiated precursor, we further improved the original method, by labelling with radioactive leucine individual bursts (or their constitutive subunits) and analyzing the globin synthesized after 18–24 hrs of incubation by a sensitive isoelectricfocusing (IEF) procedure (1), that distinguishes α , ζ, ε ,Gγ ,Aγ 'and β globin chains. We soon realized, however, that the growth of different bursts and of individual subcolonies is rather asynchronous, and that inconsistent results are obtained in different experiments if bursts at non standardized stages of maturation are analyzed. We therefore took as a maturation parameter the apparent degree of hemoglobinization , and analyzed globin synthesis in the most mature bursts only. Representative patterns of globin synthesis in single bursts from progenitors at different developmental stages are shown in fig.1.

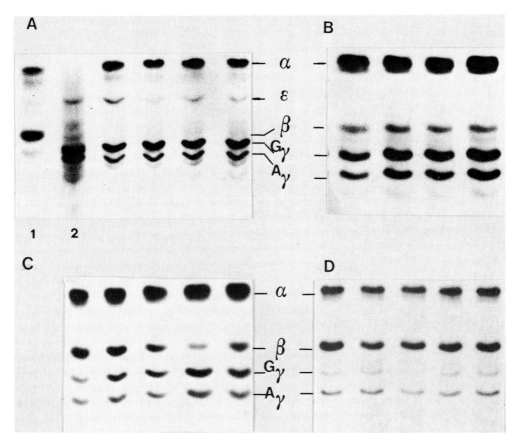

Fig.1. IEF analysis of labelled globin chains from single bursts from: (A),early fetal liver; (B) ,fetal liver; (C),cord blood; (D), adult bone marrow.1: α and β globin chains marker. 2: ε,Gγ and Aγ globin chains from K562 cells.

It is clear that the synthetic pattern in different bursts is very homogeneous at the embryonic, fetal and adult stages, although it is very heterogeneous in bursts obtained from undifferentiated precursors from cord blood. At each stage globins are produced in proportions which are roughly appropriate for the developmental stage; thus late embryonic bursts synthesize mainly α and γ globin chains, plus small proportion of ε and even smaller, barely detectable, but consistently found, amount of β chains (fig.1 and unpublished data). At more advanced stages, ε chains synthesis disappears, while β chain synthesis is increased; finally, in adult age, predominant α and β globin production is observed, with only a small amount of γ globin synthesis, mainly of the A γ type. The data are consistent (2,3,7,10,11) with the idea that a single cell lineage exists from the embryonic to the adult age, that is modulated at birth to switch from fetal to an adult program; indeed, globin synthetic values for cord blood bursts are spread at random between typically fetal and typically adult ratios. It is of interest that a linear relationship exists (2) between the Gγ/Aγ and the γ/β synthetic ratios in cord blood bursts; since the transcriptional order of non α globin genes is 5'- ε-Gγ-Aγ-δ-β, it seems that a 'polarity' exists in the activation of the γ-δ-β cluster, suggesting a precise simultaneous modulation of these linked genes. The ε gene might also participate in this phenomenon; preliminary comparisons of bursts from different fetal livers suggest that ε/γ and β/γ ratios may be inversely correlated.

A rather unexpected result has emerged from these studies, namely the consistent presence of a low, but significant level of γ globin synthesis in all adult bursts tested (10); this is in contrast with the heterogeneous distribution of HbF in adult red cells (18). This finding raises the possibility that in our experiments we were looking at bursts deriving from a selected class of progenitors that did not complete the 'switching' process (thus retaining some potential for HbF synthesis). While in the previously described series of experiments we had studied the progeny of the so called 'mature' (or intermediate type)BFU-E (M-BFU-E) (4,5), we then analyzed both a set of less (primitive BFU-E, P-BFU-E) and a set of more differentiated progenitors (CFU-E), in order to cover the whole spectrum of erythroid progenitors. Bursts deriving from these different progenitors can be distinguished on the basis of their size, day of appearance and erythropoietin sensitivity (4,5,12). This analysis (3,11) indicates that different clusters of progenitors exhibit similar Hb synthetic programs and that all types of adult progenitors are programmed for at least some HbF synthesis (fig.2). The results with CFU-Es, the in vivo undifferentiated precursor that is closest to the erythroblast stage are also consistent with previous data (10) obtained with subcolonies (possibly, although not certainly of clonal origin) from adult bursts, that can be regarded as originating from in vitro precursors fairly closely related to the CFU-E.

The conclusion from these studies is that the heterogeneous distribution of HbF in adult erythrocytes must be generated at a level distal to the undifferentiated precursor (BFU-E, CFU-E); for this reason, we investigated the globin synthetic pattern during maturation of erythroid cells. Well hemoglobinized bursts, containing reticulocytes and late erythroblasts, synthesize a lower proportion of γ globin chains than poorly hemoglobinized ones (containing early erythroblasts) from the same dish at the same day of incubation, although the latter type of burst will eventually decrease its γ globin chain production upon maturation, two days later (7). Thus, both in fetal and adult bursts (fig.3) γ globin declines relative to β globin synthesis during erythroid maturation (7,9); in adult bursts, this decline is linked to a significant decrease of Gγ/Aγ ratios (11), similar to that observed in cord blood colonies (2). Thus, a similar type of effect holds true for both the developmental and the maturational pathways, underlying a possible similarity of molecular mechanisms regulating γ globin gene expression in fetal and adult erythroblasts.

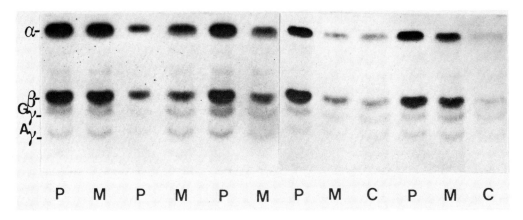

Fig.2. IEF analysis of labelled globin chains from bursts derived from P-BFU-E (P), M-BFU-E (M) and CFU-E (C).

Taken together, our data identify a source of heterogeneity at the level of erythroblasts, rather than at the level of the program of progenitor cells, and provide the basis for a hypothesis linking the presence of HbF (in vivo) in some erythrocytes only to asymmetric cell divisions occurring past the CFU-E stage and/or past the first generation of erythroblasts (11). In the former case, two lines of erythroblasts would be generated, one of which would retain the ability to synthesize some HbF during its early maturation stages; in the alternative case, all erythroblasts would be initially able to synthesize some HbF, but few only would retain this ability at more advanced stages. A corollary to this hypothesis is that successive cell divisions would eventually dilute the small amount of HbF initially synthesized to undetectable levels in most erythrocytes. While asymmetric divisions are an attractive mechanism, this idea leads to the dilemma which rules govern the decision process selecting those few cells in which γ globin genes are kept active; do extrinsic (hormones, cell to cell interactions) rather than intrinsic factors regulate asymmetric cell divisions and selective γ globin chains synthesis in erythroid cells? Further research is necessary to identify these putative extrinsic factors (if any); we wish now to discuss an alternative hypothesis that states that the restriction of HbF to few adult red cells only is a necessary consequence of : (a) the activity of γ globin genes in all adult early erythroblasts (10,11) (or the active configuration of γ globin genes in all adult erythroid progenitors); (b) the mechanism of chromatin replication and of nucleosome segregation. A scheme summarizing this hypothesis is shown in fig.4. The basic assumption (a) is that separate factors (proteins,RNAs ?) exist which associate with , and

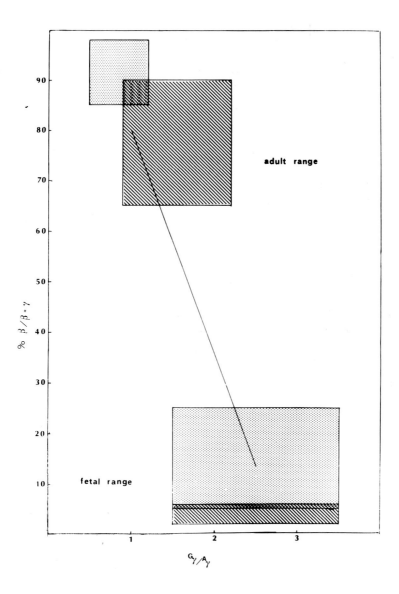

Fig.3. Relationship between $G\gamma / A\gamma$ and $\beta/\beta + \gamma$ ratios in single bursts from fetal liver, cord blood and adult BFU–Es. Shaded area: data for well hemoglobinized bursts. Hatched area: data for poorly hemoglobinized bursts. Straight line refers to average cord blood values.

regulate the activity of, the fetal (G γ and A γ) and adult (δ β) clusters. Factors activating γ globin genes are assumed to be synthesized in all erythroblasts (from adult individuals) at the very early stages only of their maturational pathway, while factors activating the $\delta\beta$ cluster are supposed to be synthesized both at early and advanced maturational stages. The second main assumption (b) derives from experimental data reported by Weintraub and his colleagues; active genes (in nuclei or chromatin) are characterized by a high degree of DNAseI sensitivity (14) which is conferred upon them by unknown tissue specific factors allowing some'high motility group' (HMG) proteins to bind to nucleosomes lying on them, thus making these genes 'accessible' to the nuclease (17); both nucleosomes and the DNAse sensitivity property appear to segregate at chromatin replication to only one of the two DNA strands (the old template active strand, + strand) , while newly synthesized nucleosomes segregate to the old – strand (and the newly synthesized + strand)(13). If this mechanism applied to the human globin gene system during erythroblast maturation, given the premises at paragraph (a), it would follow that (see fig.4):

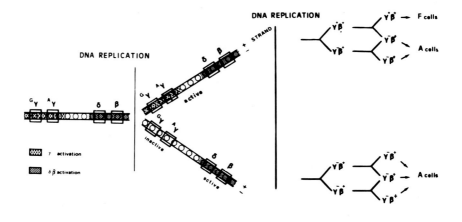

Fig. 4

the + strands of the active γ globin genes would segregate together with their old nucleosomes to one of the daughter cells, and would retain their active configuration, while the newly synthesized γ globin + strand would receive the newnucleosomes devoid of 'factors' required to activate genes, and would become repressed. This process would be repeated at each division round; however, from now on, inactive γ globin genes and those derived from them at each cell division would remain inactive, while the repetition of the process leading to inactivation at mitosis of only one of the daughter + strands, deriving from replication of the active γ globin genes, would eventually result in the appearance of only a small proportion of cells retaining at least one of the two originally active γ globin genes for the whole maturational process: we assume that these cells will give rise to F cells. The hypothesis described above does not require extrinsic factors to give rise to heterogeneity in HbF synthesis in erythroblasts; however, it should be noticed that extrinsic interactions might still be important by modulating either the relative level of synthesis of the putative γ and β activator factors, or the duration of their synthesis. DNAse sensitivity experimets and immunofluorescence studies of Hb distribution in F cells might allow to test these possibilities.

AKNOWLEDGEMENTS

This work was supported by CNR grants n. 80.01133.83 (Progetto Finalizzato Medicina Preventiva) to S.O.; n. 80.01560.96(Progetto Finalizzato Controllo Crescita Neoplastica) to A.M.G.; n. 80.01615.96 (Progetto Finalizzato Controllo Crescita Neoplastica) to C.P;from Euratom, Bruxelles (n. 159–76–7–BIOI), Volkswagen Foundation, Hannover to C.P.

REFERENCES

1.   Comi,P,Giglioni,B.,Ottolenghi,S.,Gianni,A.M.,Ricco,G.,Mazza,U., Saglio,G.,Camaschella,C.,Pich,P.G.,Gianazza,E. and Righetti,P.G. (1979):Biochem.Biophys.Res.Commun., 87:1–8.

2.   Comi,P.,Giglioni,B.,Ottolenghi,S.,Gianni,A.M.,Polli,E.,Barba,P., Covelli,A.,Migliaccio,G.,Condorelli,M., and Peschle,C. (1980) Proc.Natl.Acad.Sci.U.S.A.,77:362–365.

3.   Comi,P.,Giglioni,B.,Pozzoli,M.L.,Ottolenghi,S.,Gianni,A.M., Migliaccio,A.R.,Migliaccio,G.,Lettieri,F.,and Peschle,C.(1981) Exp.Cell Res.(in press).

4.   Eaves,C.J.,and Eaves,A.C.(1978) Blood 52:1196–1210.

5.   Eaves,C.J.,Humphries,R.K., and Eaves,A.C.(1979):in:Cellular and molecular regulation of hemoglobin switching, edited by G. Stamatoyannopoulos and A.W.Nienhuis, pp.251–278. Grune and Stratton, New York.

6.   Gale,R.E.,Clegg,J.B.,and Huehns,E.R. (1979): Nature 280:162–164.

7.   Gianni,A.M.,Comi,P.,Giglioni,B.,Ottolenghi,S.,Migliaccio,A.R., Migliaccio,G.,Lettieri,F.,Maguire,Y.P.,and Peschle,C.(1980): Exp.Cell Res. 130:345–352.

8.   Papayannopoulou,T.,Brice,M.,and Stamatoyannopoulos,G.(1977): Proc.Natl.Acad.Sci.U.S.A. 74:2923–2927.

9.   Papayannopoulou,T.,Kalamantis,Th.,and Stamatoyannopoulos,G.(1979): Proc.Natl.Acad.Sci.U.S.A. 76:6420–6424.

10.   Peschle,C.,Migliaccio,G.,Covelli,A.,Lettieri,F.,Migliaccio,R., Condorelli,M.,Comi,P.,Pozzoli,M.L.,Giglioni,B.,Ottolenghi,S., Cappellini,M.G.,Polli,E.,and Gianni,A.M.(1980) Blood 56:218–226.

11.   Peschle,C.,Migliaccio,A.R.,Migliaccio,G.,Lettieri,F.,Maguire,Y.P., Condorelli,M.,Gianni,A.M.,Ottolenghi,S.,Giglioni,B.,Pozzoli,M.L.,and Comi,P.,in:Second Conference on Hemoglobin Switching(1980) , edited by G.Stamatoyannopoulos and A.W.Nienhuis (in press).

12. Peschle,C.,Migliaccio,A.R.,Migliaccio,G.,Lettieri,F.,Quattrin,S., Russo,G., and Mastroberardino,G. Blood (in press).

13. Seidman,M.M.,Levien,A.J., and Weintraub ,H.(1979) : Cell 18:439–449.

14. Stalder,J.,Larsen,A.,Engel,J.B. ,Dolan,M.,Groudine,M.,and Weintraub,H.(1980):Cell 20:451–460.

15. Stamatoyannopoulos,G.,and Papayannopoulou,T.(1978):in Cellular and Molecular Regulation of Hemoglobin Switching, edited by G.Stamato- yannopoulos and A.W.Nienhuis, pp.323–349.Grune and Stratton,N.Y.

16. Weatherall,D.J. and Clegg,J.B.(1972):The Thalassemia Syndromes, Second Edition, Blackwell Scientific Publications, Oxford.

17. Weisbrod,S.,and Weintraub ,H.(1979)Proc.Natl.Acad.Sci.U.S.A. 76:630–634.

18. Wood,W.G.,Stamatoyannopoulos,G.,Lim,G.,and Nute,P.E.(1975) Blood ,46:671–682.

Expression of Differentiated Functions in Cancer Cells, edited by R. F. Revoltella et al., Raven Press, New York © 1982.

A Three Loci Model for the Control of the Small (Beta) Subunit of Human Ia Molecules

Rosa Sorrentino, Giorgio Corte, Franco Calabi, Nobuyuki Tanigaki, and *Roberto Tosi

*Gruppo di Microbiologia e Patologia Generale, Facoltà di Scienze, Università di Roma, 00185 Roma, Italy; Istituto di Chimica Biologica, 16132 Genova, Italy; Roswell Park Memorial Institute, Buffalo, New York 14263; *Laboratory of Cell Biology, C.N.R., 00196 Roma, Italy*

INTRODUCTION

The genetics of human Ia has advanced mainly through the analysis of large numbers of alloantisera by the classical C'-dependent cytotoxicity assay . Ten alloantigenic specificities , each recognized by a defined "cluster" of antisera , have been sorted out by the cooperative programs of the last two International Histocompatibility Workshops . Population data and segregation analysis in families support the contention that these specificities (numbered from 1 to w10) are controlled by alleles at a single locus , called HLA-DR .

However , besides antisera recognizing single ("subtypic") specificities , clusters of antisera were found which apparently reacted against more than one DR antigen , thus defining so-called "supertypic" specificities . Subsequent studies (1, 2) , based on the reaction of the same antisera on isolated Ia molecules rather than on whole cells , have revealed that two of these supertypic specificities , namely DC1 (which "includes" DR1, 2 and w6) and BR4X7 (which "includes" DR4, 7 and 7J) , actually reside on separate subsets of Ia molecules , different from those carrying the DR determinants . The observed strong association of DC1 and BR4X7 with some DR alleles must then be attributed to an extreme degree of linkage disequilibrium , presumably taking place between very closely linked loci.

It was further shown (1, 2) that all these determinants , both DR and non-DR , reside on the small (beta) subunit of Ia molecules. Thus the above data suggested the existence of <u>at least</u> two HLA-linked loci controlling the small Ia subunit . However , if the two non-DR specificities DC1 and BR4X7 are not allelic to each other , a third locus must be assumed .

In this study , molecules carrying DC1 and BR4X7 were isolated and their peptide patterns were compared . The data obtained are better interpreted in terms of a three loci model .

MATERIALS   AND   METHODS

An outline of the adopted procedure is schematically shown in Table 1 .

Detailed experimental conditions have been described in previous publications , as follows :
- purification and labelling with ^{125}I of Ia molecules : ref. 1
- specificity of alloantisera used . DC1 antisera : ref. 1 , 3 , 4
      BR4X7 antisera : ref. 2 , 5 ; DR antisera : ref. 6 .
- SDS-PAGE , pepsin digestion and microfingerprinting : ref. 7 , 8 .

RESULTS

Migration in SDS-PAGE of Ia subunits

Fig. 1 shows the autoradiographic pattern of a 10 % SDS-PAGE run of immune-complexes eluted from Staf. A bacterial bodies . Antigen-alloantiserum combinations have been chosen according to previously defined specificities . Alpha chains show similar migrations , whereas beta chains exhibit appreciable differences . As compared with DR4, 7 and w6 beta chains , DC1 beta chains have a distinctly higher mobility . Instead BR4X7 beta chains migrate less than either DR4 or DR7 and also exhibit a double band pattern (more evident in the original autoradiogram).

Table 1

Immunochemical analysis of human Ia molecules

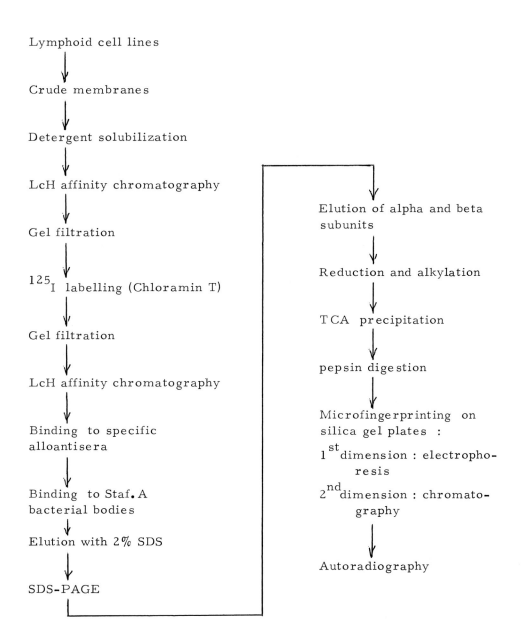

Lymphoid cell lines

↓

Crude membranes

↓

Detergent solubilization

↓

LcH affinity chromatography

↓

Gel filtration

↓

^{125}I labelling (Chloramin T)

↓

Gel filtration

↓

LcH affinity chromatography

↓

Binding to specific alloantisera

↓

Binding to Staf. A bacterial bodies

↓

Elution with 2% SDS

↓

SDS-PAGE

Elution of alpha and beta subunits

↓

Reduction and alkylation

↓

TCA precipitation

↓

pepsin digestion

↓

Microfingerprinting on silica gel plates :

1st dimension : electrophoresis

2nd dimension : chromatography

↓

Autoradiography

Peptide maps of beta subunits

The results shown in Fig. 2 indicate in agreement with previous data (7) , marked differences between DR allelic products. Also DC1 and BR4X7 exhibit differences in their peptide patterns. BR4X7 beta chains , whether isolated from a DR4-positive cell line (U698M) or from a DR7-positive cell line (Chevalier) show identical patterns .

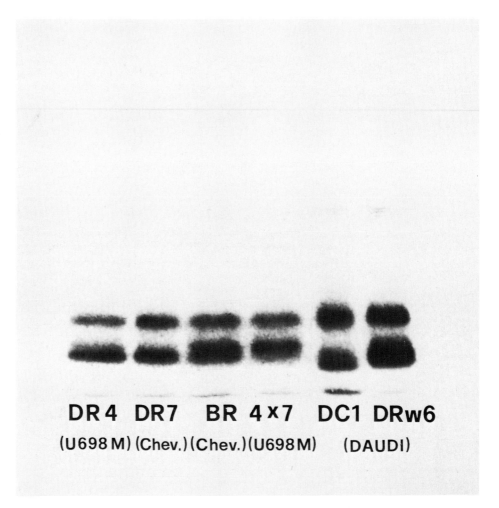

Fig. 1 . Autoradiographic pattern of 10 % SDS-PAGE of Ia molecules of different alloantigenic specificities . The following cell lines were used : U698M (DR2, 4 ; DC1 ; BR4X7) , Chevalier (DR3, 7 ; BR4X7) , Daudi (DRw6 ; DC1) . Alloantisera used were as follows (their specificity has been described in the indicated references) : DR4 : 8W477 (5, 6) ; DRw6 : Fe88/37 (1) ; DC1 : Fe131/6 (1) ; BR4X7 from Chevalier cell line : 8W613 (5) ; BR4X7 from U698M cell line : 8W1075 (5) .

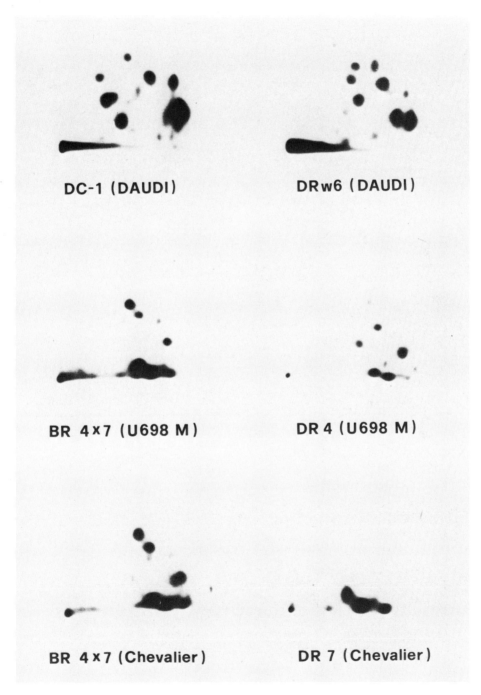

Fig. 2 - Microfingerprinting after pepsin digestion of beta subunits

Peptide maps of alpha subunits

Maps of alpha chains from DR molecules show a distinctive
feature : most of the radioactivity resides in a group of 5-6 peptides
(poorly resolved in the autoradiograms at the adopted exposure time)

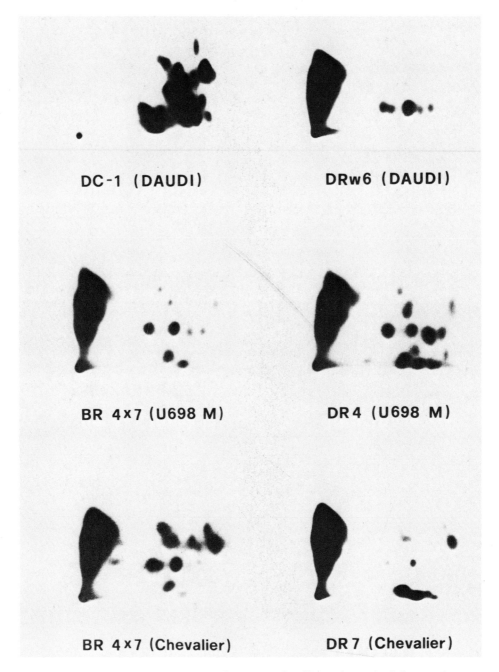

Fig. 3 - Microfingerprinting after pepsin digestion of alpha subunits

of slow chromatographic migration . These are most likely to be glycopeptides . In fact , in this kind of maps , known glycopeptides have
been shown to move only slightly in chromatography because of their
hydrophylic character . The heavy iodine labelling of these spots
may be explained by their being more accessible to the labelling of
the intact molecule . The "butterfly" pattern is totally absent in
DC1 , but it is clearly present in BR4X7 .

The remaining spots show marked differences between both
DR and non-DR molecules . BR4X7 chains isolated from U698M and
from Chevalier exhibit some peptide differences .

DISCUSSION

Taking from granted from previous data that DC1 and BR4X7
are non-DR specificities , the issue considered in the present study
was whether or not DC1 and BR4X7 are allelic specificities controlled by a single non-DR locus . Evidence on this problem can be evaluated by three kinds of comparison :
- comparison of migration (size) of the whole subunits
- " of the fingerprinting pattern of beta chains
- " " " " of alpha chains

The first criterium offers some indication in favour of marked
differences between DC1 and BR4X7 molecules , such as would be
more likely expected from products of different loci . In fact , beta
chains of DC1 molecules migrate more and beta chains of BR4X7
molecules migrate less than beta chains of DR molecules . However
this cannot be an absolute criterium , since differences in the migration of beta chains of different DR specificities have also been observed (9) . The significance of such variations is not easy to judge in
view of the contribution of the carbohydrate moiety and of the possibility of post-translational modifications of the latter . Also the
"double band" pattern shown by BR4X7 beta chains is difficult to
interpret , as discussed by Strominger (10) .

More detailed information can be obtained by comparison of
peptide maps . The fingerprinting technique has a high resolving pow-
er and , in a sense , it amplifies differences between molecules .
In fact , a single aminoacid substitution may determine the shift of
one peptide . However , it must be considered that the peptides visualized by this technique are not representative of the whole molecule.
Firstly , only tyrosine-containing peptides are detected. Secondly ,
since molecules are labelled in non denaturing conditions , tyrosine
residues which occupy internal positions in the molecule may not be
accessible to iodination . Conformational differences may thus influence the peptide pattern .

With these limitations in mind , it is clear that the beta chain peptide maps of DC1 and BR4X7 reveal marked differences between each other . However these differences are not more conspicuous than differences between DR allelic products . Multiple allelic variations (complex allelism) appear to be a common property of MHC loci . Thus these differences are not per se indicative of either allelism or non allelism between DC1 and BR4X7 .

On the other hand , the identity of the beta chain maps of BR4X7 molecules from either a DR4-positive or a DR7-positive cell line is a confirmation that the so called 4X7 "cross-reactivity" is due to a distinct gene product which is associated to DR4 and to DR7 only by virtue of linkage disequilibrium . Such conclusion had been previously reached exclusively on the basis of cross-absorption and cross-inhibition experiments (2) .

The comparison of alpha chain maps offers several points of interest . Firstly , DC1 is totally distinct , not possessing the "butterfly" pattern , which is present in DR allelic products and also in BR4X7 alpha chains . This finding may be explained in different ways : DC1 glycopeptides may not be labelled because of the absence of tyrosine residues in the proximity of carbohydrate attachment or because tyrosine residues are removed from the carbohydrate-containing peptides by pepsin digestion . Whichever the case , since Ia alpha chains possess two carbohydrate chains (10) , the absence of the "butterfly" pattern indicates rather basic structural differences . Two additional possible explanations appear to be ruled out by the available data : a) different accessibility to ^{125}I labelling of tyrosine residues in DC1 molecules . In fact , DC1 molecules labelled in 10 % SDS also showed the complete absence of labelled glycopeptides (11) . b) Lack of carbohydrate moyety in DC1 alpha chains . In fact , these chains have been shown to be LcH-retarded (R. Tosi and D. Centis , unpublished data) .

Differences between DR allelic specificities in the spots outside the "butterfly" area seem to be more marked than those previously found by unidimensional analysis after trypsin digestion (12 , 13) and by two-dimensional analysis after pepsin digestion (7). This may be due to differences in the labelling conditions , as discussed above . The conditions adopted in the present study may be such to evidentiate more clearly an alpha chain polymorphism (which , on the other hand , has been repeatedly suggested on the basis of "minor" structural differences) .

BR4X7 alpha chains from DR4-positive and from DR7-positive cell lines are similar but not isentical . It is difficult to assess at present the significance of this findind . It must be recalled that the alloantigenic determinant BR4X7 has been shown to reside on beta chains (.2) .

BR4X7 alpha chains are in any case markedly different from DC1 alpha chains both for possessing the "butterfly" pattern and also in the number and position of the remaining spots . A genetic interpretation of this finding must take into account the possible homologies with the murine system , which has been more throughly analyzed . Structural data , including aminoacid sequence data , have shown that the two major classes of Ia molecules in the mouse , namely I-A and I-E molecules , differ substancially in their beta chains (in which most of the structural polymorphism resides) and also in their alpha chains . Little sequence homology was in fact found between A_{alpha} and E_{alpha} chains (14) . The phenomenon of the non-interchangeability of alpha chains in their association with beta chains controlled by different loci appears to be a peculiarity of the Ia system . If this rule holds true also in the human situation, the observed strong differences between DC1 and BR4X7 alpha chains are hardly compatible with their beta chains being allelic . Therefore, regardless of the genetic control of alpha chains , by either HLA-linked or non-HLA-linked loci , concerning beta chains the most likely genetic arrangement is that which assumes three tightly linked loci : the first coding for DR specificities , the second coding for the DC1 specificity and the third coding for the BR4X7 specificity . Other alleles of the last two loci remain to be discovered .

When considering human Ia antigens as "differentiation antigens" , the presence of different loci products and the possibility of different functions and tissue distribution being associated with products of each locus should be taken into consideration .

REFERENCES

1. Tosi,R., Tanigaki , N. , Centis , D. , Ferrara , G.B. and Pressman , D. (1978) : J. Exp. Med. , 148 : 1592-1611

2. Tanigaki, N., Tosi , R. , Pressman , D. and Ferrara , G.B. (1980) : Immunogenetics , 10 : 151-167

3. Tosi , R. and Tanigaki , N. (1980) : In: Histocompatibility Testing 1980 , edited by P.I. Terasaki , UCLA , p.917

4. Tosi , R. and Tanigaki , N. (1980) . In : Histocompatibility Testing 1980 , edited by P.I. Terasaki , UCLA , pp. 558-563.

5. Tosi , R. (1980) . In : Histocompatibility Testing 1980 , edited by P.I. Terasaki , UCLA , p.568 .

6. Tosi , R. , Tanigaki , N. and Centis , D. (1980) . In : Histocompatibility Testing 1980 , edited by P.I. Terasaki , UCLA pp.903-905 .

7.   Corte , G. , Damiani , G. , Calabi , F. , Fabbi , M. and Bar-
     gellesi , A. (1981) : Proc. Natl. Acad. Sci. USA , 78 : 534-538.

8.   Corte , G. , Tonda , P. , Cosulich , E. , Milstein , C.P. ,
     Bargellesi , A. and Ferrarini , M. (1979) : Scand. J. Immunol.
     9 : 141-149 .

9.   Shackelford , D.A. and Strominger , J.L. (1980) : J. Exp. Med.
     151 : 144-165

10. Strominger , J.L. (1980) : In : Immunology 80 , edited by M.
     Fougereau and J. Dausset , pp. 541-554 . Academic Press ,
     London

11. Corte , G. , Calabi , F. , Damiani , G. , Bargellesi , A. ,
     Tosi , R. , and Sorrentino , R. (1981) : Nature (in press) .

12. Silver J. and Ferrone , S. (1979) : Nature , 279 : 436-437 .

13. Silver , J. and Ferrone , S. (1980) Immunogenetics , 10 : 295-298.

14. Cook, R.J., Siegelman , M.H., Capra, J.D., Uhr, J.W. and
     Vitetta , E.S. (1979) : J. Immunol., 122 : 2232-2237

Expression of Differentiated Functions in Cancer Cells, edited by R. F. Revoltella et al., Raven Press, New York © 1982.

Murine Cell Surface Glycoproteins: Macrophage Differentiation Antigens Identified and Purified with Monoclonal Antibodies

J. T. August, E. N. Hughes, and G. Mengod

Department of Pharmacology and Experimental Therapeutics, The Johns Hopkins University School of Medicine, Baltimore, Maryland 21205

Monoclonal antibodies that react with antigens of the plasma membrane have been prepared by fusion of mouse myeloma cells and spleen cells of rats immunized with NIH/3T3 plasma membranes. The antigenic targets of these monoclonal antibodies included three major cell membrane proteins of 150,000, 130,000 and 92,000 daltons that were differentiation antigens of macrophage and related phagocytic cells. One of these newly identified glycoprotein antigens, a molecule of about 92,000 daltons in leucocytes, and 80,000 daltons in NIH/3T3 cells, have been extensively characterized and was noteworthy in several respects. 1) It was a differentiation antigen of mesenchymal cells, including macrophages, monocytes, granulocytes, fibroblasts, and myoblasts, and was absent in other lymphoid and nonlymphoid cells. 2) It was a major plasma membrane component, with about 10^6 antibody binding sites per cell, and was distinguished as the predominant iodinated cell surface polypeptide. 3) The molecule on the cell surface was remarkably sensitive to proteolytic cleavage and treatment of intact cells yielded a water soluble, antigenically active fragment of about 65,000 daltons. 4) It was genetically polymorphic, with the antigenic determinant present on cells of A/J, AKR/J, C3H/HeJ, C57BL/6J, C58/J, NZB, RF/J, SJL/J, SWR/J and 129/J inbred mice, but absent on cells of BALB/cJ, DBA/1J, DBA/2J, and CBA/J mice. 5) A single co-dominant gene controlling antigen expression was located on chromosome 2. This glycoprotein has now been preparatively purified by immunoaffinity chromatography. The procedure was simple, rapid and yielded large amounts of the pure glycoprotein. The molecule was purified about 1700-fold and comprised 0.06 of the total soluble cell protein.

INTRODUCTION

Many of the differentiated functions of eukaryotic cells are believed to be mediated through proteins of the cell surface. Extensive studies have defined some of the biological functions of such proteins, especially with respect to some hematopoietic cells. Nevertheless, aside from the red blood cell, the great majority of cell surface proteins identified by vectorial labeling procedures remain unidentified. The major difficulty in characterizing these proteins is the absence of known functional properties upon which to develop specific assay procedures. Moreover, the purification of the

protein by classical procedures has proven difficult due to the
heterogeneity in size and charge of many glycoproteins.

TABLE 1. Rat monoclonal antibodies against mouse cell surface proteins

Hybridoma (AMF:)	Ig subclass	Apparent Mr of protein immunoprecipitated (kd)	
		3T3	Macrophage
1	IgG_{2a}	220	
25	IgG_{2a}	140	
26	IgG_{2a}	140	
14	IgG_{2a}	105	150
24	IgG_{2a}	105	150
9	IgG_{2a}	100	130
4	IgG_{2a}	90	
5	IgG_{2a}	90	
6	IgG_{2a}	90	
7	IgG_{2a}	90	
17	IgG_{2a}	90	
18	IgG_{2a}	90	
19	IgG_{2a}	90	
20	IgG_{2a}	90	
21	IgG_{2a}	90	
22	IgG_{2a}	90	
23	IgG_{2a}	90	
8	IgG_1	80	92
12	IgG_{2a}	80	92
15	IgG_{2a}	80	92
16	IgG_1	80	92
13	IgG_{2a}	72	
2	IgM	55	

We have undertaken a study of the major surface proteins of murine
mesenchymal cells (7). This work has been greatly facilitated by the
use of monoclonal antibodies to identify, characterize and purify the
components (19). Antibodies that reacted with cell surface antigens
of NIH/3T3 cells were generated by immunizing rats with intact NIH/3T3
cells or with an NIH/3T3 plasma membrane fraction. Spleen cells of
the immune rats were fused with mouse myeloma cells, and the cell
population was propagated under selective conditions. Hybridomas that
produced antibodies which reacted with surface antigens of NIH/3T3
cells were detected by antibody binding to the surface of intact cells.
The antibodies were further tested for immunoprecipitation of polypeptides labeled at the cell surface by ^{125}I or biosynthetically with
$[^{35}S]$methionine. The hybridomas that secreted immunoprecipitating
antibodies were cloned in soft agar. All others were discarded. In

this manner, a large number of monoclonal antibodies that immunoprecipitated eight different polypeptides have been obtained (Table 1).
These antibodies have allowed us to study a number of previously
uncharacterized mouse cell surface glycoproteins.

A remarkable finding was that three of these newly identified,
major cell surface glycoproteins were of restricted tissue expression
and may be categorized as differentiation antigens of the phagocyte
cell surface that distinguished macrophages, monocytes, and
granulocytes from other lymphoid cells (Table 2). Specifically, the
antigenic determinants defined by the AMF-14 and AMF-15 monoclonal
antibodies were expressed on most cells of the phagocyte compartment,
such as macrophages, monocytes, and polymorphonuclear neutrophils; the
antigen recognized by the AMF-9 monoclonal antibody was distributed
more narrowly over the spectrum of phagocyte differentiation, marking
the mononuclear cell lineage.

The importance of the identification of differentiation antigens
lies in the premise that the molecules themselves may be involved in
tissue-specific functions. We therefore are proceeding with the
purification and characterization of the glycoproteins. One of the
most extensively studied is a molecule that is noteworthy as the major
surface component of macrophages, is polymorphic, and is remarkably
sensitive to proteoyltic cleavage. This report summarizes our finding
with this glycoprotein and provides an example of our approach for the
use of monoclonal antibodies in the analysis of cell surface
glycoproteins.

TABLE 2. Rat monoclonal antibodies against mouse cell surface
glycoproteins

| Monoclonal | Tissue distribution[a] | | | | | | | | |
	3T3	Macro phages	Poly- morphs	Thymo- cytes	Lympho- cytes	RBC	Brain	Kidney	Liver
AMF-14	+	+	+	-	-	-	-	+	-
AMF-9	+	+	-	-	-	-	+	-	-
AMF-15	+	+	+	-	-	-	-	-	-

[a]The tissue distribution of the antigenic determinants recognized
by the monoclonal antibodies was determined by inhibition of radioimmunoassays, by immunoprecipitation from radiolabeled cells, or by
fluorescence-activated cell-sorting.

RESULTS

Characterization of a Major Cell Surface Glycoprotein As A Polymorphic Differentiation Antigen of Macrophages and Other Phagocytic Cells

Chemical properties of the glycoprotein.
The protein target of the AMF-8, 12, 15 and 16 monoclonal antibodies
was identified by immunoprecipitation (7). The molecule was intensely
labeled at the cell surface by vectorial labeling with ^{125}I and was
biosynthetically labeled with $[^{35}S]$methionine or $[^{3}H]$fucose. The
apparent M_r of the glycoprotein in fibroblast was about 80,000 daltons;
and in macrophages, about 92,000 daltons. The basis for this difference in apparent molecular weight may be attributed to differences in

glucosylation or other post translation modifications; however, differences in the amino acid composition cannot be ruled out. The glycoprotein migrated to the acidic limit of an isoelectric focusing gel, at a pH of 5.5. Chemical characterization confirmed that the molecule was a polypeptide. The antigen remained active as a soluble fraction extracted from cells at pH 9.2 with 0.4 M KCl and 1% Triton X-100, and was not extracted by acetone. The determinant was stable to heat, retaining about 80% of the antigenic activity after treatment at 100° per 10 min. On the other hand, the molecule was highly trypsin sensitive; as shown below, and was preferentially cleaved from the cell surface. Solubilization of the glycoprotein was achieved with 0.2% Triton X-100 detergent, but not with a variety of chaotropic reagents. Thus, the glycoprotein may be operationally defined as an integral plasma membrane component.

Protein polymorphism.
A remarkable and valuable property of this glycoprotein was its structural polymorphism (9). Polymorphism is a property of a number of cell surface proteins, including all of the known proteins of the major histocompatibility complex genes and several lymphocyte cell surface differentiation proteins. The importance of these alloantigens is that they identify proteins that have been implicated in a number of cell recognition, receptor, and differentiation phemomena. In addition, the polymorphism provided a basis for the genetic mapping of the genes controlling expression of the protein. The antigenic determinant of this polymorphic protein that was recognized by the monoclonal antibodies was present in tissues of several strains of mice (NIH Swiss, C3H/HeJ, A/J, C58/J, RF/J, C57BL/6J, C57BR/cdJ, AKR/J, SWR/J, SJL/J, 129/J) but was not detected in tissues of BALB/cJ, DBA/1J, DBA/2J or CBA/J mice. This difference in antigen reactivity between the strains may be attributed to genetic polymorphism, rather than lack of gene expression, as a major iodinated protein of identical electrophoretic mobility, isoelectric point and iodinated tryptic peptide compositon was present in BALB/3T3 cells. The glycoprotein appeared to be different from all other murine cell surface alloantigens identified by polyclonal and monoclonal alloantisera. None of the above other alloantigens showed the same distribution of antigen expression among different strains of mice as did the gp80 and none has been assigned to a molecular species of 80,000 or 92,000 daltons.
     Genetic analysis has shown that the gene controlling the expression of this protein, Pgp-1 (phagocyte glycoprotein-1), is on chromosome 2 of the mouse (5). The tenative gene order was Hc--Pgp-1--Ly-m11--a. Pgp-1 was about 11.8 map units proximal from Ly-m11, closely linked to Ea-6.

Four independent monoclonal antibodies react with the same polymorphic antigenic site.
Among the more than 50 independent cloned hybridomas that we have characterized, 4 produced antibodies that immunoprecipitated the 80,000-dalton glycoprotein of 3T3 cells. These four antibodies were each found to act on the same or a closely associated antigenic determinant of the glycoprotein (12). (1) The antigenic site reactive with each antibody showed the same pattern of genetic expression in different strains of mice. (2) There was a competitive cross-

reactivity of binding between the four antibodies. (3) The four antibodies each reacted with peptide fragments of the 80,000-dalton glycoprotein that had the same apparent electrophoretic mobility. (4) The kinetics of heat inactivation of the antigenic site were the same with each antibody. The only difference among the four antibodies was precipitation of additional proteolytic cleavage fragments by the AMF-15 antibody; possibly, the AMF-15 bound to a distinct antigenic site which overlapped that recognized by the other three antibodies.

The apparent dominance of a single antigenic site reactive with monoclonal antibodies from several cell fusion experiments was remarkable as the antibodies were derived from the xenogeneic immunization of rats with murine cell proteins. Such xenogeneic immunizations usually elicit responses to a variety of antigenic determinants and the detection of polymorphic antigens by monoclonal xenogeneic antibodies has been uncommon. The data suggest a specificity in the immune response to this antigen, either at the level of antigen recognition and response in the animal, or at the level of antibody production by the hybridoma.

The glycoprotein was a major constituent of the cell plasma membrane.

The 80,000 and 92,000-dalton glycoproteins of 3T3 and macrophage cells, respectively, were distinguished as major cell surface components. The glycoproteins were the major iodinated components of the cells, following external labeling with lactoperoxidase. The high concentration was confirmed by saturation binding of the monoclonal antibodies to the cell surface, which showed that there were about 10^6 antibody-binding sites per cell. This concentration is comparable to that of Thy-1, the major cell surface glycoprotein of thymocytes, with 6×10^5 molecules per cell. In addition, as calculated by immunoassay using purified glycoprotein as a standard, the glycoprotein constituted about 0.1% of the total protein of the cell. The data indicated that the polymorphic glycoprotein, with is relatively large mass and high concentration, was one of the major components of the plasma membrane. As shown by immunoelectromicroscopy, the glycoprotein appeared to be uniformly distributed throughout the surface of NIH/3T3 cells, except for coated pits (4).

The glycoprotein is a differentiation antigen of macrophages and other phagocytic cells.

The specificity of cellular expression of the glycoprotein was studied by the binding of purified, ^{125}I-labeled antibody to extracts of 21 different cultured cell lines (8). Significant antibody binding occurred only with NIH/3T3 (NIH mouse embryo fibroblast), G8-1 (Swiss Webster myoblast) and IC-21 (C57BL/6 SV40 transformed macrophage) cells. The antibody did not react with extracts of several other cell lines derived from mouse strains that were positive for spleen tissue expression of the antigen; these included Lewis lung (C57BL/6 carcinoma), EL4 (C57BL/6 T-cell lymphoma), Sarc 180 (Swiss Webster sarcoma), OTTF1 (129 embryonal carcinoma) and S-26 (A/J neuroblastoma). None of the antibodies bound to extracts prepared from any cell line of DBA/2 or BALB/c origin, such as S49.1 (BALB/c T-cell lymophoma), D2N (DBA/2 erythroid leukemia), J774 (BALB/c macrophage line), P388D1 (DBA/2 macrophage line), P815 (DBA/2 mastocytoma) and WEHI-3 (BALB/c myelomonocytic leukemia).

These results obtained with cell lines were confirmed by analysis of mouse cells and tissues. The antigen was found on several cells of the phagocyte compartment, such as resident and activated macrophages, monocytes and polymorphonuclear leukocytes. It was the predominant iodinated protein of the macrophage cell surface and accounted for at least 7.5% of the total radioactivity incorporated into the polypeptide fraction by the lactoperoxidase catalyzed reaction with about 10^6 antibody binding sites per cell. The expression of the antigen was not limited to mature cells of the myelomonocytic lineage, as a population of bone marrow cells also bound the AMF-15 monoclonal antibody. Studies with the fluorescence-activated cell sorter showed that the monoclonal antibody stained 50% to 60% of bone marrow cells, mainly those of larger size and a major fraction of adherent, resident, peritoneal cells. The concentration of the alloantigen was markedly lower in other lymphoid and nonlymphoid tissues, as shown both by antigen and the saturation of antigen sites by antibody. The majority of antigen in the spleen was present on a minor population of large, adherent and membrane immunoglobulin negative cells. The antigen was greatly reduced in thymocytes, brain, liver, kidney and skeletal muscle. Nevertheless, the antigen may mark other pathways of mesenchymal development, as this antigenic determinant was also expressed on the surface of the NIH/3T3 and the G8-1 myoblast cell lines.

Molecular characterization of the antigen on cell surfaces.
The identity of the cell surface antigen recognized by the AMF-15 monoclonal antibody was determined by immunoprecipitation from extracts of cells labeled externally with ^{125}I. The apparent molecular weight of the cell surface polypeptides immunoprecipitated from bone marrow cells, polymorphonuclear neutrophils, and peritonal macrophages was the same for each cell type, 85,000-90,000 (Fig. 1). The protein immunoprecipitated from the NIH/3T3 cell surface distinctly different, corresponding to an apparent molecular weight of 80,000 to 85,000. This difference in apparent molecular wieght between the fibroblast and phagocyte cell antigens may be attributed either to post-translational modification, such as glycosylation, or to tissue specific expression of distinct, but immunichemically related, gene products. The electrophoretic mobility of the immunoprecipitated antigen was the same under reducing and nonreducing conditions, indicating that the polypeptide was not linked by intermolecular disulfide bonds.

Proteolytic cleavage of the 92,000-dalton glycoprotein from the macrophage surface.
One property of macrophage cell surface glycoproteins that may be related to biological function is sensitivity to proteolytic cleavage. Recently, mild trypsin treatment of surface-labeled guinea pig peritoneal macrophages was shown to preferentially cleave one surface glycoprotein of 160,000 daltons (14). Likewise, the 92,000-dalton component characterized here was unique among the major iodinated components of the murine macrophage surface in its sensitivity to mild trypsin treatment. A heterogeneous 65,000-dalton glycopeptide fragment that carried the polymorphic antigenic determinant was rapidly and completely released from the cell surface as a water-soluble peptide. The trypsin-solubilized peptide was stable to subsequent proteolytic

cleavage, indicating that the reaction was specific and limited to one or a few sites of the native glycoprotein. This selective proteolytic cleavage is consistent with a biological correlate the activation of a precursor molecule. Examples of such physiological regulatory mechanisms include the cleavage activations of pancreatic zymogens and hormones, and the amplification of the blood coagulation and complement systems (for review, 13). One hypothesis is that this 92,000 dalton polymorphic antigen is identical to factor B of the alternate complement pathway. There are two findings that support this possibility. 1) It was reported that the major iodinated polypeptide of the macrophage surface comigrated with the membrane-associated factor B (20). 2) The enzymatically active B-fragment, generated in mixtures of purified B, D, and C3b, had an apparent

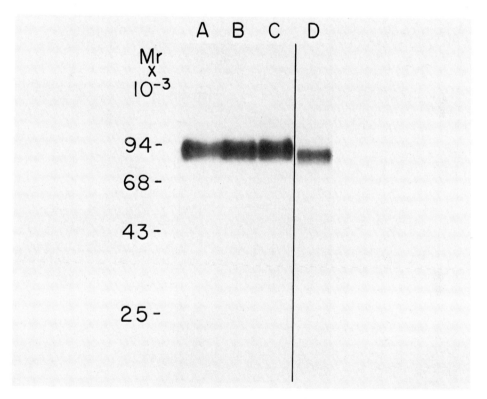

FIG. 1. Immunoprecipitation of the 92,000-Dalton Polypeptide from Different Cells.
Intact cells from (BALB/cJ x C57BL/6J)F1 mice were labeled with ^{125}I by the lactoperoxidase catalyzed reaction and the plasma membrane proteins were extracted with Nonidet P-40. Aliquots (1-3 x 10^6 cpm of acid-insoluble radioactivity) were immunoprecipitated with the AMF-15 monoclonal antibody and analyzed by electrophoresis in a linear 7.5-15 percent polyacrylamide gel gradient in the presence of 0.1 percent sodium dodecyl sulfate, as described in Figure 1. Each immunoprecipitate contained 8 x 10^4 cpm of radioactivity. (A) bone marrow cells; (B) polymorphonuclear neutrophils; (C) thioglycollate-induced peritoneal macrophages, (D) NIH/3T3 cells.

molecular weight of 63,000 (6) and this cleaved form of factor B was not present on the macrophage surface (20). Nevertheless, other findings do not support the identification of the 92,000 dalton glycoprotein as factor B. 1) We did not detect the antigenic activity in fresh plasma by quantitative absorption studies, whereas factor B was found in mouse plasma at a concentration of 120 µg/ml (20). 2) None of the four different monoclonal antibodies reactive with the polymorphic antigen inhibited murine factor B activity (Dr. V. Brade, personal communication). 3) In man, the structural gene for factor B is linked to the major histosompatibility complex (1) and a similar genetic linkage in the mouse would be expected. In contrast, the strain distribution pattern of the polymorphic antigen determinant of the 92,000-dalton glycoprotein did not correlate with any specific haplotype of the major histocompatibility complex of the mouse (9) and analysis of recombinant inbred lines indicated that the gene controlling polymorphic antigen expression was located on mouse chromosome 2 (5).

These data may be compared with other reports describing macrophage cell surface components with similar properties. A 90,000-dalton cell surface protein, accounting for 10 to 15 of the total acid insoluble ^{125}I incorporated into proteins by the lactoperoxidase catalyzed reaction, was immunoprecipitated from the J774 macrophage cell line by the 2D2C monoclonal antibody (10). The latter component may be identical with the 92,000-dalton glycoprotein described in this study. Another cell surface antigen shared by macrophages, granulocytes and fibroblasts has been previously described, but not characterized (17). The strain distribution, tissue expression, and molecular characteristics of the 92,000-dalton glycoprotein distinguished this polymorphic antigen from other murine cell surface antigens that specifically marked the myelomonocytic differentiation pathway. The Mph-1 antigen, defined by alloantisera reactive with a population of peritoneal exudate cells, had a different strain distribution and was associated with chromosome 7 (2), whereas the gene controlling the expression of the 92,000-dalton antigen was present on chromosome 2 (5). Other macrophage-specific cell surface antigens detected by monoclonal antisera, the Mac-2 and Mac-3 antigens, were not expressed on granulocyte precursors and had different molecular weights (15). The 92,000-dalton glycoprotein also differed in apparent molecular weight from other glycoprotein antigens expressed on the macrophage and identified by monoclonal antibodies, including the Fc receptor (14,18) and the Mac-1 antigen (16).

Suspected homology of the 3T3 cells line and macrophage glycoproteins.

A surprising finding in these studies was the relationship of the major 3T3 cell surface antigens to those of macrophages and other myeloid cells of the mouse. The monoclonal antibodies used in these studies were developed from splenocytes of rats immunized with the NIH/3T3 cells and the monoclonal antibodies were selected by antibody binding to target NIH/3T3 cells. Thus, all of the cell and tissue antigens detected should be cross-reactive with NIH/3T3 cell surface antigens. We may add that two other major cell surface glycoproteins that are differentiation antigens of the macrophage, in addition to the 92,000-dalton glycoprotein, are immunoprecipitated by antibodies of the AMF collection. The structural and functional homology between the fibroblast and macrophage proteins is unknown. Our experience to date indicates that polypeptides immunoprecipitated by the same monoclonal antibody from different cells commonly differ in apparent molecular weight. Moreover, the expression of the polypeptide on the plasma membrane, as indicated by lactoperoxidase-mediated iodination, may change among different cells. Although it may be speculated that such differences represent post-translational modification of the same polypeptide, it remains possible that there are differences in the amino acid structure of homologous proteins, or that there is a shared antigenic determinant among nonhomologous proteins. Resolution of these problems will require extensive characterization of the structure of these proteins. Nevertheless, our present data indicate that the 3T3 80,000-dalton and the phagocytic cell 92,000-dalton glycoproteins are closely related, as both are polymorphic and show the same sensitivity to mild proteolytic treatment.

Large scale purification of the glycoprotein.
A simple and rapid immunoaffinity chromatography procedure that yielded large amounts of the pure glycoprotein has been developed.
In a typical purification procedure, packed NZB ME cells were homogenized in a loose-fitting Dounce pestle with a 10-fold volume of cell lysis buffer [5 mM Tris-HCl, pH 9.2, 400 mM KCl, 1 mM EDTA, 1% (w/v) Triton X-100 and 1 mM phenylmethylsulfonyl fluoride]. The volume of cell lysis buffer was adjusted to yield an approximately 2:1 ratio of nonionic detergent to protein. The cell suspension was 3 times frozen in solid CO_2/methanol and thawed at 37°C, and then centrifuged in the Sorvall SS-34 rotor at 5000 rpm (3000 x g) for 5 min at 4°C. The supernatant was collected, dialyzed for 15 h against 4000 ml of column buffer containing 50 mM Tris-HCl, pH 7.6, 0.2% Triton X-100) with 3 changes of dialysate, and clarified by centrifugation in the Sorvall T-865 rotor at 37,000 rpm (100,000 x g) for 1 h at 4°C. Virtually 100% of the antigenic activity and 75% of total cell protein were solubilized by this procedure. This step was not designed to achieve purity, but rather to extract the antigen in high yield. The 100,000 x g supernatant was then applied to a column containing nonderivatized Sepharose CL-4B (5 ml packed bed volume per 100 ml of supernatant) in order to adsorb our aggregated and nonspecifically adherent materials.
AMF-15 rat monoclonal antibody, in a buffer solution containing 500 mM NaCl and 200 mM sodium citrate, pH 6.5, was coupled to cyanogen bromide activated Sepharose CL-4B (200 mg of cyanogen bromide per ml of packed beads) at a ratio of 3 mg of protein per ml of packed beads. The protein content of the filtrates indicated that 96% of the antibody preparation was coupled. A 1.5 x 7.5 cm column, containing 5 ml of monoclonal antibody-Sepharose CL-4B, was pre-eluted with 30 ml of a buffer solution containing 100 mM diethylamine, pH 11.5, 30 ml of a buffer solution containing 1 M Tris-HCl, pH 7.6, and 30 ml of column buffer. The 100,000 x g supernatant from the NZB cell extract was then applied to the column at a rate of 0.25 ml/min. Most of the protein in the extract was not retained in the column. After the protein sample was loaded, the column was washed with 50 ml of the column buffer, followed by 50 ml of a borate-salt buffer, pH 8.5 [1 M NaCl, 100 mM boric acid, 25 mM sodium borate, 0.2% (w/v) Triton X-100], in order to remove proteins adsorbed nonspecifically to the column (26). None of the antigenic activity was eluted by this wash

buffer. The column was then eluted at a rate of 0.5 ml/min with 40 ml of a buffer solution containing 100 mM diethylamine and 0.2% (w/v) Triton X-100, pH 11.5. Fractions of 2 ml were collected in tubes containing 0.5 ml of a neutralizing buffer (2 M Tris-HCl, pH 7.6). The antigen eluted as a single, sharp peak of activity together with a small protein peak. Virtually all of the antigen applied to the column was recovered. The active fractions were pooled and concentrated at 4°C by use of a negative pressure dialysis-concentrating apparatus (Micro-Pro Di Con; Bio-Molecular Dynamics, Beaverton, OR). The vacuum dialysis buffer (2000 ml) contained 20 mM sodium phosphate, 100 mM NaCl and 0.2% (w/v) Triton X-100, pH 8.0.

The concentrated antibody affinity fraction was further purified by molecular seive chromatography on Sephacryl S300 (Pharmacia) in the dialysis buffer as above. The antigenic activity was recovered as a single symmetrical peak, and the fractions containing the antigen were pooled and concentrated as above.

The purity of the glycoprotein was determined by sodium dodecyl sulfate/polyacrylamide gel electrophoresis followed by staining for protein with Coomassie Brilliant Blue R-250 (Figure 2). A single band of about 80,000 apparent molecular weight was present as the major molecular species in the eluates of both the antibody affinity and S300 columns. The purified glycoprotein represented a very small fraction of the total soluble cell proteins and was not detected among the other polypeptides of similar molecular weight in the crude extract. The diffuse pattern of the glycoprotein may be attributed to heterogeneity in glycosylation and the amount of purified protein, 16 μg, applied to the gel. Analysis of the individual fractions from the Sephacryl S300 column showed that this glycoprotein co-purified with the antigenic activity. An immunologically unreactive polypeptide of 38,000 daltons present in the affinity column eluate was removed by Sephacryl S300 chromatography.

A summary of this procedure is shown in Table 3. The quantity of glycoprotein in the crude extract and antibody affinity fractions was measured by radioimmune assay, standardized with the pure glycoprotein. The yield of the purification appeared to be virtually 100%. There was no detectable loss of antigenic activity in either of the two steps. The concentration of the glycoprotein in crude extracts calculated from these data was 0.06%, with an overall purification of about 1700-fold.

TABLE 3. Purification of a 80,000-dalton differentiation antigen of mouse mesenchymal cells.

Purification Fraction	Volume	Total Protein	Protein[a]	Antigen Fraction of Total	Yield
	ml	mg	mg	%	%
Crude extract	196	725	0.4	.06	---
Antibody affinity	1.4	0.8	0.4	50	95+
Sephacryl S-300	1.5	0.4	0.4	(100)	95+

[a]Antigen protein was measured by the solid phase radioimmunoassay, standaridized with the pure protein, whose concentration was determined by the Lowry procedure.

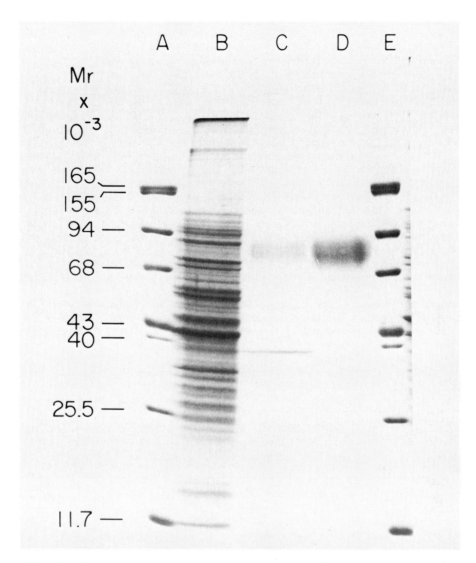

FIG. 2. Electrophoretic analysis of the purified polymorphic glycoprotein.
The polymorphic glycoprotein antigen was purified by monoclonal antibody affinity and molecular sieve chromatography in the presence of Triton X-100, as described in the text. The samples were analyzed by electrophoresis in a linear 5 to 20% polyacrylamide gel gradient in the presence of 0.1% sodium dodecyl sulfate. The gel was stained with Coomassie Brilliant Blue R-250. A, standard proteins: Escherichia coli RNA polymerase β', β subunits (Mr = 165,000, 155,000); phosphorylase a (Mr = 94,000), bovine serum albumin (Mr = 68,000), ovalbumin (Mr = 43,000); Escherichia coli RNA polymerase α-subunit (Mr = 40,000), chymotrypsinogen (Mr = 25,500), and cytochrome c (Mr = 11,700). B, 125 μg of NZB ME crude extract; C, 15.6 μg of antibody column eluate; D, 16 μg of Sephacryl S300 eluate; E, standard proteins as in lane A.

This procedure also has been applied with equal success to a number of mouse cell surface glycoproteins recognized specifically by other monoclonal antibodies. We have used the same experimental protocol and the same cell extract to purify three different plasma membrane glycoproteins shared by mouse macrophages and 3T3 cells. In several cases, complete purifications were achieved with a single affinity column step. Moreover, the affinity columns were used several times without detectable loss of antigen binding capacity.

A major advantage of using monoclonal antibody affinity chromatography as an early step in the purification of the polymorphic plasma membrane glycoprotein was to bypass the more traditional procedures of ion-exchange and molecular sieve chromatography. The charge and size heterogeneity of the glycoprotein restricted the efficacy of such methods. The need for the continued presence of detergents to maintain the glycoprotein in a soluble form also appeared to handicap the application of conventional procedures. Another advantage of the affinity column was the ease of application to large scale purification. The effective capacity of the AMF-15 monoclonal antibody affinity column was remarkedly high, and chromatography of even larger quantities of cell extract resulted in a correspondingly greater amount of purified glycoprotein. In other studies, approximately 2 mg of the purified 80,000-dalton glycoprotein was obtained by passing 3 g of crude extract through the same AMF-15 antibody column. All of the antigenic activity of the extract was recovered in the purified fraction, indicating that the functional capacity of the antibody column had not been exceeded. As the column contained about 15 mg of monoclonal antibody, this amount of antigen approached the maximal capacity. Such high capacity may not be attainable uniformly with all monoclonal antibodies, however, as the capacity of the column can be expected to differ depending upon the affinity of the antibody and the effect of antibody coupling. The reported antigen-binding capacities of other monoclonal antibody affinity columns appeared to differ widely.

The purified glycoprotein was a single component of about 80,000 daltons, which was greater than 95% pure by sodium dodecyl sulfate/polyacrylamide gel electrophoresis. The glycoprotein co-purified with the antigenic activity and was quantitatively immunoprecipitated by the antibody; it thus constituted the structure carrying the antigenic determinant recognized by the monoclonal antibody. The preferential solubilization of the antigen by use of detergent was consistent with the characterization of the glycoprotein as an integral membrane component.

The preparative purification of the polymorphic glycoprotein showed that the molecule was a major cell surface component, constituting 0.06% of the total soluble proteins in the cell. Assuming a purification of 1700-fold, it can be calculated that there were about 1.97×10^6 molecules of the glycoprotein per 3T3 cell. This value is in agreement with the number of antibody molecules bound per 3T3 cell in saturation binding studies (8). Equivalent amounts of the polymorphic glycoprotein were found on thioglycollate-induced macrophages. As plasma membrane proteins as a group comprise less than a few percent of total cell protein, it may be presumed that the polymorphic glycoprotein accounted for a substantial fraction of plasma membrane protein.

CONCLUSION

With its high concentration and restricted tissue expression, the polymorphic glycoprotein probably makes an important contribution to the molecular architecture and function of the phagocyte cell surface. The purification and characterization of the polymorphic glycoprotein is an important first step in understanding its cell surface organization and its role in the biology of phagocytic cells. Several tools, including a genetic system, the purified glycoprotein, monoclonal antisera, and monospecific polyclonal antisera, are now available for studies of the biological function of this molecule.

REFERENCES

1. Allen, F.M., Jr. (1974): Vox Sang. 27:382-384.
2. Archer, J.B. and Davies, D.A.L. (1974): J. Immunogenetics 4:113-123.
3. Bitter-Suerman, D., Burger, R., Brade, V. and Hadding, V. (1976): J. Immunol. 117:1799-1804.
4. Bretscher, M.S., Thomson, J.N. and Pearse, B.M.F. (1980): Proc. Natl. Acad. Sci. USA 77:4156-4159.
5. Colombatti, A., Hughes, E.N., Taylor, B.A., and August, J.T. (1981): in press.
6. Gotze, O., Bianco, C. and Cohn, Z.A. (1979): J. Exp. Med. 149:372-386.
7. Hughes, E.N. and August, J.T. (1981): J. Biol. Chem. 256:664-671.
8. Hughes, E.N., Colombatti, A., and August, J.T. (1981): in press.
9. Hughes, E.N., Mengod, G. and August, J.T. (1981): J. Biol. Chem. 256: 7023-7028.
10. Mellman, I.S., Steinman, R. M., Unkeless, J.C. and Cohn, Z.A. (1980): J. Cell Biol. 86:712-722.
11. Mellman, I.S. and Unkeless, J.C. (1980): J. Exp. Med. 152:1048-1069.
12. Mengod, G., Hughes, E.N. and August, J.T. (1981): Arch. Biochem. Biophys., in press.
13. Reich, E., Rifkin, D.B. and Shaw, E. (1975): Proteases and Biological Control. Cold Spring Harbor Laboratory, New York.
14. Remold-O'Donnell, E. (1980): J. Exp. Med. 152:1699-1708.
15. Springer, T. (1980): In: Monoclonal Antibodies, edited by R. Kennett, T. McKearn, and K. Bechtol, pp. 185-217. Plenum Press, New York.
16. Springer, T., Galfre, G., Secher, D.S. and Milstein, C. (1979): Eur. J. Immunol. 9:301-306.
17. Tiller, G.E., McGiven, A.R. and Phil. E. (1973): Aust. J. Exp. Biol. Med. Sci. 51:793-798.
18. Unkeless, J. (1979): J. Exp. Med. 150:580-596.
19. Williams, A.F., Galfre, G. and Milstein, C. (1977): Cell 12:663-673.
20. Yin, H.L., Aley, A., Bianco, C. and Cohn, Z.A. (1980): Proc. Natl. Acad. Sci. USA 77:2188-2196.

Expression of Differentiated Functions in Cancer Cells, edited by R. F. Revoltella et al., Raven Press, New York © 1982.

Biochemical Analysis of Human T Lymphocyte Antigens

Cox Terhorst, André van Agthoven, Jannie Borst, Kenneth LeClair, and Peter Snow

Sidney Farber Cancer Institute and Department of Pathology, Harvard Medical School, Boston, Massachusetts 02115

ABSTRACT

Eight monoclonal reagents, anti-T1, -T3, -T4, -T5, -T6, -T8, -T9, -T10, which define stages of differentiation of human thymus derived lymphocytes, were used for biochemical analysis of their target antigens. By comparing these cell surface markers with murine markers, the following homologues are proposed: T1/Lyt-1, T5 and T8/Lyt-2 and -3, T6/TL, and T10/Qa2. The antigens T3 and T8 are involved in functions which are specifically programmed in T lymphocytes (T3) or the T cytotoxic subset (T8). T9 is involved in the receptor site for transferrin.

INTRODUCTION

Cell mediated immunity encompasses a wide range of observable phenomena in a variety of regulatory and effector systems. The most common forms of cell mediated responses studied, i.e., delayed type hypersensitivity, allograft rejection, tumor rejection, graft-versus-host reactions, all involve thymus derived lymphocytes (T cells). Moreover, it has become increasingly clear from both animal and human studies that synergistic interactions of different subsets of T cells dictate the control mechanisms of the immune response.

A number of antibody reagents have been developed which enable us to define T cell subsets which are endowed with different functional programs (6). Such antibodies also permit a better understanding of the stages of maturation of lymphocytes within the thymus gland. Thus, using eight monoclonal reagents, anti-T1, -T3, -T4, -T5, -T6, -T8, -T9, -T10 (Table I), Reinherz and Schlossman (21) have proposed that in man at least three stages of intrathymic differentiation can be defined. The earliest stage was shown to be restricted to 10% of thymocytes which were identified by reactivity with anti-T9 and anti-T10. Subsequently, human thymocytes acquire the antigen T6, and begin to express reactivity with anti-T4, -T5, and -T8. The $T4^+$, $T5^+$, $T8^+$ "common" thymocyte population therefore represents the majority of thymocytes (75%). With further maturation, thymocytes lose T6 reactivity, segregate into $T4^+$, $T5^-$, $T8^-$ and $T4^-$, $T5^+$, $T8^+$ subsets, and acquire reactivity with anti-T1 and anti-T3. Lastly, it appears that as the thymocyte is exported into the

93

TABLE I. Monoclonal antibodies to human T cell surface antigens (21)

Monoclonal Antibody	Cell Surface Expression (% Reactivity with antibodies)		
	Thymocytes	T cells	Bone Marrow
anti-T1	10	100	< 5%
anti-T3	10	100	< 5%
anti-T4	75	60	< 2%
anti-T5	80	25	< 2%
anti-T8	80	30	< 2%
anti-T6	70	0	0
anti-T9	10	0	0
anti-T10	95	5	< 20%

peripheral T cell compartment, it loses the T10 marker, since this antigen is lacking on virtually all peripheral T lymphocytes. The exported $T1^+$, $T3^+$, $T4^+$ and $T1^+$, $T3^+$, $T5^+$, $T8^+$ subsets represent the T lymphocyte inducer and cytotoxic/suppressor populations, respectively (21).

The cell surface markers T1, T3, T4, T5, T6, T8, T9, and T10 are also extremely useful markers for studying T cell malignancies (22). With the monoclonal reagents specific for these antigens, a large number of acute lymphocytic leukemias and lymphoblastic lymphomas have been studied (18). The results of these studies are consistent with the notion that heterogeneity of T cell malignancies, for the most part, reflects stages of normal T cell differentiation.

A detailed analysis of the structure and biosynthesis of these cell surface antigens should therefore facilitate investigations that, 1) develop our understanding of the differentiative pathways of human thymus derived lymphocytes, 2) aid in the molecular description of T cell functions, and 3) allow further classification of T cell malignancies. This paper summarizes the first steps taken in that direction.

All eight cell surface markers were found to be glycoproteins. Preliminary experiments indicate that these markers are indeed amphiphilic proteins (29), suggesting that they are integral membrane proteins. Using the preliminary biochemical descriptions and their tissue distribution, the human T cell markers were compared with known murine markers. We propose the following possible homologues: T1/Lyt-1, T5 and T8/Lyt-2 and -3, T6/TL, and T10/Qa2. The possible biological functions of some of the cell surface glycoproteins will be discussed.

MATERIALS AND METHODS

The starting materials for these studies were obtained from human peripheral blood T lymphocytes, thymocytes and from T leukemic cell lines HPB-ALL, MOLT-4, CCRF-CEM.

Cells were labeled metabolically with $[^{35}S]$-L-methionine and cell surface labeling was primarily done using $Na[^{125}I]$ and lactoperoxidase or

$NaB[^3H]_4$ after treatment with galactose oxidase/neuraminidase or dilute periodate. Immunoprecipitation techniques and all other methods are described in detail elsewhere (14,28,29,32).

RESULTS AND DISCUSSION

T1

Although the cellular expressions of T1 and T3 antigens were similar on peripheral T cells and thymocytes, several lines of evidence suggested that these antigens are not identical. First, the T1 antigen was expressed on the majority of T cell lines, while the T3 antigen was expressed on a minority (32). Second, functional studies showed that the purified anti-T3 immunoglobulin (Ig) by itself induced both a T cell proliferative response, as measured by tritiated thymidine uptake after three days in *in vitro* culture, and could block the proliferative responses of human T lymphocytes to soluble and cell surface antigens. In contrast, anti-T1 did not affect these responses (23).

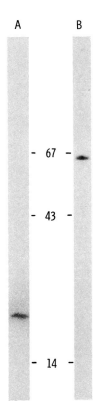

A   B

- 67 -

- 43 -

- 14 -

FIG. 1. *Analysis by SDS-PAGE of immunoprecipitates prepared from ^{125}I-labeled T lymphocyte lysates. a) ^{125}I-labeled T cell lysate precipitated with anti-T3; b) ^{125}I-labeled T cell lysate precipitated with anti-T1.*

Analysis of the immunoprecipitates of lysates of ^{125}I-labeled human T lymphocytes showed that the molecular weight of the T1 antigen was estimated at 69K, T3 antigen at 20K, both under reducing and nonreducing conditions (Figure 1) (32). In order to further investigate the glycoprotein nature of the thymic differentiation marker T1, human peripheral blood T lymphocytes were labeled with tritiated sodium borohydride after mild oxidation. In one experiment, the lymphocytes were treated with diluted sodium periodate, which oxidizes sialic acid specifically (11). In another experiment, T cells were labeled with $NaB[^3H]_4$ after treatment with neuraminidase and galactose oxidase. By this method, the penultimate galactose residues of sugar side chains are labeled with tritium. Because the antigen T1 is labeled with tritium using these methods, T1 is judged to be a glycoprotein (Figure 2).

After treatment with periodate and tritiated sodium borohydride, the target antigen for anti-T1 was found to be on a 160K glycoprotein, in

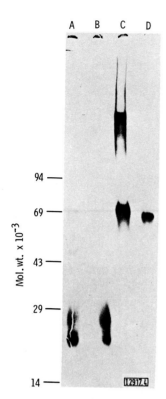

A   B   C   D

Mol. wt. x 10^{-3}

94 —

69 —

43 —

29 —

14 —

[12917.4]

FIG. 2. *SDS-PAGE of immunoprecipitates prepared with anti-T3 and
anti-T1 of tritiated human peripheral blood T lymphocytes. Lanes A
and C were precipitated after treatment with periodate and sodium borohydride. Lanes B and D show precipitates after treatment with
neuraminidase/galactose oxidase and
NaB[^{3}H]$_4$. a) anti-T3; b) anti-T3;
c) anti-T1; d) anti-T1.*

addition to the 69K protein found
with other labeling techniques (Figure 2c). In contrast, after treatment with galactose oxidase and
neuraminidase, no 160,000 mol wt
band was observed on SDS-PAGE (Figure 2d). This indicates that the
T1 antigen may exist on the cell
surface in complex with another
protein, or as a dimer which can be
detected only after cross-linking
on the cell surface. Such a cross-
linking event could occur via a
Schiff's base between the aldehyde
function of an oxidized sialic acid
residue and a neighboring amino
group, which may account for the
observation that the 160K protein
was detected only after treatment
with periodate, and not after oxidation with galactose oxidase.

The antigen T1 is not only expressed on thymocytes and T cells,
but can be detected on chronic lymphocytic leukemia cells (CLL's) and
lymphomas of B cell origin (18).
Both cell distribution and molecular
weight suggest that T1 could be
similar to the target antigen of
some monoclonal anti-Lyt-1 reagents
in the murine system (15).

T3

A chemical characterization of the differentiation antigen T3 appears
to be of great interest, since T3 is involved in a function which is in-
dispensible for T lymphocyte responses.

T3 was found as a 20K protein in ^{125}I-labeled immunoprecipitates (Figure 1) and could also be precipitated from NP-40-solubilized membrane
fractions isolated from human phytohemagglutinin (PHA)-activated T lymphocytes or human thymocytes metabolically labeled with [^{35}S]-L-methio-
nine (32). However, after labeling with NaB[^{3}H]$_4$ we have observed a
smear from 25K to around 29K, in addition to the 20K glycoprotein in

immunoprecipitates made with anti-T3 (Figure 2). More recently, the same "smear" has been detected after labeling with [125]I (4). This smear consists of a number of glycoproteins if analyzed by two-dimensional gel electrophoresis (Figure 3).

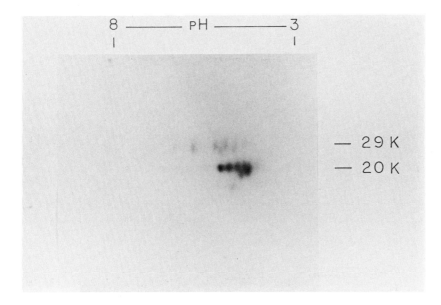

FIG. 3. *Two-dimensional gel of T3.*

If analyzed by two-dimensional gel electrophoresis, T3 itself appears as a complex set of spots around 20K (Figure 3). The complexity of this pattern can be reduced to one spot after extensive treatment with neuraminidase. Treatment with endoglycosidase-H and neuraminidase demonstrated that T3 contains at least one high mannose glycan moiety and one complex oligosaccharide (4). After endoglycosidase-H treatment, the 20K polypeptide chain is converted to a 17K polypeptide. This observation is in line with pulse chase experiments in which a 15K and a 17K precursor of T3 were detected.

Preliminary pulse chase experiments indicate that the 25-29K protein is not a precursor of T3. Peptide mapping and N-terminal aminoacid sequencing will be necessary to confirm this. The 25-29K protein may be tightly associated with T3, perhaps in a protein complex which is of importance for the function of T3.

In our opinion, no murine counterpart of T3 has been described to date. Thy-1, which has been reported to be a glycoprotein (18,700 mol wt) with a protein molecular weight of 12,500, the rest being carbohydrate, is expressed on all rodent thymocytes, T lymphocytes, glial cells and some neuron cells. In contrast, T3, which is in the same molecular weight category, is limited to cells of T lineage. Moreover, unlike anti-T3 antibodies, no functional activity of anti-Thy-1 antisera has been reported (5).

T4

The antigen T4 which identifies the helper/inducer subset of human T cells, was immunoprecipitated from a Nonidet P-40 lysate of human thymocytes labeled with tritiated sodium borohydride after a mild oxidation with a low concentration of sodium periodate (28). The glycoprotein detected by anti-T4 has a molecular size of 62K daltons (Figure 4-1).

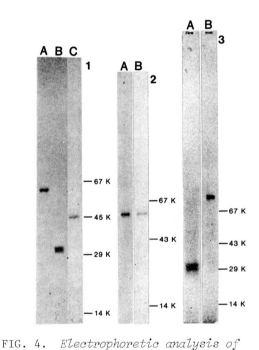

FIG. 4. *Electrophoretic analysis of immunoprecipitates made with monoclonal antibodies to T4, to T5, and β2-microglobulin.*
4-1. [³H]-labeled thymocyte lysate.
a) anti-T4; b) anti-T5; c) anti-β2m
4-2. [³⁵S]-labeled T cells.
a) anti-T4 reduced; b) anti-T4 nonreduced.
4-3. [³⁵S]-labeled T cells.
a) anti-T5 reduced; b) anti-T5 nonreduced.

The target antigens detected by anti-T4 can also be precipitated from a NP-40 solubilized membrane preparation of human peripheral blood T lymphocytes. T cells purified on a nylon wool column were activated with phytohemagglutinin and cultured in the presence of [³⁵S]-L-methionine. Electrophoresis on SDS-polyacrylamide gel shows that T4 has the same molecular size under reducing and nonreducing conditions (Figure 4-2).

Since the T4 antigen is uniquely present on those human T cells which are programmed for T helper/inducer functions, a comparison with the Lyt-1 antigen was of interest. Alloantiserum to Lyt-1.1 precipitated a 67K dalton glycoprotein and a 87K dalton glycoprotein that could be labeled with tritiated sodium borohydride and galactose oxidase but not with the ^{125}I (8). A monoclonal antiserum (termed 53-7.3) detected a 70K dalton glycoprotein on ^{125}I-labeled C57Bl/6 thymocytes (15). Although the original anti-Lyt-1 antisera in the presence of complement would lyse only 33% of Thy-1 positive cells, the monoclonal reagents react with all T cells. As the Lyt-1 marker was detected on all T lymphocytes, and since the target antigens are larger than those of anti-T4, the relationship between T4 and Lyt-1 is not clear. In some ways Tl seems more similar to Lyt-1 than does T4. The possibility that the original alloantisera (anti-Lyt-1) contain antibodies which react with a murine homologue of T4 has not been excluded. In any case, further protein chemical data are required for more definitive comparisons between Lyt-1, Tl and T4.

T5 and T8

The monoclonal reagents anti-T5 and anti-T8 define the suppressor/ cytotoxic T cell subset in man (21), as do anti-Lyt-2 and anti-Lyt-3 in mice. Target antigens for anti-T5 and anti-T8 are glycoproteins of 33K daltons (Figure 4) which are sometimes found as two bands (30K and 32K daltons) (28). Under nonreducing conditions, both T5 and T8 form dimers of 76K daltons (Figure 4-3).

Murine Lyt-2 and Lyt-3 antigens were found on cell surface glycoproteins from thymocytes ^{125}I-labeled with lactoperoxidase (7,15). Immune precipitations carried out with alloantisera to Lyt-2 and Lyt-3 detected a 35K dalton protein for each marker on C57Bl/6 thymocytes (7). However, in contrast, a monoclonal rat xenoantibody (53-6.7) precipitated a 65K glycoprotein that was resolved into subunits of 30K and 35K under reducing conditions (15). Therefore, a similar situation exists as for T5 and T8.

Since inhibition of cell mediated lympholysis (CML) by antisera directed at the Lyt-2 and Lyt-3 differentiation markers had been reported (9,12,19,24,25), we tested whether anti-T5 and anti-T8 reagents would inhibit CML. These experiments were conducted using a continuously growing T cell clone JR-2-3 which was derived from a continuously growing cytotoxic T cell line JR-2 (27). The cytolytic activity of JR-2-3 is specific for HLA-A2-containing target cells and can be inhibited by monoclonal antibodies directed at β2-microglobulin or the heavy chain of the HLA-complex (W6/32).

As shown in Table II, anti-T8$_{11}$ inhibits killing completely and anti-T8$_1$ inhibits partially, whereas anti-T5 has no detectable effect in this reaction. This supports the notion that the different monoclonal antibodies (anti-T5, -T8$_1$, -T8$_{11}$) detect different antigenic determinants. Whether these determinants are located on different polypeptide chains is currently under investigation (26).

These experiments not only indicate that the target antigens for anti-T5 and anti-T8 share several properties with the Lyt-2,3 antigens, but they strongly suggest that the differentiation antigen T8 is involved in the function of the cytotoxic T cell.

TABLE II.   Inhibition of CML by monoclonal antisera specific for thymo-
            cyte differentiation antigens (26)

Monoclonal Reagent Added	Dilution	Percentage ^{51}Cr Release at E/T of 1:2
--	--	50.3
anti-HLA-DR (279)	1/25	42.6
	1/200	44.6
	1/400	38.5
anti-HLA-DR (TM-11)	1/25	50.1
	1/200	52.1
	1/400	51.0
anti-β2-microglobulin (A88)	1/25	-2.8
	1/200	3.8
	1/400	12.5
anti-T5	1/25	27.5
	1/200	43.4
	1/400	42.5
anti-T8ı	1/25	5.1
	1/200	8.8
	1/400	15.6
anti-T8ıı	1/25	-4.9
	1/200	-12.4
	1/400	-8.3

T6

The T6 antigen is a marker which appears to be specific for human thymocytes and thymus derived leukemias (22). The only nonthymic cells which have shown positive reactivity with some, but not all of the anti-T6 monoclonals are Langerhans cells (3). SDS-polyacrylamide gel electrophoresis revealed that the T6 antigen is a protein with an apparent molecular weight of 49K under both reducing and nonreducing conditions (Figure 5 lanes A and B).

If thymocytes were radioactively labeled with tritiated sodium borohydride after mild treatment with 1 mM sodium periodate, a similar band

of 49K daltons was observed after SDS-polyacrylamide gel electrophoresis
of the immunoprecipitate, indicating that the target antigen for anti-T6
is a glycoprotein (29). A smaller protein of 12K daltons was detected
in experiments starting with ^{125}I-labeled lysates (Figure 5 lane A).
This protein was not seen after tritium labeling (Figure 5 lane C) and
is therefore not a glycoprotein. This suggests that T6 might be associated with the small subunit of HLA-A/B antigens, β2-microglobulin,
which is known not to be a glycoprotein.

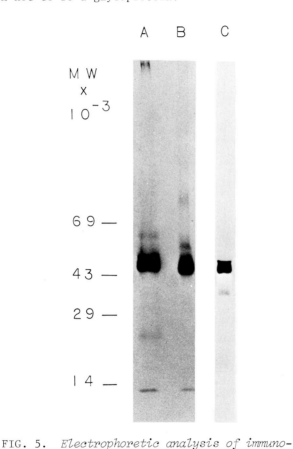

FIG. 5. *Electrophoretic analysis of immunoprecipitates made with monoclonal antibody to
T6 of lysate from ^{125}I-labeled or ^{3}H-labeled
human thymocytes.*
*a) ^{125}I-labeled thymocytes, sample prepared in
the presence of 2-mercaptoethanol (reducing).*
*b) ^{125}I-labeled thymocytes, sample prepared in
the absence of 2-mercaptoethanol (nonreducing).*
*c) ^{3}H-labeled thymocytes, sample prepared in
the presence of 2-mercaptoethanol (reducing).*

Two approaches were used to study a possible association of T6 cell-
surface antigens with β2-microglobulin. First, a thymus preparation

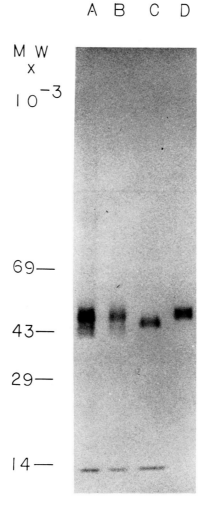

FIG. 6. *Electrophoretic comparison of immunoprecipitates made with monoclonal antibody to T6 and to HLA-A, -B, and -C antigens (W6/32) of lysate from ^{125}I-labeled human thymocytes.*

a) Immunoprecipitate with anti-β2-microglobulin.

b) Eluate from lane A, prepared with β2-microglobulin.

c) Immunoprecipitate made with monoclonal antibody to HLA-A, -B, and -C antigens (W6/32) from lane B.

d) Immunoprecipitate made with monoclonal antibody by T6 from lane B.

labeled with ^{125}I was solubilized in NP-40 and divided into two parts. One half was treated with a preformed complex made with an anti-β2-microglobulin reagent and rabbit anti-mouse IgG. As a control, the other half was incubated with a preformed complex of rabbit anti-mouse IgG and a nonimmune ascites. Following removal of immunoprecipitated material, additional immunoprecipitations were performed on both lysates with either anti-T6, -T9, or -T10. In the case of the lysate that was pretreated with the anti-β2-microglobulin reagent, significantly less material could be precipitated with anti-T6 (11,000 cpm) than after pre-clearing with nonimmune ascites (60,000 cpm). Both anti-T9 and anti-T10 precipitated the same amount of radioactive material. This indicates that on thymocytes at least 80% of the T6 is associated with β2-micro-globulin. Comparison of an anti-β2-microglobulin and an anti-T6 immuno-precipitate by SDS-polyacrylamide gel electrophoresis demonstrated that the smaller subunit of the T6 antigen migrates as β2-microglobulin on a 5-15% gradient gel.

In order to investigate the possible association of T6 with β2-micro-globulin, another experiment was designed. First, all proteins assoc-iated with β2-microglobulin were isolated from an NP-40 lysate of ^{125}I-labeled human thymocyte membrane proteins by immunoprecipitation with a preformed complex of rabbit anti-mouse IgG and mouse anti-β2-microglob-ulin. Subsequently, the immune complex was eluted with purified β2-microglobulin. In previous studies, it was shown that such an elution does not disrupt the tight interactions between the rabbit antibodies and the mouse IgG (14). Using this technique, 80% of the β2-microglob-ulin-associated proteins are eluted from the immunoprecipitate. These eluted β2-microglobulin-associated proteins were then treated with anti-T6 or the monoclonal reagent W6/32 (2). This experiment clearly showed that anti-T6 could precipitate a 49K dalton protein out of the mixture of β2-microglobulin-associated proteins (Figure 6). HLA-A and -B anti-gens are slightly smaller (45K daltons) than the T6 antigen (49K daltons), and both bands could be observed in the original precipitate with the anti-β2-microglobulin reagent (Figure 6 lane A). These experiments demonstrate that the antigen T6 is indeed associated with β2-microglob-ulin.

The β2-microglobulin band is barely visible in immunoprecipitations with anti-T6 (Figure 6 lane D). This can be explained in several ways. First, T6 probably contains a much larger number of tyrosine residues, which are reactive with ^{125}I-sodium iodine in the presence of lactoper-oxidase and H_2O_2. Second, the anti-T6 antibody may dissociate the two polypeptide chains. Third, part of the polypeptide chains recognized by anti-T6 may be expressed on the cell surface not associated with β2-microglobulin. In an earlier report, a 49K dalton polypeptide chain (NA1/34) had been found on MOLT-4 cells that was not associated with β2-microglobulin but with a slightly larger protein termed βt. Our studies (29) prove that NA1/34 and anti-T6 precipitate identical glyco-proteins. Although T6 is associated with β2-microglobulin in all pre-cipitations, we have now found an additional nonglycosylated polypep-tide of 12K with an isoelectric point of pH = 7.0 (Figure 7) (31). This may be identical to the βt antigen detected by Ziegler and Milstein (34).

We have analyzed T6 antigens from thymuses of 20 individuals using the

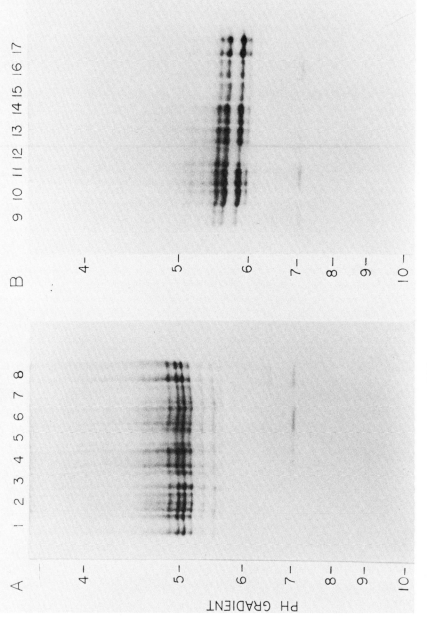

FIG. 7. *Isoelectric focussing of* ^{125}I*-labeled immunoprecipitates from 9 separate thymuses.*

technique of isoelectric focussing (31). An example of such an analysis of nine separate thymus preparations is given in Figure 7. After treatment with neuraminidase, the complexity of T6 is greatly reduced, but this treatment does not completely remove all sialic acids. We estimate that T6 contains at least three complex oligosaccharide side chains. No charge heterogeneity was found in T6 immunoprecipitates from 20 thymus preparations, other than in the band at pH = 7.0 (Figure 7). This finding is in agreement with the limited polymorphism found in murine TL antigens (10). When a number of leukemic cell lines were analyzed by the same technique, the T6 antigens from one cell line (MOLT-4) proved different from all the other cell lines and thymuses. This difference disappeared after neuraminidase treatment (31). T6 on MOLT-4 may therefore contain a deviating oligosaccharide side chain.

Our results concerning the tissue distribution of T6 and its association with β2-microglobulin strongly suggest that this antigen is the human homologue of the murine TL antigens (1,10,33).

T9 and T10

Although the markers T9 and T10 proved to be useful in recognizing early thymic cells, their expression is not limited to the T cell lineage (21). Both markers have been detected on lectin-activated T lymphocytes (29), cells from non-T lymphoid malignancies, and fetal liver cells (18,20).

SDS-polyacrylamide gel electrophoresis of anti-T9 immunoprecipitates prepared from ^{125}I-labeled thymocyte lysates showed that the target antigen for anti-T9 is a 94K dalton protein under reducing conditions. When the gels were run under nonreducing conditions, the protein migrated at 190,000. Furthermore, T9 antigen can also be isolated after tritiation of sialic acid residues or galactose residues.

Recently, Trowbridge and Omary (30) have implicated T9 as the receptor for transferrin. Surprisingly, the monoclonal antibody anti-T9 does not inhibit binding of ^{125}I-labeled transferrin to human reticulocytes, but inhibits significantly the $^{59}Fe_2^+$ uptake (14). LeClair and colleagues found that transferrin can be cross-linked to a 90K dalton protein using a heterobifunctional cross-linker FAPB-imidate (16). The receptor for transferrin present in the cross-linked complex could indeed be identified as T9.

The target antigen for anti-T10 was found to be a glycoprotein of molecular weight 45K. If immunoprecipitates prepared with anti-T10 were analyzed by SDS gel electrophoresis under nonreducing conditions, a band with apparent molecular weight of 37K was seen. This may indicate that the T10 protein contains intrachain sulfhydryl bridges that stabilize the folding of the polypeptide chain. In some experiments, a weak nonglycosylated protein of 12K daltons was found in anti-β2-microglobulin reagents (29), but is the 12K, pH 7.05 protein, which is also found in anti-T6 precipitates (31).

The tissue distribution and molecular properties of T10 are reminiscent of the murine Qa2 antigens (13,17).

TABLE III.   Characterization of human T cell surface antigens.

Antigen	Molecular weight		Glyco-protein	Possible Murine Equivalent
	Reduced	Non-reduced		
T1	69,000	69,000	+	Lyt-1
T3	20,000	20,000	+	--
T4	62,000	62,000	+	Lyt-1 ?
T5	33,000	76,000	+	Lyt-2 or Lyt-3
T8	33,000	76,000	+	Lyt-2 or Lyt-3
T6	{ 49,000 + 12,000	{ 49,000 + 12,000	+ − }	TL
T9	94,000	190,000	+	--
T10	46,000	37,000	+	Qa2

CONCLUSIONS

A series of monoclonal reagents which were previously found to define stages of differentiation of human thymocytes and which were shown to be useful in the classification of thymus derived malignancies, has been used for a preliminary description of their target antigens (Table III). All antigens are cell surface glycoproteins, some of which have been shown to be amphiphilic proteins. The T3, T4, T5 and T8 antigens are exclusively expressed on cells of the T lineage, whereas T1, T6, T9 and T10 are not. The T1, T6 and T10 antigens exhibit a restricted distribution, whereas T9 appears on a large number of proliferating cells (20).

Preliminary biochemical analysis in conjunction with the tissue distribution patterns were used in comparing these markers with murine cell surface markers. The following homologues are proposed: T1/Lyt-1, T5 and T8/Lyt-2 and Lyt-3, T6/TL, and T10/Qa2. The antigens T3 and T8 are involved in functions which are specifically programmed in T lymphocytes (T3) or the T cytotoxic subset (T8). T9 identifies the cell surface receptor for transferrin.

A detailed analysis of the structure of these glycoproteins, their biosynthesis, and their *in situ* vectorial organization should provide more information about their function. A chemical description of these antigens is of paramount importance for studies of the molecular genetics of T cell differentiation.

ACKNOWLEDGEMENTS

We thank Dr. Peter Schrier for critically reading the manuscript. This research was supported by grants from the National Institutes of Health (AI-15066 and AI-17651).

REFERENCES

1. Anundi, H.L., Rask, L., Ostberg, L., and Peterson, P.A. (1975): *Biochemistry*, 14:5046-5056.
2. Barnstable, C.J., Bodmer, W.F., Brown, G., Galfré, G., Milstein, C., Williams, A.F., and Ziegler, A. (1978): *Cell*, 14:9-20.
3. Bhan, A.K., Reinherz, E.L., Poppema, S., McClusky, R., and Schlossman, S.F. (1980): *J. Exp. Med.*, 152:771-782.
4. Borst, J., and Terhorst, C. (1981): (manuscript in preparation).
5. Campbell, D.G., Williams, A.F., Bayley, P.M., and Reid, K.B.M. (1979): *Nature*, 282:341-343.
6. Cantor, H., and Boyse, E. (1976): *Cold Spring Harbor Symp. Quant. Biol.*, 41:23-32.
7. Durda, P.J., and Gottlieb, P.D. (1976): *J. Exp. Med.*, 144:476-483.
8. Durda, P.J., Shapiro, C., Gottlieb, P.D. (1978): *J. Immunol.*, 120:53-61.
9. Fan, J., Ahmed, A., and Bonavida, B. (1980): *J. Immunol.*, 125:2444-2453.
10. Flaherty, L. (1981): In: *The Major Histocompatibility Complex*, edited by M. Dorf. Garland Press, New York. pp. 33-57.
11. Gahmberg, C.G., and Andersson, L.C. (1978): *Ann. NY Acad. Sci.*, 312:240.
12. Hollander, N., Pillemer, E., and Weissman, I.L. (1980): *J. Exp. Med.*, 152:674-687.
13. Kincade, P.W., Flaherty, L., Lee, G., Watanabe, T., and Michaelson, J. (1980): *J. Immunol.*, 124:2879-2885.
14. LeClair, K.L., van Agthoven, A., and Terhorst, C. (1981): *J. Immunol. Meth.*, (in press).
15. Ledbetter, J.A., and Herzenberg, L.A. (1979): *Immunol. Rev.*, 47:65.
16. Maasen, J.A., and Terhorst, C. (1981): *Eur. J. Biochem.*, 115:153-158.
17. Michaelson, J., Flaherty, L., Vitetta, E.A., and Poulik, M.D. (1977): *J. Exp. Med.*, 145:1066-1070.
18. Nadler, L.M., Ritz, J., Griffin, J., Todd, R., Reinherz, E., and Schlossman, S.F. (1981): *Progress in Haematology*, Vol. 12.
19. Nakayama, E., Shiku, H., Stockert, E., Oettgen, H.F., and Old, L.J. (1979): *Proc. Nat. Acad. Sci. (USA)*, 76:1977-1981.
20. Omary, M.B., Trowbridge, I.S., and Minowada, J. (1980): *Nature*, 286:888-891.
21. Reinherz, E.L., and Schlossman, S.F. (1980): *Cell*, 29:821-827.
22. Reinherz, E.L., Kung, P.C., Goldstein, G., Levey, R.H., and Schlossman, S.F. (1980): *Proc. Nat. Acad. Sci. (USA)*, 77:1588-1592.
23. Reinherz, E.L., Hussey, R.E., and Schlossman, S.F. (1980): *Eur. J. Immunol.*, 10:758-762.
24. Sarmiento, M., Glasebrook, A.L., and Fitch, F.W. (1980): *J. Immunol.*, 125:2665-2672.
25. Shinohara, N., Hämmerling, U., and Sachs, D.H. (1980): *Eur. J. Immunol.*, 10:289-594.
26. Snow, P., Spits, H., LeClair, K., and Terhorst, C. (1981): (manuscript in preparation).
27. Spits, H., DeVries, J., and Terhorst, C. (1981): *Cell Imm.*, (in press).
28. Terhorst, C., van Agthoven, A., Reinherz, E.L., and Schlossman, S.F. (1980): *Science*, 209:520-521.
29. Terhorst, C., van Agthoven, A., LeClair, K., Snow, P., Reinherz, E.L., and Schlossman, S.F. (1981): *Cell*, 23:771-780.
30. Trowbridge, I.S., and Omary, M.B. (1981): *Proc. Nat. Acad. Sci. (USA)*, (in press).
31. van Agthoven, A., and Terhorst, C. (1981): submitted for publication.

32. van Agthoven, A., Terhorst, C., Reinherz, E.L., and Schlossman, S.F. (1981): *Eur. J. Immunol.*, 11:18-21.
33. Vitetta, E.S., Uhr, J.W., and Boyse, E.A. (1975): *J. Immunol.*, 114: 252-258.
34. Ziegler, A., and Milstein, C. (1979): *Nature*, 279:243-244.

Expression of Differentiated Functions in Cancer Cells, edited by R. F. Revoltella et al., Raven Press, New York © 1982.

Properties of the Epidermal Growth Factor Receptor-Kinase

*†Graham Carpenter, *†Christa Stoscheck, and *Stanley Cohen

Department of Biochemistry and Division of Dermatology, †Department of Medicine, Vanderbilt University School of Medicine, Nashville, Tennessee 37232

Epidermal growth factor (EGF) is a small polypeptide (molecular weight = 6000) which stimulates the proliferation of mammalian cells in vivo and in vitro (see reference 3 for review). The mechanism of growth factor interaction with responsive cells grown in culture has been studied intensively in recent years. The results of these investigations have defined a pathway for growth factor binding and metabolism by intact cells (Figure 1). There is experimental data to support steps 1 through 10 which depict the binding of EGF to specific receptors on the cell surface (5,16), the clustering or aggregation of EGF:receptor complexes (13,19), internalization of the complexes in endocytotic vesicles (2,12,13,18,19), fusion of the vesicles with multivesicular bodies, presumably lysosomes (13,18), and extensive degradation of EGF within the lysosome (2,18) with the subsequent release of low molecular weight (^{125}I-labeled monoiodo-tyrosine from ^{125}I-EGF) degradation products into the extracellular miliue (2). The fate of internalized receptors is not clear. Receptor replacement in the plasma membrane may occur either by recycling of internalized receptors, steps 11, 12 and 15, or by de novo biosynthesis, steps 13-15. The data of Das and Fox (10) indicate that, in fibroblasts, at least a small portion of the internalized receptors (Mr = 190,000) are converted to lower molecular weight products (Mr = 62,000 to 37,000).

The binding of EGF to its surface receptors produces, in sensitive cell populations, a series of cellular activities culminating with increased DNA synthesis and cell division. To understand how interactions at the cell surface initiate cell proliferation, it is necessary to define the pathway shown in Figure 1 in terms of a series of biochemical reactions which produce intracellular signals that influence the nucleus and perhaps other growth controlling sites within the cell.

It is reasonable to expect that many of the biochemical reactions initiated by the formation of EGF:receptor complexes will be difficult to detect. If the intact cell is employed there will be many "background" reactions; moreover, it will be difficult to separate direct and indirect responses. Perhaps an even greater obstacle is that these reactions, or reaction products, may be too low to detect and measure quantitatively. For these reasons we have sought a cell-free system to detect biochemical responses to EGF:receptor formation.

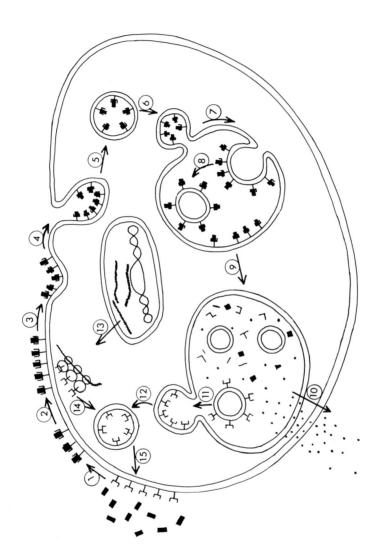

FIG. 1. Schematic outline of the formation of EGF:receptor complexes on intact cells and the intracellular metabolism of the cell-bound complexes.

The tumor cell line A-431, derived from a human epidermoid carcinoma, contains a high concentration of EGF receptors - 2×10^6 receptors per cell (12) - compared to other cell types which generally have about 1×10^5 receptors per cell. Believing that higher receptor concentrations might serve to amplify direct biochemical responses to the formation of EGF:receptor complexes, this cell line was chosen for investigation. Morphologic studies have indicated that this cell line is sensitive to the addition of EGF (8). Within 5 minutes of exposure to EGF at 37° the A-431 cells exhibited extensive ruffling and extension of filopodia. During this time fluid pinocytosis also was stimulated, as indicated by a 10-fold increase in the uptake of horseradish peroxidase (14). Other studies of the interaction of fluorescein or ferritin-EGF conjugates with A-431 cells have established that these cells bind and metabolize EGF as shown in steps 1 through 9 of Figure 1 (13,14,18). Interestingly, the effects of EGF on membrane ruffling and the uptake of horseradish peroxidase are transient in nature and correlate temporally with the initial binding of EGF to A-431 cells. Both effects are observed within 1 minute after the addition of EGF, last for approximately 15 minutes, and are not detectable 20 minutes after EGF addition.

STUDIES OF EGF INTERACTION WITH MEMBRANES PREPARED FROM A-431 CELLS

Growth Factor Binding

Membranes were prepared from A-431 cells by the procedure of Thom et al. (20) as detailed elsewhere (4). The vesicular membrane preparations had a specific ^{125}I-EGF binding capacity of 16 picomoles per mg protein - approximately 6-fold higher than the binding capacity of intact A-431 cells (4). The binding of ^{125}I-EGF to these membranes is rapid - reaching equilibrium within 10 minutes at room temperature or 5°. The binding is specific for EGF and is saturated at approximately 1.6×10^{-8} M total EGF. Half-maximal binding occurs in the presence of 1.2×10^{-9} M growth factor (4).

EGF-Stimulated Protein Phosphorylation

The incubation of A-431 membranes with γ-^{32}P ATP resulted in the incorporation of radioactivity into trichloroacetic acid insoluble, organic solvent nonextractable material as shown in Figure 2 (14). The data in this figure also show that following the addition of EGF to the membrane preparation at 0° the phosphorylation of endogenous membrane proteins was increased approximately 3-fold. EGF-enhanced phosphorylation was observed at higher temperatures, but the increased activity of phosphatases or other hydrolytic enzymes (eg. ATPases) and the rapidity of the reaction made assays more convenient to perform at 0°.

Certain characteristics of the phosphorylation reactions have been described (4). The basal and EGF-stimulated protein phosphorylation reactions required a divalent cation - either Mn^{+2} (2 mM) or Mg^{+2} (50 mM). Phosphorylation was not affected by Ca^{+2} and was not sensitive to cyclic nucleotides. Maximal stimulation occurred in the presence of approximately 3×10^{-8} M EGF. Human EGF and derivates of mouse EGF, including fluorescein-EGF and EGF lacking the

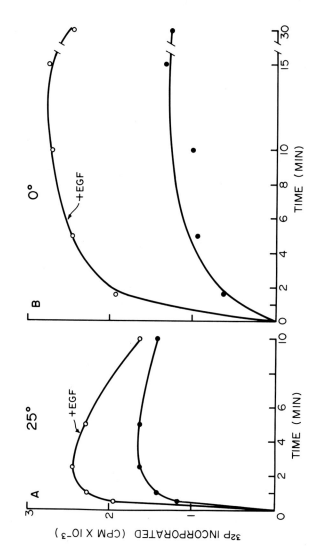

FIG. 2. Stimulation by EGF of the incorporation of $[^{32}P]$phosphate from $[\gamma-^{32}P]ATP$ into A-431 cell membranes (from Carpenter, et al., 1979, reference 4).

COOH-terminal two amino acids (EGF$_{1-51}$) or five amino acids (EGF$_{1-48}$) were effective in stimulating phosphorylation. A wide variety of other peptide hormones were tested for their ability to stimulate phosphorylation in this system, but none were effective. The A-431 membrane phosphorylation system affects the phosphorylation of both endogenous and certain exogenous substrates. Histones were a good exogenous substrate while casein was not. The EGF-stimulated phosphorylation activity is similar in several respects to the protein kinase associated with sarcoma tumor viruses, the src kinase. For example, both kinases produce phosphorylated tyrosine residues on protein substrates (21). Also the EGF-sensitive kinase from A-431 cells is able to recognize and phosphorylate antibodies to the viral kinase (7).

The nature of the phosphorylated endogenous proteins in A-431 membranes was examined by SDS-gel electrophoresis and autoradiography (17). The data show that (1) EGF increased the phosphorylation of many membrane components, particularly those having apparent molecular weights of 170,000, 150,000 and 80,000, (2) proteins phosphorylated in the presence of EGF were also labeled, but to lesser extent, in the absence of the growth factor, and (3) there was no correlation between the intensity of Coomassie Blue staining and the amount of phosphorylation. The extent of EGF-stimulation of individual bands in the gel was approximately 2 to 3-fold.

These studies do not reveal the mechanism by which EGF binding to its receptor is coupled to activities affecting protein phosphorylation. However, experimental evidence (4,9) demonstrates that (1) substrate (ATP) availability does not become a limiting factor and is not affected by EGF, (2) the activation process is reversible upon the removal of EGF, and (3) the rate and extent of dephosphorylation is not affected by EGF. It would appear, therefore, that the stimulatory effect of EGF, in this system, is to increase protein kinase activity.

EGF stimulates protein phosphorylation in cells other than the A-431 tumor cell line. Activation of phosphorylation has been observed in placental membranes (6) and in membranes prepared from cultured human fibroblasts (17). In each case EGF increased phosphorylation of a protein having an approximate molecular weight of 170,000.

CO-PURIFICATION OF RECEPTOR AND PROTEIN KINASE

To understand the biochemical details of the mechanism by which EGF binds to receptors and thereby activates a protein kinase, it is necessary to isolate the component molecules of this system--the EGF receptor, the EGF-sensitive protein kinase, and the endogenous substrate(s) of the phosphorylation reaction. Purification of these membrane components obviously required solubilization as a first step. Although it has not been possible to solubilize the EGF receptor with retention of binding activity from sources such as the placenta, the receptor has been extracted in an active form from A-431 cells with the non-ionic detergent Triton X-100 (1). The solubilized receptor preparation has protein kinase activity which can be increased by the formation of EGF:receptor complexes (9). In the solubilized extract, as in the particulate membranes, EGF-sensitive phosphorylation is especially evident on endogenous proteins that have molecular

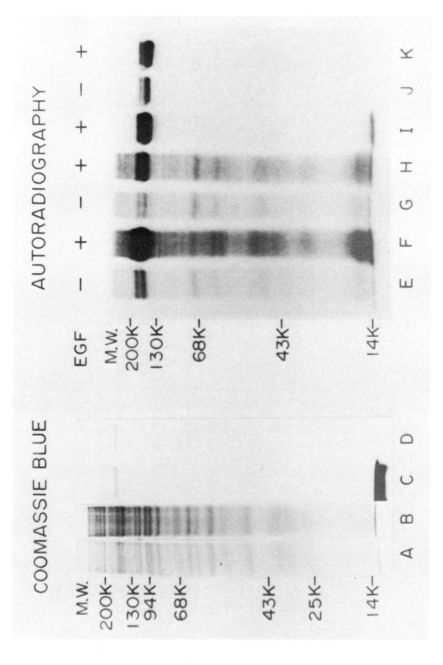

FIG. 3. SDS gel electrophoresis, Coomassie Blue staining, and autoradiography of solubilized and affinity purified A-431 membranes. Lanes A, E and F-original detergent solubilized membranes. Lanes B, G and H-material not adsorbed on the EGF-agarose. Lanes C and I-material eluted from the affinity resin with EGF. (The highly stained band at the bottom of lane C is EGF.) Lanes D, J and K-material eluted from the affinity resin with ethanolamine (from Cohen, et al., 1980, reference 9).

weights of 170,000 and 150,000 (9). Therefore, the hormone-receptor-effector system remains intact and active after detergent solubilization. Gel filtration of the solubilized preparation on Sephacryl S-300 showed that ^{125}I-EGF binding activity and EGF-enhanced protein phosphorylation activity penetrated the gel matrix and eluted at a position indicating a micellar-protein molecular weight less than ferritin (440,000), but larger than catalase (232,000).

In view of the complex composition of the detergent extract and the limited quantities of membrane available, affinity chromatography was employed to attempt purification of the EGF receptor. Triton extracts of A-431 membranes were mixed in a "batch" procedure with EGF covalently attached to agarose beads. The beads were then washed exhaustively and finally a high concentration of free EGF was added to elute material bound to the EGF-agarose. Since it was not feasible to measure ^{125}I-EGF binding activity in the eluted material due to the high concentration of unlabeled EGF present, only phosphorylation activity could be assayed. Elution of the EGF-agarose with EGF resulted in the recovery of about 37% of phosphorylation activity present in the original solubilized extracts. To assay the eluted material for EGF receptor activity, an alternate means was sought to effect elution from the EGF-agarose. The most effective procedure for elution involved incubation of the extract absorbed to EGF-agarose with 5 mM ethanolamine, pH 9.7. Approximately 39% of the binding activity present in the original solubilized extract was recovered in the ethanolamine eluate. Recovery of phosphorylation activity by ethanolamine elution of the affinity column was low (14%). This may reflect the fact that not all of the kinase activity is associated with the receptor or that some of the endogenous membrane substrates are removed by this purification step.

The data presented in Figure 3 demonstrate the protein composition by SDS-gel electrophoresis and Coomassie Blue staining, of the original and affinity purified receptor-kinase preparations. Also shown in Figure 3 are comparisons, by SDS gel electrophoresis and autoradiography, of the endogenous components which are phosphorylated in the original and affinity purified preparations. The Coomassie Blue staining patterns of the original solubilized extract (Lane A) and the material which did not absorb to the affinity column (Lane B) are nearly identical. Elution of the affinity resin with EGF (Lane C) or with ethanolamine (Lane D) results in identical staining patterns which consist of one major band (molecular weight approximately 150,000) and several trace bands, including one of about 170,000 daltons. The data in Figure 3 indicate a substantial purification of the receptor-kinase by this affinity chromatography step.

The results shown in Figure 3 also demonstrated that the affinity purified material has phosphorylation activity which is sensitive to the addition of EGF and that the phosphorylated endogenous substrates are proteins having molecular weights of approximately 150,000 and 170,000 (compare Lanes J and K).

The time course of ^{125}I-EGF binding to the highly purified receptor is shown in Figure 4 and the dependence on growth factor concentration is demonstrated in Figure 5. These properties of the purified receptor are similar to the characteristics of the receptor in the intact membrane (4). Binding equilibrium is reached with 10 minutes and saturation occurs at 2×10^{-8} M. The binding is half maximal at

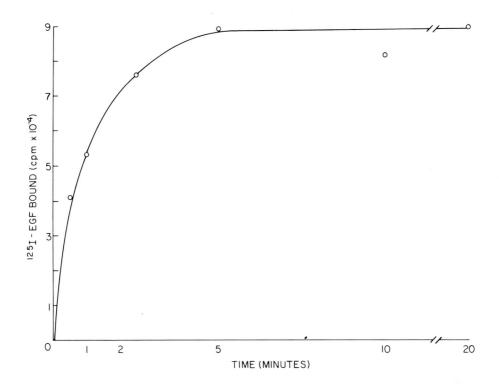

FIG. 4.   Time course of ^{125}I-EGF binding to purified EGF receptor. Affinity purified receptor (9) was incubated at room temperature with 3.3×10^{-8} M ^{125}I-EGF.   At the indicated times the amount of radioactivity bound to the receptor was determined by polyethylene glycol precipitation (1).

TABLE 1.   Effect of temperature on the binding of ^{125}I-EGF to affinity purified receptor.

| Temperature | ^{125}I-EGF Binding (cpm) | |
	1 min	20 min
0°	8,042	14,029
25°	22,049	32,050
37°	37,399	42,814

Affinity purified EGF receptor prepared from A-431 membranes (9) were incubated with 3.3×10^{-8} M ^{125}I-EGF at the indicated temperatures for 1 min or 20 min times.   The receptor-bound radioactivity was determined by rapid polyethylene glycol precipitation and filtration (1).

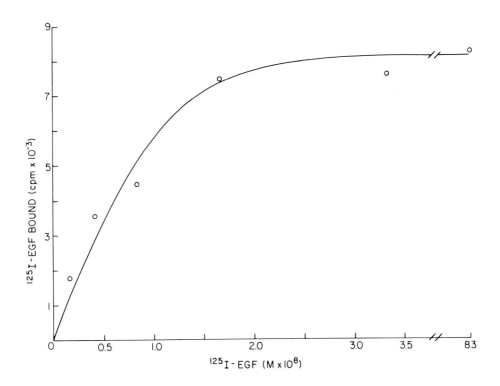

FIG. 5. Effect of increasing concentrations of ^{125}I-EGF on binding to the purified receptor. Affinity purified EGF receptor (9) was incubated at room temperature for 30 min with indicated concentrations of ^{125}I-labeled EGF. Receptor-bound radioactivity was determined by polyethylene glycol precipitation (1).

approximately 6 x 10^{-9} M. At the lowest concentration of ^{125}I-EGF, 0.16 x 10^{-8} M, 23% of the total radioactivity was bound to the receptor. At saturating concentrations less than 10% of the total ^{125}I-EGF was bound to the receptor. The data in Table 1 show that the binding of ^{125}I-EGF to the purified receptor is temperature dependent - more so than observed with the receptor in particulate membrane preparations. Both the initial binding rate, approximated by the 1 min time point, and the equilibrium level of ^{125}I-EGF binding to the receptor are decreased at low temperatures. The data in Figure 6 show that the binding of ^{125}I-EGF to the purified receptor is reversible. Purified receptor was incubated with ^{125}I-EGF for 20 minutes and an excess of unlabeled EGF was added, t = 0 in Figure 6. The bound ^{125}I-EGF rapidly dissociated from the receptor with a half-life of approximately 11 minutes.

The affinity purified EGF receptor has been used as an immunogen to inject rabbits. Sera collected from these animals have a high titer of anti-EGF receptor activity. The binding of ^{125}I-EGF to human fibroblasts is inhibited by 100% at sera dilutions of 1:1000.

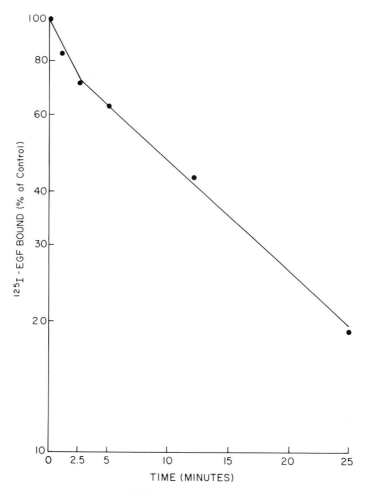

FIG. 6. Dissociation of ^{125}I-EGF from purified receptor. Affinity
purified EGF receptor (9) was incubated at room temperature with
^{125}I-EGF (3.3×10^{-8} M) for 20 min. At this time (t = 0) radioactivity
specifically bound to receptor was determined by polyethylene glycol
precipitation and that value was considered to be 100% binding.
The remaining tubes received a 100-fold molar excess of unlabeled
EGF (3.3×10^{-6} M) and radioactivity remaining bound to the receptor
was measured at the indicated times. After 50 min. the bound radioactivity was 6% (data not shown).

The antibodies block induction of DNA synthesis by EGF and block
EGF-stimulation of protein phosphorylation in vitro. None of these
immune sera block the basal kinase activity. Further studies are
being conducted to determine the exact nature of the antigen(s)
recognized by these antisera and to determine their utility in understanding receptor metabolism and receptor activation of protein kinase
activity.

CONCLUDING REMARKS

Several groups have attempted to identify the EGF receptor by covalent crosslinking of ^{125}I-EGF to the surface of cultured cells or to crude membrane preparations. Wrann and Fox (22) and Das, et al. (11) report a molecular weight for the EGF receptor of 175,000 in A-431 cells and 190,000 in 3T3 cells, respectively. Hock, et al. (15) obtained molecular weights of 180,000 and 160,000 for the EGF receptor in placental membranes. The major protein species obtained by affinity chromatography of the EGF receptor on EGF-agarose has a molecular weight of approximately 150,000 and this is in close agreement with the estimates described above of the receptor molecular weight. The 150,000 dalton band described in Figure 3 most likely is the EGF receptor.

The co-purification of the EGF receptor and EGF-stimulated phosphorylation activity by affinity chromatography suggests that the two activities are closely associated in the membrane. At present it is not possible to resolve the question of whether kinase activity is also located in the 150,000 dalton band in the affinity purified material or whether it is present as one of the trace bands.

The results suggest that the EGF receptor may, in fact, be a substrate for EGF-sensitive protein kinase activity. This does not preclude the possibility that, in the intact cell, other membrane or even non-membrane proteins also may be substrates for this phosphorylation activity. One would predict, based on these in vitro results, that subsequent to the binding of EGF to its receptor the phosphorylated state of the receptor is increased. The significance of the coupling of protein phosphorylation to the formation of EGF:receptor complexes in the intact cell is not clear at present, but the early events of hormone:receptor aggregation on the cell surface might be affected by phosphorylation of the receptor. Also it is intriguing to think that the growth factor-sensitive kinase is able in the intact cell to phosphorylate cytoplasmic proteins which act as second messengers for EGF.

ACKNOWLEDGMENTS

The authors acknowledge the support of the American Cancer Society BC-294 (G.C.), National Cancer Institute CA24071 (G.C.), United States Public Health Service HD00700 (S.C.), and an American Cancer Society Research Professorship (S.C.).

REFERENCES

1. Carpenter, G. (1979): Life Sci. 24: 1691-1698.

2. Carpenter, G. and Cohen, S. (1976): J. Cell Biol. 71: 159-171.

3. Carpenter, G. and Cohen, S. (1979): Ann. Rev. Biochem. 48: 193-216.

4. Carpenter, G., King, L. and Cohen, S. (1979): J. Biol. Chem. 254: 4884-4891.

5. Carpenter, G., Lembach, K. J., Morrison, M. M. and Cohen, S. (1975): <u>J. Biol. Chem.</u> 250: 4297-4304.

6. Carpenter, G., Poliner, L. and King, L. (1980): <u>Molec. and Cell. Endocrinol.</u> 18: 189-199.

7. Chinkers, M. and Cohen, S. (1981): <u>Nature</u> (in press).

8. Chinkers, M., McKanna, J. A. and Cohen, S. (1979): <u>J. Cell Biol.</u> 83: 260-265.

9. Cohen, S., Carpenter, G., and King, L. (1980): <u>J. Biol. Chem.</u> 255: 4834-4842.

10. Das, M. and Fox, C. F. (1978): <u>Proc. Natl. Acad.Sci. U.S.A.</u> 75: 2644-2648.

11. Das, M., Miyakawa, T., Fox, C. F. and Pruso, R. M. (1977): <u>Proc. Natl. Acad. Sci. U.S.A.</u> 74: 2790-2794.

12. Haigler, H. T., Ash, J. F., Singer, S. J. and Cohen, S. (1978): <u>Proc. Natl. Acad. Sci. U.S.A.</u> 75: 3317-3321.

13. Haigler, H. T., McKanna, J. M. and Cohen, S. (1979): <u>J. Cell Biol.</u> 81: 382-395.

14. Haigler, H. T., McKanna, J. A. and Cohen, S. (1979): <u>J. Cell Biol.</u> 83: 82-90.

15. Hock, R. A., Nexo, E. and Hollenberg, M. D. (1979): <u>Nature</u> 277: 403-405.

16. Hollenberg, M. D. and Cuatrecasas, P. (1973): <u>Proc. Natl. Acad. Sci. U.S.A.</u> 70: 2964-2968.

17. King, L., Carpenter, G. and Cohen, S. (1980): <u>Biochemistry</u> 19: 1524-1528.

18. McKanna, J. A., Haigler, H. T. and Cohen, S. (1979): <u>Proc. Natl. Acad. Sci. U.S.A.</u> 76: 5689-5693.

19. Schlessinger, J., Shechter, Y., Willingham, M. C. and Pastan, I. (1978): <u>Proc. Natl. Acad. Sci. U.S.A.</u> 75: 2659-2663.

20. Thom, D., Powell, A. J., Lloyd, C. W. and Rees, D. A. (1977): <u>Biochem. J.</u> 168: 187-194.

21. Ushiro, H. and Cohen, S. (1980): <u>J. Biol. Chem.</u> 255: 8363-8365.

22. Wrann, M. M. and Fox, C. F. (1979): <u>J. Biol. Chem.</u> 254: 8083-8086.

Expression of Differentiated Functions in Cancer Cells, edited by R. F. Revoltella et al., Raven Press, New York © 1982.

Basal Lamina and the Control of Proliferation of Malignant and Normal Cells

D. Gospodarowicz, D. K. Fujii, and I. Vlodavsky

Cancer Research Institute, University of California, Medical Center, San Francisco, California 94143

A number of in vitro studies demonstrate that the substrate upon which cells are cultured can alter both the cellular shape and proliferative response to various mitogens in an interrelated manner (14, 15, 23, 37, 41, 48). In the present review, we describe the use of the basal lamina (BL) produced by cultured corneal endothelial cells (21, 24, 36, 67) as a substrate on which to culture both transformed and normal cells of various origins.

I. Effect of Basal Lamina on Tumor Cell Attachment, Migration and Proliferation

A central issue in tumor biology is the understanding of the interactions between tumor cells and their environment. It is of interest in this regard to study the tumor cells' interaction with extracellular matrices and BL's, since this could throw light on the need for stromal and fibroblastic support for tumor cell growth (1, 45); on the ability of tumor cells to reorganize their local environment in order to grow and invade (47, 56); and on the mechanisms through which various artificial substrates that are introduced in vivo into the animal result in the production of malignant mesothelioma and fibrosarcoma (66). We have therefore studied the use of the BL produced by cultured corneal endothelial cells as a substrate on which to culture human cells originating from solid tumors (colon carcinoma and Ewing's sarcoma).

1. Tumor cell attachment, migration, morphology, and organization when maintained on plastic versus basal lamina-coated dishes. In the case of either colon carcinoma cells (Fig. 1) or Ewing cells, as many as 50-80% of the cells seeded on BL-coated dishes attached firmly within 30 min, and 70-90% by one hour, as compared to only about 5-10% of the cells on plastic. Even after 24 hr, no more than 25% of the seeded cells attached to plastic (71). The looser attachment of either the colon carcinoma or Ewing cells to plastic than to BL was easily demonstrated by subjecting the cultures to a gentle pipetting. This released up to 95% of the cells grown on plastic, while no more than 5% of the cells cultured on the BL were released. An even looser attachment of the Ewing cells maintained on plastic could be observed at confluence, since in this case only a gentle shaking of cultures was required to release the cells from the dish. The rapid attachment of colon carcinoma cells and Ewing's sarcoma cells was

shown in subsequent studies (70) to be mediated by different adhesion factors present in the BL. While colon carcinoma cells attached to the BL through their interaction with laminin, the Ewing's cells interacted with fibronectin. The presence of specific adhesion factors in basal lamina, as well as the ability or inability of tumor cells to produce and/or interact with such factors, may determine the localization of given tumor cell types to specific matrices. Such specific cell-matrix interaction may then direct the growth, migration, as well as the invasiveness and metastasis of tumor cells.

Tumor cell migration was studied qualitatively by seeding cell aggregates rather than single cells on plastic or BL and observing the extent of cell migration out of the aggregates. Cell aggregates that were seeded at low or high densities into plastic dishes retained their previous morphology (71). The Ewing cells remained mostly in the form of floating and loosely packed cell aggregates, while the colon carcinoma cells remained as tightly packed, ball-like aggregates, mostly attached to the plastic. In neither case, and even after 10 days in culture, did cells migrate out of the cell aggregates (71). In contrast, seeding of the same cell aggregates on BL-coated dishes was associated with spreading and migration of cells that could be observed within 5 to 15 min after seeding. Migratory activity was best observed in the cells located at the periphery of the aggregates (71). Small aggregates flattened out in less than one hour, leading to the formation of colonies composed of flat and non-overlapping cells. Depending on the size of the initial aggregate, cell overlapping could be seen in the center of some of these colonies, but as time proceeded the cells reorganized and adopted a monolayer configuration (71). Since cell migration is observed prior to cell proliferation, it can be regarded as a specific cellular response to the mere contact between cells and the BL. This may reflect the preferential adhesion of the cells to the BL components such as laminin or fibronectin (70). These interactions of cells with BL adhesion factors can be stronger than the interaction between cells and are obviously much stronger than the interaction between cells and plastic.

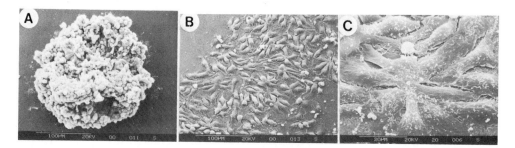

Fig. 1. Scanning electron microscopy of colon carcinoma cells maintained in tissue culture on either a plastic substratum (A) or a BL (B, C). While on plastic cells grew as an aggregate of cells which did not adhere to the substratum (A), when maintained on ECM the cells flattened and grew as a monolayer (B, C).

Both the colon carcinoma and the Ewing cells adopt a flattened morphology only on BL. At confluence on BL, both cell types develop as a continuous monolayer of organized, non-overlapping cells (71). The morphological configuration of confluent cultures of the Ewing cells was similar to that of a confluent vascular endothelial cell monolayer, thereby corroborating the initial impression of Ewing (12) with regard to the cellular source of the disease.

2. <u>Effect of the basal lamina on tumor cell growth.</u> Normal human epithelial cells are difficult to grow using conventional culture techniques. This applies even to malignant cells of epithelial origin (52), some of which, when maintained in culture, have an extremely long doubling-time (10-20 days). Since cell shape has been shown to be a major factor in regulating cell growth (15, 48, 49, 52), we compared the growth rate of cells plated on plastic (spherical configuration) to that of cells plated on BL which adopt a flattened morphology. Although differences in growth rate were observed, both the Ewing and colon carcinoma cells proliferated in either configuration. This observation therefore demonstrated that adhesion of the cells to the BL and their subsequent flattening imposed no restriction on their proliferation. On the contrary, when cells flattened out a stimulation of cell growth which depended on the cell type and culture conditions was observed. This stimulation was particularly evident with the colon carcinoma cells which, when seeded on plastic, showed a lag period of 3 to 4 days before resuming a logarithmic growth rate (16 hr doubling time). In contrast, seeding of the same cells on BL resulted in an active cell migration concomitant with an immediate resumption of proliferation, so that after 3 to 4 days the cell density of cultures maintained on an BL was 4- to 10-fold higher than that of cultures maintained on plastic (71).

An increased growth-rate of cells maintained on BL was also observed with the Ewing cells. Since these cells showed a very loose attachment to plastic, both attached and floating cells had to be counted in order to reach a meaningful conclusion regarding an effect on the total number of cells. When the cultures were maintained on BL, the number of firmly attached and floating cells exceeded by 2- to 4-fold that of cultures maintained on plastic. If only the number of firmly attached cells was compared while the floating cells were ignored, active proliferation of the attached cells was observed only in dishes coated with a BL. This resulted in an infinite increase in the final density of attached cells in cultures maintained on a BL versus those attached on plastic, since cells did not proliferate on the latter substrate. Similar studies with human choroidal melanoma cells have also demonstrated that cells maintained on BL proliferate rapidly (71). This contrasts with a very slow rate of proliferation of these cells (12 to 18 days average doubling time) when maintained on plastic. Effects similar to those of the BL as far as cell attachment and proliferation are concerned were not observed when tumor cells were seeded on plastic dishes coated with purified preparations of collagen types I, III, or IV (71).

The above results therefore demonstrate that cultured tumor cells can proliferate both when they are highly flattened and firmly attached to the substrate and when they are loosely attached or in suspension. Cell adhesion to the BL, however, results in a stimulation of cell growth, which is best observed when the cell fractions grow in the anchorage-dependent configuration, but not in the floating configuration, thereby indicating the need for actual contact.

II. Effect of Basal Lamina on the Attachment, Migration, Proliferation, and Differentiation of Nerve Cells

Nerve cells do not have the ability to produce a BL <u>in vivo</u> and therefore rely on that produced by other tissues during the early steps of embryogenesis for both their migration and neurite outgrowth. This is shown by the very firm attachment of neurites and of their growth cones to the BL <u>in vivo</u>. The interaction of nerve cells with a proper substrate could therefore be important insofar as nerve cell migration and differentiation are concerned. Likewise, a close contact with the BL seems to be important in the control of nerve cell proliferation. In both the cortex and spinal cord, dividing nerve cells can only be found in close contact with the BL which forms the inner lining of the cortex or which is located along the central cavity of the spinal cord. Following division, nerve cells can migrate to the outer part of the cortex or of the spinal cord and differentiate.

To study the interaction of nerve cells with the BL, we first used as a model the PC12 cell line, which is derived from a pheochromocytoma and has been shown to respond to nerve growth factor (NGF) by extending neurites on collagen-coated dishes. When the rate of firm attachment of PC12 cells to plastic versus collagen- and BL-coated dishes is compared, it was found to be 5%

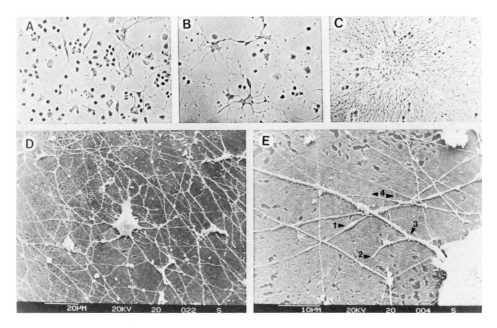

Fig. 2. (A-C) Phase contrast micrographs of unfixed PC12 cells cultured on extracellular matrix in the absence of NGF for 3 days (A), and in the presence of NGF for 3 days (B) and 13 days (C). (D-E) Scanning electron micrographs of PC12 cells on extracellular matrix in the presence of NGF for 12 days. (E) Arrows point to (1) a varicosity in a neurite; (2) the end of a neurite; (3) a branching point; and (4) fine projections extending from a neurite.

for plastic, 20% for collagen-coated dishes, and 90 to 95% for BL-coated dishes in 24 hours (16). Following their attachment to the BL, the cells, which on either plastic or collagen substrata remained rounded, became flattened and began to emit fine neurites characterized by branching, varicosities, and growth cones (Fig. 2). This outgrowth of neurites is only temporary and by day 3 they start to regress unless NGF is present. In its presence, however, extensive thin neurite outgrowth can be seen, and apparent fasciculation of some neurites is observed (16). In contrast, no neurites are extended by NGF-treated cells on plastic, and those cells on collagen-coated dishes extend thick, straight neurites poorly attached to the substrata at only a few points and with little branching or varicosities. Thus, BL may be permissive for neurite outgrowth, and the trophic effects of NGF are necessary for long-term differentiation (16).

The ability of the BL to support extensive cell differentiation is not its only biological effect, since it can affect nerve cell migration and proliferation. While on plastic or collagen-coated dishes single cells will eventually aggregate and give rise to ball-like clumps of cells, single cells on BL will grow as a monolayer of flattened cells. Only when cultures are kept for extended periods of time at confluence will cells eventually overgrow each other. Moreover, whereas the rate of proliferation of cells maintained on plastic is very slow, that of cultures maintained on BL is faster and can be improved by the addition of EGF to the medium (16).

III.   Effect of BL on the Proliferation of Normal Cells Maintained in the Presence of Plasma

Culture of most cells in vitro requires the presence of serum (8). Consequently, investigators have spent much effort in a search to identify the various factors in serum that stimulate cell growth in vitro. An important step in the search for serum growth factors has been the finding that one of the most potent mitogenic factors present in serum, baptized platelet-derived growth factor (PDGF), is in fact derived from platelets (3, 4). While plasma was unable to support the growth of aortic smooth muscle cells (58) or that of BALB/c 3T3 cells (42), serum made from the same pool of blood stimulated their proliferation. Addition of a platelet extract to cell-free plasma or that of PDGF restored the growth-promoting activity (42, 58, 59). One could therefore conclude that one of the principal mitogens responsible for the induction of DNA synthesis present in whole blood serum is derived from platelets (42, 59). However, all studies have thus far used cells maintained on plastic rather than on BL. This difference in the substrate upon which the cells are maintained could have prevented their response to factors present in plasma, thereby creating the difference in mitogenic activity between plasma and serum. To explore the possibility that the serum factors to which cells maintained on BL become sensitive are also present in plasma, we have compared the mitogenic activity of plasma versus serum, using as target cells vascular smooth muscle cells (VSM) maintained on either plastic or an BL (26).

VSM cells maintained on plastic proliferate in response to serum but not to plasma (26, 59). In contrast, when cells were maintained on BL and exposed to either plasma or serum, they proliferated actively under both conditions and plasma was observed to be even more mitogenic for cells maintained on an BL than was serum for cells maintained on plastic. When the growth rate and the final cell density of cultures maintained on BL and exposed to either plasma or serum were compared, they were found to be the same (26) (Fig. 3). When the final cell density of cultures maintained on BL was analyzed as a function of the serum or plasma concentration to which they were exposed, it was found to be a direct function of the serum or plasma concentration. It is therefore likely that the proliferation of vascular smooth muscle cells is controlled by factor(s) present in plasma and that the BL has only a permissive role (26).

These results emphasize how drastically one can modify the proliferative response of a given cell type to serum factors by modifying the substrate upon which the cells are maintained (26). It is possible that the lack of response of various cell types maintained under tissue culture conditions to plasma factors

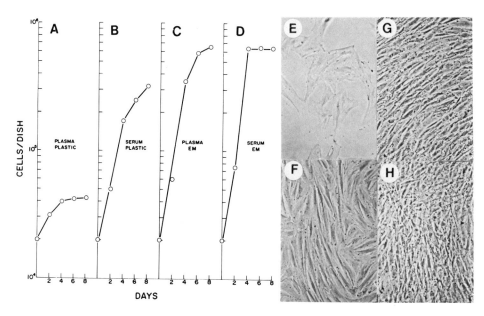

Fig. 3 (A-D). Proliferation of bovine vascular smooth muscle (VSM) cells maintained on plastic or dishes coated with basal lamina and exposed to either plasma or serum. VSM cells were seeded at 2×10^4 cells per 35 mm dish and maintained in the presence of DMEM supplemented with either 10% plasma (A, C) or serum (B, D). The cells were maintained on either plastic (A, B) or BL (C, D). (E-H) Morphological appearance of vascular smooth muscle cells maintained on plastic (E, F) or BL (G, H). Cultures were plated and maintained as described above and exposed to either 10% plasma (E, H) or 10% serum (F, G). Pictures were taken on day 8 with a phase contrast microscope (X 80).

responsible in vivo for their proliferation and differentiation could be directly attributed to the artificial substrate, whether plastic or glass, upon which the cells rest and which limits their ability to produce a BL.

IV.   The Identification of Growth-promoting Agents for Normal Cells when Maintained on a Basal Lamina instead of Plastic

1. Vascular endothelial cells. Previous studies (22, 33, 34) have shown that vascular endothelial cell cultures maintained on plastic and propagated in the presence of fibroblast growth factor (FGF) divide with an average doubling time of 18 hours when seeded at either a high (up to 1:1000) or low split ratio. Upon reaching confluence, the cells adopt a morphological configuration similar to that of the confluent culture from which they originated. In contrast, seeding of the same cells at a high split ratio in the absence of FGF results in a much longer doubling time (60-78 h), and within a few passages cultures maintained in the absence of FGF exhibit, in addition to a much slower growth rate, morphological as well as structural alterations which mostly involved changes in the composition and distribution of the BL (40, 68). This raises the possibility that the BL produced by these cells could have an effect on their ability to proliferate and to express their normal phenotype once confluent.

This is what is in fact observed when the growth of bovine vascular endothelial cells seeded at low density on plastic versus BL is compared. Regardless of the initial cell density (sparse culture, 10 cells/mm^2, or clonal density, 1 cell/cm^2) at which cells are seeded, cultures divided extremely rapidly when maintained on BL-coated dishes. Addition of FGF to such cultures did not decrease their mean doubling time, which is already at a minimum (18 to 20 hr), nor does it result in a higher final cell density, which is already at a maximum (900-1000 cells/mm^2). One can therefore conclude that, while low density cell cultures maintained on plastic proliferate poorly and therefore require FGF in order to become confluent within a few days, when the cultures are maintained on BL, they proliferate actively and no longer require FGF in order to become confluent. However, in either case (either maintained on plastic and exposed to FGF or maintained on an BL), the rate of proliferation is a direct function of the serum or plasma concentration to which cultures are exposed. It is therefore likely that, as with VSM cells, the effect of the BL is more a permissive than a direct mitogenic effect, since cells still required serum or plasma in order to proliferate (27, 35). Since vascular endothelial cells maintained on BL now respond to plasma factor(s), one is led to wonder what the nature of such factor(s) is.

Among the plasma factors which could be held directly or indirectly responsible for the active proliferation of vascular endothelial cells are the high density lipoproteins (HDL), as well as the low density lipoproteins (LDL). Earlier studies have shown that both LDL and HDL can interact specifically with vascular endothelial cells (13, 53, 61, 64, 65, 69), and others have shown that LDL could be mitogenic for vascular smooth muscle cells and dermal fibroblasts when added to lipoprotein-deficient serum (LPDS) (7, 13, 57) or to serum from abetalipoproteinemic subjects (44). Likewise, in the case of cells which have a limited ability to make cholesterol de novo, or in the case of cells maintained in the presence of compounds such as compactin which totally inhibit their ability to make cholesterol, addition of LDL to the medium leads to resumption of cell proliferation (18). In that case, LDL could act by providing an exogenous source of cholesterol to the cells, thereby obviating the block in cholesterol synthesis resulting from the presence of the inhibitor in the medium (18). We have therefore compared the respective mitogenic activities of HDL and LDL on vascular endothelial cell cultures exposed to LPDS or to serum-free medium.

Vascular endothelial cells maintained in the presence of medium supplemented with LPDS grow poorly (63). Such cultures therefore require the presence of lipoproteins in order to proliferate optimally. Of the two classes of lipoproteins (HDL and LDL) which have been studied, HDL seems to be the major factor involved in the proliferation of vascular endothelial cells. This is due primarily to its lack of toxicity when added at high concentration, as well as to its lack of dependence on LPDS in order to exhibit its mitogenic properties (63).

LDL, unlike HDL, had a biphasic effect. Although mitogenic for vascular endothelial cells when added at low concentration, once physiological concentrations are reached it becomes toxic for the cells (63). Moreover, and in contrast with HDL, the mitogenic effect of LDL was found to be a function of the LPDS concentration to which cultures were exposed. LDL at a concentration of 200 µg protein/ml did not stimulate cells to proliferate at an optimal growth-rate unless cultures were maintained in high (5% to 10%) LPDS concentration. This mitogenic effect on the part of HDL, as opposed to the cytotoxic effect of LDL, was observed regardless of the density at which cultures were seeded (clonal or high density cultures). Therefore, HDL at physiological concentrations can replace serum or plasma. This is best exemplified by our observation that cells maintained in serum-free medium on BL will proliferate at an optimal rate, provided that HDL (250 μg protein/ml) is added together with transferrin (10 μg/ml) to the medium. In contrast, in the absence of LPDS, LDL concentrations as low as 80 μg protein/ml resulted in cell death and at 30 μg protein/ml had only a small mitogenic effect in comparison to that of HDL.

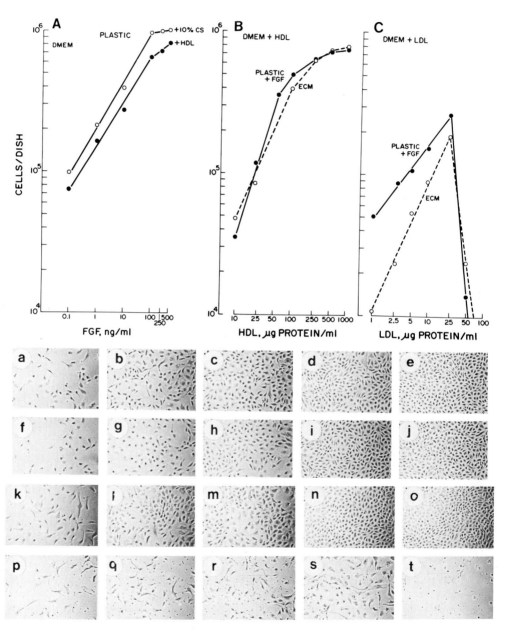

FIGURE 4

The substrate upon which cultures were maintained was found to be of crucial importance if a mitogenic effect on the part of either HDL or LDL is to be observed. When maintained on plastic, cells exposed to LPDS did not survive and therefore could not respond to either lipoprotein (63). In contrast, when maintained on BL they survived quite well, thereby making it possible to observe the mitogenic effect of either HDL or LDL. This suggests that, in vivo, the integrity of the basal lamina upon which endothelial cells rest and migrate is an important factor in determining the cells' response to lipoproteins present in plasma (63).

2. Vascular smooth muscle cells. Among the plasma components which could affect the proliferation of VSM cells are HDL and LDL, as well as somatomedin C, insulin, EGF, and FGF, since those agents have been shown to be mitogenic for a wide variety of cell types maintained under serum-free conditions (51) as well as for VSM cell cultures exposed to plasma (32, 33).

We have therefore compared the effects of the substrate (either BL or plastic) on the proliferative response of low density VSM cell cultures exposed to a synthetic medium supplemented with these various factors. We were further encouraged to take this approach by previous observations (26) which indicated that VSM cells maintained on BL-coated dishes have a much lower requirement for either serum or plasma in order to proliferate actively than when they are maintained on plastic. It is therefore possible that VSM cells, when maintained on BL-coated dishes, could survive and still be responsive to plasma factors even when maintained in a well-defined synthetic medium unsupplemented with either plasma or serum (25). Preliminary studies demonstrated that transferrin, which

Fig. 4. Comparison of the proliferation of bovine vascular endothelial cell cultures maintained on plastic and exposed to either 10% calf serum or serum-free medium supplemented with HDL (500 μg protein/ml) and increasing concentrations of FGF (A) versus that of cultures maintained either on plastic or BL-coated dishes (ECM) and exposed to serum-free medium supplemented with either increasing concentrations of HDL (B) or LDL (C). (A) Vascular endothelial cells were seeded at 2×10^4 cells per 35 mm plastic dish and exposed to medium supplemented with either 10% calf serum (o) or 500 μg protein/ml of HDL (o). FGF was added every other day at concentrations ranging from 0.1 to 500 ng/ml. After 6 days, cell cultures were trypsinized and counted. (B & C) Vascular endothelial cells were seeded at 2×10^4 cells per 35 mm dish in 10% calf serum in either plastic (o———o) or BL-coated (o-----o) dishes (ECM). Eight hours later, medium was removed and the cultures washed twice. Serum-free medium supplemented with increasing concentrations of HDL (from 10 to 1000 μ protein/ml) (A) or with increasing concentrations of LDL (10 to 100 μg protein/ml) was then added. When cultures were maintained on plastic, FGF (100 ng/ml) was added every other day. On day 6 the cultures were trypsinized and the cells counted. Morphological appearance of bovine vascular endothelial cell cultures maintained either in plastic dishes (a-j) or BL-coated dishes (k-t). Cells were exposed to DMEM supplemented with increasing concentrations of HDL (a & k = 25 μg; b & l = 50 μg; c & m = 100 μg; d & n = 250 μg, and e & o = 500 μg protein/ml), DMEM supplemented with 500 μg protein/ml of HDL (f-j), or DMEM supplemented with increasing concentrations of LDL (p = 1 μg; q = 5 μg; r = 10 μg; s = 25 μg; t = 50 μg protein/ml). In the case of plastic dishes, FGF was added every other day at different concentrations (f = 0.1 ng, g = 1.0 ng, h = 10 ng, i = 100 ng, and a-e and j = 250 ng/ml). Pictures were taken on day 6 (phase contrast, X 85).

is the main iron-carrying protein in the bloodstream, must be present if any mitogenic response to plasma factors on the part of VSM cells seeded and maintained in total absence of serum is to be observed. It is likely that this absolute requirement for transferrin either reflects its role in delivering iron to the cells or its ability to detoxify the medium by removing toxic traces of metals (5).

When low density VSM cell cultures were maintained on BL-coated dishes and exposed to a synthetic medium supplemented with transferrin (10 µg/ml), HDL (250 µg protein/ml), insulin (2 µg protein/ml), and FGF (100 ng/ml), cells proliferated as actively as when they were exposed to optimal serum concentration. The single omission of HDL, insulin, or FGF resulted in a lower growth-rate of the cultures, as well as in a lower final cell density (25) (Fig. 5). This indicates that all of these factors have an additive effect upon one another and must be present simultaneously in order to induce optimal cell growth. Neither FGF nor insulin, either singly or in combination, had a significant effect on cell growth. When the ability of EGF (50 ng/ml) to substitute for FGF was tested, it was found to be as potent as FGF. Likewise, somatomedin C at low concentration (10 ng/ml) can fully substitute for insulin (25).

Since HDL, as well as insulin and EGF, are all normally present in plasma, these factors may reflect the plasma constituents involved in the control of the proliferation of VSM cells when such cells are maintained on BL-coated dishes and exposed to plasma. The concentrations at which insulin was mitogenic are clearly pharmacological. However, since insulin can be replaced by somatomedin C, and since it is known to have a low affinity for somatomedin binding sites, it may be that the high concentrations of insulin required are due to its weak interaction with the somatomedin binding sites. If this is the case, the mitogenic activity of insulin on VSM cells is not directly mediated through its interaction with high affinity insulin binding sites but rather through its weak interaction with somatomedin C binding sites. In contrast, the effect of EGF, which was further documented by the identification on the cell surface of EGF receptor sites, is probably due to a direct interaction of EGF with the cells (25).

The use of a synthetic medium supplemented with HDL, insulin, and EGF has allowed VSM cells not only to proliferate actively in the total absence of serum but also to be passaged repeatedly. This therefore makes realization of the goal of serial passage in a totally defined medium possible.

The substrate upon which VSM cells are maintained is an important factor in their response to the various factors to which they are exposed. When cells are maintained on plastic and exposed to a synthetic medium, they will not proliferate. The addition of FGF, which in previous studies has been shown to replace the requirement for a BL, will allow the cells to proliferate and to respond to either HDL or LDL. Yet, the lifespans of the cultures are far from impressive, since even when exposed to HDL and FGF cells senesce after undergoing 23 generations. In contrast, when cells are maintained on BL-coated dishes, even when exposed to a synthetic medium unsupplemented with any factor, cells can undergo 15 generations before senescing and, while the addition of FGF to the medium no longer has any effect on the lifespan of the cultures, that of HDL, insulin, and FGF or EGF will allow the cells to undergo 46 generations before senescing (25). The effect of the BL in delaying cell senescence is even more impressive if one considers the case of cells exposed to synthetic medium supplemented with optimal concentration of serum. While

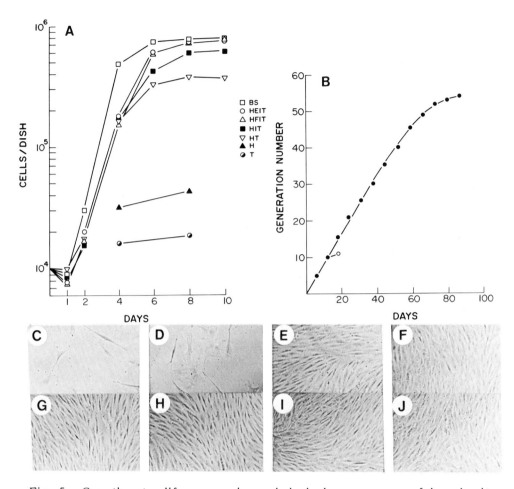

Fig. 5. Growth-rate, lifespan, and morphological appearance of low density VSM cell cultures seeded on BL-coated dishes (or extracellular matrix = ECM) and passaged in the total absence of serum. (A) VSM cells were seeded at 1 X 10⁴ cells per 35 mm dish coated with BL, as described in ref. 25. Cells were exposed to 10% bovine serum (BS □); transferrin (10 µg/ml, T, ◑); HDL (250 µg/ml, H ▲); HDL and transferrin (HT ▽); HDL, insulin (2.5 µg/ml), and transferrin (HIT ■); HDL, FGF (100 ng/ml), insulin, and transferrin (HFIT △); or HDL, EGF (50 ng/ml), insulin, and transferrin (HEIT ○). (B) Lifespan of VSM cell cultures seeded in the absence of serum and passaged repeatedly at low cell density. Cultures were passaged at 10⁴ cells per 35 mm dish (●). Cultures were exposed to DMEM supplemented with HDL (250 µg/ml), insulin (2.5 µg/ml), FGF (100 ng/ml), and transferrin (10 µg/ml). Similar lifespans were observed when cultures were passaged in the presence of EGF (50 ng/ml) instead of FGF (25). As soon as transferrin was omitted from the medium, cells no longer proliferated (○) and cultures therefore could no longer be passaged. (C-J) Morphological appearance of bovine VSM cells seeded as described above on BL-coated dishes and exposed to (C) transferrin (10 µg/ml); (D) HDL (250 µg protein/ml); (E) HDL and transferrin (10 µg/ml); (F) HDL, transferrin, and insulin (2.5 µg/ml); (G) HDL, transferrin, and EGF (50 ng/ml); (H) HDL, transferrin, and FGF (100 ng/ml); (I) HDL, transferrin, insulin, and FGF; or (J) HDL, transferrin, insulin, and EGF.

cultures maintained on plastic and exposed to serum can be maintained at best for 16 generations, cultures maintained on BL have now undergone 70 generations and have as yet shown no sign of senescence (25). It may therefore be concluded that the BL upon which VSM cells are maintained not only makes cells sensitive to factors present in plasma but also delays to a considerable extent the ultimate senescence of the cells when they are exposed to a synthetic medium supplemented either with well-defined factor(s) or with serum.

   3.   Corneal endothelial cells.   The corneal endothelium forms the inner lining of the cornea.   Like the vascular endothelium, this tissue consists of a single cell monolayer composed of highly flattened, closely apposed, and contact inhibited cells endowed with a cell surface polarity.   While the apical cell surface is a nonthrombogenic surface and is exposed to the aqueous humor, the basal cell surface is involved in the secretion of a highly thrombogenic basement membrane called Descemet's membrane, upon which it rests.

   Previous studies have shown that both FGF and EGF can support the proliferation of bovine corneal endothelial cells when maintained on plastic and exposed to serum (31).   In contrast, when that same cell type is maintained on a BL, neither FGF nor EGF is required in order to induce the cells to proliferate. Exposure to plasma or serum alone is enough to insure an optimal growth rate of the cultures, regardless of the cell density at which cultures are seeded initially (28, 38).   Further analysis of the plasma factors involved in the control of proliferation of corneal endothelial cells (17) demonstrated that these factors are similar to those supporting the proliferation of VSM cells and consist of transferrin (10 μg/ml), HDL (250 μg/ml), FGF (100 ng/ml) or EGF (20 ng/ml), and insulin (2.5 μg/ml).   Using such a combination of factors, one can induce low density corneal endothelial cell cultures to proliferate with a growth-rate similar to that observed when cells are exposed to optimal serum concentration (17) and to continue to be able to be passaged repeatedly at low cell density and in the total absence of serum.   As with other cell types, the substrate upon which cells are maintained is crucial if such an effect on the part of transferrin, HDL, insulin, and FGF or EGF is to be observed, since cultures maintained on plastic will not proliferate when exposed to similar conditions (17).   Also in accord with observations with other cell types is the fact that the longevity of corneal endothelial cell cultures maintained in serum-free conditions and on BL-coated dishes is greatly improved.   These conditions also result in a cell model which more closely mimics the in vivo situation, since in vivo the corneal endothelium is exposed to the aqueous humor which, depending on the species considered, has a protein concentration that is only 0.1% to 1% that of plasma.

   4.   Granulosa and adrenal cortex cells.   Both of these cell types in vivo have the ability to produce steroids.   Earlier studies done on the control of proliferation of bovine granulosa cells have shown that this cell type, when maintained on plastic and exposed to optimal serum concentration, proliferates slowly or not at all (29).   The addition of either EGF or FGF to the media could trigger substantial cell proliferation, since low density cell cultures exposed to either mitogen can have an average doubling time as low as 18 hours (29). Addition of either mitogen also delays the ultimate senescence of the cultures (29).   With adrenal cortex cells, on the other hand, although they do divide extremely slowly and rapidly senesce when maintained on plastic and exposed to serum, the addition of FGF, but not that of EGF, results in both a shortening of the average population doubling time and in the prevention of their precocious senescence in culture (30).   In contrast, maintaining either granulosa or adrenal

cortex cells on an BL renders the requirement for growth factors obsolete, and the addition of plasma alone is enough to insure an optimal growth-rate of the cultures (20). However, the plasma factor(s) to which granulosa and adrenal cortex cells respond when maintained on BL were found to be quite different from those to which endothelial or smooth muscle cells responded. In particular, HDL, which was shown to be mitogenic for endothelial or vascular smooth muscle cells over a wide range of concentrations, was cytotoxic for granulosa cells when present at concentrations above 50 µg protein/ml (60). With adrenal cortex cells, cytotoxicity was observed at a concentration above 30 µg protein/ml (19). Insulin was observed to be the main mitogen for both granulosa and adrenal cortex cells, and both cell types responded to concentrations as low as 30 ng/ml by proliferating actively, reaching a final cell density which was 60% that of cultures exposed to optimal serum or plasma concentrations. Addition of either EGF or FGF helped the cultures to reach a final cell density similar to that observed when cells were maintained in the presence of either plasma or serum. As with other cell types, the importance of the substrate in supporting the proliferative response to insulin of both granulosa and adrenal cortex cells was demonstrated by the fact that such response could be observed only with cultures maintained on BL-coated dishes but not with those maintained on plastic (19, 60).

Both of these cell types when cultured in the absence of serum and in the presence of insulin, HDL, and FGF were still capable of producing steroids in response to dibutyryl cyclic AMP. In the case of granulosa cells, exposure to FSH improved the ability of the cells to produce steroids, and in the case of adrenal cells exposure to ACTH also stimulated steroid production above its normal level. Addition of either LDL or HDL to the culture medium of confluent cultures grown in the absence of serum improved the ability of the cells to produce steroids.

Therefore, not only can one grow both adrenal cortex and granulosa cell cultures in a defined medium, but the differentiated properties of these cells are also preserved, as shown by their ability to respond to stimuli provided by their trophic hormones.

V. The Nature of the Factors Present in Basal Lamina which are Involved in Cell Attachment versus Cell Proliferation

The intricate nature of the BL is exemplified by the difficulties encountered in identifying its composition and by the complex interaction of its known components (6) (collagen, glycoproteins, proteoglycans, and glycosaminoglycans) which form a highly stable scaffolding upon which cells rest in vivo. Because the reconstitution of this unique structure from its known constituents would be a formidable task, we have examined the role that these components play in cell proliferation by indirect methods which rely on selective inactivation by chemical, enzymatic, or heat treatment of intact BL produced by cultured corneal endothelial cells. Although all of the treatments we have used are known to affect glycoproteins, and specifically proteoglycans, only three were effective in inactivating the BL's ability to support cell proliferation. Exposure of BL-coated dishes to 14M NH_4OH (pH 13.8), which results in the cleavage of proteoglycoproteins or glycopeptides at the O-glycosidic bond between the protein and carbohydrate moieties (2, 50) inhibited the rate of proliferation of vascular endothelial cells by 97%. Likewise, treatment of BL-coated dishes with 4M Guanidine-HCl, which extracts up to 80% of the GAG's, caused a 92% reduction in cell growth. Treatment of BL-coated dishes with nitrous acid

(HNO$_2$), which results in the degradation of heparin or heparin sulfate into sulfated disaccharides and non-sulfated oligosaccharides (9, 10, 43, 46), affected cell proliferation by 90% and led to the release of $^{35}SO_4$-labeled macromolecules, 50% of which were disaccharides. Although the effect of HNO$_2$ on intact BL is not known, its specific degradation of isolated heparan and heparan sulfate could indicate that it has a similar effect on BL, and this may correlate with its adverse effect on the ability of the BL to support cell growth. Chemical treatment of the BL with a reducing agent such as dithiothreitol (from 0.1 mM to 100 mM), which has been reported to destroy the biological activity of platelet-derived growth factor completely, did not affect its ability to support growth, nor did treatment with sodium dodecyl sulfate (2%) or urea (2M or 8M). Specific enzymatic treatment of the BL with collagenase, pepsin, trypsin, chymotrypsin, or neuraminidase, did not inhibit cell proliferation. It is therefore doubtful that any of the substrates of these enzymes plays a direct role in cell proliferation. The lack of effect of either hyaluronidase or chondroitinase ABC, as well as the presence of chondroitinase-resistant material in extracts of BL which affect cell proliferation, would tend to rule out a role for hyaluronic acid or chondroitin sulfates in the permissive effect of the BL on cell proliferation (39).

The importance of cell shape in proliferation suggests that attachment factors present within the BL which, because of their direct contact with the cell membrane, could modify cell shape, could also play a dual role in controlling cell proliferation.

To investigate the relationship between growth and attachment, we have compared the ability of vascular endothelial cells to attach to BL following treatment by alkaline pH and heat. In the absence of serum, only 10% of the cells attach to plastic after one hour, and maximal cell attachment (40%) is not reached before 18 h. In contrast, cells seeded on BL-coated dishes rapidly attach and spread and most (90%) have attached by 1 h. No significant difference is seen in the rate of cell attachment after treatment of the BL at pH 13.8, which destroys 97% of the ability of the BL to support cell proliferation. In fact, initial cell attachment (1 h) was slightly enhanced by alkaline treatment. It therefore appears unlikely that the component of the BL which is removed or destroyed by high pH treatment is involved in cell attachment (39).

In contrast to the results obtained after treatment of the BL with alkaline pH, thermal treatment of the collagen bed, which results in its denaturation, had the opposite results. Treatment of the BL at 70°C, which has no effect on cell proliferation, greatly reduces the rate of cell attachment. The rate of cell attachment is reduced even further after treatment of the BL at 90°C, although cell growth is reduced by only 60%. This indicates that the BL component(s) implicated in cell growth is probably distinct from those involved in cell attachment. Thermal disruptions of the BL also revealed the importance of the spatial geometry of the BL component responsible for cell proliferation (39). The present study provides evidence regarding the nature of the components of the BL which are responsible for conveying the permissive effect of the BL on cell proliferation. It is likely that the active component is a sulphated glycoprotein or proteoglycan that is susceptible to extraction by 4M Guanidine-HCl, is degraded by nitrous acid, and contains an O-glycosidic bond and glucosamine and/or galactosamine. Its resistance to hyaluronidase and chondroitinase ABC suggests that neither hyaluronic acid nor chondroitin sulfates are involved (39). Identification of the active component, however, must await a detailed analysis of the BL and of the material extracted from the BL under conditions which inhibit cell proliferation. Although cell attachment and proliferation appear to be separate processes mediated through different mechanisms, the role of the component of the BL responsible for cell proliferation and cell differentiation has yet to be examined. It is well known that cell proliferation precedes many differentiated steps during embryogenesis, and numerous BL components have been shown to be important in differentiation. It will be of interest to compare the component of the BL which is active in cell proliferation to the alkaline-labile component of demineralized bone matrix described by Reddi and Huggins (54, 55) as inducing differentiation of fibroblasts. It may very well be that it will turn out to be calcium, which, in the form of microcrystalline precipitate, has been shown to be as good a commitment factor as FGF or PDGF (62). In that regard, it is of interest to note that, in vivo, basement membranes in all types of organs are rich in calcium deposits which are bound to the numerous cationic groups present within the GAG's and proteoglycans, particularly in heparan sulfate. The ability of basement membrane to accumulate calcium is reflected by its ability to stain with alizarin red and may represent an evolutionary mechanism through which the commitment factors are automatically incorporated into the substrate upon which cells will migrate, proliferate, and differentiate.

VI. CONCLUSION

The ways in which the BL exerts its permissive effect on cell proliferation can only be the object of speculation. One possible effect is to modify the cell shape in order to make it responsive to factor(s) to which the cells do not respond unless they adopt an appropriate shape. Recently, Folkman and Moscona (15), using vascular endothelial cells maintained on tissue culture dishes coated with an agent which modifes the adhesiveness of the cells to the dish, were able to control procisely the cellular shape in morphologies ranging from highly flattened to almost spheroidal. When the extent of cell spreading was correlated with DNA synthesis or cell growth, it was found to be highly coupled. Whereas highly flattened cells responded to serum factors, spheroidal cells no longer responded and intermediate degrees of response could be observed, depending on how flattened the cells were. Likewise, with corneal epithelial cells, changes in cell shape which depend on the substrate upon which the cells are maintained correspond to drastically altered sensitivities of the cells to EGF versus FGF (23, 37). An attractive hypothesis proposed by Yaoi and Kanaseki (72) is that the BL could play a key role in mitosis and facilitate cytokinesis. This hypothesis was based on their observation that, while both high and low density cultures maintained on BL exhibit a high rate of DNA synthesis and a high mitotic index, only high density cultures maintained on plastic have both a high rate of DNA synthesis and a high mitotic index. In contrast, low density cultures maintained on plastic, although they have a high rate of DNA synthesis, have a low mitotic index, thus suggesting that cells do not enter into mitosis. It is therefore likely that, while plastic provides a foreign substrate upon which cells can attach tenaciously and spread in a vain attempt to phagocytose it, the BL provides a natural substrate that cells recognize as their own and upon which they can undergo their characteristic changes in morphology (rounding up) occurring at mitosis. These morphological changes probably reflect the hydrolysis of specific components of the BL leading to the disruption of the microfibrillar system and the rearrangement of the cellular cytoskeleton, so that cells can go through the cleavage steps, giving rise to two progeny cells instead of undergoing endomitosis.

REFERENCES

1. Aaronson, S.A., Todaro, G.J., and Freeman, A.E., (1970): Exp. Cell Res. 61:1-5.
2. Anderson, B., Hoffman, P., and Meyer, K. (1965): J. Biol. Chem. 240:156-167.
3. Balk, S.D. (1971): Proc. Natl. Acad. Sci. USA 68:271-275.
4. Balk, S.D., Whitfield, J.F., Youdale, T., and Braun, A.C. (1973): Proc. Natl. Acad. Sci. USA 70:675-679.
5. Barnes, D. and Sato, G. (1980): Cell 22:649-655.
6. Bornstein, P. and Sage, H. (1980): Ann. Rev. of Biochem. 49:957-1003.
7. Brown, G., Mahley, R., and Assmann, G. (1976): Circ. Res. 39:415-424.
8. Carrel, A. J. (1912): Exp. Med. 15:516-536.
9. Castenalli: A.A., Balduinia, D., and Brovelli, A. (1970): In:Chemistry and Molecular Biology of the Intercellular Matrix, v. 2 edited by E. Balazs, pp. 945-957.
10. Cifonelli, J.A. (1968): Carbohydr. Res. 8:233-242.
11. Dulbecco, R. and Elkington, J. (1975): Proc. Natl. Acad. Sci. USA 72:1584-1588.
12. Ewing, J. Proc. N.Y. Pathol. Soc. (1921): 21:17-24.
13. Fielding, P.E., Vlodavsky, I., Gospodarowicz, D., and Fielding, C.J. (1979): J. Biol. Chem. 254:749-755.
14. Folkman: J. (1977) In: Recent Advances in Cancer Research: Cell Biology, Molecular Biology, and Tumor Virology, vol. 1, edited by R.C. Gallo, pp. 119-130, CRC, Cleveland.
15. Folkman, J. and Moscona, A. Nature 273:345-349.
16. Fujii, D.K., Massoglia, S., Savion, N., and Gospodarowicz, D. (1981): Cell, submitted.
17. Giguere, L., Cheng, J., and Gospodarowicz, D. (1981): J. Cell. Physiol., in press.
18. Goldstein, J.L., Helgeson, J.A.S., and Brown, M.S. (1979): J. Biol. Chem. 254:5403-5409.
19. Gospodarowicz, D., Cheng, J., and Ill, C.R. (1981): Endocrinology, in press.
20. Gospodarowicz, D., Delgado, D., and Vlodavsky, I. (1980): Proc. Natl. Acad. Sci. USA 77:4094-4098.
21. Gospodarowicz, D. and Gonzalez, R. (1981): J. Cell Physiol., submitted.
22. Gospodarowicz, D., Greenburg, G., Bialecki, H., and Zetter, B. (1978): In Vitro 14:85-118.
23. Gospodarowicz, D., Greenburg, G., and Birdwell, C. (1978): Cancer Research 38:4155-4171.
24. Gospodarowicz, D., Greenburg, G., Foidart, J.-M., and Savion, N. (1981): J. Cell. Physiol., in press.
25. Gospodarowicz, D., Hirabayashi, K., Giguere, L., and Tauber, J.-P. (1981): J. Cell Biol., in press.
26. Gospodarowicz, D. and Ill, C.R. (1980): Proc. Natl. Acad. Sci. USA 77:2726-2730.
27. Gospodarowicz, D. and Ill, C.R. (1980): J. Clin. Inv. 65:1351-1364.
28. Gospodarowicz, D. and Ill, C.R. (1980): Exp. Eye Res. 31:181-199.
29. Gospodarowicz, D., Ill, C.R., and Birdwell, C.R. (1977): Endocrinology 100:1108-1120.
30. Gospodarowicz, D., Ill, C.R., Hornsby, P.J., and Gill, G.N. (1977): Endocrinology 100:1080-1089.

31. Gospodarowicz, D., Mescher, A.L., and Birdwell, C.R. (1977): Exp. Eye Res. 25:75-89.
32. Gospodarowicz: D., Mescher, A.L., and Birdwell, C.R. (1978): In:Gene Expression and Regulation in Cultured Cells, Third Decennial Review Conference, National Cancer Institute Monographs, no. 48, pp. 109-130.
33. Gospodarowicz, D., Moran, J.S., and Braun, D. (1977): J. Cell Physiol. 91:377-385.
34. Gospodarowicz, D., Moran, J.S., Braun, D., and Birdwell, C.R. (1976): Proc. Natl. Acad. Sci. USA 73:4120-4124.
35. Gospodarowicz, D. and Tauber, J.-P. (1980): Endocrine Reviews 1:201-227.
36. Gospodarowicz, D., Vlodavsky, I., Greenburg, G., Alvarado, J., Johnson, L.K., and Moran, J. (1979): Rec. Progr. in Hormone Res. 35:375-448.
37. Gospodarowicz: D., Vlodavsky, I., Greenburg, G., and Johnson, L.K. (1979): In: Cold Spring Harbor Conferences on Cell Proliferation, v. 6: Hormones and Cell Culture, edited by R. Ross and G. Sato, pp. 561-592, Cold Spring Harbor, New York.
38. Gospodarowicz, D., Vlodavsky, I., and Savion, N. (1980): Vision Res. 21:87-103.
39. Greenburg, G. and Gospodarowicz, D. (1981): J. Cell Biol., in press.
40. Greenburg, G., Vlodavsky, I., Foidart, J.-M., and Gospodarowicz, D. (1980): J. Cell Physiol. 103:333-347.
41. Grobstein, C. (1967): Cancer Inst. Monograph 26:279-299.
42. Kohler, N. and Lipton, A. (1974): Exp. Cell Res. 87:297-301.
43. Kosher, R.A. and Searls, R.L. (1973): Dev. Biol. 32:50-68.
44. Layman, D.L., Jelen, B.J., and Illingworth, D.R. (1980): Proc. Natl. Acad. Sci. USA 77:1511-1515.
45. Leighton, J. (1957): Cancer Res. 17:929-935.
46. Lindahl: V. and Roden, L. (1972): In:Glycoproteins, v. 45, edited by A. Gottschalk, pp. 491-515.
47. Liotta, L.A., Abe, S., Robey, P.G., and Martin, G.R. (1979): Proc. Natl. Acad. Sci. USA 76:2268-2272.
48. Maroudas, N.G. (1973): Nature 244:353-354.
49. Maroudas, N.G., O'Neill, C.H., and Stanton, M.R. (1973): Lancet 1:807-809.
50. Marshall, R.D. and Neuberger, A. (1972): In:Glycoproteins, v. 45 edited by A. Gottschalk, pp. 322-336.
51. Mather, J.P. and Sato, G.H. (1979): Exp. Cell Res. 124:215-222.
52. Rafferty, K.A. (1975): Adv. Cancer Res. 21:249-292.
53. Reckless, J.P.D., Weinstein, D.B., and Steinberg, D. (1978): Biochim. Biophys. Acta 529:475-487.
54. Reddi, A.H. and Huggins, C.B. (1974): Proc. Soc. Exp. Biol. Med. 145:475-486.
55. Reddi: A.H. (1976): In:Biochemistry of Collagen, edited by G.N. Ramachadran and A.H. Reddi, pp. 449-477.
56. Rifkin, D.B., Loeb, J.N., Moore, G., and Reich, E. (1974): J. Exp. Med. 139:1317-1328.
57. Ross, R. and Glomset, J.A. (1973): Science 180:1332-1339.
58. Ross, R., Glomset, J., Kariya, B., and Harker, L. (1974): Proc. Natl. Acad. Sci. USA 71:1207-1210.
59. Ross, R. and Vogel, A. (1978): Cell 14:203-210.
60. Savion, N., Lui, G.-M., Laherty, R., and Gospodarowicz, D. (1981): Endocrinology, in press.
61. Stein, O. and Stein, Y. (1976): Biochim. Biophys. Acta 23:563-568.

62. Stiles, C.D., Capne, G.T., Scher, C.D., Antoniades, H.M., Van Wyk, J.J., and Pledger, W.J. (1979): Proc. Natl. Acad. Sci. USA 76:1279-1283.
63. Tauber, J.-P., Cheng, J., and Gospodarowicz, D. (1980): J. Clin. Inv. 66:696-708.
64. Tauber, J.-P., Goldminz, D., and Gospodarowicz, D. J. Cell. Physiol., in press (1981).
65. Tauber, J.-P., Goldminz, D., Vlodavsky, I., and Gospodarowicz, D. (1981): J. Clin. Inv., in press.
66. Thomassen, M.J., Buoen, L.C., and Brand, K.G. (1975): J. Natl. Cancer Inst. 54: 203-207.
67. Tseng, S.C., Savion, N., Gospodarowicz, D., and Stern, R. (1981): J. Biol. Chem., in press.
68. Vlodavsky, I., Fielding, P.E., Fielding, C.J., and Gospodarowicz, D. (1978): Proc. Natl. Acad. Sci. USA 75:356-360.
69. Vlodavsky, I. and Gospodarowicz, D. (1980): Nature 289:304-306.
70. Vlodavsky, I., Johnson, L.K., Greenburg, G., and Gospodarowicz, D. (1979): J. Cell Biol. 83:468-486.
71. Vlodavsky, I., Lui, G.-M., and Gospodarowicz, D. (1980): Cell 19:607-616.
72. Yaoi, Y. and Kanaseki, T. (1972): Nature 237:283-285.

Expression of Differentiated Functions in Cancer Cells, edited by R. F. Revoltella et al., Raven Press, New York © 1982.

Properties of Sarcoma Growth Factors Produced by Sarcoma Virus Transformed Cells

Joseph E. De Larco and George J. Todaro

Laboratory of Viral Carcinogenesis, National Cancer Institute, Frederick Cancer Research Facility, Frederick, Maryland 21701

Murine sarcoma virus (MSV) transformed cells have been characterized by a loss of measurable cell surface receptors for the growth stimulating polypeptide, epidermal growth factor (EGF) [6,24]. The apparent loss of cell surface receptors occurs in both fibroblastic and epitheloid cells transformed by MSV [7]. The MSV-transformed cells release polypeptides into the medium that stimulate cell growth and initiate a phenotypic change in the morphology of untransformed monolayer cell cultures and also induce anchorage independent cell growth [4]. Several of these polypeptide, growth factors compete with EGF for its membrane receptors. These factors are specific for sarcoma virus-transformed cells in that neither supernatants from untransformed cells nor cells transformed by DNA tumor virus have detectable quantities of these EGF competing polypeptide growth factors. The major soft agar growth stimulating activity, sarcoma growth factor (SGF), has an apparent molecular weight of approximately 8,500 and will not stimulate the growth of cells lacking active EGF receptors. Radiolabeled SGF is purified and characterized using human carcinoma cells that have a large number of EGF receptors. The EGF receptors are used as affinity sites for binding SGF. These studies show that the binding to and eluting from the EGF receptors yields a specific radiolabeled peptide as well as agar growth stimulating activity [3]. The specific binding to the EGF receptors rose from 0.1% of the input counts for the crude material to approximately 25% of the input counts for the twice cycled material. Cycling also provides a single isoelectric focusing band at pH 6.8 for the ^{125}I-SGF, whereas uncycled material had a heterogenous isoelectric profile. Cells lacking EGF receptors are unable to respond to the growth stimulating effects of this partially purified SGF [8]. It appears, therefore, that SGF released by MSV-transformed cells elicits it biologic effects via specific interaction with EGF membrane receptors.

To determine whether the SGF is a product of the sarcoma virus genome or a product of a cellular origin, the SGF-like peptide growth

139

factor from a temperature sensitive Kirsten sarcoma virus transformed
cell was investigated (ts-371 cl 5) [22]. At the temperature permissive for transformation (32°C), these cells display the transformed
phenotype, lack measurable EGF receptors as determined by ^{125}I-EGF
binding, grow in soft agar, and release SGF-like peptides; whereas
at the nonpermissive temperature they display a flat morphology, have
EGF receptors, and neither grow in soft agar nor release SGF-like
peptides. The SGF-like growth factors released at the permissive
temperature by cells transformed with this ts-sensitive mutant is
compared with the cells transformed by the wild type sarcoma virus.
Neither of these growth factors are temperature sensitive under the
conditions of assay (65°C X 120 min.).

MATERIALS AND METHODS

Serum-Free Conditioned Media

The cells were grown in roller bottles (Falcon #3027; 850 cm^2)
containing Dulbecco's modification of Eagle's medium (DMEM) [10]
with 10% calf serum (Colorado Serum Co.). The cells were washed
once for 1 hour and again for 16 hours with 100 ml of serum-free
Waymouth's medium [14] (GIBCO, MD705/1). These washes were discarded and two subsequent serum-free 48-hour collections were
harvested and are referred to as "conditioned media". The viability of the cells maintained either in a medium containing 10%
serum or in serum-free for 5 days with 4 changes of medium was
greater than 80%, as determined by trypan blue exclusion. The
"sarcoma-conditioned media" were clarified by centrifugation at
100,000 X g for 45 minutes. The supernate was concentrated 20-fold
in a hollow fiber apparatus (Amicon; DC2) and dialyzed against 5
changes consisting of 5 volumes each of 1% acetic acid. This
material was lyophilized and extracted with 1 M acetic acid. One
percent of the volume of the starting conditioned media was used.
The extract was clarified by centrifugation at 100,000 X g for 30
minutes. Approximately 90% of this 1 M acetic acid extract was
chromatographed through a Bio-Gel P-60 column (5 X 90 cm) that had
been equilibrated in and eluted with 1 M acetic acid. The column
was run at 4°C at a flow rate of 15 ml/hr and 15 ml fractions were
collected unless otherwise stated. Aliquots were lyophilized for
protein determinations [16], EGF competition, stimulation of thymidine incorporation, and soft agar growth activity.

The EGF was isolated from male mouse salivary glands [19]. This
peptide was labeled with ^{125}I using a modification of the original
chloramine-T method [13]. Between 10 and 20 µg of lyophilized
protein were dissolved in 50 µl of 0.4 M sodium phosphate, pH 7.5,
and 2 mCi of ^{125}I, as the sodium salt, were added. The reactions
were initiated by adding 5 µl of chloramine-T solution (100 µg/ml);
2 minutes later an additional 5 µl aliquot was added, and after an
additional 1.5 minutes the third and last 5 µl aliquot of chloramine-
T was added. One minute after the last addition of chloramine-T, the
iodinations were stopped by adding 100 µl of saturated tyrosine in
0.01 M Tris-HCl, pH 8.4. The iodinated proteins were separated from
the reagents by passing the mixtures over columns (0.7 X 14 cm) of
Sephadex G-15 equilibrated in and eluted with phosphate buffered

saline (PBS). Bovine serum albumin (Pentex-Crystallized) (BSA) was added to the peak tubes to give a final concentration of 5 mg/ml, the fractions were pooled, and small aliquots were stored frozen at -20°C.

Assays for EGF Bindings and for Radioreceptor Competitions

The ^{125}I-EGF binding assays were performed on subconfluent cell cultures of Mv-1-Lu (CCL64, American Type Culture Collection). Cells were seeded at 2.5 X 10^4 cells per 16 mm well (Linbro Cat. No. 76-033-05) in DMEM containing 10% calf serum. After 24 hours the medium was removed and the cells were washed twice with binding buffer (DMEM containing 1 mg/ml BSA and 50 mM N, N-bis-(2-hydroxyethyl)-2-amino-ethane-sulfonic acid (BES), adjusted to pH 6.8) [7]. ^{125}I-EGF bindings were initiated by adding 200 µ liters of ^{125}I-EGF solution (2 ng/ml). The bindings were continued for 1 hour at room temperature. The unbound radiolabeled EGF was removed and the monolayers were washed three times with binding buffer to remove traces of unbound labeled EGF. The radiolabeled ligand bound was quantitated by lysing the cells (0.01 M Tris-HCl, pH 7.4 containing 0.5% sodium dodecyl sulfate and 0.005 M EDTA) and counting the lysate in a gamma counter. Nonspecific binding was estimated by determining the amount of cell-bound radioactivity in the presence of a large excess of unlabeled EGF (10 µg/ml). The specific binding is obtained by subtracting the nonspecific binding from the total binding.

Assay for Growth-Promoting Activity

Serum-deprived, subconfluent normal rat kidney cells were prepared for this assay by trypsinizing the fibroblastic clone 49F [5]. They were seeded at 2.5 X 10^4 cells per 16 mm well (Linbro Cat. No. 76-033-05) in DMEM containing 10% calf serum. After 24 hours the medium was removed; the cells were washed with fresh serum-free medium and then incubated with 1 ml per well of Waymouth's medium containing 0.1% calf serum. Three days later, 0.1 ml of binding buffer containing the sample to be tested was added. Sixteen hours after the addition, the cells were exposed for 8 hours to 2.5 µCi of ^{3}H-thymidine (NEN; NET-027.6.7 Ci/mM). The medium containing the radio-labeled thymidine was removed, and the cultures were washed twice with 1 ml of DMEM containing 100 µg/ml unlabeled thymidine and incubated for 30 min. After the incubation, the monolayers were washed three times, the cells were disrupted with lysing buffer, and the DNA was precipitated by adding the lysate to 3 vol. of cold 10% trichloroacetic acid. The precipitated DNA was removed by filtration (Millipore; HA, 0.45 µM); the filters were dried and added to counting vials with 5 ml of toluene/Liquifluor (NEN, NEF 903), and the radio-activity measured in a liquid scintillation counter (Beckman, LS-250).

Soft Agar Growth Assay

Soft agar assays were performed using the NRK fibroblastic clone 49F. Agar plates were prepared in 60-mm tissue culture dishes (Falcon, 3003) by first applying a 2 ml base layer of 0.5% agar (Difco, Agar Noble) in DMEM containing 10% calf serum. Over this basal layer, an additional 2 ml layer of 0.3% agar was added to the above medium

containing the appropriate concentration of protein, and 1 X 10^4 indicator cells. These dishes were incubated at 37°C in a humidified
atmosphere of 5% CO_2 in air. Colonies were measured unfixed and
unstained using an inverted microscope. Colonies with greater than
50 cells were scored as positive unless otherwise stated.

Receptor Affinity Purification of EGF-like Molecules

The human carcinoma line, A431, which is known to have a large
number of EGF receptors, was used in order to preferentially bind
EGF-like molecules from an iodinated stock containing SGF. The A431
cells were fixed to tissue culture dishes by treating them with a 5%
solution of formaldehyde in PBS for 5 minutes. The formaldehyde
solution was removed from the cells, which were then washed four
times with PBS, and twice with binding buffer. The Bio-Gel P-60
pool II was radioiodinated to a specific activity of 73 mCi/μg.
The iodinated material was diluted in binding buffer and bound to
fixed A431 cells for 90 minutes at 22°C. The unbound material was
removed and saved for further binding. The cells were washed four
times with binding buffer and the bound material was eluted from the
cells using three 1 ml washes of 0.1% acetic acid. The acetic acid
was lyophilized. The bound and eluted material(s) were reconsti-
tuted in binding buffer. The three fractions, (1) untreated, (2)
unbound, and (3) bound and eluted, were tested for their ability to
bind to A431 cells using the standard binding conditions.

Heat Treatment

Lyophilized pools of the materials to be tested for tempeature
sensitivity were dissolved and diluted in binding buffer that had
been neutralized with 0.5 $\underline{M}$ trisodium phosphate. Two aliquots of
one ml were taken from each sample and placed in a plastic capped
tube (Falcon #2063). One tube of each, the control, was kept on
ice while the other aliquot of each was heated in a 65°C water bath
for 2 hours.   After heating, these tubes wre placed in an ice
bath. The bioassays were run on all samples simultaneously.

RESULTS

The human carcinoma cell line, A431, has an exceptionally large
number of epidermal growth factor (EGF) receptors [11]. A
Scatchard plot for EGF binding to A431 cells generates a linear
plot, and at saturating EGF concentrations these cells bind
approximately 2.2 X 10^6 molecules of EGF per cell. In contrast,
Scatchard plots obtained using a fibroblastic normal rat kidney
(NRK) clone show they only bind approximately 2.4 X 10^4 molecules
of EGF per cell at saturating concentrations of EGF [8]. Taking
advantage of these findings and those previously described which
show that SGF acts through the EGF receptor [8], we decided to
test whether SGF could be purified using formalin-fixed A431
human carcinoma cells to selectively enrich for this growth
factor. The starting material or crude SGF used in this purification was the 8,500 molecular weight peptide pool obtained
from a Bio-Gel P-60 chromatography [6].

The A431 cells were fixed with formaldehyde in tissue culture dishes and then used to specifically bind either mouse salivary gland EGF or SGF produced by MSV-transformed cells. The unbound material from these preparations was removed, the cells washed several times, and the bound growth factors dissociated from their receptors with dilute acid. The materials released retain their biological activities and can rebind to their receptors.

Table 1 shows the ability of different radiolabeled SGF preparations to bind to and be eluted from A431 cells. After two cycles of binding and eluting, the remaining counts bound with a much higher efficiency to A431 cells. In the case of the twice-cycled material, approximately 24% of the input counts bound specifically to the A431 cells; whereas only 0.12% of the input counts from the crude SGF bound specifically to the A431 cells. The ratio of specific to nonspecific binding for SGF also increased with cycling from 0.18 for the uncycled material to 18.7 in the case of the twice cycled material. The recycled radiolabeled-SGF did not bind to a clone of mouse 3T3 cells which lack EGF receptors [18] (data not shown).

TABLE 1
Purification of ^{125}I-SGF Using Binding and Elution
from an EGF Receptor-Rich Cell

Material	Specific Binding / Nonspecific Binding	Percent of input dpm Bound
Bio-Gel P-60 pool II	0.18	0.12
After the first cycle	5.6	2.8
After the second cycle	18.7	23.9

When 12 μg of unlabeled crude SGF was cycled over fixed A431 cells in a 100-mm tissue culture dish as described in Materials and Methods, the receptors were able to bind and release the biological activity. Table 2 shows that the portion which was bound to and eluted from the fixed cells contained over 90% of the activity found in the untreated SGF preparation. If one assumes the percentage of unlabeled peptides which bound to the fixed A431 cells is similar to that for the radiolabeled peptides (Table 1), then there was considerably less than 5 ng per ml of peptide from SGF pool II in the soft agar assay of the bound and eluted material. In the controls, which consisted of binding buffer cycled over fixed A431 cells, neither the "unbound" nor the "bound" materials had any soft agar growth stimulating activity.

To contrast the differences in homogeneity of the radiolabeled peptide preparations prior to and after cycling over fixed A431 cells, isoelectric-focusing was performed. The isoelectric focusing columns run on ^{125}I-labeled EGF and iodinated preparations of crude SGF before and after cycling on fixed A431 cell monolayers. Isoelectric focusing of the ^{125}I-labeled EGF preparation prior to purification pI of 3.8 and the larger peak has a pI of 4.4. The labeled EGF that

had been bound to and eluted from fixed cells gave a single sharp
peak upon isoelectric focusing which had a pI of 4.4; this value is
consistent with that previously published for EGF [23]. In contrast,
isoelectric focusing of iodinated crude SGF gave a heterodisperse
profile with the majority of the labeled material having acidic pI's.
The radiolabeled peptide(s) from crude SGF which was bound to and
eluted from the fixed A431 cells, however, gave a sharp peak upon
isoelectric focusing which had a pI of between 6.8 and 7.0.

TABLE 2
Soft Agar Growth Stimulation
By Cycled Bio-Gel P-60 Pool II SGF Preparations

Preparation	Percent of seeded Cells Forming Colonies With Greater than 50 Cells
Untreated Pool II at a final concentration of 1.2 µg/ml	60
Pool II unbound to fixed A431 cells	4
Pool II bound to and eluted from fixed A431 cells	55
Binding buffer unbound to fixed A431 cells	0
Binding buffer bound to and eluted from fixed A431 cells	0

Ten milliliters of either binding buffer or binding buffer containing 12 µg/ml of Pool II SGF was bound to fixed A431 cells for 45 min
at room temperature. The unbound material was then transferred to
another dish of fixed A431 cells and bound for an additional 45 min.
The plates were each washed twice with serum-free Waymouth's medium
and PBS before eluting the "bound materials" from the fixed cells.
The eluted materials were lyophilized and redissolved in a volume
of binding buffer equal to that of the unbound material. Soft agar
assays were set up using the above materials at a 1:10 dilution
and read after 13 days.

To test if isoelectric focusing could be used preparatively to
purify the growth stimulating activity, an experiment was performed
in which unlabeled crude SGF was isoelectric focused with carrier
^{125}I-SGF that had been purified by cycling on EGF receptor-rich
human carcinoma cells. The fractions were tested for their ability
to stimulate both the colony formation in soft agar and cell division
growth arrested fibroblastic NRK cell monolayers. These major growth

activities co-migrated with the radioactivity from the cycled ^{125}I-SGF and is found in a narrow region with a pI of between 6.8 and 7.0. Isoelectric focusing, then, can be used to further purify the growth factor from crude preparations with the retention of biological activity.

The SGF obtained by two cycles of binding to and eluting from A431 receptors was compared with the original crude material and with EGF on 10-30% polyacrylamide gradient gels. There was no detectable difference in the migration patterns of the untreated EGF, and the EGF that had been bound to and eluted from fixed A431 cells. There was, however, a marked difference between the migration pattern of the uncycled SGF and SGF that had been cycled on fixed A431 cells. The uncycled SGF migrated as a broad diffuse band that appeared as a doublet on the original X-ray film, whereas the cycled SGF migrated as a sharp band centered with the diffuse band seen in the uncycled pool II material. Both purified EGF and EGF cycled on A431 cells ran as slightly heavier than SGF. This result is in contrast to their behavior on the Sephadex G-50 gel filtraton system, where SGF appears to be heavier than EGF. Using Bio-Gel P-60 chromatography (a polyacrylamide gel), SGF elutes as a peptide with an apparent molecular weight of approximately 10,000, while EGF adsorbs to the column and is eluted after the salt peak [19]. In each of these systems, however, it is clear that the active component of SGF is not mouse salivary gland EGF, but is a recognizably different peptide.

To test whether EGF receptors are required for the biologic activity of SGF, clones derived from 3T3 cells that lack EGF receptors were tested. These clones were generously provided by Dr. Harvey Herschman (UCLA). They had been selected by stimulating the highly passaged 3T3 culture in the presence of colchicine [18]. While 3T3 itself is responsive to the mitogenic action of EGF, the selected clone, NR6/6, was neither responsive to the mitogenic action of EGF nor did it have detectable EGF receptors [23]. 3T3 cells and the NR6/6 clone were tested in parallel for their response to calf serum and to a number of purified growth factors, including mouse EGF [1, 19] and SGF. The parental clone, 3T3/8, responded to all of the growth factors tested, as determined by ^{3}H-thymidine incorporation into DNA (Table 3). The NR6/6 clone, on the other hand, responded to all of the growth factors except EGF and SGF. DNA synthesis was stimulated in both clones when they were treated with calf serum, fibroblast growth factor (FGF) [12], multiplication stimulating activity (MSA) derived from rat liver cells [9,17], or the MSA-like activity released from a human fibrosarcoma line [5]. The cells were also tested for their ability to grow in soft agar in the presence of SGF. In the soft agar assay, the 3T3/8 cells responded readily by developing a high percentage of large colonies (>50%) when treated with SGF, whereas the EGF receptor negative cell, NR6/6, did not respond at all. The above results suggest EGF receptors are required for SGF to exert its biologic effect in mouse 3T3 cells.

TABLE 3
Effect of Various Growth Factors on the Induction of DNA Synthesis
in Resting Mouse 3T3 Clones with and without EGF Receptors
^{3}H-Thymidine Incorporation
$(X\ 10^{-3})$

Test Cells Additions	3T3/8 (EGF-R$^+$)	NR6/6 (EGF-R$^-$)	Ratio of ^{3}H-Thymidine Incorporation (EGF-R$^-$/EGF-R$^+$)
None	2.4	2.8	1.2
EGF (10 ng/ml)	33.5	3.1	0.09
SGF (1 µg/ml)	63.7	2.9	0.05
Calf serum (600 µg/ml)	55.3	63.7	1.2
FGF (10 ng/ml)	31.5	47.3	1.5
MSA (10 ng/ml)	18.2	14.3	0.8
H-MSA (200 ng/ml)	23.5	16.2	0.7

Table 4 shows that the sarcoma virus-transformed cells, transformed
by the Kirsten sarcoma virus mutant, Ts371 clone 5, show rapid
alterations in their available cell surface receptors when shifted
from permissive to nonpermissive temperatures. The cells were grown
for several days at a permissive temperature, 36°C, and then sifted
for a 24-hour period to 32°C, 36°C, and 39°C, the latter being
nonpermissive for expression of the transformed phenotype [5]. After
24 hours, the cells were assayed for EGF receptors, as previously
described. Whereas the cells transformed by wild type virus show
essentially no receptors at any of the temperatures, the cells
transformed by the mutant viruses show a greatly increased number of
receptors at 39°C, comparable, in fact, to those found on the
untransformed parental cells. At 32°C, however, they show only 10 to
20% the number of receptors shown at 39°C, and cells maintained at
36°C have repeatedly expressed an intermediate number of available
EGF receptors. The conclusion from these experiments is that the
transformed cells have the capability of producing EGF cell surface
receptors. The shift to the nonpermissive temperature, then, would
involve the rapid inactivation or disappearance of a product, presumably a protein, that blocks EGF receptor availability.

TABLE 4
Effect of Temperature at which Cells have Grown
on ^{125}I-EGF Binding

	Previous Day At	EGF Bound
TS371 cl5	32°	1,470
	36°	3,940
	39°	10,970
Untransformed NRK	32°	8,700
	36°	9,500
	39°	8,300
KiSV transformed NRK	32°	350
	36°	200
	39°	260

Table 5 shows that the temperature-sensitive mutant-transformed cells are able to respond to SGF at the nonpermissive temperature. In soft agar assays they are comparable to their untransformed parental cells in their ability to respond to SGF. This experiment shows that the defect at the nonpermissive temperature is not the lack of ability to respond to SGF.

To determine whether SGF-like growth factors released by MSV-transformed cells are a product of the sarcoma virus genome or the host cell genome, the SGF-like peptides from a wild type Kirsten sarcoma virus transformed NRK cell (KNRK) was compared with that from a temperature-sensitive Kirsten sarcoma virus transformed NRK cell (ts-371 cl 5). Serum-free conditioned media were collected from these sarcoma virus transformed clones at their permissive temperatures, and their acid soluble peptides were separated over an acidic Bio-Gel P-60 column [6]. The main SGF-like activity found in the serum-free media conditioned by each of these clones eluted from the columns with apparent molecular weights of approximately 8,500. In each case this peak contained the main soft agar growth stimulating activity as well as EGF radioreceptor competing activity and mitogenic activity as measured by stimulating ^{3}H-thymidine incorporation into serum depleted NRK cells.

To determine if the major growth activity present in the media conditioned by NRK cells transformed with a temperature sensitive sarcoma virus (ts-371 cl 5) is itself temperature sensitive, and therefore potentially responsible for the ts-properties of this transformed cell, the 8,500 molecular weight activity present was pooled and tested along with the equivalent pool of activity present

TABLE 5
Growth Stimulation by SGF of Normal and TS Mutant
Transformed Cells at the Nonpermissive Temperature

	Temperature	Agar Colony Formation
TS371 c15	32°	>500
	36°	>500
	39°	5
+ SGF (20 µg/ml	39°	150
NRK	32°	0
	36°	0
	39°	0
+ SGF (20 µg/ml)	39°	70
KiSV transformed NRK	32°	>500
	36°	>500
	39°	>500

in the media conditioned by NRK cell transformed by a wild type
Kirsten sarcoma virus (KNRK). The results of these experiments are
found in Table 6. In comparing ts-371 cl 5 heated and unheated
aliquots for their ability to stimulate thymidine incorporation, it
appears there are little if any differneces at either dilution. The
soft agar growth stimulating activity was also insensitive to this
heat treatment step as performed (samples were heated in a 65°C water
bath for 120 min at pH 7.0). The results from the heat treatment of
the equivalent factor(s) obtained from KNRK were quite similar,
indicating the "SGF" obtained from the cell transformed by the
temperature sensitive sarcoma virus is no more "temperature sensitive",
under the conditions tested, than that obtained from the cell
transformed by the wild type sarcoma virus.

DISCUSSION

A model consistent with these observations is the production and
release by MSV-transformed cells of an EGF-like peptide factor or
factors which are able to bind to and block cellular EGF receptors,
and act as mitogens either on the cells producing them or on other
cells having functional receptors capable of binding these factors.
This could account for both the lack of measurable EGF receptors on
the MSV-transformed cells as well as for the lowered serum requirement
for MSV-transformed cells.

TABLE 6
Effects of Heating on the Biological Activity of Growth Factors
Released by Cells Transformed by Either a Wild Type KiSV
or a Temperature-Sensitive (ts-371) KiSV

Source of Growth Factor	Stimulation of ^{3}H-Thymidine Incorporation cpm Above Control		Percent of 49F Cells That Formed Soft Agar Colonies[a]	
ts-371	dilution		dilution	
	1.4	30,651	1:1	75
	1:16	4,758	1:4	62
ts-371 heated[b]	1:4	28,588	1:1	76
	1:16	6,119	1:4	61
KNRK	1:3	135,721	1:3	70
	1:15	28,892	1:15	52
			1:75	4
KNRK heated[b]	1:3	129,766	1:3	66
	1:15	26,552	1:15	40
			1:75	8

[a]Colonies were scored 10 days after seeding. Those colonies larger than approximately 20 cells were scored as positive.

[b]Heat treatment was carried out for 120 min in a water bath maintained at 65°C. The samples were adjusted to pH 7.0 before heating.

The data presented in this communication are consistent with the above model in that MSV-transformed cells produce at least one EGF-like peptide (SGF) which is capable of binding to and blocking EGF receptors. Using the EGF receptor to purify this peptide(s), the biological activity co-purifies with the EGF receptor-binding activity. This factor from MSV-transformed cells has both similarities and differences when its properties are compared to mouse submaxillary gland EGF. It binds to EGF receptors with an affinity similar to EGF, and they both stimulate cell division in serum-depleted cells. They differ in that EGF has a more acidic pI (4.4) than SGF (6.8), they migrate differently in both SDS polyacrylamide gel electrophoresis and acetic acid (gel permeation) chromatography, and EGF will not stimulate anchorage independent growth while SGF will.

The above results demonstrate that SGF can be purified by taking advantage of its ability to reversibly interact with EGF membrane receptors on fixed cells. The purified peptide(s) has EGF receptor-competing activity as well as growth stimulating activity. The fixed human carcinoma cells, then, could be used to purify yet unknown growth factors that interact with the EGF receptor system.

The temperature sensitive MSV virus-transformed cells maintained at the permissive temperature of 32°C exhibit the transformed phenotype and either lack or have a greatly decreased number of available EGF receptors. If the media is changed and the cells are then incubated at the nonpermissive temperature (39°C), they begin to flatten out and their available EGF receptors begin to reappear within a day.

The release of SGF-like growth factors by these transformed cells is also temperature dependent. The cells maintained at the permissive temperature release the SGF-like peptides whereas those maintained at the nonpermissive temperature do not. An obvious question arising from these studies is the origin of the growth factors released by sarcoma virus transformed cells. Are they direct viral products or are they host cell gene products that are controlled by the product of the sarcoma gene? If the growth factors which are able to confer the transformed phenotype on untransformed cells are viral gene products, one might expect them to be temperature sensitive when obtained from cells that are transformed by a sarcoma virus which is temperature sensitive with respect to transformation. If they are products of the host cell, they would be no more temperature sensitive than the growth factors isolated from cells transformed by the wild type virus. The regulation of their expression would, however, be temperature dependent and at the nonpermissive temperature the ts-sarcoma gene product would be inactivated and therefore unable to stimulate the host's expression of these growth factors. Recently, several groups have shown the src products from both avian and mammalian sarcoma virus exhibits an unusual protein kinase activity and, when kinase activities of temperature sensitive viruses were examined, they were shown to be more readily heat-inactivated than the kinases of the wild type viruses [2,15,20, and 21]. The SGF-like factor released by the ts-sarcoma virus transformed cells is extremely heat stable compared to the kinases and is no more temperature sensitive, under the conditions assayed, than the SGF-like factor released by cells transformed by the wild type sarcoma virus. This data suggests the SGF-like peptides produced and released by sarcoma virus transformed cells are not direct products of the murine sarcoma genomes, but rather the expression of cellular genes that are normally suppressed.

REFERENCES

1. Cohen, S., Taylor, J. M., Murakami, K., Michelakis, A. M., and Inagami, T. (1972): Biochemistry, 11:4286-4292.

2. Collett, M. S. Erikson, R. L. (1978): Proc. Natl. Acad. Sci. USA 75:2021-2024.

3. De Larco, J. E., Reynolds, R., Carlberg, K., Engle, C., and Todaro, G. (1980): J. Biol. Chem. 255:3685-3690.

4. De Larco, J. E. and Todaro. (1976): Cell 8:365-371.

5. De Larco, J. E. and Todaro, G. J. (1978): Nature 272:356-358.

6. De Larco, J. E. and Todaro, G. J. (1978): Proc. Natl. Acad. Sci. USA 75:4001-4005.

7. De Larco, J. E. and Todaro, G. J. (1978): J. Cell. Physiol. 94: 335-342.

8. De Larco, J. E. and Todaro, G. J. (1980): J. Cell Physiol. 102: 267-277.

9. Dulak, N. C. and Temin, H. M. (1973): J. Cell Physiol. 81:153-170.

10. Dulbecco, R. and Freeman, G. (1959): Virology 8:396-397.

11. Fabricant, R. N., De Larco, J. E., and Todaro, G. J. (1977): Proc. Natl. Acad. Sci. USA 74:565-569.

12. Gospodarowicz, D., Greene, G., and Moran, J. S. (1975): Biochem. Biophys. Res. Commun. 65:778-787.

13. Greenwood, F. C., Hunter, W. M., and Glover, J. S. (1963): Biochem. J. 89:114-123.

14. Kitos, P. A., Sinclair, R., and Waymouth, C. (1962): Exp. Cell Res. 27:335-342.

15. Levinson, A. D., Oppermann, H., Levintow, L., Jarmus, H. E., and Bishop, J. M. (1978): Cell 15:561-572.

16. Lowry, O. H., Rosebrough, N. J., Farr, A. L., and Randall, R. J. (1951): J. Biol. Chem. 193:265-275.

17. Nissley, S. P. and Reekler, M. M. (1976): In: NCI Monograph: The Association Research Conference, Lake Placid, NY, pp. 167-172.

18. Pruss, R. M. and Herschman, H. R. (1977): Proc. Natl. Acad. Sci. USA 74:3918-3921.

19. Savage, C. R. and Cohen, S. (1972): J. Biol. Chem. 247:7609-7611.

20. Sefton, B. M., Huntner, T., and Beemon, K. (1980): J. Virol. 33: 220-229.

21. Sen, A., Todaro, G. J., Blair, D. G., and Robey, W. G. (1979): Proc. Natl. Acad. Sci. USA 76:3617-3621.

22. Shih, T. Y., Weeks, M. O., Young, H. A., and Scolnick, E. M. (1979): J. Virol. 31:546-556.

23. Taylor, J. M., Cohen, S., and Mitchell, W. M. (1970): <u>Proc. Natl. Acad. Sci. USA</u> 67:164-171.

24. Todaro, G. J., De Larco, J. E., and Cohen, S. (1976): <u>Nature</u> 264:26-31.

Expression of Differentiated Functions in Cancer Cells, edited by R. F. Revoltella et al., Raven Press, New York © 1982.

Effects of Interferon and Tumor Promoters on Terminal Cell Differentiation

Leila Diamond, Livia Cioé, Debra Laskin, and Thomas G. O'Brien

The Wistar Institute, Philadelphia, Pennsylvania 19104

Tumor promoters are substances that can enhance tumor formation initiated by subeffective doses of a carcinogen but that are not themselves carcinogenic or mutagenic (reviewed in 2). In the two-stage, initiation and promotion, model of mouse skin carcinogenesis, the most effective tumor promoters are diesters of the diterpene alcohol, phorbol (Fig. 1), isolated from seeds of the plant Croton tiglium (reviewed in 18). In recent years, a series of naturally occurring and synthetic phorbol esters has become available, and it has been found that there is in general a positive correlation between the tumor-promoting activity in mouse skin of these compounds and their induction of a wide variety of biochemical and biological effects in vivo and in cell culture (3, 10, 12, 32, 38). In the latter case, they may affect the transport of small molecules, macromolecular synthesis, the expression of characteristics associated with neoplastic transformation, and the spontaneous and induced expression of differentiated phenotypes by normal and neoplastic cells. In some cell types, phorbol ester tumor promoters inhibit terminal cell differentiation whereas in other cell types, they can stimulate terminal differentiation.

The cellular glycoprotein(s), interferon, in addition to its antiviral activity, can also modulate cellular functions and properties (16, 17, 37). For example, it affects progression through different phases of the cell cycle in several types of cells and, in Friend erythroleukemia cells, has inhibitory or stimulatory effects on terminal differentiation, depending on dose.

The mechanisms by which phorbol esters and interferon exert their pleiotropic effects on cells are not understood, and we are using two differentiating cell culture systems as models to try to elucidate these mechanisms. One cell system is a clone of BALB/c 3T3 fibroblasts which undergoes "adipose conversion" (11) in a manner similar to that described by Green and colleagues for Swiss 3T3 cells (14, 15). The second cell system is the C3H/10T1/2 cell line which can be induced to express multiple new phenotypes by treatment with the

153

nucleoside analog, 5-azacytidine (aza-CR) (5, 6, 36). This paper
describes the reversible inhibition of expression of the differentiated phenotype in these cells by phorbol ester tumor promoters and
interferon (4, 11, 25).

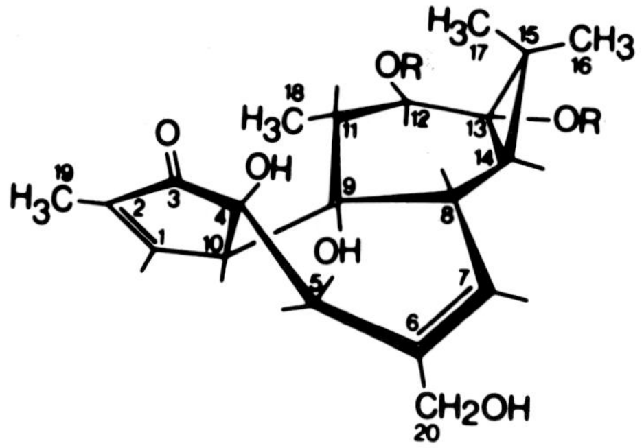

FIG. 1. Structure of phorbol-12,13-diesters as described by Hecker
(18). Phorbol, an alcohol with the carbon skeleton tigliane, is
the parent alcohol of the tumor-promoting phorbol-12,13-esters
found in croton oil (reviewed in 10, 18). The most potent promoter
in the series is 12-O-tetradecanoylphorbol-13-acetate (TPA), also
designated phorbol myristate acetate or PMA in the literature.

MATERIALS AND METHODS

The preadipose clone, A31T, of BALB/c 3T3 cells was established in
this laboratory (11). C3H/10T1/2 clone 8 cells (28) were obtained at
passage 8 from Dr. Sukdeb Mondal, University of Southern California.
Both cell lines were grown in Eagle's minimum essential medium
(Auto-Pow, Flow Laboratories) supplemented with vitamins as formulated
for Eagle's basal medium and 10% fetal bovine serum. The cultures
were grown in stoppered flasks or in petri dishes incubated in a humidified atmosphere of 5% CO_2 in air. Routinely, after stock cultures
had been grown approximately 10 passages, new sublines were initiated
from frozen stocks.

For experiments, BALB/c 3T3 cells were inoculated into 60-mm tissue
culture dishes at a density of 2.4×10^4 cells/cm^2. Experiments were
started when the monolayers were confluent (zero time) and the cultures
were refed at 2-3-day intervals thereafter with medium containing 1
µg insulin per ml (referred to as "standard medium") or with medium
without insulin. The number of lipid-positive cells was scored at
intervals by microscopic observation without staining or after
staining with the fat-soluble dye, oil red O. During the course of
differentiation, the amount of visible lipid per cell increased
progressively from undetectable (microscopically) to lipid-engorged
cells containing one to six large lipid droplets. A lipid-positive or
lipid-filled cell is defined arbitrarily as one having progressed
approximately halfway through this sequence of lipid accumulation.

C3H/10T1/2 cells were seeded, for experiments, into 60-mm dishes at a
density of 50 cells/cm^2 and, 24 hr later, aza-CR was added at a final

concentration of 2×10^{-6}M. The cultures were washed after 24 hr and refed twice weekly thereafter with control medium or medium containing the test agent. At the termination of an experiment, the cells were fixed in methanol, stained with Giemsa, and the average number of myotubes (multinucleated cells with two or more nuclei per cell) per dish (2-3 dishes per group) was scored at 100X magnification.

Interferon was prepared by infecting mouse L-cell cultures with Newcastle disease virus; mock interferon was prepared from uninfected cultures. The uninfected and infected cultures were incubated in serum-free medium for 18 hr; the supernatant fluids were harvested and adjusted to pH 2.0, stored at 4°C for 5 days and readjusted to pH 7.4. The antiviral titer was determined by comparison with that of a highly purified interferon preparation. This was obtained from Dr. P. Lengyel, Yale University, and had a specific activity of 2.1×10^9 units/mg protein. At equivalent antiviral doses, the purified and unpurified interferon preparations had similar effects on cell differentiation.

12-0-tetradecanoylphorbol-13-acetate (TPA) was purchased from Chemical Carcinogenesis, Eden Prairie, MN; stock solutions (1.6×10^{-4}M in acetone) were stored at -20°C. Fresh stock solutions (1000X) of aza-CR (Sigma) were prepared in phosphate-buffered saline pH 7.4, as needed, and sterilized by filtration.

Uptake of 2-deoxyglucose (2-DG) was measured by the procedure of Lee and Weinstein (23). Lactic acid was determined on deproteinized samples of culture medium by the procedures of Hohorst (19) and O'Brien et al. (27). The pH of culture medium was determined under paraffin oil on samples (at 22°C) that had equilibrated in a CO_2 incubator overnight.

RESULTS

Adipose Conversion of BALB/c 3T3 Fibroblasts

Confluent cultures of BALB/c 3T3 clone A31T cells with a reduced growth rate gradually accumulate triglyceride, which appears as lipid droplets in the cytoplasm (Fig. 2). The accumulation of triglyceride is enhanced by insulin and results finally in fully differentiated adipose cells with no proliferative potential. As adipose conversion proceeds, the cells develop biochemical profiles characteristic of adipocytes (9). There is a several hundred-fold increase in the activity of NAD^+-linked α-glycerophosphate dehydrogenase, a key enzyme in the triglyceride synthetic pathway since its action provides the only source of the triglyceride precursor, glycerol-3-phosphate. Lipoprotein lipase activity is also increased during adipose conversion although these cells probably do not require this enzyme for triglyceride synthesis; under the usual culture conditions, they utilize exogenous glucose as the source of the carbon atoms for both the fatty acid and glycerol moieties. After the preadipose cells have differentiated, they are responsive to lipolytic agents and can be stimulated by isoproterenol to hydrolyze triglyceride to free glycerol.

Effects of the Tumor Promoter TPA on Adipose Conversion

Treatment of preadipose BALB/c 3T3 cells with the potent tumor promoter, TPA, at concentrations $\geq 10^{-8}$M, or with other phorbol ester tumor promoters, inhibits adipose conversion (Fig. 2). There is no

TABLE 1. Effect of TPA on lactate production in BALB/c 3T3 cells
following the first and fourth exposures to TPA[a]

| Hours after treatment | μmoles lactate/5 ml medium | | | |
| | First exposure | | Fourth exposure | |
	-TPA	+TPA	-TPA	+TPA
0	0	0	0	0
3	0.56	0.68	-	2.70
6	1.25	1.50	-	6.1
9	1.72	2.52	1.05	9.7
16	2.70	4.35	1.35	20.1
24	3.79	6.25	1.45	24.9
48	4.23	9.82	1.45	39.9
72	5.83	12.9	1.90	39.9

[a]Cells were plated at 5×10^5 cells/60-mm dish in 5 ml standard medium and refed 4 days later without TPA or refed 2, 4 and 7 days later with standard medium with or without TPA (1.6×10^{-7}M). After an additional 3 days in both cases, the cultures were washed twice with warm phosphate-buffered saline and refed with 5 ml medium containing 10% dialyzed fetal bovine serum with or without TPA (1.6×10^{-7}M). Media were harvested from duplicate dishes at the indicated times and lactate concentration determined.

TABLE 2.   Effect of organic acids on adipose conversion of
BALB/c 3T3 cells[a]

| Treatment | Percent adipose cells | | | | | |
	Day 12		Day 14		Day 21	
Control	2.5	(0.8)	17	(0.6)	60	(0.3)
L-Lactic acid	0	(12.7)	0	(14.0)	0	(19.3)
D-Lactic acid	0	(3.5)	0	(4.5)	0	(4.5)
Acetic acid	0	(3.8)	0	(6.2)	0	(9.6)

[a]Cells were seeded in Eagle's minimum essential medium + 10% fetal bovine serum. Beginning 4 days later, when the cultures were confluent, they were refed at 3-4 day intervals with standard medium and the indicated additions at 10 mM final concentrations. The numbers in parentheses indicate the L-lactate concentrations (mM) in the spent medium.

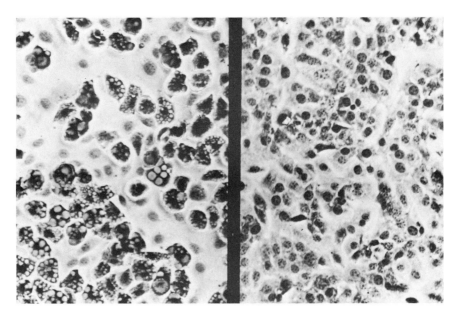

FIG. 2. Adipose conversion in BALB/c 3T3 cells. Confluent
cultures were refed every 2-3 days with control (left) or TPA (1.6
x 10⁻⁷M)-containing (right) Eagle's minimum essential medium.
After 32 days the monolayers were fixed with 10% formalin and
stained with oil red O. More than 70% of the cells in the control
contained many large lipid droplets. (X 300).

accumulation of triglyceride and no increase in α-glycerophosphate
dehydrogenase or lipoprotein lipase activity (11, 24). The inhibition
of differentiation by TPA is reversed when the cells are refed with,
or subcultured into, medium that does not contain the tumor promoter.

At those concentrations that inhibit adipose conversion of BALB/c
3T3 cells, TPA stimulates lactate production from glucose, with maximum stimulation occurring 4-7 days after the start of treatment with
TPA (Table 1). The cells at this time are capable of converting more
than 80% of the glucose in the medium (5.5 mM at zero time) to lactate
in 48 hr. This results in a decrease in medium pH from 7.4-7.5 to
7.1-7.2. If such cultures are then changed to medium that does not
contain TPA, the high rate of lactate production stops, the medium pH
does not fall, and the cells begin to differentiate.

The increased lactate production in response to TPA treatment is
not the result of enhanced cell growth because the promoter is only
mitogenic for these cells the first time they are exposed to it (11).
Thereafter, repeated treatment with TPA does not result in further
increases in cell number, and the cell density plateaus at a level
approximately twice that of control cultures (see Fig. 2).

The consistently observed correlation between enhanced lactate production by TPA and inhibition of adipose conversion suggested to us
that the inhibitory effect of the promoter on differentiation was due

to its reduction of the pH of the culture medium (27). This idea has
been supported by subsequent experiments in which the medium pH was
artificially manipulated (26). For example, organic acids such as D-
and L-lactic acid or acetic acid were added to the culture medium
(final concentration 10 mM, medium pH 7.1-7.2) and shown to mimic the
effects of TPA: there is stimulation of cellular L-lactic acid production with lowering of the medium pH and an inhibition of adipose
conversion (Table 2). The differentiation process can also be modulated by varying the $NaHCO_3$ concentration in the medium and keeping
the percent CO_2 in the atmosphere constant (Table 3). In the absence
of TPA, adipose conversion proceeds normally at medium pH levels
greater than 7.5, is delayed slightly at pH 7.35 and inhibited at pH
7.15. In TPA-treated cultures, adipose conversion is inhibited at pH
7.35, as expected, but at the higher pH levels, conversion is slightly
delayed and then proceeds rapidly. At these higher pH levels, TPA
does not stimulate lactate production nor lower the pH of the medium.

Thus, we conclude that the medium pH is an important factor in the
regulation of adipose differentiation in BALB/c 3T3 cells and is the
basis for the modulation of the differentiation process by TPA. The
promoter can inhibit differentiation in these cells if its stimulation
of lactate production and glycolysis results in a lowering of the pH
of the culture medium; the promoter does not inhibit conversion if the
buffering capacity of the medium prevents a decrease in medium pH.

The effects of TPA on hexose transport activity in these cells may
explain, at least in part, how the cells are able to sustain the high
rate of lactate production required for generating and maintaining a

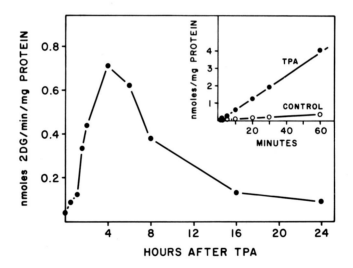

FIG. 3. Time course of TPA-stimulated 2-DG uptake in preadipose
BALB/c 3T3 cells. Post-confluent cultures containing very few differentiated cells were treated with TPA ($1.6 \times 10^{-7}M$) dissolved in
conditioned medium. Uptake of 2-DG was measured at the indicated
times in a 10-min assay using the procedure of Lee and Weinstein
(23). <u>Inset</u>: Uptake of 2-DG was assayed for the indicated lengths
of time in cells treated with TPA for 4 hr or left untreated.

TABLE 3. The effect of pH on adipose conversion of BALB/c 3T3 cells[a]

	Percent adipose cells			
	Day 12	Day 14	Day 18	Day 20
Control				
pH 7.15	0	0	1-5	5-10
pH 7.35	< 1	1-5	70-80	65-75
pH 7.52	1-5	20-30	55-65	60-70
pH 7.90	1-5	25-35	55-65	60-70
TPA				
pH 7.35	0	0	0	0
pH 7.52	0	0	65-75	75-85
pH 7.90	0	0	70-80	75-85

[a]Cells were seeded and grown to confluence in Eagle's medium + 10% serum at pH 7.5. They were refed 4 days later with control or TPA $(1.6 \times 10^{-7}M)$-containing standard medium adjusted to the indicated pH levels with $NaHCO_3$. Cells treated with TPA in medium at pH 7.15 eventually degenerated because of the low pH (6.8) that the medium attained.

TABLE 4. Effect of low doses of interferon and TPA on the adipose conversion of BALB/c 3T3 cells[a]

Day	Number of lipid-positive cells/4 mm^2			
	Control	TPA	Interferon	TPA + Interferon
0	2	2	2	2
7	65	43	14	0
10	93	116	24	11
14	168	208	71	44
17	248	252	137	66
20	290	299	155	95
23	> 300	> 300	199	115

[a]Confluent cultures were refed twice weekly beginning at zero time with either fresh medium alone or fresh medium containing $1.6 \times 10^{-9}M$ TPA, 50 units/ml interferon, or $1.6 \times 10^{-9}M$ TPA + 50 units/ml interferon.

lowered medium pH. TPA stimulates hexose transport in both undifferentiated and differentiated cells (9; unpublished data). The maximum stimulation of 2-DG uptake occurs at 4 hr after exposure of confluent cultures of preadipose cells to TPA for the first time (Fig. 3). There may at this time be a 10- to 20-fold increase in transport activity, with the effect of TPA being predominantly on the V_{max}. TPA also stimulates transport of the non-metabolizable glucose analog, 3-0-methylglucose (unpublished data).

The comparative effects of TPA on hexose transport in cultures of undifferentiated cells exposed acutely or chronically to the promoter are shown in Fig. 4. In cultures exposed to TPA for the first time, either at confluence or 4 days post-confluence when the cells are just starting to differentiate, TPA increases 2-DG uptake 10- to 20-fold. However, if the cells have been chronically treated with TPA for 7 days prior to measuring transport activity and are not differentiating, the basal level of activity is extremely high and there is very little further stimulation by TPA.

EFFECT OF TPA ON 2-DEOXYGLUCOSE UPTAKE IN CONFLUENT, 4 DAY POSTCONFLUENT AND CHRONICALLY TPA-TREATED CELLS

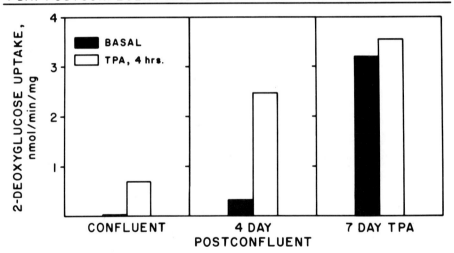

FIG. 4. Effect of acute versus chronic TPA treatment on 2-DG uptake in undifferentiated BALB/c 3T3 cells. Cells seeded in 60-mm dishes were grown to confluence and some cultures were assayed for 2-DG uptake (left panel). Some cultures were refed with standard medium 2 days later and assayed two days after that for 2-DG uptake (middle panel). The third group (right panel) was refed every 2-3 days with standard medium containing TPA (1.6×10^{-7}M) and assayed for 2-DG uptake after 7 days. With this chronically TPA-treated group, the uptake assay was done 2 days after the last refeeding so that the TPA which had been added then was completely metabolized (unpublished data). For the uptake assays, cells were pretreated with TPA for 4 hr, at which time 2-DG uptake by undifferentiated cells in response to TPA is maximal (see Fig. 3). Values are the averages of duplicate dishes assayed for 5 min. Solid bars, basal levels; open bars, TPA-treated for 4 hr.

Thus, it is not the initial transient stimulation of hexose transport activity by TPA, but rather the persistently high transport activity that accompanies chronic exposure which may generate the high rate of lactic acid production. These findings do not, however, rule out the possibility that other TPA-induced changes in cellular metabolism may be more directly responsible for the observed high rate of glycolysis in these cells than the transport effect. The mechanism that enables the cells to maintain the high levels of transport activity in the presence of TPA is currently being explored.

Effect of Interferon on Adipose Conversion

Mouse interferon also is a reversible inhibitor of adipose conversion in BALB/c 3T3 cells (4). It is effective at concentrations that do not affect cell growth or survival but may delay the $G_1 \rightarrow S$ transit. In cultures treated with low doses of interferon and TPA, the two compounds act synergistically to inhibit differentiation (Table 4). Interferon does not stimulate 2-DG uptake or lactic acid production in BALB/c 3T3 cells and does not affect the stimulation of these activities by the promoter (unpublished data).

Myotube Formation in C3H/10T1/2 Cells

When C3H/10T1/2 cells are treated at low density with $2 \times 10^{-6}M$ aza-CR, they become elongated and cell growth is slightly inhibited.

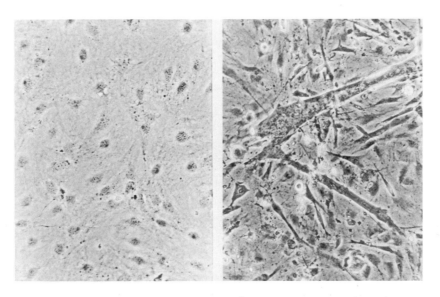

FIG. 5. Myotube formation in C3H/10T1/2 mouse cells. (Left) control cultures. (Right) cultures treated for 24 hr with aza-CR and then refed twice weekly with fresh medium. The cultures were photographed after 10 days. Phase contrast. (X 120).

Subsequently, treated and untreated cells grow out in isolated foci and divide at approximately the same rate. The aza-CR-treated cultures reach confluence after 8-10 days, forming a monolayer of fibroblast-like cells that differ in morphology from the epithelioid cells of untreated cultures at confluence. In the treated cultures at this time, foci of long, broad, multinucleated cells can be seen within the background monolayer (Fig. 5). These multinucleated cells arise from the fusion of bipolar mononucleated cells (6) and contain on the average 3 to 30 nuclei per cell. The formation of multi-nucleated myotubes reaches a maximum after 14-16 days and seldom involves more than 1% of the total cell nuclei; most myotubes atrophy soon after they are formed and disappear (5). It has been shown (5, 6) that the myotubes that develop in response to aza-CR treatment will contract in response to acetylcholine, possess acetylcholine receptors that bind α-bungarotoxin and have myosin ATPase activity which can be detected histochemically.

Effects of Interferon and TPA on Myotube Formation

Continuous exposure of aza-CR-treated C3H/10T1/2 cells to interferon (20-100 units/ml) inhibits myotube formation (Fig. 6). The few myo-

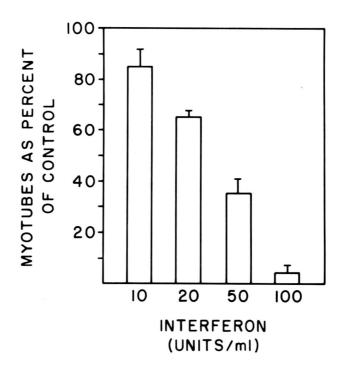

FIG. 6. Effect of interferon on aza-CR-induced myotube formation in C3H/10T1/2 cells. Cultures were treated with aza-CR for 24 hr and, beginning 24 hr later, refed twice weekly with fresh medium containing interferon. Myotube formation was scored after 10 days. The data from 3 experiments have been pooled. The average number of myotubes in control cultures was 750/60-mm dish.

tubes that develop with the higher concentrations of interferon are smaller and contain fewer nuclei per cell than those that form in control cultures. Interferon does not inhibit myotube formation if present only during the aza-CR treatment period. It is most effective as an inhibitor if added to the cultures within 24 hr after aza-CR treatment and becomes progressively less effective with increasing delays in the start of treatment; it is ineffective if first added to the cultures 4-5 days after aza-CR treatment. The inhibitory effect of interferon on myotube formation is reversible by refeeding the cultures with medium that is interferon-free. When cultures have been treated with 100 units/ml interferon for 10 days, myotubes begin to appear 24 hr after the removal of interferon and, 4 days later, there are almost twice as many myotubes as in cultures that have never been exposed to interferon.

Both interferon and mock interferon prepared in serum-containing media have a stimulatory effect on the growth of C3H/10T½ cells. However, interferon prepared in serum-free medium does not enhance cell growth at the concentrations used in the experiments reported here and mock interferon prepared in serum-free or serum-containing medium has no effect on myotube formation.

In agreement with Mondal and Heidelberger (25), we find that TPA also reduces the number and size of the myotubes formed in aza-CR-treated C3H/10T½ cells.

DISCUSSION

TPA and interferon belong to a unique class of diverse agents that also includes growth-promoting hormones and the src gene product: these agents have the ability to exert multiple and varied effects on cells. Depending on the cell type and its physiologic state, they can enhance or inhibit a broad range of cell functions. Both TPA and interferon can affect cell growth, the synthesis of specific cellular products, and the properties of cell membranes (3, 10, 12, 16, 17, 32, 37, 38). Some effects occur rapidly and may result from an initial interaction with the cell surface. Other effects occur later and may result from the modification of cell synthetic processes.

Sensitivity to the antiviral effect of interferon is dependent on the presence of surface receptors (7, 24), but it has not yet been clearly demonstrated that interferon's interaction with similar receptors leads to its effects on cell growth and functions. Because of the extremely high lipophilicity of phorbol ester tumor promoters, it was difficult to obtain firm evidence for specific binding (i.e., receptors) of these compounds. Recently, however, Driedger and Blumberg (13) were able to demonstrate specific saturable binding of phorbol esters to cell particulates by using phorbol-12,13-dibutyrate, one of the less lipophilic and less biologically active promoters in the series. Subsequently, others have obtained evidence for high-affinity specific receptors on the membranes of intact live or glutaraldehyde-fixed cells (20, 34). It has been proposed (reviewed in 10) that the primary action of the phorbol esters is mediated through interaction with these binding sites (8), and that the promoters are binding to and usurping the receptors normally used by some endogenous growth factor (38). However, there is as yet no direct evidence for either of these suggestions, and the chemical identity and functional significance of the phorbol ester receptors are not known.

There are now a number of examples of modification of cell functions by interferon (16, 17, 37). It does not appear to inhibit overall protein synthesis in these systems but does inhibit or enhance the synthesis of specific cell products, some of which may be crucial to cell growth. In Friend erythroleukemia cells, for example, high concentrations of interferon inhibit both cell growth and dimethylsulfoxide-induced erythroid differentiation (31). In contrast, interferon inhibits differentiation in BALB/c 3T3 preadipose and aza-CR-treated C3H/10T1/2 cells, but not cell growth.

Sreevalsan et al. (35) found that high concentrations of interferon (1000 units/ml) inhibit the synthesis of DNA and the induction of ornithine decarboxylase in Swiss 3T3 cells stimulated by polypeptide growth factors or TPA. It seems unlikely that interferon inhibits adipose conversion of BALB/c 3T3 cells through effects on cell growth for the concentrations of interferon that inhibit conversion (50-200 units/ml) do not inhibit TPA-stimulated ^{3}H-thymidine incorporation or ornithine decarboxylase activity (unpublished data). Furthermore, interferon also inhibits adipose conversion of Swiss 3T3-L1 cells with no apparent effect on cellular DNA content or protein synthesis (22).

Rossi et al. (30) found that in Friend cells interferon affects both the transcription and translation of globin mRNA. In the case of interferon suppression of steroid-inducible glutamine synthetase in chick neural retina, Shirasawa and Matsuno (33) found that interferon reduced the level of enzyme mRNA on polysomes. Since both adipose conversion in BALB/c 3T3 cells and myotube formation in C3H/10T1/2 cells require switching of complete differentiation programs, it probably will be difficult to determine the primary molecular mechanism involved in the inhibition of their differentiation.

Jones and Taylor (21) have shown that aza-CR is incorporated into the DNA of C3H/10T1/2 cells and is an efficient inhibitor of cytosine methylation. They propose that the incorporation of the cytosine analog into DNA can lead to erasure of previously established DNA methylation patterns and is, thus, related to the analog's effects on differentiation in these cells. The model does not require the continued presence of aza-CR for the effects on differentiation to be apparent and is, therefore, consistent with the long interval between aza-CR-treatment and the appearance of myotubes, a time of extensive cell division and consequently the diluting out of aza-CR from cell nuclei. A possible mechanism for the inhibition of myotube formation by interferon and/or TPA is that these agents alter the extent or pattern of remethylation that occurs after removal of the analog (21).

Our observations indicate that environmental (medium) pH has a critical role in the conversion of BALB/c 3T3 preadipose cells to adipocytes. It is an important determinant in the required "rearrangement" of the intracellular metabolism program from one geared to a relatively high rate of lactic acid production (glycolysis) and little triglyceride synthesis to one in which there is enhanced glucose utilization for fatty acid and triglyceride synthesis and no lactic acid production (see 1, 14). TPA can apparently inhibit adipose conversion by "locking in" the intracellular metabolism program of the preadipocyte phenotype. Through its stimulation of hexose transport activity and lactate production, it creates an environment (low pH) unfavorable for differentiation. This explanation for the mechanism of TPA's inhibition of differentiation is consistent with the fact that conversion can be inhibited by lowering the medium pH by means other than

TPA, and that conversion is not inhibited when TPA-induced decreases in pH are prevented. The adverse environment created by the low environmental pH could be affecting any of the many steps in the triglyceride biosynthetic pathway, either by blocking the development of some key enzyme(s) or by inhibiting the activity of key enzymes after they do develop.

The striking effect of TPA on hexose transport activity probably plays a major role in the mechanism of TPA inhibition of adipose conversion. It is paradoxical that, although most of the carbon atoms comprising the triglyceride that accumulates during differentiation come from glucose, the stimulation of glucose transport by TPA has an inhibitory rather than a stimulatory effect on triglyceride synthesis. This is because TPA creates a permanently high glycolytic rate in cells that have not yet acquired the differentiation-specific metabolic pathways that channel glycolytic intermediates into triglyceride. An analogous effect is seen with insulin: this hormone does not stimulate hexose transport in undifferentiated cells but, as the cells differentiate during the post-confluent period, they gradually acquire an insulin-responsive hexose transport system and the capacity to use the increased amounts of glycolytic intermediates for triglyceride synthesis (29; unpublished data).

It is important to note that, in contrast to the transient effect of TPA on hexose transport activity seen after initial exposure of the cells, after continuous exposure to TPA the basal levels of transport activity become extremely high. This suggests that the critical effect of TPA may be on the intracellular mechanism(s) that regulates transport activity in response to environmental conditions and cellular requirements. By uncoupling normal control mechanisms that are based on "supply and demand," TPA enables the cells to permanently maintain high levels of transport which, in turn, generate high rates of lactate production.

The mechanism by which TPA affects the differentiation of preadipose cells may be unique to these cells or may also be relevant to TPA's inhibition of myotube formation in C3H/10T1/2 cells. In both cases, the promoter may, for example, be affecting the synthesis or function of regulatory proteins involved in the biosynthetic pathways leading to differentiation. Interferon does not stimulate glycolysis in preadipose 3T3 cells and, thus, may appear not to be acting through the same mechanism as TPA. However, it too could be affecting some regulatory protein(s) in this or the C3H/10T1/2 cell system. Further studies in these cell systems with these two chemically distinct agents, TPA and interferon, applied alone or in combination, may help to elucidate the regulatory mechanism(s) for expression of the differentiated phenotype.

ACKNOWLEDGEMENTS

This work was supported, in part, by grants CA-23413, CA-09171 and CA-10815 awarded by the National Cancer Institute, DHHS.
We thank Dr. Peter Lengyel for the gift of purified interferon.

REFERENCES

1. Ailhaud, G., editor (1979): INSERM Symposia Series, Vol. 87. Institut National de la Sante et de la Recherche Medicale, Paris.

2. Boutwell, R.K. (1964): Prog. Exp. Tumor Res., 4:207-250.
3. Boutwell, R.K. (1974): CRC Crit. Rev. Toxicol., 2:419-443.
4. Cioé, L., O'Brien, T.G., and Diamond, L. (1980): Cell Biol. Int. Rep., 4:255-264.
5. Constantinides, P.G., Jones, P.A., and Gevers, W. (1977): Nature, 267:364-366.
6. Constantinides, P.G., Taylor, S.M., and Jones, P.A. (1978): Develop. Biol., 66:57-71.
7. Cox, D.R., Epstein, L.B., and Epstein, C.J. (1980): Proc. Natl. Acad. Sci. USA, 77:2168-2172.
8. Delclos, K.B., Nagle, D.S., and Blumberg, P.M. (1980): Cell, 19:1025-1032.
9. Diamond, L., and O'Brien, T.G. (1980): In: Carcinogenesis: Fundamental Mechanisms and Environmental Effects, edited by B. Pullman, P.O.P. Ts'o, and H. Gelboin, pp. 335-346. D. Reidel Publishing Co., Holland.
10. Diamond, L., O'Brien, T.G., and Baird, W.M. (1980): Adv. Cancer Res., 32:1-74.
11. Diamond, L., O'Brien, T.G., and Rovera, G. (1977): Nature, 269:247-249.
12. Diamond, L., O'Brien, T.G., and Rovera, G. (1978): Life Sci., 23:1979-1988.
13. Driedger, P.E., and Blumberg, P.M. (1980): Proc. Natl. Acad. Sci. USA, 77:567-571.
14. Green, H. (1978): In: 10th Miami Symposium on Differentiation and Development, edited by F. Ahmad, pp. 13-36. Academic Press, New York.
15. Green, H., and Kehinde, O. (1974): Cell, 1:113-116.
16. Gresser, I., De Maeyer-Guignard, J., Tovey, M.G., and De Maeyer, E. (1979): Proc. Natl. Acad. Sci. USA, 76:5308-5312.
17. Gresser, I., and Tovey, M.G. (1978): Biochim. Biophys. Acta, 516:231-247.
18. Hecker, E. (1978): In: Carcinogenesis, Vol. II, Mechanisms of Tumor Promotion and Cocarcinogenesis, edited by T.J. Slaga, A. Sivak, and R.K. Boutwell, pp. 11-48. Raven Press, New York.
19. Hohorst, H.O. (1963): In: Methods of Enzymatic Analysis, edited by H.U. Bergmeyer, pp. 226-270. Academic Press, New York.
20. Horowitz, A.D., Greenebaum, E., and Weinstein, I.B. (1981): Proc. Natl. Acad. Sci. USA, (in press).
21. Jones, P.A., and Taylor, S.M. (1980): Cell, 20:85-93.
22. Keay, S., and Grossberg, S.E. (1980): Proc. Natl. Acad. Sci. USA, 77:4099-4103.
23. Lee, L.-S., and Weinstein, I.B. (1979): J. Cell. Physiol., 99:451-460.
24. Lin, P.-F., Slate, D.L., Lawyer, F.C., and Ruddle, F.H. (1980): Science, 209:285-287.
25. Mondal, S., and Heidelberger, C. (1980): Cancer Res., 40:334-338.
26. O'Brien, T.G., and Saladik, D. (1980): J. Cell. Physiol., 104:35-40.
27. O'Brien, T.G., Saladik, D., and Diamond, L. (1979): Biochem. Biophys. Res. Commun., 88:103-110.
28. Reznikoff, C.A., Brankow, D.W., and Heidelberger, C. (1973): Cancer Res., 33:3231-3238.

29. Rosen, O.M., Smith, C.J., Fung, C., and Rubin, C.S. (1978): J. Biol. Chem., 253:7579-7583.
30. Rossi, G.B., Dolei, A., Cioé, L., Benedetto, A., Matarese, G.P., and Belardelli, F. (1977): Proc. Natl. Acad. Sci. USA, 74:2036-2040.
31. Rossi, G.B., Matarese, G.P., Grappelli, C., Belardelli, F., and Benedetto, A. (1977): Nature, 267:50-52.
32. Scribner, J.D., and Suss, R. (1978): In: International Review of Experimental Pathology, edited by G.W. Richter, and M.A. Epstein, Vol. 18, pp. 137-198. Academic Press, New York.
33. Shirasawa, N., and Matsuno, T. (1979): Biochim. Biophys. Acta, 562:271-280.
34. Shoyab, M., and Todaro, G.J. (1980): Nature, 288:451-455.
35. Sreevalsan, T., Rozengurt, E., Taylor-Papadimitriou, J., and Burchell, L. (1980): J. Cell. Physiol., 104:1-9.
36. Taylor, S.M., and Jones, P.A. (1979): Cell, 17:771-779.
37. Taylor-Papadimitriou, J. (1980): In: Interferon 2, edited by I. Gresser, pp. 13-46. Academic Press, New York.
38. Weinstein, I.B., Wigler, M., and Pietropaolo, C. (1977): In: The Origins of Human Cancer, edited by H.H. Hiatt, J.D. Watson, and J.A. Winsten, pp. 751-772. Cold Spring Harbor Laboratory, New York.

Expression of Differentiated Functions in Cancer Cells, edited by R. F. Revoltella et al., Raven Press, New York © 1982.

Lineages in Cell Differentiation and in Cell Transformation

H. Holtzer, M. Pacifici, S. Tapscott, G. Bennett, R. Payette, and A. Dlugosz

Department of Anatomy, School of Medicine, University of Pennsylvania, Philadelphia, Pennsylvania 19104

Though the concept of lineage is an old one, its profound implications for modern biology are rarely appreciated. If they were, many
proposals regarding the action of specific exogenous molecules in
inducing "undifferentiated" cells to "differentiate" would require
considerable revision (17). To understand how only one type of precursor yields progeny which differentiate into red blood cells, whereas only another type of precursor yields progeny which differentiate
into muscle cells requires an understanding of those mechanisms that
initiate and maintain lineages. Knowledge of how lineages function
on a molecular level is equally crucial to the understanding of how
only cells in the chondrogenic, melanogenic or lymphogenic lineages
have the option to yield, respectively, chondroma, melanoma and
lymphoma cells. The constraints that lineages impose on the metabolic
options of cells also account for the observation that chondroma,
melanoma, and lymphoma cells have more in common with their respective
normal precursor cells than with one another or with other types of
malignant cells.

Cell lineages account for the generation of new phenotypes between
generations of cells on the one hand, and the maintainance of phenotypic constancy between generations of cells on the other. The basic
paradigm of any lineage is illustrated in Fig. 1. This scheme is a
statement of the observation - as well as a prediction - that no exogenous molecule, no cell-cell interaction will induce a zygote, or
blastula cell, or embryonal carcinoma cell, or any primitive "stem
cell" to transform directly into a definitive red blood, nerve, or
muscle cell. Only after a minimal number of "quantal cell cycles"
will such precursors yield blood, nerve, or muscle cells (17,19,11).
In this regard it is misleading to view any cell as phenotypically
"undifferentiated", "totipotent", "undetermined", "unprogrammed" or
even as "multipotential". Exogenous molecules, such as hormones,
cAMP, EGF, collagen chains, fibronectin, GAGS, DMSO or cell-cell
interactions may be required to permit the expression of the inherited
differentiation program of a given cell, but such exogenous molecules
cannot be the primary mechanism for the generation of the differentiation program of that cell type. The phenotypic options - the

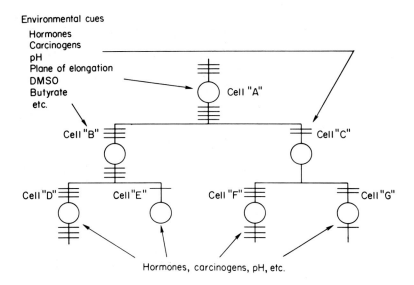

Fig. 1. A SIMPLE LINEAGE SCHEME. Whether cells acquire new phenotypic
options or retain those of their mother depends upon whether they undergo a quantal or proliferative cell cycle. In this Figure the proliferative cell cycles are indicated by horizontal bars. If Cell "A" or
"C" replicates, yielding two Cell "A's" or two "C's" the cell cycle is
a proliferative one, maintaining phenotypic constancy. These occur
in most cell cultures and in regulative developmental systems. Alternatively, if "A" or "C" replicates, yielding, respectively, daughters
"B" and "C", or daughters "F" and "G", the cycle is quantal, one that
generates phenotypic diversity. Cells "B" and "C" are differentiated,
but transitory, phenotypes. The molecular consequences of "traversing"
a quantal cell cycle is that genomic sites not available for transcription in the mother cell become available for transcription in the
daughter cells. Rules of this simple lineage are: (1) Cell "A" cannot
directly transform into phenotype "B" or "C", or "D", or "E", etc.
(2) Only daughters of "A" possess the prerequisite chromosomal structures that will permit its daughters to transcribe coordinately linked
sets of genes that activate the differentiation programs of Cells "B"
and "C". Similarly only the daughters of "B" have the option to
differentiate into "D" and "E". (3) Cell "B" cannot yield daughters
with the option to differentiate into "F" or "G". This scheme sets
limits to the response of cells to exogenous molecules. For example,
some cell-cell interactions might induce Cell "B" to divide, not
asymmetrically, but symmetrically, yielding either two "D's" or two
"E's"; alternatively, some cell-cell interactions might kill Cell "B".
Lastly, the metabolic consequences of treating cells with carcinogens
or cocarcinogens depend upon the phenotypic status of the responding
cell. Transformed "B" cells will have different phenotypic options
from transformed "D" or "E" or "A" cells (see Text).

differentiation program - of a zygote, embryonal carcinoma cell, presumptive myoblast, myoblast, hepatoma or lymphoma cell are the cumulative products of a precisely defined succession of quantal cell cycles.

Early Sequential Formation of Lineages in Chick Embryos

To determine when cells in a mesenchymal lineage become independent of putative exogenous molecules or complex tissue-tissue interactions, somites or limb buds of different ages were dissociated and cloned (10,17). Single cells from 3 day limb buds or somites yielded one of two types of clones: (1) myoblast-fibroblast clones, or (2) chondroblast-fibroblast clones. Mixed clones of both myoblasts and chondroblasts were never observed. From this study it was concluded that the readily-clonable cells in early limb buds had already bifurcated into a myoblast-fibroblast lineage and a chondroblast-fibroblast lineage. It was further inferred that the founder cell common to both lineages was probably a transitory phenotype that had bifurcated during the second day of development, prior to the morphological appearance of the limb bud. Others (5,29) using quail-chick grafts in vivo have also concluded that the founder cells of the future myogenic and chondrogenic cells of the limb bud are irreversibly shunted into one or the other lineage between the 25th and 40th hours of development.

More recently we asked whether cells from the 15-18 hour chick blastodisc had entered any of the more readily-recognizable lineages. The procedures for rigorously cloning somite or limb bud cells proved less successful when applied to early blastodisc cells. However, even in the absence of strict cloning, dissociated cells from 18 hour blastodiscs grown at low density already had, or shortly would, segregate into founder cells of the (1) erythrogenic, (2) neurogenic, (3) trunk melanogenic, (4) retinal melanogenic, and (5) cardiogenic lineages. Both entry into, and transit through, these lineages occur in the total absence of morphogenesis, of massive cell movements (eg. gastrulation, neurulation, etc.) of directed migration, of complex tissue-tissue interactions, as well as in the absence of putative specific inducing molecules (34,36).

The evidence for the early shunting of blastodisc cells into at least 5 major lineages is as follows: Many dissociated cells settle to the substrate and spread in 3 to 4 hours. Virtually all of the attached cells are full of yolk granules. Over the next several weeks most of these yolk-laden cells die. Approximately 30%, however, proliferate and yield progeny that lose their yolk. By day 2 - 3, islands of 20-30 small, yolk-free cells are detected among the large yolk-rich cells. The yolk-free cells increase in number between days 2 and 8.

Within 24 to 48 hours small cells, lightly adherent to the substrate or floating in the medium, emerge in these cultures. They are benzidine positive and identical to the primary and secondary erythroblasts described by Weintraub, et al. (19,40). These cells replicate and by day 5 display the features of erythroblasts in the penultimate and ultimate compartments of the embryonic erythrogenic lineage.

In day 4 cultures modest numbers of cells with neurite-like processes are also observed. They lie on the surface of the epithelioid islands of yolk-free cells. By day 6 or 7 nests of definitive neurons

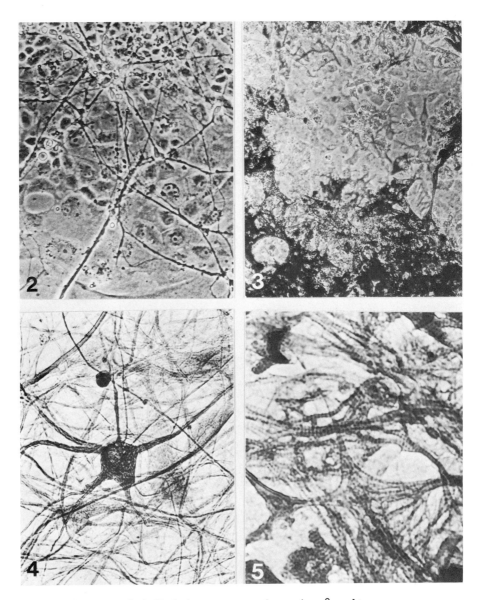

Fig. 2.   Cluster of definitive neurons in a day 8 culture.
Fig. 3.   Dense clusters fo dendritic melanoblasts from a day 7 culture.
Fig. 4.   A neuron from a day 8 culture treated with antibody against
neurofilament protein (anti-NIF) and visualized with the immunoperoxidase technique.   Note the absence of stain in the underlying presumptive neuroblasts and glial cells.   Fig. 5.   A day 10 culture treated
with antibody against muscle-specific myosin and visualized by the
immunoperoxidase technique.   The branched, striated stuctures are
characteristic of heart cells and are clearly distinguishable from
skeletal myoblasts which have never been seen in these cultures.

with repeatedly branching processes are present (Fig. 2). Neural processes are characterized by 10nm filaments known as "neurofilaments".
In the chick they consist of at least 3 proteins with MWs of 180, 160
and 70 kd (3,38). Antibodies have been prepared against these neuroal-
specific 10nm filaments. Figure 4 illustrates a region from an 8 day
culture treated with the antiserum to the 180 kd filament protein, using
the immunoperoxidase technique.

Trunk pigment cells appear in day 6-7 cultures. These melanoblasts
proliferate, forming scattered masses of individual cells with overlapping dendritic processes. Morphologically these pigment cells are
indistinguishable from those derived from the trunk neural crest (Fig.
3). A distinctly different pigmented phenotype also appears in these
cultures. These pigmented cells form epithelioid patches of 50-300
cells aand are indistinguishable from retinal pigment cells.

In occasional cultures prepared from dissociated 18 hour blastodiscs
we observed the spontaneous contractions characteristic of muscle in
vitro. Accordingly a total of 14 cultures were stained with an anti-
myosin IgG known to bind exclusively to the A-bands of both skeletal
and cardiac myoblasts (8,11,23). Nine of the 14 cultures stained with
anti-myosin in revealed patches of striated, branched cardiac myoblasts
(Fig. 5). The number of cells/patch varied from 10-80 and the number
of patches per dish varied from 1 to 6.

The Terminal Quantal Cell Cycle In A Neurogenic Lineage

That quantal cell cycles are obligatory for the movement of cells
from one compartment to the next in a lineage derives largely from the
analysis of cells in the myogenic, chondrogenic, and erythrogenic lineages (10,16,17,19,20). For example, replicating presumptive myoblasts
synthesize the "constitutive" myosin heavy and light chains and beta-
and gamma-actins found in many types of cells. In contrast, following
the quantal cell cycle which separates replicating presumptive myoblasts
from their daughters, the postmitotic myoblasts, the latter initiate
the synthesis of the muscle-unique myosin heavy and light chains, alpha-
actin and myoglobin. We have now localized an analogous quantal cell
cycle which separates replicating presumptive neuroblasts from their
postmitotic daughters, the definitive neuroblasts (3,38). Virtually 100%
of the precursor cells in the early 3 day spinal cord cycle and synthesize the fibroblast-type of 10nm (Fig. 6) filaments (FIF). These
replicating precursor cells do not bind antibody against the 180kd subunit of the 10nm neurofilaments (NIF). During the next 24 hours many
of these presumptive neuroblasts traverse their terminal quantal cell
cycle and enter mitosis. If treated with Colcemid the cells that enter
mitosis are arrested in metaphase. In addition to arresting cells in
metaphase, Colcemid also induces 10nm filaments to aggregate into cables
(1,7,14,23,26). In metaphase-arrested cells these Colcemid-induced
cables encircle the condensed chromosomes All of these cables in the
metaphase-arrested cells bind the anti-FIF (Figs. 9 and 10). However, a
small percentage of the arrested cells bind both anti-FIF and anti-NIF
(Fig. 11). It has been shown (38) that normal postmitotic neuroblasts
for a short period following their terminal mitosis contain both types
of 10nm filaments, but with maturation the FIF protein disappears,
leaving only the NIF proteins. In summary: The

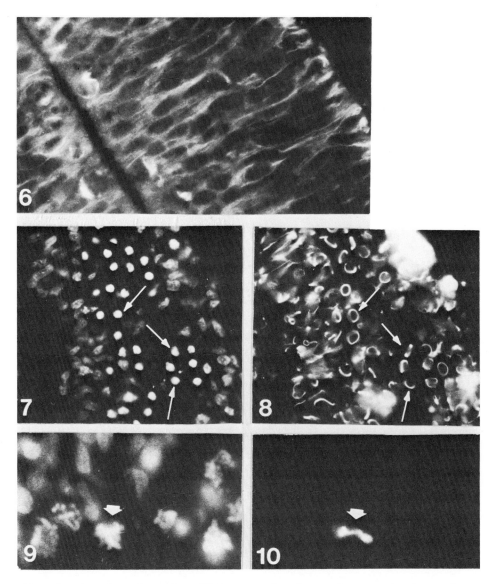

Fig. 6. Section through a 48 hr neural tube, prior to the formation of post-mitotic neuroblasts, stained with anti-FIF, demonstrating its presence in neuroepithelial cells.

Figs. 7 and 8. Two exposures of the same microscopic field of a 48 hr Colcemid-treated neural tube following staining with the fluorescent chromatin stain Bisbenzamid-H (Fig. 7) and anti-FIF (Fig. 8). The metaphase cells appear as brightly staining areas of condensed chromatin, each with an associated FIF positive ring (arrows).

Figs. 9 and 10. Two exposures of the same microscopic field of a Colcemid-treated 72 hr neural tube stained with Bisbenzamid (Fig. 9) and anti-NIF (Fig. 10). At this stage, neurons are withdrawing from the cell cycle. Arrows indicate a metaphase-arrested cell adjacent to the neurocoel with an associated NIF-positive ring.

evidence suggests that during the terminal quantal cell cycle presumptive neuroblasts initiate the synthesis of the 10nm neurofilaments; upon further maturation these new postmitotic neuroblasts lose their FIF.

Ts-RSV Reversibly Blocks Terminal Differentiation

Elsewhere we have suggested that the mechanisms responsible for the functioning of lineages also control the transformation of normal cells into malignant cells (21). We reported that the differentiation programs of myogenic, chondrogenic and melanogenic cells were reversibly blocked by transformation with a ts-RSV. At permissive temperature many of these cells cannot be distinguished morphologically from one another nor distinguished from transformed fibroblasts (4,18, 21,32). From a histological point of view these 3 different types of transformed cells would have to be classified as "undifferentiated". If, however, after 10-20 generations at permissive temperature the 3 types of cultures are shifted to non-permissive temperature, they develop many terminally differentiated postmitotic muscle, or cartilage, or pigment cells, respectively (see also 13,30).

A more careful recent analysis demonstrates that many of the transformed myogenic cells at permissive temperature are more "leaky" with regard to expressing portions of their terminal differentiation program than was first reported. In our original report (18) the criterion for terminal differentiation was the formation of many postmitotic, multinucleated, striated, myotubes. However, staining with antibodies against muscle-specific light meromyosin (anti-LMM) and against the MIF, reveals that approximately 5-8% of the transformed cells express their terminal differentiation program in an atypical fashion at permissive temperature. These striking differences in the expression of the terminal differentiation program between ts-transformed myogenic cells at non-permissive and permissive temperature, both under phase and fluorescence microscopy are illustrated in Figs. 11-16. The binding of the labelled anti-LMM in myotubes at non-permissive temperature is limited exclusively to the edges of the A-bands that make up the well-defined striated myofibrils (Fig. 12). These myofibrils run the entire length of the myotube. The spotty binding of the anti-MIF in these myotubes (Fig. 13) is characteristic of the distribution of this type of 10 nm filament in myotubes at an intermediate stage of maturation. Upon further maturation, the MIF localizes in the I-Z region (see 2 and 23 for changes in distribution of FIF and MIF in maturing myotubes). What had been underestimated in our earlier work are the modest number of atypical, small, abortive myotubes that appear and presumably die at permissive temperatures (Figs. 14-16). These atypical myotubes are irregular in outline, and bind the anti-LMM diffusely in the perinuclear region (Fig. 15). Striated myofibrils are not present and the myotubes do not contract spontaneously. The intense binding of the anti-MIF throughout the myotube is characteristic of very immature myotubes (2,12,23). These atypical myotubes do not change appreciably, though they have been maintained in culture for over 2 weeks.

In summary, the effect of the pp60 src kinase on the terminal differentiation program of myogenic cells is not "all or none" on the level of the individual cell. In keeping with this observation, Tate and co-workers (personal communication) have recently found that the

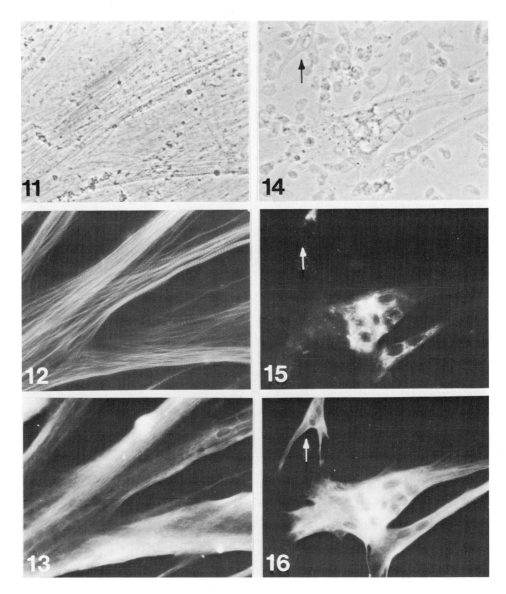

Phase and fluorescent micrographs of the same fields of RSV-transformed myogenic cells grown at non-permissive (Figs. 11-13) and permissive (Figs. 14-16) temperatures. Cells were double-stained with fluorescein -conjugated anti-LMM (Figs. 12 and 15) and rhodamine-conjugated anti-MIF (Figs. 13 and 16). The cells grown at non-permissive temperature are indistinguishable from control cells. Note that the presumptive myoblasts and fibroblasts do not bind either antibody. At permissive temperature the myotubes are small, flat and irregularly shaped. The anti-myosin antibody localized to a perinuclear region (Fig. 15); the anti-MIF antibody distributed throughout the myotube, as in a normal immature myotube (Fig. 16). Note the MIF positive muscle cell that binds very little anti-myosin (arrows).

expression of the differentiation program of ts-transformed myogenic cells reared at permissive temperature varies considerably, depending upon culture conditions. It will be of interest to determine whether the culture conditions that favor terminal differentiation affect the activity of the pp60 src kinase. It will also be important to determine whether altered culture conditions may be able to modulate expression of the transformed phenotype of infected chondrogenic or melanogenic cells as well. Terminally-differentiated myotubes are permanently postmitotic, in contrast to terminally-differentiated chondroblasts and melanoblasts. Either the fate of the integrated viral DNA and/or the frequency of transcription of the pp60 src gene in postmitotic cells may differ from that in cells that continue to cycle.

TPA Reversibly Blocks Terminal Differentiation

The pleiotropic effects of the cocarcinogen 12-0-tetradecanoyl-phorbol-13-acetate (TPA) has been thoroughly reviewed (9,24,41). That TPA affects the differentiation program of many types of cells is unquestioned. What is perplexing is how it affects these programs. For example, with respect to pigmented cells alone it has been demonstrated that TPA (a) enhances pigmentation but kills human melanoma cells (25); (b) retards (31) or blocks (27) pigmentation of murine melanoma cells; (c) reversibly blocks pigmentation in melanoblasts derived from chick neural crest (24,35); (d) enhances (37) or reversibly blocks (15) pigmentation in melanoblasts from quail neural crest. Some of these contradictory observations are due to species and culture conditions. Nevertheless pigmentation of chick neural crest that was reversibly blocked in our culture medium was also blocked in the medium Sieber-Blum and Sieber (37) used for quail cells (24). On the other hand, dissociated chick retinal pigment cells did not pigment in either medium in the presence of TPA. The state of the pigment cells is also important. TPA had no discernible effect on non-replicating retinal pigment cells, whereas it not only blocks pigmentation in replicating retinal cells, but it alters the cell morphology as well. TPA reversibly transforms epithelial retinal pigment cells into overlapping "fibroblastic-like" cells (35).

TPA rapidly but reversibly affects the cell surface and morphology of chondroblasts and blocks the synthesis of the chondroblast-specific sulfated proteoglycan (28,33). It also markedly inhibits the synthesis of the cartilage-specific Type II collagen chains. TPA blocks chondrogenesis in limb buds grown in medium consisting of 10% calf serum and MEM, but will not block chondrogenesis in limb buds reared in medium consisting of embryo extract, horse serum and MEM (17; Pacifici and Holtzer, unpublished observations).

TPA reversibly blocks two very different events regulated by the terminal differentiation program of postmitotic myoblasts: (a) it reversibly blocks the fusion of postmitotic myoblasts into multi-nucleated myotubes (6); and (b) it reversibly, but selectively, dismantles the striated myofibrils assembled in myotubes (8,23,39). This effect is remarkably specific for the myofibrillar contractile proteins; there are no obvious effects on the beta- or gamma-actins of the microfilaments subtending the sarcolemma or on the constitutive contractile proteins in non-muscle cells. This rapid and dramatic depletion of the striated myofibrils in myotubes is readily reversible

and is associated with the failure of the treated cells to accumulate
Ca^{2+}. It is to be stressed that TPA has no obvious effect on the con-
stituive contractile proteins in presumptive myoblasts or fibroblasts,
nor on the beta- or gamma-actins making up the microfilaments subtending the sarcolemma. In brief, somehow TPA selectively induces the
degradation not of the cell's household contractile proteins, but of
the muscle cell's "luxury" contractile proteins (8,19).

Conclusions

The central theme of this paper can be re-stated in the form of a
thought question: do embryonic cells have greater degrees of freedom
regarding phenotypic choices than more mature cells or malignant cells?
If they do, then clearly (a) the microenvironment plays a major role in
the determination of phenotypic types, and (b) the genetic control of
phenotypic options in embryonic cells must be qualitatively different
from those operating in more mature cells. The view that embryonic
cells are phenotypically more versatile than mature cells stems from
classical embryology. This literature often confused morphogenesis
and cytogenesis, and even more, confused the metabolic options of a
given embryonic cell for the metabolic options acquired by its progeny
generations later. For example, consider the experiments claiming
that embryonic cells are labile and depend upon "inducing" molecules
for the determination of their cytological fate. Such experiments
involved the transplantation of blocks of tissue often containing 10^4
cells, from one site to another. Weeks later, and after as many as 10
cell divisions, the descendants of the original 10^4 cells were categorized cytologically. If these descendants formed cell types they
would have formed if left in situ, the original cells were adjudged
"determined" or "committed". Alternatively, if the descendants formed
a different phenotype in the new location, it was concluded that the
original cells were "undifferentiated" and that specific molecules in
the new site induced the original cells to become types they would not
otherwise have formed. A simpler explanation is that both the grafted
cells and the ones they replaced were equivalent, and in some early
stage of a lineage that subsequently branched many times. For example,
consider a graft consisting of Type "A" cells in Fig. 1. In its
original location the microenvironment influences, say, the plane of
cell division, thereby segregating cytoplasmic factors so that all "A"
cells gave rise to two "B" cells. In the foreign location a different
microenvironment determines a different plane of cell division thereby
segregating the cytoplasmic factors in a different way so that all "A"
cells now yield two "C" cells. In the original location the terminal
descendants of "A" are "D" and "E" cells. In the grafted site the
terminal descendants of "A" are "F" and "G" cells. These results,
which are in harmony with the data of classical embryology, completely
bypass the notion that specific exogenous molecules in one step convert "undifferentiated" cells to differentiate terminally. The lineage
concept does not minimize the importance of the microenvironment, it
redefines its role. As suggested in Fig. 1, the microenvironment plays
an important role in affecting the binary decision (11,17,19) cells
must make during a quantal cell cycle.
The above considerations regarding lineages provide a model for the
observation that chondromas typically are derived from cartilage cells,
whereas hepatomas or mammary tumors are the progeny of liver or

mammary cells. In keeping with this fundamental fact is the observation that though pp60 src and TPA block the expression of the differentiation program of many cell types, they do not cancel such programs. Neither virus nor TPA nor BudR (17,19,24) render the responding cells more embryonic or less differentiated. The phenotypic status of the ts-transformed or TPA-treated cells remains constant. This must mean that generation after generation these blocked cells transmit with great fidelity their respective differentiation programs to their daughter cells. More will be known about differentiation, transformation and cell lineages when more is known of how chromosomal structures transmit differentiation programs to successive generations whether or not the programs are expressed.

This research was supported in part by the National Institutes of Health Grants HL-18708, HL-15835 (to the Pennsylvania Muscle Institute) CA-18194, GM-20138, the Muscular Dystrophy Association, a John A. Hartford Foundation Fellowship (R. P.), and a Medical Scientist Insurance Scholarship (S. T.).

BIBLIOGRAPHY

1. Bennett, G. S., Fellini, S. A., Croop, J. M., Otto, J. J., Bryan, J. and Holtzer, H. (1978): Proc. Nat. Acad. Sci. U.S.A., 75: 4364-4368.
2. Bennett, G. S., Fellini, S. A., Toyama, Y. and Holtzer, H. (1979): J. Cell Biol., 82:577-584.
3. Bennett, G. S., Tapscott, S. J., Kleinbart, F. A., Antin, P. B. and Holtzer, H. (1981): Science, (in press).
4. Boettiger, D., Roby, K., Brumbaugh, J., Biehl, J. and Holtzer, H. (1977): Cell, 11:881-890.
5. Christ, B., Jacob, H. J. and Jacob, M. (1979): Experientia, 35: 1376-1378.
6. Cohen, R., Pacifici, M., Rubinstein, N., Biehl, J. and Holtzer, H. (1977): Nature, 266:538-540.
7. Croop, J. M. and Holtzer, H. (1975): J. Cell Biol., 65:271-285.
8. Croop, J. M., Toyama, Y., Dlugosz, A. and Holtzer, H. (1980): Proc. Nat. Acad. Sci. U.S.A., 77:5273-5277.
9. Diamond, L., O'Brien, T. G. and Baird, M. W. (1980): Adv. Cancer Res., 32:1-74.
10. Dienstman, S., Biehl, J., Holtzer, S. and Holtzer, H. (1974): Dev. Biol. 39:83-95.
11. Dienstman, S. and Holtzer, H. (1975): In: The Cell Cycle and Cell Differentiation, edited by J. Reinert and H. Holtzer, pp. 1-25, Springer-Verlag, Heidelberg and New York.
12. Fellini, S. A., Bennett, G. S., Toyama, Y. and Holtzer, H. (1978): Differentiation, 12:59-69.
13. Fiszman, M. Y. and Fuchs, P. (1975): Nature, 254:429-431.
14. Franke, W. W., Schmid, E., Osborn, M. and Weber, K. (1978): Proc. Nat. Acad. Sci. U.S.A., 75:5034-5038.
15. Glimelius, B. and Weston, J. A. (1981): Dev. Biol., 82:95-101.
16. Groudine, M., Scherrer, K. and Holtzer, H. (1974): Cell, 3:243-247.
17. Holtzer, H. (1978): In: Stem Cells and Tissue Homeostasis, edited by B. I. Lord, C. S. Potten and R. J. Cole, pp. 1-28, Cambridge University Press.

18. Holtzer, H., Biehl, J., Yeoh, G., Meganathan, N. and Kaji, A. (1975): Proc. Nat. Acad. Sci. USA, 72:4051-4055.
19. Holtzer, H., Rubinstein, N., Fellini, S., Yeoh, G., Birnbaum, J. and Okayama, M. (1975): Quart. Rev. Biophysics, 8:523-557.
20. Holtzer, H., Okayama, M., Biehl, J. and Holtzer, S. (1978): Experientia, 34:281-283.
21. Holtzer, H., Biehl, J., Pacifici, M., Boettiger, D., Payette, R. and West, C. (1980): IN: Results and Problems in Cell Differentiation, Vol. II, edited by R. G. McKinnell, M. A. DiBerardino, M. Blumenfeld and R. D. Gerard, pp. 166-174, Springer-Verlag, Heidelberg and Berlin.
22. Holtzer, H. Croop, J. M., Toyama, Y., Bennett, G. S., Fellini, S.A. and West, C. (1980): IN: Plasticity of Muscle, edited by D. Pette, pp. 133-146, Walter de Gruyter, Berlin
23. Holtzer, H., Bennett, G. S., Tapscott, S. J., Croop, J. M., Dlugosz, A. and Toyama, Y. (1981): IN: Proceedings of the 2nd International Symp. of Cell Biology, Berlin, Springer-Verlag, Heidelberg.
24. Holtzer, H., Pacifici, M., Payette, R., Croop, J. M., Dlugosz, A. and Toyama, Y. (1981): IN: Symposium on cocarcinogenesis and Biological Effectos of Tumor Promoters, Berlin, Raven Press, New York.
25. Huberman, E., Heckman, C. and Langenbach, R. (1979): Cancer Res., 39:2618-2624.
26. Ishikawa, H., Bischoff, R. and Holtzer, H. (1969): J. Cell Biol., 43:312-330.
27. Lotan, R. and Lotan, D. (1980): J. Cell Physiol., 106:179-189.
28. Lowe, M. E., Pacifici, M. and Holtzer, H. (1974): Cancer Res. 38:2350-2356.
29. Mauger, A. and Kieny, M. (1980): Wilhelm Roux's Archives, 189:123-134.
30. Moss, P. S., Honeycutt, N., Pawson, J. and Martin, G. S. (1979): Exp. Cell Res., 123:95-106.
31. Mufson, R. A., Fisher, P. B. and Weinstein, I. B. (1979): Cancer Res., 39:3915-3919.
32. Pacifici, M., Boettiger, D., Roby, K. and Holtzer, H. (1977): Cell, 11:891-899.
33. Pacifici, M. and Holtzer, H. (1980): Cancer Res., 40:2461-2464.
34. Payette, R., Biehl, J. and Holtzer, H. (1979): Anat. Rec., 193:647-648.
35. Payette, R., Biehl, J. Toyama, Y., Holtzer, S and Holtzer, H. (1980): Cancer Res., 40:2465-2474.
36. Payette, R., Biehl, J., Toyama, Y. and Holtzer, H. (1981): (in press).
37. Sieber-Blum, M. and Sieber, F. (1980): European J. Cell Biol., 22(1):407.
38. Tapscott, S. J., Bennett, G. S., Toyama, Y., Kleinbart, F. A. and Holtzer, H. (1981): Dev. Biol., (in press).
39. Toyama, Y., West, C. M. and Holtzer, H. (1979): Am. J. Anat. 156:131-137.
40. Weintraub, H., Campbell, G. L. and Holtzer, H. (1971): J. Cell Biol., 50:652-658.
41. Weinstein, I. B., Wigler, M. and Pietropaolo, C. (1977): In: Origins of Human Cancer, edited by H. H. Hiatt, J. D. Watson, and J. A. Winsten, pp. 751-772, Cold Spring Harbor Press, New York.

Expression of Differentiated Functions in Cancer Cells, edited by R. F. Revoltella et al., Raven Press, New York © 1982.

Clonal Differentiation of Hemopoietic Multipotential Cells *In Vitro*

G. R. Johnson

Cancer Research Unit, Walter and Eliza Hall Institute of Medical Research, P. O. Royal Melbourne Hospital, 3050 Victoria, Australia

It is generally accepted that all of the mature hemopoietic cells can arise from a single cell, the multipotential hemopoietic stem cell. Although a murine assay for this cell has existed for many years (20) the events leading to the commitment and differentiation of multipotential cells have remained obscure. The murine assay involves the injection of hemopoietic cells into lethally-irradiated recipients and subsequent examination of the hemopoietic clones that arise within the spleen. The earliest regulatory events occurring during the development of these spleen colonies are not readily accessible due to the in vivo nature of the assay and thus several theories have been proposed to account for the hemopoietic differentiation that is observed. It has been proposed that external factors mediated by non-hemopoietic microenvironmental cells induce multipotential cells to differentiate along particular hemopoietic lineages, the hemopoietic lineage that arises being dependent upon the particular microenvironment the initiating multipotential cell inhabits (22,23). An alternative theory based upon observations of spleen colony growth, proposes that multipotential cell differentiation is stochastic and that different probabilities can be assigned to each of the hemopoietic lineages to determine the likelihood of commitment to any specific lineage (13,21). More recently, it has been proposed that humoral regulators determine which hemopoietic lineages will differentiate from multipotential cells (2).

In vitro assays for hemopoietic progenitor cells and more recently multipotential cells provide an alternative means to study the events leading to multipotential cell commitment and differentiation. The present report will, in part, review the patterns of differentiation observed when multipotential cells are grown in vitro and provide some data from experiments designed to determine the factors required to initiate these differentiation sequences.

181

MATERIALS AND METHODS

All experiments have been performed with adult or fetal cells obtained from either CBA, C57BL/6 or crosses between these two mouse strains. Cultures of cells were established in the presence of fetal calf serum and agar-medium and colonies were scored by criteria as described previously (7,10,17). Methylcellulose cultures containing fetal calf serum were established using the method of Iscove et al (6). All cultures were maximally stimulated, as determined by dose-response curves with pokeweed mitogen-stimulated spleen cell conditioned medium (SCM). Procedures for the production of SCM have been published elsewhere (17). The preparation of erythropoietin used in all experiments was obtained from Connaught Laboratories, Ontario (Step III, 12.6 Units Epo/mg). Due to its impure nature it will be referred to throughout the text as the erythropoietin preparation or "erythropoietin."

The morphology of smeared colony cells was determined by the use of benzidine and Giemsa staining as described previously (10). Intact cultures were stained with the megakaryocyte specific staining procedure for acetylcholinesterase as described by Melchner and Lieschke (15).

A Model of Multipotential Hemopoietic Stem Cell Differentiation Based Upon the Characteristics of Colony Growth In Vitro

When cultures of either CBA fetal or adult hemopoietic cells are maximally stimulated by SCM a number of different, morphologically distinct, colony types develop. Individual colonies may contain neutrophils, neutrophils and macrophages, macrophages, eosinophils, megakaryocytes or erythrocytes. When a single hemopoietic lineage (or in the case of neutrophils and macrophages, two lineages) are detected within a single clone, the initiating cell is believed to be a committed progenitor cell for that lineage (for review, 16). The presence of each of the different colony types in cultures stimulated with SCM indicates that each of the factors required for progenitor cell differentiation is present in this source of conditioned medium. Cultures stimulated by SCM also contain clones expressing three or more hemopoietic lineages and in every case examined one of these lineages has always been erythroid (11). These colonies have been termed mixed-erythroid colonies and represent the differentiation of multipotential cells in vitro. As well as expressing multiple hemopoietic lineages, mixed-erythroid colonies contain cells capable of producing secondary mixed-erythroid colonies and in vivo spleen colonies (4,19). The cells initiating mixed-erythroid colonies in vitro have the two properties attributed to multipotential hemopoietic cells, i.e. capacity for multiple differentiation and self-renewal.

The constant presence of erythroid cells in multipotential colonies in vitro is unexpected in that other combinations of hemopoietic cells without erythropoiesis may be expected based upon the theories of multipotential cell commitment (2,13,21,22,23). Since the SCM used in all experiments may contain factors selectively promoting the differentiation of erythroid committed progeny in multipotential clones, the patterns of differentiation obtained when alternative stimuli are used have been examined. Cultures initiated under serum-free conditions stimulated with GM-CSF produced clones which upon transfer to SCM-containing cultures produced multipotential colonies (8). In every case however these

colonies contained erythroid cells, indicating that the earliest commitment events in the development of these clones could not be altered by
these alternative culture conditions.

The observation that erythroid cells are always present in in vitro
multipotential clones has been made primarily on the basis of morphology.
Since the different committed progenitor cells cannot be distinguished
upon the basis of morphology the possibility exists that clones expressing single hemopoietic lineages may have arisen from multipotential cells
but only a limited number of the committed progenitor cells developing in
the clone may continue to differentiate.   The reculturing of primary
clones to determine the types of secondary clones produced should in part
answer this question.   When such experiments have been performed, only
primary mixed-erythroid colonies have been found to produce secondary
multipotential and committed progenitor-derived clones (19).   With each
of the other clone types believed to have arisen from committed progenitor cells, the limited numbers of secondary clones obtained have contained cells of the same morphological type as the parent colony.   Thus with
primary granulocyte-macrophage colonies, all secondary colonies have contained only neutrophils and/or macrophages (19).   A similar situation
has been observed upon reculturing of primary eosinophil colonies and
erythroid colonies and no secondary colonies have been observed upon re-
culture of primary megakaryocyte colonies (8,12).

These data have been taken into account and a theory of multipotential
cell differentiation proposed in which erythropoiesis is an obligatory
part (8).   Such a model differs from those proposed previously in that as
a consequence of being committed to differentiate, fixed and relatively
constant proportions of each of the different committed progenitor cells
(with erythroid progenitor cells always being produced) arise from each
multipotential cell.   The factors required to initiate this fixed sequence
of events from multipotential cells however remain unknown.

Factors Initiating Differentiation of Multipotential Cells In Vitro

Although SCM presumably contains the factors necessary to promote the
differentiation of multipotential cells, these activities have not yet
been biochemically separated from those factors acting upon committed
progenitor cells.   It still remains possible therefore that the regulators promoting differentiation of committed progenitor cells also interact with multipotential cells to induce their commitment to progenitor
cells.   Some evidence for this has come from experiments with the
granulocyte-macrophage progenitor cell regulator GM-CSF (18).   Although
apparently pure by biochemical parameters, GM-CSF not only stimulates
the development of granulocytes and macrophages from the appropriate
committed progenitor cell, but is also capable of initiating in vitro
multipotential cell differentiation (18).

An alternative approach to defining the regulatory factors required to
initiate differentiation from multipotential cells is to investigate differences between mouse strains.   With CBA mice, the presence of SCM and
fetal calf serum is sufficient to allow mixed-erythroid colony formation.
The low levels of erythropoietin present in the fetal calf serum being
sufficient to allow the terminal stages of erythroid differentiation to
occur.   With C57BL/6 cells however mixed-erythroid colonies are absent
or occur at a very low frequency in cultures containing SCM and fetal
calf serum.   The frequency of C57BL/6 mixed-erythroid colonies can be

increased however by the deliberate addition of preparations containing erythropoietin (Table 1).

TABLE 1.   Effect of "erythropoietin" upon colony formation from CBA and C57BL/6 bone marrow cells [a]

"Erythropoietin"	CBA colonies		C57BL/6 colonies	
	Total	%Mixed-eryth	Total	%Mixed-eryth
-	96	17	79	0
+	102	17	111	11

[a] Methylcellulose cultures contained 5×10^4 bone marrow cells, 20% fetal calf serum and maximally stimulated by SCM.   Erythropoietin preparation (Connaught Step III) addition to cultures at concentration of 1 Unit Epo per culture.   Data means of 4 replicate cultures in each instance, determined after 7 days' incubation.

To determine the responsiveness of CBA or C57BL/6 bone marrow mixed-erythroid colony-forming cells to "erythropoietin," cultures containing varying dilutions of SCM and the erythropoietin preparation have been established.   At all concentrations of the erythropoietin preparation (0.1 - 2.0 Units Epo) and in the presence of maximal stimulation by SCM, maximal numbers of CBA-derived mixed-erythroid colonies were obtained. However with C57BL/6 cells, at the lowest concentrations of "erythropoietin"used no mixed-erythroid colonies were obtained, but their numbers increased with increasing concentrations of the erythropoietin preparation (9).   The effect of adding 1 Unit of the erythropoietin preparation on C57BL/6 mixed-erythroid colony formation is shown in Table 1. Although CBA and C57BL/6 mixed-erythroid colony formation appears to have a differential sensitivity to the erythropoietin preparations used in these studies, the mixed-erythroid colony-forming cells from both mouse strains appear to be equally responsive to SCM (9).

The absence of mixed-erythroid colony formation with C57BL/6 cells in the absence of the erythropoietin preparation could be due to several mechanisms.   The mixed-erythroid colony-forming cell may not differentiate at all and simply remain as a single cell in the culture dish. Alternatively, the multipotential cell may differentiate but not express the erythroid component.   To test for this latter possibility cultures of CBA or C57BL/6 cells were cultured in methylcellulose and maximally stimulated by SCM.   After 7 days of incubation all of the colonies were removed, smeared and stained with Giemsa stain.   When examined microscopically, 8 of the 70 CBA colonies examined were mixed-erythroid colonies and no examples of multiple differentiation without erythropoiesis were observed.   With C57BL/6 cells only 1 mixed-erythroid colony was observed from 72 sequential colonies sampled (Table 2).   Careful examination of the remaining colonies showed that they contained only neutrophils, neutrophils and macrophages, macrophages or megakaryocytes and presumably had arisen from committed progenitor cells for these lineages (Table 2).   No examples of multiple differentiation without erythropoiesis have been observed previously with C57BL/6 mice and the present data confirm this.

An alternative procedure to determine whether C57BL/6 multipotential cells differentiate without expressing erythropoiesis in the absence of "erythropoietin" is provided by the observed high proportion of multipotential clones that include megakaryocytes.   Previous studies with CBA cultures have demonstrated that between 40 and 50 percent of mixed-erythroid colonies contain acetylcholinesterase-positive megakaryocytes (7,8). Similar findings have been made by others using either C57BL/6 (14) or C57BL/6 x C3H$_{F1}$ cells (3).

TABLE 2. Morphological characterization of colonies stimulated by spleen conditioned medium[a]

| Mouse strain | Total sequential colonies examined | Percent colonies | | | | | |
		Neut.	Neut-macro.	Macro.	Meg.	Eryth.	Mixed-eryth.
C57BL/6	72	22	43	33	1	0	1
CBA	70	13	34	36	0	6	11

[a]Methylcellulose cultures contained 10^4 bone marrow cells, 20% fetal calf serum and were maximally stimulated by SCM. Colonies sequentially removed from replicate cultures at day 7 of incubation, smeared and Giemsa-stained for microscopic examination.

Cultures of CBA or C57BL/6 bone marrow cells have been established and maximally stimulated by SCM. After seven days' incubation intact cultures were stained for the presence of acetylcholinesterase and entire culture dishes examined microscopically. With CBA cultures, in addition to the expected numbers of megakaryocytc colonies, megakaryocytes were also observed mixed with erythroid and other cells (Table 3). These latter colonies, containing acetylcholinesterase-positive megakaryocytes correspond to the mixed-erythroid colonies observed after Giemsa staining.

TABLE 3. Presence of megakaryocytes mixed with other hemopoietic cells in cultures without erythropoietin [a]

Mouse Strain	Meg colonies	"Mixed" meg colonies
CBA	10 ± 2	6 ± 2
C57BL/6	12 ± 2	0

[a]Agar cultures contained 5 x 10^4 cells, 20% fetal calf serum and maximally stimulated by SCM. After 7 days' incubation intact cultures stained for acetylcholinesterase, dried and mounted for microscopic examination of entire culture. Data means from 3 replicate cultures of either CBA or C57BL/6 cells.

With C57BL/6 cultures stimulated with SCM but without addition of the erythropoietin preparation expected numbers of megakaryocyte colonies were observed in stained intact cultures (Table 3). However despite careful observation of these cultures no examples of colonies containing acetylcholinesterase-positive cells mixed with other recognizable hemopoietic cells (e.g. neutrophils, macrophages) were observed (Table 3). These data suggest that in the absence of exogenously added preparations containing "erythropoietin," commitment and differentiation of C57BL/6 multipotential cells does not occur. Additional evidence for this is obtained when C57BL/6 cultures containing the erythropoietin preparation are examined. If C57BL/6 multipotential cells do not differentiate in the absence of "erythropoietin" then upon addition of the erythropoietin preparation to cultures maximally stimulated by SCM, extra colonies should be formed. Conversely, if in the absence of the erythropoietin preparation C57BL/6 multipotential cells differentiate without expressing the erythroid lineage then no additional colonies should form when the "erythropoietin" is added to these cultures. As shown in Table 1, additional colonies are obtained when "erythropoietin" is added to C57BL/6 cultures. These additional colonies contained erythroid cells mixed with other hemopoietic cells when examined morphologically and were indistinguishable from CBA mixed-erythroid colonies.

Differentiation of multipotential colony-forming cells in CBA, C57BL and backcross individuals

To further examine the requirements for mixed-erythroid colony formation in vitro, cells obtained from individual 12 day fetal livers were cultured in the presence of SCM. Previous experiments with CBA and C57BL/6 fetal liver cells have demonstrated strain differences in the responsiveness of multipotential cell differentiation to SCM and "erythropoietin" (7). In the present study, 12 day fetal liver cells obtained from matings between CBA x CBA, C57BL/6 x C57BL/6, CBA x (C57BL/6 x CBA)F_1 or C57BL/6 x (C57BL/6 x CBA)F_1 mice were cultured in methylcellulose cultures containing fetal calf serum and optimal concentrations of SCM. After 7 days' incubation both total and erythroid colony numbers were counted. Preliminary experiments showed that in all cases between 45% and 55% of colonies containing erythroid cells were mixed-erythroid colonies. For each individual fetal liver culture therefore, the degree to which mixed-erythroid colony formation occurs has been assessed by expressing the number of colonies containing erythroid cells as a percent of the total number of colonies. These data are shown in Figure 1. With fetal livers obtained as a result of mating CBA individuals, between 39% and 70% of all colonies contained erythroid cells (mean 54%). By comparison, with C57BL/6 individuals, in some instances no colonies containing erythroid cells were observed and at most 13% of colonies contained erythroid cells, the mean percent of erythroid-containing colonies being 3% (Figure 1). Cultures of 12 day fetal livers resulting from backcrossing between parental and F_1 individuals also showed great variation in the percentage of erythroid colonies. However a mean of 33% (range 11 - 57%) was observed with CBA x F_1 cells compared with a mean of 17% (range 4 - 50%) with C57BL/6 x F_1 12 day fetal liver cells (Figure 1).

DISCUSSION

The earliest cellular events occurring during the commitment and differentiation of multipotential hemopoietic stem cells remains unknown. The present work using an in vitro clonal assay that allows differentiation from multipotential cells to occur, demonstrates that, at least in vitro, different factors are required to initiate the differentiation sequence depending upon the mouse strain used. When only "erythropoietin" is added to cultures of either CBA or C57BL/6 hemopoietic cell differentiation does not occur (7,10). The addition of SCM however produces colonies expressing multiple hemopoietic lineages with either CBA fetal liver or adult bone marrow cells (7,10). The development of these mixed-erythroid colonies displays a sigmoid dose dependence upon the concentration of SCM added to the cultures. With C57BL/6 cells however, clones expressing multiple hemopoietic differentiation occur very infrequently when only SCM is added to cultures. The number of mixed-erythroid colonies obtained with C57BL/6 cells increases in a dose dependent manner when "erythropoietin" is added to cultures containing

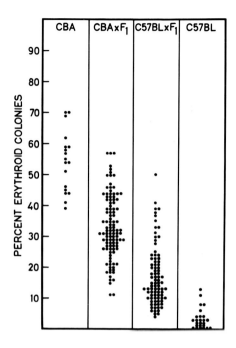

Figure 1:   Methylcellulose cultures of cells obtained from individual 12 day fetal livers contained 20,000 cells, 20% fetal calf serum and were optimally stimulated by SCM.   Each point from a single culture in which the percent of colonies containing erythroid cells was determined after 7 days' incubation.

SCM (1,5,9).   The deliberate addition of erythropoietin preparations to CBA cultures stimulated with SCM does not increase the number of mixed-erythroid colonies obtained but can increase the degree of hemoglobin-isation within the erythroid progeny (7,10).
    These observations suggest that with CBA cells, the factor(s) required for multipotential cell commitment are present in SCM, but that either the same or additional factors are present in the erythropoietin pre-parations used to stimulate C57BL/6 mixed-erythroid colony formation. The presence of additional factors in the erythropoietin preparation appears to be the most favourable alternative, since mixed-erythroid colony development from C57BL/6 cells displays an identical dose depend-ence upon SCM stimulation when compared to CBA mixed-erythroid colony development (9).   In the C57BL/6 cultures however, the addition of an erythropoietin preparation at a concentration of 1 Unit or greater was required to test the dose responsiveness of these cells to SCM (9).
    The requirement for erythropoietin in C57BL/6 cultures deserves comment.   In almost all instances impure preparations of erythropoietin have been used and for this reason in the present work it is not suggest-ed that it is actually erythropoietin that initiates commitment of C57BL/6 multipotential cells.   Experimental evidence for this has been obtained by others using delayed addition experiments.   Cultures of C57BL/6 cells have been initiated with SCM and erythropoietin prepara-tions have been added after various days of culture, the delayed addit-ion of erythropoietin leading to apparently normal colony development

(1,5).   Two points need to be mentioned about these experiments however, impure erythropoietin preparations were used at relatively high
concentrations and although apparently normal colony development occurred
within the expected culture period the cultures were not examined prior
to the erythropoietin addition.   The possibility still exists therefore that multipotential cell differentiation did not commence until
after the erythropoietin preparation was added to the cultures.

The present work and that previously published demonstrate that in
vitro cultures can be used to study the factors required to initiate
commitment and differentiation of multipotential hemopoietic stem cells.
The observed differences between CBA and C57BL/6 individuals and the
results obtained with backcross individuals indicate that genetic factors
may determine the responsiveness of multipotential cells to differentiation factors.   Further experiments are required to determine the exact
nature of these differentiation factors and whether the same factors or
multiple factors determine the observed differences between CBA and
C57BL/6 cells.

ACKNOWLEDGEMENTS

This work was supported by the Carden Fellowship Fund of the Anti-
Cancer Council of Victoria, The National Health and Medical Research
Council, Canberra, and the National Cancer Institute, Bethesda, Grant
No. CA 25972.   The author is indebted to Mr. G. Lieschke for acetyl-
cholinesterase staining of intact cultures.

REFERENCES

1. Axelrad, A. A., Mcleod, D. L., Suzuki, S., and Shreeve, M. M. (1978):
   In: Differentiation of Normal and Neoplastic Hematopoietic Cells,
   edited by B. Clarkson, P. A. Marks, and J. E. Till, Cold Spring
   Harbor Conferences on Cell Proliferation, 5:155-163.

2. Frindel, E. (1979):In: Cell Lineage, Stem Cells and Cell Determination, INSERM Symposium No. 10, edited by N. Le Douarin, pp 227-239.
   Elsevier/North-Holland, Biomedical Press.
3. Humphries, R. K., Eaves, A. C., and Eaves, C. J. (1979):
   Blood, 53:746-763.
4. Humphries, R. K., Jacky, P. B., Dill, F. J., Eaves, A. C., and
   Eaves, C. J. (1979): Nature, 279:718-720.
5. Iscove, N. N. (1978): In: Hemopoietic Cell Differentiation, edited
   by D. W. Golde, M. J. Cline, D. Metcalf, and C. F. Fox, (ICN-UCLA
   Symposium on Molecular and Cellular Biology, Vol.X, Academic Press,
   New York.
6. Iscove, N. N., Guilbert, L. J., and Weyman, C. (1980):
   Exp.Cell.Res., 126:121-126.
7. Johnson, G. R. (1980): J.Cell.Physiol., 103:371-383.
8. Johnson, G. R. (1981): In: Experimental Hematology Today 1981,
   edited by S. J. Baum, G. D. Ledney, and A. Khan, pp 13-20.
   S. Karger, Basel.
9. Johnson, G. R. (1981): In: Hemoglobin Switching, Edited by
   G. Stamatoyannopoulos, and A. W. Nienhuis. Grune and Stratton,
   New York (in press).
10.Johnson, G. R., and Metcalf, D. (1977): Proc.Nat.Acad.Sci. (USA)
   74:3879-3882.

11. Johnson, G. R., and Metcalf, D. (1979): In: Cell Lineage, Stem Cells and Cell Determination, INSERM Symposium No. 10, edited by N. Le Douarin, pp 199-213, Biomedical Press, Elsevier/North-Holland.
12. Johnson, G. R., and Metcalf, D. (1980): Exp.Hematol. 8:549-561.
13. Korn, A. P., Henkelman, R. M., Ottensmeyer, F. P., and Till, J. E. (1973): Exp.Hemat., 1:362-375.
14. McLeod, D. L., Shreeve, M., and Axelrad, A. A. (1976): Nature, 261:492-494.
15. Melchner, Von H., and Lieschke, G. (1981): Blood (in press).
16. Metcalf, D. (1977): Hemopoietic Colonies. In Vitro Cloning of Normal and Leukemic Cells. Springer-Verlag, Berlin-Heidelberg-New York.
17. Metcalf, D., and Johnson, G. R. (1978): J.Cell.Physiol., 96:31-42.
18. Metcalf, D., Johnson, G. R., and Burgess, A. W. (1980): Blood, 55:138-147.
19. Metcalf, D., Johnson, G. R., and Mandel, T. (1978): J.Cell.Physiol., 98:401-420.
20. Till, J. E., and McCulloch, E. A. (1961): Radiation Res., 14:213-222.
21. Till, J. E., McCulloch, E. A., and Siminovitch, L. (1964): Proc. Nat.Acad.Sci., 51:29-36.
22. Trentin, J. J. (1970): In: Regulation of Hematopoiesis, edited by A. S. Gordon, pp 161-186, Appleton-Century-Crofts, New York.
23. Trentin, J. J. (1976): In: Stem Cells of Renewing Cell Populations, edited by A. B. Cairnie, P. K. Lala, and D. G. Osmond, pp 255-264. Academic Press, New York.

Expression of Differentiated Functions in Cancer Cells, edited by R. F. Revoltella et al., Raven Press, New York © 1982.

Effects of the Human T-Cell Lymphoma (Leukemia) Virus and T-Cell Growth Factor on Human T-Cells

Robert C. Gallo, Mikulas Popovic, Francis W. Ruscetti, V. S. Kalyanaraman, Marvin S. Reitz, Jr., *Ivor Royston, **Samuel Broder, and Marjorie Robert-Guroff

*Laboratory of Tumor Cell Biology, National Cancer Institute, National Institutes of Health, Bethesda, Maryland 20205; *Department of Medicine, Division of Hematology/Oncology, University of California, San Diego, California 92023; **Metabolism Branch, National Cancer Institute, National Institutes of Health, Bethesda, Maryland 20205*

ROLE OF RETROVIRUSES IN ANIMAL LEUKEMIAS

Retroviruses are causative agents of leukemia and lymphoma in several animal species including chickens, mice, cats, cows and gibbon apes (see reference 1 for a summary). The types of disease induced in animals by these agents include most of the forms seen in man and especially, leukemias and lymphomas of T-cells. The mechanism(s) by which animal retroviruses transform cells in vitro and cause disease in vivo is of obvious interest. Understanding the process of viral carcinogenesis may also help elucidate the process of carcinogenesis in general including chemical- and radiation-induced neoplasms as well as the apparently spontaneous neoplastic transformations. The basis for this potential understanding arises from the current knowledge of transforming and non-transforming animal retroviruses. The transforming retroviruses, those that are capable of transforming cells in vitro and which generally cause acute disease in vivo, carry a transforming gene, variously called "src," "onc," "leuk," etc. Molecular biological studies indicate that these transforming genes were derived from normal host cell DNA in the past, presumably by recombination events between viral and host DNA. Because these genes are present in retroviruses, it becomes much easier to isolate them for analysis and characterization of the gene product. The counterparts of these transforming genes are present in normal host cell DNA. Perhaps these cellular genes are occasionally "turned on" by any of a variety of possible inducers, and the resulting cellular gene product causes abnormal growth. Therefore, a study of the viral transforming genes may help elucidate a more general type of carcinogenesis.

The non-transforming retroviruses, in contrast, are responsible for most of the naturally occurring animal leukemias. They do not

transform cells in vitro and generally require a long induction
period before leukemogenesis occurs in vivo. These viruses
apparently do not have a transforming gene, and hence, cannot code
directly for a transforming protein. One of the more attractive
hypotheses for leukemogenesis by these viruses is a viral promoter
insertion model (9). In this model, integration of proviral DNA
into the host chromosome results in the switching on of cellular
genes involved with cell proliferation. Only a portion of the
proviral DNA may be necessary to act as promoter. The cellular
genes turned on can apparently be the same genes picked up by the
transforming viruses in the past (see W. Hayward elsewhere in this
book). Once again, understanding this process may have more general
applicability to other types of carcinogenesis, not simply that
which is viral-induced.

HUMAN LEUKEMOGENESIS AND GROWTH OF HUMAN T-CELLS

The first step in determining whether retroviruses are involved
in leukemias and lymphomas of human T-cells in ways analogous to
animal models, is the isolation of a human virus. Some putative
human retroviruses have been reported, although the identification
of these agents as truly human has been very ambiguous, due to
varying degrees of relationship to known primate viruses (see
reference 19 for a summary). A new opportunity for the analysis of
human T-lymphocytes for retroviruses was provided by the discovery
of human T-cell growth factor (TCGF) in phytohaemagglutinin (PHA)
-stimulated lymphocyte conditioned media (8, 18). This factor has
allowed the routine long-term growth in vitro of of both normal and
neoplastic human T-cells. In addition to providing a system for
studying the biology of normal and neoplastic T-cells, TCGF can be
used for the regular propagation in culture of malignant T-cells
for use in detection of a human retrovirus produced at low levels,
or by rare cell types.

T-Cell Growth Factor

The purification of human TCGF from serum free conditioned medium
has been reported (7). Following a procedure involving ammonium
sulfate precipitation, ion exchange chromatography, gel filtration,
and preparative SDS polyacrylamide gel electrophoresis, the factor
was approximately 800-fold purified compared to the starting material.
Some of the biochemical properties of the purified material are
listed in Table 1.

T-Cell Proliferation

The normal route for proliferation of mature T-cells appears to
involve three major steps (see reference 17 for a review): 1) the
activation of a subset of T-cells by an antigen or lectin resulting
in acquisition of TCGF receptors; 2) the interaction of the antigen
or lectin with an adherent cell and a different subset of T-cells
(TCGF producer precursors) leading to a TCGF-producing T-cell and
3) the interaction of the activated T-cell possessing receptors
with TCGF resulting in T-cell proliferation. Following the purification of TCGF with a resulting preparation free of lectin activators

TABLE 1. Biochemical Properties of Human TCGF

1.	Sensitivity to Treatments:	
	a. Boiling	+
	b. RNase	−
	c. DNase	−
	d. Trypsin	+
	e. Freezing	−
	f. N-ethylmaleimide	−
	g. Dithiothreitol	−
	h. $HgCl_2$	−
2.	Stabilized by:	
	a. Polyethylene glycol	+
	b. Albumin	+
	c. Glycerol	−
3.	Molecular weight:	
	a. SDS-polyacrylamide gel electrophoresis	12-13,000
	b. Gel filtration	20,000
4.	Isoelectric point	6.8

and growth inhibitors, a difference was observed in the growth requirements of normal and neoplastic T-cells. While the response of both types of cells was markedly stronger to the purified TCGF compared to crude TCGF, neoplastic T-cells responded to TCGF without prior lectin activation, whereas normal T-cells still required the initial activation (11). This result suggests that the neoplastic T-cells had been activated in vivo by some mechanism and already possessed TCGF receptors. A summary of the properties of cultured normal and neoplastic T cells is presented in Table 2. In both cases the cultured cells are relatively mature T-cells which form E-rosettes, lack terminal deoxyribonucleotidyl transferase, and may possess functional specificity.

The finding that many neoplastic mature T-cells respond directly to TCGF without prior lectin activation has a practical advantage, as it allows the culturing of the transformed cells without the proliferation at the same time of normal T-cells. At the same time, the in vivo activation of the neoplastic T-cells has greater interest with regard to the control of T-cell proliferation and the mechanism of cell transformation. One or more possible mechanisms could account for the in vivo activation of neoplastic T-cells: 1) chronic antigen exposure, 2) changes occurring in the cell membrane after neoplastic transformation resulting in exposure of previously cryptic TCGF receptors, and 3) possession of TCGF receptors by a rare subset of normal T-cells which are actually the targets for transformation. Some of the neoplastic T-cell lines established using TCGF have subsequently become constitutive producers of TCGF. As these cells also possess TCGF receptors, a possible mechanism for chronic self-stimulation of cell proliferation is provided.

RELEASE OF RETROVIRUS BY CULTURED HUMAN NEOPLASTIC T-CELLS

Some of the cultured neoplastic T-cell lines have been found to release a type-C retrovirus called human T-cell lymphoma (leukemia)

TABLE 2. Comparative Properties of Human Mature T-cells Cultured Using TCGF

	Requirements for Growth		
Cell Source	No Additions	TCGF Alone	PHA Initiation + TCGF
Normal	-	-	+
CTCL[a]	-(rarely +)	+	+

	Morphologic and Cytochemical Characteristics		
	Morphology	Acid Phosphatase	Non-specific Esterase
Normal	Normal lymphoblasts	+	-
CTCL	Heterogenous, giant multinucleated cells and other smaller lymphoblasts, mono- or bi-nucleated; some with convoluted nuclei	+++ (diffuse intense reaction)	+ diffuse intense reaction in a few cells; most with small para-nuclear cyto-plasmic granule

	Marker Studies and Chromosome Analysis				
	TdT[b]	EBV[c]	IgG[d]	E-Rosettes	Chromosomes
Normal	-	-	-	+	normal diploid
CTCL	-	-	-	+	variable and like primary cells

[a] CTCL means cutaneous T-cell leukemia or lymphoma (Sezary syndrome, mycosis fungoides, and related diseases).
[b] TdT means terminal deoxyribonucleotidyl transferase.
[c] Tests for EBV were assays for the EBV specific nuclear antigen.
[d] IgG refers to tests for surface immunoglobulins.

virus (HTLV) (10, 12). The first isolate, $HTLV_{CR}$, was obtained from a lymph node derived T-cell line from a patient (C.R.) with cutaneous T-cell lymphoma (10). HTLV was subsequently isolated from two additional blood samples obtained from patient C.R. and a second cell line, CTCL-3 was established (10). In addition, T-cells from patient C.R. were cultured independently by Dr. S. Broder in Dr. T. Waldmann's laboratory and a cell line, CR-CTC, resulted which expresses HTLV proteins and possesses integrated HTLV DNA sequences (unpublished results). A second isolate, $HTLV_{MB}$, was obtained from T-cells established in culture from a patient (M.B.) with cutaneous T-cell leukemia (Sezary syndrome) (12). A summary of these virus isolations is presented in Table 3.

All the analyses carried out on the two HTLV strains have indicated that they are highly related to each other and unique from other known retroviruses. The analyses have included nucleic acid

TABLE 3. Isolation of HTLV from Cells of Patients with Cutaneous
T-Cell Lymphoma and Leukemia

Specimen Source	Cell Growth		Virus Production	
	Cell Line Established	Requirement for TCGF	Requirement for IdU Induction[a]	Constitutive
Cutaneous T-cell lymphoma				
Patient C.R. lymph node	HUT-102			
	passages 4-50	±	+	-
	passages >56	-	-	+
Patient C.R. fresh blood leukocytes	None[b]	N.A.[c]	-	+
Patient C.R. fresh blood leukocytes	CTCL-3	+	-	+
Patient C.R. fresh blood leukocytes	CR-CTC	+	-	+
Cutaneous T-cell leukemia (Sezary syndrome)				
Patient M.B. fresh blood leukocytes	CTCL-2	-	-	+

[a] IdU means iododeoxyuridine.
[b] No attempt was made to culture these cells continuously.
[c] N.A. means not applicable.

hybridization studies (14), immunologic studies on the major core protein (p24) of HTLV (5) and studies on the immunologic relatedness of the HTLV reverse transcriptase to that of other retroviruses (15). No significant relationship to any other retrovirus has been detected.

HTLV is Acquired by Infection

Nucleic acid hybridization data have indicated that HTLV is an acquired human retrovirus. HTLV sequences are not present in the DNA of the normal human donors examined (14). If HTLV were an endogenous, germ-line transmitted retrovirus, one would expect HTLV proviral sequences to be integrated in all cells of those individuals harboring the virus. That this is not the case has been shown by experiments in which HTLV ^{3}H-cDNA was hybridized to DNA extracted from both T-and B-cells of patient C.R. While the ^{3}H-cDNA probe hybridized specifically to the T-cell DNA, hybridization to B-cell DNA was indistinguishable from that to normal human liver DNA (Figure 1). Thus, these experiments lend further support to the acquired nature of HTLV.

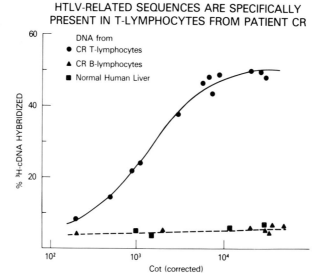

FIG. 1. HTLV-related sequences are specifically present in T-
lymphocytes from patient C.R. Percent hybridization is
expressed as percent of input acid-precipitable counts resistant
to S1 nuclease digestion and is corrected for time = 0. The
^{3}H-HTLV-cDNA was prepared as previously described (14). The
purification of cellular DNA has been described (3) as have the
conditions for annealing ^{3}H-cDNA to cell DNA (14).

Specific Antibodies to HTLV in Human Sera

Evidence suggesting that HTLV infection is correlated with human
disease has been sought in a sero-epidemiological survey of patients
with cutaneous T-cell lymphomas and leukemias. Initially, a group
of 17 coded patient sera were examined for natural antibodies to
HTLV by two techniques: a solid phase radioimmunoassay using disrupted HTLV and a radioimmunoprecipitation assay using iodinated
proteins of HTLV. These studies revealed that two patients possessed
natural antibodies to HTLV internal core proteins p24 and p19 (13).
The positive patient sera were obtained from patient C.R., the person
from whom HTLV was isolated, and from patient M.J., the latter an
individual with Sezary syndrome. No natural antibodies were seen
in sera from 55 random normal donors. The specificity for HTLV of
the antibodies detected in patient sera was confirmed in competition experiments carried out in both systems. In addition, specificity of the natural antibodies for HTLV p24 has been demonstrated
by a radioimmunoprecipitation assay using iodinated homogeneous HTLV
p24 (4). Table 4 summarizes the specificity tests and shows that
these natural antibodies recognize only proteins of HTLV. No other
retroviral proteins compete for the antibody activity nor do normal
cellular proteins. Among the cells tested, only lysates of those
producing HTLV competed.

TABLE 4. Specificity of Natural Antibody in Patient Sera for Proteins of HTLV

| | Competition of Reactivity in Patient Sera | | | |
| | to HTLV$_{CR}$ Proteins by Solid Phase RIA[a] | | to HTLV p24 by RIP[b] | |
	Patient C.R.	Patient M.J.	Patient C.R.	Patient M.J.
Viral Lysates				
HTLV$_{CR}$	+	+	+	+
HTLV$_{MB}$	+	N.D.[c]	N.D.	N.D.
Bovine leukemia virus	-	-	-	-
Gibbon ape leukemia virus	-	-	N.D.	N.D.
Simian sarcoma (woolly monkey) virus				
Rauscher murine leukemia virus	-	-	-	-
Feline leukemia virus	-	-	-	-
Baboon endogenous virus	-	-	-	-
Avian myeloblastosis virus	-	-	N.D.	N.D.
Mason-Pfizer monkey virus	N.D.	N.D.	-	-
Squirrel monkey retrovirus	N.D.	N.D.	-	-
Cell Lysates				
HTLV-producing cells (HUT102)	+	+	+	+
Transformed T-cells not producing HTLV (HUT78)	-	-	-	-
PHA stimulated normal T-cells	-	-	N.D.	N.D.
T-cell lines (immature or pre-T)	-	-	N.D.	N.D.
B-cell lines	-	-	N.D.	N.D.

[a] RIA means radioimmunoassay.
[b] RIP means radioimmunoprecipitation.
[c] N.D. means not done.

BIOLOGIC ACTIVITY OF HTLV

Having evidence that HTLV is an acquired retrovirus and having some suggestive serologic evidence for the presence of HTLV in patients with cutaneous T-cell lymphomas and leukemias, we next attempted to demonstrate infectivity of HTLV. Initial attempts to infect a variety of cell types of different species were unsuccessful. It was only when we used T-cells of relatives of a patient with acute lymphocytic leukemia that successful transmission of HTLV was achieved. The transmission experiments were carried out using T-lymphocytes obtained from peripheral blood and infected with 100 virus particles per cell. The T-cells were subsequently cultured in medium containing PHA for five days. Thereafter, cell growth was maintained using medium containing TCGF. This result has been recently extended to other families; i.e., transmission of HTLV in vitro was achieved with T-cells from the blood of other normal people. In all positive cases the people were closely related to a patient with an HTLV positive T-cell neoplasia.

Expression of HTLV p19 in Virus-producing Cells

Transmission attempts were monitored using an indirect immune fluorescent assay and a monoclonal antibody to HTLV p19 (16). Both radioimmune precipitation assays using iodinated proteins of HTLV and affinity chromatography of iodinated HTLV proteins on columns of monoclonal antibody coupled to Sepharose have shown the specificity of this antibody for HTLV p19. Assays of a large number of both patient cells, cells of normal donors and established cell lines of various types and species have shown that only cells known to produce HTLV express the p19 antigen. Table 5 summarizes these studies.

In Vitro Transmission of HTLV

As described above, transmission of HTLV to T-cells of relatives of a patient with acute lymphocytic leukemia as indicated by expression of HTLV p19 in the infected cells is summarized in Table 6. Cells of the father and one sister became clearly positive for the antigen suggesting productive infection with HTLV had occurred. Cells of the father have been monitored for six months and still continue to express p19. A second sample of blood cells was obtained from the father and the experiments were repeated. This second sample also showed expression of p19 but following a longer lag period.

A comparison of the fluorescence of the prototype HUT102 cells and the HTLV-infected cells of the father is shown in Fig. 2. Both cell types show a characteristic surface fluorescence. The immune fluorescence assay utilizes cells fixed in methanol:acetone (1:1) rather than living cells. The fact that living cells do not stain with the monoclonal antibody to p19 supports the notion that p19 is an internal viral component. While with conventional antisera, one might expect to see the cytoplasm also fluoresce, the anti p19 only stains the cells when virus is assembled at the cell membrane. Evidently, the single antigenic site recognized is only presented in the proper configuration at this time.

TABLE 5.   Specificity of Expression of HTLV p19 by Immune Fluorescence Assay Using Monoclonal Antibody to p19

Cell Type	Number Tested	Number Expressing HTLV p19
Cutaneous T-Cell Lymphomas and Leukemias		
Mycosis fungoides	17	3[a]
Sezary syndrome	9	1[b]
Other Lymphomas and Leukemias		
Acute lymphocytic leukemia	10	0
T-cell lymphomas	6	0
Chronic lymphocytic leukemia	4	0
T-cell chronic lymphocytic leukemia	2	0
Hairy cell leukemia	3	0
Acute myelogenous leukemia	1	0
Miscellaneous Solid Tumors	5	0
Normal Peripheral Blood Lymphocytes	9	0
T-Cells of Normal Relatives of		
Leukemia-Lymphoma Patients	11	0
Human Cell Lines		
B-cell lines	5	0
T-cell lines	12	0
Miscellaneous	7	0
Animal Retrovirus-Infected Cell Lines	13	0

[a]The positive cells include HUT102 cells from which HTLV, strain CR,
was first isolated (10), CTCL-3 cells, derived from a second blood
sample of the same patient, CR (10), and CR-CTC cells derived by
Dr. T. Waldmann from an independent blood sample of patient C.R.
[b]The positive cells were CTCL-2 cells from which a second strain of
HTLV was isolated, $HTLV_{MB}$ (12).

Because of the limited availability of TCGF, we have not been
able to culture all the cells of interest. Pursuing the transmission
experiments described above, we have followed cells of the father
closely. Reverse transcriptase activity was present in early passage
cells but then fell to undetectable levels. This is not totally
unexpected considering previous demonstrations of loss of reverse
transcriptase activity following viral infection (6). Other parameters monitored and found positive in the HTLV-infected cells have
included the presence of viral particles by electron microscopy and
the presence of HTLV p24 as shown by a competition radioimmunoassay
for the p24 antigen (5).

Induction of a Membrane Protein Following Lectin Activation of Human Lymphocytes

HTLV can induce expression of a lymphocyte antigen on T-cells of
normal donors. This phenomenon is not restricted to certain families.
Before describing this effect, some background information on this
antigen is summarized here. A mouse monoclonal antibody (L22) recognizes an antigen on activated human T-cells. The induction of this
human activation antigen (HAA) on T-cells by PHA is illustrated in
Fig 3.

TABLE 6.   <u>In Vitro Transmission of HTLV to T-cells of Relatives of a</u>
           <u>Patient with Acute Lymphoblastic Leukemia</u>

Relationship of Cell Donor to Patient	Number of Weeks Post-HTLV Infection	Expression of HTLV p19 by Immune Fluorescence (% Positive)
Sister (#80-49)	1	0
	8	50
	10	55
	11	36
Father (#80-50)	1	10
	3	20
	5	34
	9	25
	10	28
	11	19
	32	17
(#80-84)[a]	1	0
	6	0
	8	13
Mother (#80-51)	1	0
Sister (#80-52)	1	3

[a]A second blood sample (#80-84) was obtained from the father and the experiments were repeated.

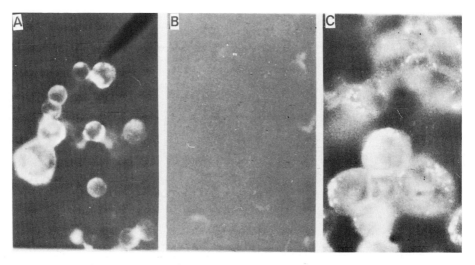

FIG. 2.   Immune fluorescence of HTLV-producing cells using a
monoclonal antibody to HTLV p19. The indirect immune
fluorescent assay has been described (16).

A.   HTLV-infected 80-50 cells of the father of a patient
     with ALL.
B.   Uninfected 80-50 cells of the father.
C.   HTLV-producing HUT102 cells.

   HAA has not been isolated; but some experiments suggest that
it may be related to the TCGF receptor. Fig. 4 shows the blocking
of detection of HAA when activated T-cells are first treated with
TCGF. This blocking effect is species specific, as human TCGF
is an effective blocker while rat and mouse TCGF are not. While
HAA can be detected on B-cells, B-cells do not have TCGF receptors
and TCGF does not block detection of HAA on B-cells. A definitive
answer concerning whether HAA is related to the TCGF receptor must
await isolation of the receptor.

INTERACTION OF HTLV WITH HUMAN T-CELLS

   One of the striking findings which arose in our studies of
T-cells from people with leukemias and lymphomas involving mature
T-cells was that these cells can be cultured directly with TCGF
while mature normal T-cells must first be activated with antigen
or lectin before they can respond to the growth factor. This result
suggests that neoplastic T-cells are already activated _in vivo_. In
order to test whether HTLV plays any role in this _in vivo_ activation,
fresh peripheral blood lymphocytes or thymocytes were incubated with

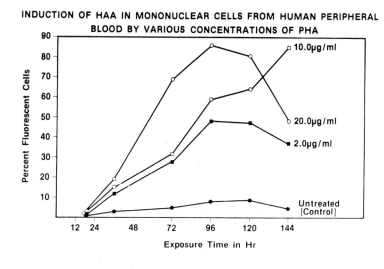

FIG. 3.   Induction of human human activation antigen by
          phytohemagglutinin. HAA induction was monitored by
          indirect immune fluorescence using the L22 monoclonal
          antibody.

retroviral preparations for 1 hour and then cultured with TCGF.
Three to five days later, they were examined for the presence of
HAA. Fig. 5 presents the results.

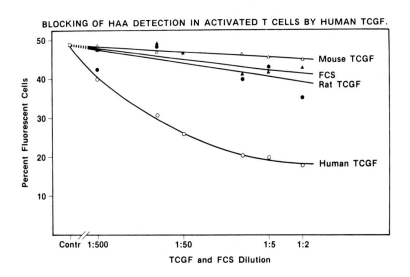

FIG. 4. Blockage of detection of HAA by TCGF. HAA-expressing
T-cells were incubated for 60 min at 37^{0}C with 200 µl of
the indicated factors serially diluted two-fold in RPMI-
1640 medium containing 20% fetal calf serum. The cells
were then processed for immune fluorescence using the L22
monoclonal antibody. The TCGF preparations used all had
similar titers on either mouse (for rat or mouse factor)
or human (for human factor) T-cells and included: rat
TCGF kindly provided by Dr. K. Smith, Norris Cotton Cancer
Center, Hanover, New Hampshire; mouse TCGF (BRL, Rock-
ville, MD); and human TCGF prepared in our laboratory
from PHA-stimulated lymphocyte conditioned medium (7).
The undiluted solution of fetal calf serum (FCS) used
was 36 mg/ml protein. The protein concentrations of
undiluted factors, and their titers (the dilutions of
growth factor giving 50% maximal growth of target T-
cells) were as follows:
Human TCGF: 2.2 mg/ml protein; 1:16
Mouse TCGF: 1.5 mg/ml protein; 1:12
Rat TCGF: 2.0 mg/ml protein; 1:12

   While slight induction of HAA was obtained with all the retroviruses tested, HTLV was the best inducer, especially taking into
account that 10 fold less viral particles were used. This result
is consistent with a model we have proposed concerning the process
of possible viral leukemogenesis of mature T-cells (2). This model

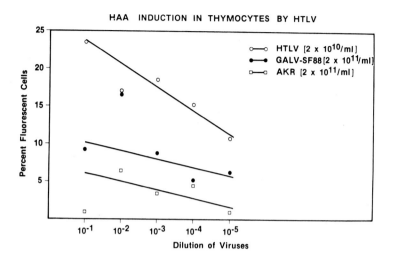

FIG. 5. <u>Induction of HAA by Retrovirus</u>. Human thymocytes
(5x10⁶) were incubated for 60 minutes with occasional
shaking at 37°C with the indicated dilutions of retroviruses in a total volume of 0.5 ml. The cells were then
centrifuged, washed with RPMI-1640 medium containing 20%
fetal calf serum, and resuspended in 5 ml of the same medium. Thymocytes were cultured for 3 days before examining
by immune fluorescent assay for the induction of HAA using
the L22 antibody.

involves several steps: 1) a virus, e.g., HTLV, interacts with
mature human T-cells resulting in activation and the appearance of
TCGF receptors. 2) The virus or a portion of it is subsequently
integrated into the T-cell genome. 3) The integrated proviral DNA
activates the TCGF gene in the infected cell leading to T-cell proliferation. 4) Autostimulation results as the cells producing TCGF
also possess TCGF receptors. This model is presented schematically
in Fig. 6.

The evidence favoring this model includes the already mentioned
difference in growth of normal and neoplastic T-cells, the presence
of a retrovirus, HTLV, in some neoplastic T-cells, the finding that
several cultured lines of relatively mature neoplastic T-cells have
become constitutive TCGF producers, the data showing that HTLV is
an acquired, not endogenous virus, the demonstration that HTLV can
infect certain T-cells, that HTLV can induce specific antibody production, and that HUT102 cells, an HTLV-producing cell line, do
produce TCGF (Gootenberg, Ruscetti, Gazdar and Gallo, in press).
These results are all necessary to the model. Moreover, some other
T-cell leukemic lines also appear to produce and respond to TCGF.
It must be pointed out, however, that to date only about 10% of the
neoplastic mature T-cell lines established eventually become inde-

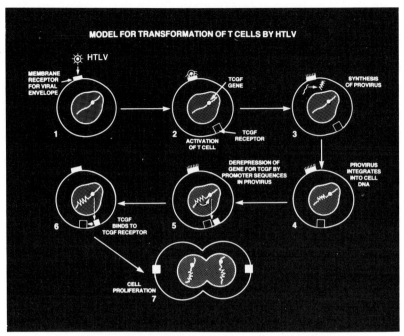

FIG. 6.   A schematic model for the first stage of T-cell
          leukemic transformation. We propose that the target cell
          is a mature T-cell with an antigen receptor site, which
          in the case of a proposed viral induced disease, recog-
          nizes an envelope protein of HTLV. This leads to the
          development of receptors for TCGF. Concomitantly, nucleic
          acid sequences contained in the HTLV genome which are
          integrated into the host cell DNA leads to an abnormal
          expression of the gene for TCGF. Available data indicate
          that separate subsets of T-cells usually make and respond
          to TCGF under normal circumstances. The above model of a
          cell both making and responding to TCGF may lead to uncon-
          trolled proliferation. In turn, this may subsequently
          lead to an increase in the likelihood of mutational events
          which "fix" the transformed state. Later in the progres-
          sion of leukemogenesis, cells which express virus may be
          selected against by immune mechanisms, making finding them
          rare by the time of frank disease.

pendent of exogenous TCGF. This argues against the proposed model
and suggests that TCGF production and subsequent autostimulation is
a phenotypic variation which occurs in these neoplastic cell lines
and gives the cells a selective advantage for in vitro growth. On
the other hand, we have recent evidence that the neoplastic T-cells
produce an altered TCGF. An altered TCGF or one produced at very
low levels could explain the low percentage of mature T-cell lines
which become TCGF-independent. Experiments are currently underway
to verify the authenticity of the proposed model.

REFERENCES

1. Gallo, R.C. (1978): In: <u>Viruses and Environment</u>, pp. 43-78. Academic Press, New York.
2. Gallo, R.G.: In: Third Annual Bristol-Myers Symposium on Cancer Research, edited by H.S Kaplan and S.A. Rosenberg, in press. Academic Press, New York.
3. Gallo, R.C., Gallagher, R.E., Wong-Staal, F., Aoki, T., Markham, P.D., Schetters, H., Ruscetti, F., Valerio, M., Walling, M.J., O'Keefe, R.T., Saxinger, W.C., Smith, R.G., Gillespie, D.H., and Reitz, M.S. (1978): <u>Virology</u>, 84:359-373.
4. Kalyanaraman, V.D., Sarngadharan, M.G., Bunn, P.A., Minna, J.D., and Gallo, R.C.: <u>Nature</u>, in press.
5. Kalyanaraman, V.S., Sarngadharan, M.G., Poiesz, B.J., Ruscetti, F.W., and Gallo, R.C., (1981): <u>J. Virol.</u> 38:906-915.
6. Krakower, J.M., Barbacid, M., and Aaronson, S.A. (1977): J. Virol., 24:1-7.
7. Mier, J.W., and Gallo, R.C. (1980): <u>Proc. Nat. Acad, Sci. U.S.A)</u>, 77:6134-6138.
8. Morgan, D.A., Ruscetti, F.W., and Gallo, R.C. (1976): <u>Science</u>, 193:1007-1008.
9. Neel, B.G., Hayward, W.S., Robinson, H.L., Fang, J., and Astrin, S.M. (1981): <u>Cell</u>, 23:323-332.
10. Poiesz, B.J., Ruscetti, F.W., Gazdar, A.F., Bunn, P.A., Minna, J.D., and Gallo, R.C. (1980): <u>Proc. Natl. Acad. Sci. (U.S.A.)</u>, 77:7415-7419.
11. Poiesz, B.J., Ruscetti, F.W., Mier, J.W., Woods, A.M., and Gallo, R.C. (1980): <u>Proc. Natl. Acad, Sci. (U.S.A.)</u>, 77:6815-6819.
12. Poiesz, B.J., Ruscetti, F.W., Reitz, M.S., Kalyanaraman, V.S. and Gallo, R.C.: Submitted.
13. Posner, L.E., Robert-Guroff, M., Kalyanaraman, V.S., Poiesz, B.J., Ruscetti, F.W., Fossieck, B., Bunn, P.A., Minna, J.D., and Gallo, R.C. In press, <u>J. Exp. Med.</u>
14. Reitz, M.S., Poiesz, B.J., Ruscetti, F.W., and Gallo, R.C. (1981): <u>Proc. Natl. Acad. Sci., (U.S.A.)</u>, 78:1887-1891.
15. Rho, H.M., Poiesz, B.J., Ruscetti, F.W., and Gallo, R.C. In press, <u>Virology</u>.
16. Robert-Guroff, M., Ruscetti, F.W., Posner, L.E., Poiesz, B.J., and Gallo, R.C.: Submitted.
17. Ruscetti, F.W., and Gallo, R.C. (1981): <u>Blood</u>, 57:379-394.
18. Ruscetti, F.W., Morgan, D.A., and Gallo, R.C. (1977): J. <u>Immunol.</u>, 119:131-138.
19. Wong-Staal, F. and Gallo, R.C.: In: <u>Retroviruses and Leukemia</u>, edited by F. Gunz and E. Henderson, in press. Grune and Stratton, New York.

Acknowledgment: M.P. is on sabbatical leave from the Cancer Research Institute, SAS, Bratislava, Czechoslovakia and is a recipient of an Eleanor Roosevelt International Cancer Fellowship.

Expression of Differentiated Functions in Cancer Cells, edited by R. F. Revoltella et al., Raven Press, New York © 1982.

T-Lymphocyte Cell Line Production of Human Lymphokines

J. E. Groopman, A. J. Lusis, I. Nathan, R. H. Weisbart, and D. W. Golde

Division of Hematology-Oncology, Department of Medicine, UCLA School of Medicine, Los Angeles, California 90024, and Veterans Administration Hospital, Sepulveda, California 91343

The study of permanent human cell lines derived from patients with a variety of hematopoietic neoplasms has provided insights into the differentiated functions of normal and malignant human blood cells. The myeloid cell lines HL-60 and KG-1 obtained from patients with acute promyelocytic leukemia and acute myeloblastic leukemia, respectively, are capable of differentiation with expression of granulocytic and/or macrophage functions (8,9,15,23,27). Certain strains of K-562, a cell line derived from the pleural effusion of a patient with blast crisis of chronic myelogenous leukemia (18), appear to have erythroid characteristics and can be induced to synthesize human embryonic hemoglobins (1,2,14,25). Recent evidence suggests that the original K-562 line may be multipotent (19).

We have derived a T-lymphoblast cell line, Mo, from the spleen of a patient with a T-cell variant of hairy-cell leukemia. The Mo cells manifest many of the characteristics of normal activated human T lymphocytes, in that they form E rosettes with sheep erythrocytes, are lysed by anti-thymocyte serum and complement, express the Ia (DR) antigen, contain the tartrate-resistant isozyme 5 of acid phosphatase characteristic of hairy-cell leukemia, do not make immunoglobulin, and do not express markers of Epstein-Barr virus infection (26). Recently, we have employed monoclonal antibodies directed against surface antigens present on sub-populations of normal human T lymphocytes, and have found that the Mo cells belong to the "helper" or "inducer" subset of T cells (17,24). This observation is consistent with their capacity to elaborate a variety of lymphokines that have been previously believed to be of T-cell origin (Table 1).

Colony-stimulating factor (CSF) is necessary for the in vitro development of granulocyte-macrophage colonies derived from myeloid progenitors present in human bone marrow (4). Colony-stimulating factor probably is an in vivo regulator of normal granulopoiesis although the data on this point are

TABLE 1. Factors produced by Mo cell line

Colony-stimulating factor (CSF)
Erythroid-potentiating activity (EPA)
Neutrophil migration-inhibitory factor (NIF)
T-cell growth factor (TCGF)
Fibroblast growth factor (MoFGF)
γ (immune) interferon (γ IFN)

---

largely circumstantial. A variety of CSFs have been
described arising from T lymphocytes, macrophages, fibroblasts, endothelial cells, and placenta (3,5,6,7,12). The
Mo cells constitutively elaborate high titers of CSF and we
have previously reported purification of this molecule to a
specific activity of 3.5 X 10^6 units, where 1 unit is equivalent to one colony per 10^5 light density nonadherent mononuclear bone marrow cells (21). Mo CSF is an acidic
glycoprotein with an apparent molecular weight of 34,000 to
36,000 daltons. We were able to achieve this purity
starting with as little as 1.8 liters of conditioned medium
because of the high CSF specific activity found in the Mo
serum-free conditioned medium.

The Mo CSF is clearly separable from an erythroid-
potentiating activity elaborated by the cell line which
promotes the proliferation of both early and late erythroid
progenitors, BFU-E and CFU-E, respectively (11,20).
Erythroid-potentiating activity is an acidic glycoprotein
of molecular weight about 45,000 and has been purified
approximately 250-fold from serum-free conditioned medium.
It is separable from the Mo CSF not only on the basis of
molecular weight but by its remarkable heat stability. The
EPA molecule is stable to boiling for 5 minutes while the
Mo CSF is not. Both the Mo CSF and the Mo EPA resolve on
flat-bed isoelectric focusing gels with major peaks between
4.5 and 5.0; the Mo EPA has, in addition, two smaller peaks,
one between 3.5 and 4.0 and the other between 6.0 and 6.5.
It is of interest that the Mo CSF stimulates proliferation
of the human myeloid leukemia cell line, KG-1, and the Mo
EPA stimulates proliferation of the human erythroleukemia
cell line, K-562 (10,16). These cell lines may provide
convenient assays for hematopoietic cell growth factors and
may be useful in studying the regulation of proliferation of
neoplastic hematopoietic cell lines.

Human γ (type II, immune) interferon can be derived from
mitogen-stimulated T lymphocytes. The Mo cells constitutively elaborate low titers of γ interferon. Upon induction
with the T-cell mitogen, phytohemagglutinin, there is an
approximately 100-fold increase in γ interferon elaborated
into the conditioned medium after three to four days of
culture (22). Certain chemical agents, such as phorbol
diesters (TPA), sodium butyrate, and dexamethasone in
conjunction with PHA have proven to act as potentiators of
Mo γ interferon production. We have shown that the

interferon elaborated by the Mo cells is only of the γ type in that it is completely destroyed upon reduction to pH 2 and is not neutralized by antisera to human leukocyte α or β interferon. Mo cell production of γ interferon was not enhanced by Sendai virus, poly I-poly C, BUdR, or exposure to leukocyte interferon.

Mo γ interferon is a highly labile molecule which is destroyed by heating to 56° for 1 hour, incubation at acid pH, exposure to denaturing agents such as 8 M urea and 6 M guanidine hydrochloride, and detergents such as sodium dodecyl sulfate. There was nearly complete retention of biologic activity when Mo γ interferon was treated with 10 mM β-mercaptoethanol; this observation suggests that if disulfide linkages are present, they are not critical for the activity of the Mo γ interferon. Mo γ interferon is a hydrophobic molecule that can be readily purified to a specific activity of about 10^5 international units per mg protein, using a controlled pore glass (CPG) column. Mo γ interferon is a glycoprotein that binds almost completely to concanavalin A-Sepharose. The interferon can be eluted from the concanavalin A-Sepharose with α-methyl mannoside and displays less heterogeneity with respect to glycosylation than γ interferon derived from mitogen-stimulated peripheral blood mononuclear cells. Consistent with previous reports of human γ interferon, the Mo γ interferon has an affinity for polynucleotides and binds to poly U-Sepharose.

Gel filtration chromatography of serum-containing Mo-conditioned medium induced with PHA demonstrates that the Mo γ interferon separates as a major species with an apparent molecular weight of approximately 70,000 daltons and a minor species of lower molecular weight (Fig. 1). Sequential elution with 1 M NaCl and 20% ethylene glycol recovers two further peaks of γ interferon. It is not clear at this time whether this results from different gene products for γ interferon, aggregates of Mo γ interferon molecules, or binding of Mo γ interferon to carrier proteins.

A number of other lymphokines are elaborated by the Mo cell line. A neutrophil migration-inhibitory factor is elaborated both constitutively as well as upon induction with T-cell mitogens and is an acidic glycoprotein with a major molecular weight species of approximately 25,000 daltons and a second species of about 45,000 daltons (28). The neutrophil migration-inhibitory factor, like the erythroid-potentiating activity, is a highly stable molecule with respect to heat, acid pH, denaturing agents, and detergents.

We have recently identified a fibroblast growth factor derived from the Mo cells which stimulates both human and murine fibroblasts (13). The Mo fibroblast growth factor is a glycoprotein which is stable to heating at 100°C for 5 minutes and displays heterogeneity with respect to iso-electric point and molecular weight. The major species of the Mo fibroblast growth factor has an apparent molecular weight of 38,000 daltons and resolves at pH 4 to 5 on

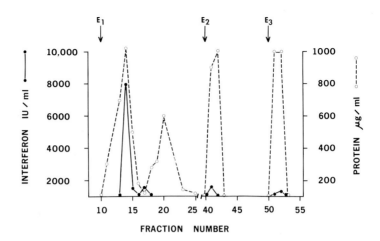

FIG. 1. Gel filtration chromatography of Mo
γ interferon on Ultrogel AcA 44 (LKB).
Sequential elution was performed with phosphate-
buffered saline pH 7.4 (E₁), 1 M NaCl in 0.02 M
phosphate buffer (E₂) and 20% ethylene glycol
in 0.02 M phosphate buffer (E₃). The interferon recovered with E₂ and E₃ may represent
ionic and hydrophobic interactions with the
Ultrogel, respectively.

preparative isoelectric focusing gels. On SDS gel electrophoresis, two major peaks of Mo fibroblast growth factor
activity were noted at 32,000 daltons and 38,000 daltons.
  The Mo cell line constitutively elaborates high titers
of T-cell growth factor (TCGF, interleukin II). This
neoplastic T-lymphoblast cell line may proliferate in vitro
in response to its own T-cell growth factor. Such autostimulation of permanent neoplastic cell lines has been
proposed as a model for the pathogenesis of some neoplasias.
  It is evident that a permanent human T-lymphoblast cell
line of neoplastic origin expresses many of the differentiated functions of normal activated inducer/helper T cells.
The Mo cell line provides a model for the study of both T-
lymphokine synthesis as well as a homogeneous cell source
for the isolation and purification of these important
regulatory molecules.

                            REFERENCES

1. Andersson, L.C., Jokinen, M., and Gahmberg, C.G. (1979):
    Nature, 278:364-365.
2. Andersson, L.C., Nilsson, K., and Gahmberg, C.G. (1979):
    Int. J. Cancer, 23:143.
3. Brennan, J.K., Lichtman, M.A., DiPersio, J.F., and
    Abboud, C.N. (1980): Exp. Hematol. 4:441-464.

4. Burgess, A.W., and Metcalf, D. (1980): Blood, 56:947-958.

5. Burgess, A.W., Metcalf, D., Nicola, N.A., and Russell, S.H.M. (1978): In: Hematopoietic Cell Differentiation. (ICN-UCLA Symposia on Molecular and Cellular Biology, Volume 10),edited by D.W. Golde, M.J. Cline, D. Metcalf, and C.F. Fox, pp. 399-416. Academic Press, New York.

6. Chervenick, P.A., and LoBuglio, A.F. (1972): Science, 178:164-166.

7. Cline, M.J., and Golde, D.W. (1974): Nature, 248:703-704.

8. Collins, S.J., Gallo, R.C., and Gallagher, R.E. (1977): Nature, 270:347.

9. Collins, S.J., Ruscetti, F.W., Gallagher, R.E., and Gallo, R.C. (1978): Proc. Natl. Acad. Sci. USA, 75: 2458.

10. Gauwerky, C.E., Lusis, A.J., and Golde, D.W. (1980): Exp. Hematol., 8 (Suppl. 8):117-127.

11. Golde, D.W., Bersch, N., Quan, S.G., and Lusis, A.J. (1980): Proc. Natl. Acad. Sci. USA, 77:593-596.

12. Golde, D.W., Finley, T.N., and Cline, M.J. (1972): Lancet, 2:1397-1399.

13. Groopman, J.E., Lusis, A.J., and Golde, D.W. (1981): J. Supramol. Struct., Suppl. 5:129.

14. Hoffman, R., Murnane, M.J., Benz, E.J., Jr., Prohaska, R., Floyd, V., Dainiak, N., Forget, B.G., and Furthmayr, H. (1979): Blood, 54:1182-1187.

15. Koeffler, H.P., and Golde, D.W. (1978): Science, 200: 1153-1154.

16. Lusis, A.J., and Koeffler, H.P. (1980): Proc. Natl. Acad. Sci. USA, 77:5346-5350.

17. Kung, P.C., Goldstein, G., Reinherz, E.L., and Schlossman, S.F. (1979): Science, 206:347-349.

18. Lozzio, B.B., Lozzio, C.B., Bamberger, E.G., and Feliu, A.S. (1981): Proc. Soc. Exp. Biol. Med., in press.

19. Lozzio, C.B., and Lozzio, B.B. (1975): Blood 45: 321-334.

20. Lusis, A.J., and Golde, D.W. (1981): In: Hemoglobins in Development and Differentiation, edited by G. Stamatoyannopoulos, and A.W. Nienhuis, in press. Alan R. Liss, New York.

21. Lusis, A.J., Quon, D.H., and Golde, D.W. (1981): Blood, 57:13-21.

22. Nathan, I., Groopman, J.E., Quan, S.G., Bersch, N., and Golde, D.W. Submitted for publication.

23. Newburger, P.E., Chovaniec, M.E., Greenberger, J.S., and Cohen, H.J. (1979): J. Cell Biol., 82:315.

24. Reinherz, E.L., Kung, P.C., Goldstein, G., and Schlossman, S.F. (1979): Proc. Natl. Acad. Sci. USA, 76:4062.

25. Rutherford, T.R., Clegg, J.B., and Weatherall, D.J. (1979): Nature, 280:164-165.

26. Saxon, A., Stevens, R.H., and Golde, D.W. (1978): Ann. Intern. Med., 88:323-326.

27.   Territo, M.C., and Koeffler, H.P. (1981): <u>Br. J.</u>
       <u>Haematol.</u>, 47:479-483.
28.   Weisbart, R.H., Billing, R., and Golde, D.W. (1979):
       <u>J. Lab. Clin. Med.</u>, 93:622-626.

Expression of Differentiated Functions in Cancer Cells, edited by R. F. Revoltella et al., Raven Press, New York © 1982.

Hemopoietic Growth Factor Production and Differentiation of a Murine Myelomonocytic Leukemia Cell Line

M. A. S. Moore and Y.-P. Yung

Department of Developmental Hematopoiesis, Sloan Kettering Institute for Cancer Research, New York, New York 10021

An increased understanding of the pathophysiology of leukemia in man and other species has come from in vitro culture studies of leukemic bone marrow and leukemic cell lines. Despite a spectrum of proliferative and maturation defects, human myeloid leukemic cells retain dependence upon myeloid colony stimulating factor (CSF) for their in vitro proliferation (29). Consistent defects in leukemia have been reported that involve negative feedback control mechanisms. For example normal monocyte-macrophage (M-CFC) and to a lesser extent granulocyte-macrophage (GM-CFC) progenitor cells are inhibited by physiological concentrations of prostaglandin E (PGE) produced by macrophages (19) whereas the progenitor cells in the bone marrow of patients with acute and chronic myeloid leukemia are resistant to PGE inhibition (30). The Iron binding proteins, lactoferrin and acidic isoferritin, appear also to play a role in negative control of hematopoiesis. Lactoferrin contained in and released by mature normal neutrophils inhibits monocyte-macrophage production of CSF thus indirectly limiting myelopoiesis (3) and while leukemic cells retain responsiveness to lactoferrin, the granulocytes of patients with myeloid leukemia are deficient in their content of this iron binding protein (5,7). Recently Broxmeyer et al (6) have identified acidic isoferritin as a possible physiological regulator of myelopoiesis since low concentrations of the molecule specifically inhibit the proliferation of normal GM-CFC. In contrast, GM-CFC in leukemic bone marrow appear to be refractory to acidic-isoferritin-mediated growth inhibitors, suggesting a mechanism for provision of a significant growth advantage to the leukemic clone.

In normal myelopoiesis, CSF is required at each step in the proliferation and differentiation sequence from GM-CFC to mature neutrophil and macrophage thus it is not possible to distinguish between a proliferation-inducing versus a differentiation-promoting action. However in the majority of acute myeloid leukemias, CSF promotes proliferation but not differentiation (29). This observation does not necessarily imply that the maturation block in leukemia is

irreversible and much attention has been paid to various myeloid leukemic cell line models that indeed can be induced to terminal differentiation. The most extensively studied has been the mouse myeloid
leukemic cell line M-1 (16,34) which can be induced to granulocyte
and/or macrophage differentiation by compounds as diverse as DMSO,
actinomycin-D, endotoxin, phorbol esters, dexamethasone and various
protein inducers (12,13,21). The human promyelocytic leukemic cell
line HL-60 (9) can likewise be induced to terminal differentiation to
granulocytes by exposure to polar compounds (9), conditioned media
(11), retinoids (2), and to macrophages, following treatment with
phorbol esters (33,21). The existence of physiological inducers of
myeloid leukemic cell differentiation has been documented in various
systems with the most consistent being the observation that serum
collected 3-6 hrs following endotoxin administration could induce
terminal differentiation of the M-1 cell line (22), and also a murine
myelomonocytic leukemic cell line WEHI-3 (8,23). Since endotoxin
induces a dramatic increase in serum CSF levels and high concentrations
of pure GM-CSF were shown to induce leukemic cell differentiation (24)
it was assumed that the differentiation-inducing protein was indeed
CSF. More recent biochemical characterization of post-endotoxin serum
has shown that the differentiation factor could be separated from
GM-CSF (MGI-1) (22) and was termed MGI-2, or could be separated from
the bulk of serum CSF but co-eluted with a minor species of CSF which
stimulated only granulocyte colony formation (8). The cellular origin
of endotoxin-induced differentiation protein is unclear, but macrophages are likely candidates and in this context, evidence is pointing
to the capacity of myeloid leukemic cells to produce their own differentiation-inducing protein (12,37). Indeed differentiation inducing agents such as endotoxin, phorbol esters, and glucocorticoids
appear to act indirectly, promoting differentiation by inducing leukemic cells to produce their own differentiation protein (12,37).

The capacity of leukemic cells to produce hematopoietic growth
regulating factors, either constitutively or following appropriate
induction is well documented and may be central to the selective
advantage of the leukemic population. To explore this possibility we
have undertaken a series of studies on growth factor production and
factor responsiveness of a murine myelomonocytic leukemic cell line
WEHI-3.

PRODUCTION OF GROWTH REGULATORY FACTORS BY WEHI-3

MYELOMONOCYTIC LEUKEMIA CELLS

The myelomonocytic leukemia, WEHI-3 originated in a Balb/c mouse
which had undergone mineral oil injections intended to induce plasma
cell tumor development (26,36). The tumor was composed of a mixed
population of monocytic and granulocytic cells. On transplantation
of the tumor, four distinct sublines developed, two of which retained
the original chloroma appearance and were distinguishable by karotype,
(one diploid and one tetroploid). The two nonchloroma sublines were
also distinguishable karyologically, because one had a hypodiploid 39
chromosome stemline. Chromosome marker studies in vivo and DNA-content
studies on cells from mice carrying the tetraploid subline confirmed
that in this leukemia both the monocytic and granulocytic cells are
neoplastic, indicating the existence of a neoplastic stem cell capable

of differentiation into both cell series. Serum and urine samples from
mice carrying this tumor contained high levels (frequently over 200
μg/ml) of lysozyme, and cell suspensions of the solid tumor also contained this enzyme. This tumor therefore fulfills all the criteria
applied to human myelomonocytic leukemia and proved a useful laboratory
model for this type of leukemia. Tumor cells could proliferate in agar
to form mixed colonies of granulocytes and macrophages, and both colony
size and plating efficiency were significantly increased in the
presence of an exogenous source of colony stimulating factor (25,26).
Individual colonies were capable of self renewal upon in vitro recloning and can be considered as leukemic stem cells, since individual
colonies implanted in vivo into the spleen or kidney produced progressively growing tumors with the same morphology as the original WEHI-3
tumor (25).

Two continuous cell lines of WEHI-3 have been developed. The first
was developed by Ralph et al (31) from the 125th passage of the WEHI-3
subline B (the hypodiploid line). This line is not inducible to
mature granulocytes or macrophages although it is Fc and C^1 receptor
positive, phagocytic, Thy-1 antigen positive and secretes plasminogen
activator and lysozyme (31). While incapable of extensive differentiation the most significant feature of the cell line is its capacity to
produce a wide spectrum of biologically relevant molecules that influence hemopoiesis and immune responses (see Table 1).

TABLE 1. Production of growth regulatory factors by the WEHI-3
          (D^-) myelomonocytic cell line

1. Produces GM-CSF (32)

2.   "   Macrophage (M)-CSF and neutrophil (G) - CSF (38)

3.   "   Eosinophil CSF (28)

4.   "   Megakaryocyte - CSF (39)

5.   "   Erythroid burst promoting activity (Iscove, N., personal
                                                    communication)

6.   "   Erythropoietin (18)

7.   "   Mast cell growth factor (35,41)

8.   "   Granulocyte precursor self-renewal factor (10)

9.   "   LAF (Interleukin I) (1)

10.   "   Endogenous pyrogen (1)

11.   "   Prostaglandin E (19)

12.   "   Lysozyme and plasminogen activator (31)

13. Has receptors for and responds to lactoferrin inhibition (4)

While it may be argued that production of these various regulatory macromolecules reflects oncogenic transformation, it should be noted that all the features of the cell line are features displayed by subpopulations of macrophages under appropriate stimulation. Indeed the most neoplastic feature of the cell line is that most of the factors are produced continuously and constitutively rather than as a result of lymphokine or adjuvant induction.

A second cell line was independently developed from WEHI-3B at an early stage of in vivo passage (Wyss, C. & Moore, M.A.S., unpublished) and in contrast to the preceding cell line, it retains its hypodiploid karytype and can be induced to terminal granulocyte and/or macrophage differentiation (23,24). To distinguish this line from that of Ralph et al we are adopting the nomenclature WEHI-3B(D$^+$) for the former and WEHI-3B(D$^-$) for the latter.

Activities in WEHI-3B(D$^-$) conditioned medium stimulated granulocyte and macrophage colony formation over an approximately 100-fold dilution of an eight fold concentrate of serum-free conditioned medium (CM) and with optional concentrations of CM approximately 40 to 50 granulocyte-macrophage colonies could be stimulated per 10^4 marrow cells plated. Partial separation of the activities stimulating the formation of granulocyte and macrophage colonies can readily be obtained by passing concentrated WEHI-3 CM through a DEAE Sephadex column (38). Semipurified neutrophil (G) CSF obtained in this manner did not induce monocyte-macrophage production and/or proliferation and was totally devoid of the capacity to induce plasminogen activator or prostaglandin E production by peritoneal macrophages.

Partially purified WEHI-3 CM is routinely used as a standard CSF source in parallel with a macrophage CSF derived from L cells. It has become apparent that significant strain differences exist with respect to myeloid cloning efficiency when WEHI-3 CM (G-CSF) is used but which are not apparent when L cell CSF was used. A particular abnormality was evident in NZB marrow cultures, since with unfractionated WEHI-3CM, GM-CFC were consistently low over a broad age span and when more purified G-CSF was obtained by passage over DEAE sephadex an even lower CFC response was observed (17). The incidence of WEHI-3 CSF-responsive cells in NZW mice was normal and (NZBxNZW)F, mice had an intermediate GM-CFC incidence that reflected the influence of both the parental strains. Certain other strains are also very poor responders to WEHI-3 CSF, for example, the NZC strain, which unlike the NZW, shares a common origin with the NZB. The C58/J strain also shows a low GM-CFC incidence in response to WEHI-3-CSF and has in common with the NZB, production of high levels of endogenous xenotropic virus and a high incidence of spontaneous leukemias and lymphomas. Horland et al (15), recently reported that the RF strain of mouse which has a high spontaneous incidence of granulocytic leukemia also has a marked defect in marrow GM-CFC. It is of significance that WEHI-3 CM was used as the source of CSF in that study.

Mast Cell Growth Factor (MCGF) Production by WEHI-3 Cells

We have reported a feeder layer-independent long-term in vitro culture system for murine mast cells (35,41). Concanavalin A activated murine splenic leukocyte conditioned medium prepared under conditions optimal for T cell growth factor production, was found also to contain a growth promoting activity for murine mast cells identified by their morphology, characteristic ultrastructure of the granules, positive reaction with toluidine blue and alcian blue, presence of receptors for IgG and IgE, as well as presence of histamine, serotonin. L-Dopa, 5-hydroxytryptophan and sulfated products within cytoplasm. Following 2 to 3 weeks of culture in the presence of the conditioned medium, mast cell lines were established from various sources devoid of initially matured mast cells. Such sources included spleen and bone marrow of athymic nude mice, long-term cultured marrow cells as well as T cell depleted normal marrow. Established mast cell lines have been maintained in exponential growth for over 9 months by passaging in the conditioned medium every 3 to 7 days. Cultured mast cells are absolutely dependent upon the conditioned medium-derived growth factor(s) for growth and viability, and cell death ensues within 24 hr in the absence of the factor(s).

MCGF is also produced by WEHI-3 cells without need for mitogen activiation (41). The possibility that MCGF was similar, if not identical, to other growth factors elaborated by the leukemic cell line was assessed following partial purification of the activities from WEHI-3 conditioned medium. Table 2 shows that MCGF activity in WEHI-3 CM exceeded that in Con-A stimulated spleen CM and that 4 can be separated from the bulk of Macrophage and GM-CSF following elution from DEAE, cellulose. However co-purification with G-type CSF was evident.

TABLE 2. Presence of MCGF in G-CSF Enriched Fractions of DEAE-Sephadex Separated WEHI-3 CM.

Source of Activity	MCGF Activity (Stimulation Index)[a]
Con-A spleen CM (50% v./v.)	245
WEHI-3 CM (10% v./v.)	531
WEHI-3 - G-CSF (20 μg protein/ml)[b]	636
WEHI-3-M-CSF (20 μg protein/ml)	6

[a]MCGF activity determined by ^{3}HTdR incorporation over 4 hours into established mast cell lines (41). The relative amounts of ^{3}HTdR incorporated were expressed as stimulation indices (S.I.) defined as: -Average cpm of test sample/average cpm of medium controls.

[b]DEAE sephadex separation of G- from M-CSF as previously reported (38).

To investigate whether MCGF action in vitro is genetically restricted and mouse strain dependent, as was shown for G-CSF, we attempted to establish long term lines of mast cells from bone marrow of NZB and C58 mice. As can be seen in Table 3, this was unsuccessful, however long term mast cell replication was obtained following the culture of bone marrow from the genetically anemic and mast cell deficient (40) WW^v and Sl/Sl^d mice and their littermate controls.

TABLE 3. Establishment and Long Term Growth of Mast Cells from Bone
of Various Mouse Stains[a]

Mouse Type	Total Mast Cells recovered by the 3rd Passage x10^6	Number of Passages
W/+	5.8	10+
W/W^V	4.4	10+
Sl/+	9.9	10+
Sl/Sl^d	7.9	10+
C58	0.4	4
NZB	0.0	1

[a]Bone marrow cells were cultured at 10^5/ml and passaged every 4-8 days
in a 50:50 mixture of Con-A mouse spleen leukocyte conditioned medium
and supplemented RPMI 1640 medium (35).

Despite sharing a number of properties with G-CSF, including low
affinity for DEAE, a molecular weight of 35,000 and unresponsiveness of
NZB marrow progenitors, preliminary analysis has revealed several distinctive properties of MCGF not shared by G-CSF, namely sensitivity to
neuraminidase and resistence to high temperature (40). Moreover,
lactoferrin, which suppresses G-CSF production by WEHI-3 cells (4) has
little effect on the concurrent production of MCGF, and MCGF purified
from splenic leukocyte CM has little G-CSF activity (41).

INDUCTION OF TERMINAL DIFFERENTIATION OF LEUKEMIC WEHI-3B (D$^+$ CELLS)

We examined the ability of mouse serum obtained 3 hours after
intravenous injection of 5 µg of endotoxin to induce differentiation of
WEHI-3B (D$^+$) leukemic cells cloned in semi-solid agar, following the
protocol of Metcalf (23). Table 4 shows that post-endotoxin serum
(5% v/v) induced all WEHI-3B (D$^+$) colonies to convert from tight ball-
like clones of immature blast cells to diffuse colonies containing
mature neutrophils and/or macrophages. Normal mouse serum was without
affect. The possibility that this differentiation-inducing activity
in post-endotoxin serum was mediated by a subspecies of CSF, possibly
of the granulocyte-specific type (8), was investigated in the following way. Partially purified G-CSF from WEHI-3B (D$^-$) conditioned
medium or macrophage-type CSF from L-cell conditioned medium was added
to agar cultures of WEHI-3B (D$^-$) and the dose response of the sources
of CSF was equated with the CSF activity in endotoxin serum. It can
be seen in Table 4 that all three preparations were capable of inducing
some differentiation of the leukemic target cells, however when assessed at an equivalent level of CSF activity (500 units per culture)
post-endotoxin serum caused 100% differentiation of the leukemic cells
with barely significant differentiation induced by the G-CSF-enriched
WEHI-3 CM and slightly more differentiation induction with L cell CM.

TABLE 4. Induction of Differentiation of WEHI-3B (D$^+$) Colonies by a
Differentiation-Inducing Activity in
Post-Endotoxin Serum

Test material[a]	% Diffuse/Differentiated WEHI-3B(D$^+$) Colonies
Saline	1
Normal mouse serum	2
Post-endotoxin serum	100
WEHI-3B G-CSF	4
LCCM M-CSF	18

[a]0.05 ml of post endotoxin or normal serum added to 1 ml agar cultures
containing 300 WEHI-3B (D$^+$) cells. An equivalent level of CSF activity
- 500 units per culture - was provided by an appropriate titrations of
WEHI-3 and L cell CM. Cultures scored for diffuse colonies at day 7.

CONCLUSION

The WEHI-3 myelomonocytic leukemic cell lines appear to possess
functional properties shared with the earliest committed myeloid
progenitor cells (GM-CFC) and their differentiated progeny. The linked
production of a wide spectrum of hemopoietic growth regulatory factors
by the leukemic cells parallels that seen following antigen or mitogen
stimulation of normal splenic or peripheral blood leukocytes (27).
A significant neoplastic feature of WEHI-3 cells is their ability to
produce growth factors constitutively and thus circumvent control net-
works involving multiple cell interactions. An additional feature
is the ability of the leukemic cells to produce growth factors to
which the leukemic cells respond, providing an opportunity for autostimulation which may be more universally applicable to the selective
advantage of neoplastic cells.

The various growth factors elaborated by leukemic cells appear to
be functionally and structurally identical to factors produced by
normal cells but a final answer must await total purification and
sequencing of the various molecules. Our preliminary data shows that
certain of the growth factors (G-CSF, M.C.G.F., megakaryocyte CSF),
are not readily separated by a number of biochemical procedures and
they share other features in common - for example the genetic unresponsiveness of NZB bone marrow to G-CSF and MCGF. We have documented
that despite these similarities, specific growth factor production
can be independently controlled as illustrated by the ability of
lactoferrin to inhibit normal and leukemic cell production of G-CSF
but not MCGF.

The ability of certain lines of WEHI-3 to undergo terminal
maturation provides yet another example to support the contention that
leukemic maturation arrest is not irreversible, provided the right
stimulus for differentiation is applied. It seems increasingly unlikely that this leukemic differentiation-inducing factor corresponds
to a known subset of myeloid CSF's even though it copurifies with
G-CSF in post-endotoxin serum (8). The results we have obtained using
post-endotoxin sera versus conditioned medium from a non-differentia-

ting line of WEHI-3, rich in G-CSF indicates either that GM-differen-
tiation protein and G-CSF are different molecules or that in the course
of leukemic transformation WEHI-3 cells began to produce an aberrant
molecule which retains a proliferative action for leukemic cells but
lacks differentiation-inducing capacity.

REFERENCES

1. Bodel, P. (1978): Journal Exp. Med.,147:1503.
2. Breitman, T., Selonick, S., and Collins, S. (1980): Proc. Natl.
   Acad. Sci.,(USA) 77:2936-40.
3. Broxmeyer, H.E. (1979): J. Clin. Invest.,64:1717-1720.
4. Broxmeyer, H.E., and Ralph, P. (1977): Cancer Res.,37:3578.
5. Broxmeyer, H.E., Mendelsohn, N., and Moore, M.A.S. (1977): Leukemia
   Research, 3:12.
6. Broxmeyer, H.E., Bognacki, J., Dorner, M.M., deSousa, M., and Lu, L.
   (1981): In "Haematology and Blood Transfusion-Modern Trends in
   Human Leukemia IV", edited by Neth, R., Gallo, R., Graaf, T.,
   Springer-Verlad, Berlin. (in press)
7. Broxmeyer, H.E., Jacobsen, N., Kurland, J., Mendelsohn, N. and
   Moore, M.A.S. (1978): J. Nat. Cancer Inst., 60:497-512.
8. Burgess, A.W., and Metcalf, D. (1980): In. J. Cancer, 26:647-654.
9. Collins, S.J., Ruscetti, F.W., Gallagher, R.E., and Gallo, R.C.
   (1978): Proc. Natl. Acad. Sci., (USA), 75:245.
10. Dexter, T.M., Garland, J., Scott, D., Scolnick, E. and Metcalf, D.
    (1980): J. Exp. Med., 152:1036.
11. Elias, L., Wogenrich, F.J., Wallace, J.M., and Longmire, J. (1980):
    Leuk. Res., 4:301-307.
12. Honma, Y., Kasukabe, T., and Hozumi, M. (1978): Exp. Cell Research,
    111:261-267.
13. Honma, Y., Kasukabe, T., Okabe, J., and Hozumi, M. (1977): Gann.
    68:241-246.
14. Honma, Y., Okabe, J., Kasukabe, T., and Hozumim, M. (1980): Gann.
    71: 543-547.
15. Horland, A.A., MacMarrow, L., and Wolman, S.R. (1980): Exp. Hematol.
    8:1025.
16. Ichikawa, Y. (1969): J. Cell Physiol., 74:223.
17. Kincade, P.W., Lee, G., Fernade, G., Moore, M.A.S., Williams, N.
    and Good, R.A. (1979): Proc. Natl. Acad. Sci.(USA), 76:3464.
18. Kubanek, B., Heit, W., and Rich, I.N. (1981): Exp. Hematol. 9
    (suppl. 9): 59.
19. Kurland, J.I., Pelus, L.M., Ralph, P., Bockman, R.S., and Moore,
    M.A.S. (1979): Proc. Natl. Acad. Sci. (USA), 76: 2326-2330.
20. Lachman, L.B., Hacker, M.P., Blyden, G.T., and Handschumacher, T.
    (1977): Cell. Immunol. 34:416.
21. Lotem, J., and Sachs, L. (1979): Proc. Natl. Acad. Sci. (Wash.)
    76:5158-5162.
22. Lotem, J., Lipton, J. and Sachs, L. (1980): Int. J. Cancer, 25:
    762-771.
23. Metcalf, D. (1980): Int. J. Cancer, 25:225-233.
24. Metcalf, D. (1979): Int. J. Cancer, 24:616-623.
25. Metcalf, D. and Moore, M.A.S. (1970): J. Natl. Cancer Inst., 44:801.

26. Metcalf, D., Moore, M.A.S., and Warner, N. (1969): <u>J. Natl. Cancer Inst.</u> 43:983.
27. Metcalf, D., Russell, S. and Burgess, A.W. (1978): <u>Transplant Proc.</u> 10:91.
28. Metcalf, D., Parker, J., Chester, H.M., Kincade, P.W. (1974): <u>J. Cell Physiol.</u> 84:275.
29. Moore, M.A.S., Spitzer, G., Williams, N., Metcalf, D., and Buckley, J. (1974): <u>Blood</u> 44:1-11
30. Pelus, L.M., Broxmeyer, H.E., Clarkson, B.D., and Moore, M.A.S. (1980): <u>Cancer Research</u>, 40:2525.
31. Ralph, P., Moore, M.A.S., and Nilsson, K. (1976): <u>J. Exp. Med.</u>, 143:1828.
32. Ralph, P., Broxmeyer, H.E., Moore, M.A.S., and Nakoinz, I. (1978): Cancer Res., 38:1414.
33. Rovera, G., O'Brien, T.G., and Diamond, L. (1979): <u>Science 204</u>:868.
34. Sachs, L., (1978): <u>Nature</u> 274:535
35. Tertian, G., Yung, Y.P., Guy-Grand, D., and Moore, M.A.S. (1981): <u>J. Immunol.</u> (in press).
36. Warner, N., Moore, M.A.S., Metcalf, D. (1969): <u>J. Natl. Cancer Inst.</u> 43:963.
37. Weiss, B., and Sachs, L. (1978): <u>Proc. Natl. Acad. Sci.</u> (Wash.) 75:1374-1378.
38. Williams, N., Eger, R.R., Moore, M.A.S., and Mendelsohn, N. (1978): <u>Differentiation</u> 11:59.
39. Williams, N., Jackson, H., Ralph, P., and Nakoinz, I. (1981): <u>Blood</u>, 57:157.
40. Yung, Y.P., and Moore, M.A.S. (1981): Submitted for publication.
41. Yung, Y.P., Eger, R., Tertian, G. and Moore, M.A.S. (1981): <u>J. Immunol.</u>(in press).

Expression of Differentiated Functions in Cancer Cells, edited by R. F. Revoltella et al., Raven Press, New York © 1982.

Expression of Lineage-Specific Surface Antigens in Human Non-Lymphocytic Leukemias

Bice Perussia, Deborah Lebman, *Beverly Lange, Jeffrey Faust, Giorgio Trinchieri, and Giovanni Rovera

*The Wistar Institute of Anatomy and Biology and *The Division of Oncology, Children's Hospital of Philadelphia, Philadelphia, Pennsylvania 19104*

SUMMARY

A panel of mouse monoclonal antibodies have been produced that are directed against surface differentiation antigens of human hematopoietic cells. These antibodies when screened against peripheral blood cells, can be grouped according to their reactivity with granulocytes, monocytes, or both; none of the antibodies reacted with T or B lymphocytes.

When tested for reactivity with bone marrow cells, four granulocyte-specific monoclonal antibodies (R1B19, B34.2, B40.1, L11.1) recognize surface antigens present on all cells of the myeloid lineage, including myeloblasts and promyelocytes, but do not react with erythroid elements. A monocyte-specific antibody (B44.1) reacts with monocytes, promonocytes, a fraction of promyelocytes, myelocytes and metamyelocytes. Two myelomonocytic-specific antibodies (B13.4 and B9.8) react with monocytes, granulocytes, metamyelocytes and a fraction of myelocytes. One antibody (L5.1) does not react with any cell in the peripheral blood but reacts specifically with immature erythroid precursor cells (proerythroblasts and erythroblasts).

The monoclonal antibodies were also tested for their reactivity with leukemic cells freshly obtained from patients with acute or chronic leukemias and against established lines of human leukemic cells. The antibodies reacting with normal immature myeloid cells were also able to detect surface antigens present on cells of patients with acute myeloid but not with acute lymphocytic leukemias. Antibodies reacting with mature myeloid cells and/or mature myelomonocytic cells reacted with the differentiated myeloid cells present in chronic myeloid leukemia. Antibodies directed against mature myelomonocytic cells (B9.8 and B13.4) reacted with myelomonocytic leukemia cells. Some of the monoclonal antibodies also reacted with established cell lines of human myeloid leukemia (HL60, KG1, ML3) and erythroleukemia (K562(S)). Surface markers of both the erythroid and myeloid lineage were present on two cell lines (HL60 and K562(S)). HL60 human promyelocytic leukemia cells reacted with all the monoclonal antibodies directed against immature myeloid cell surface antigens and with L5.1, an antibody that is directed against immature erythroid cells. The human K562(S) cell line reacted with L5.1 and with myeloid-specific antibodies (R1B19, B40.1, L11.1, B34.2).

The expression of the surface differentiation antigen recognized by monoclonal antibody R1B19, specific for myeloid cells, was not changed when promyelocytic leukemia HL60 cells were induced by 12-0-

tetradecanoyl-phorbol-13-acetate (TPA) treatment to differentiate into
macrophage-like cells. Mature myelomonocytic-specific markers
(recognized by B13.4 and B9.8) were expressed when HL60 cells were
induced to differentiate in vitro using TPA, but monocytic-specific
markers were not induced. The data indicate that TPA-induced differentiation in vitro is partially defective.

INTRODUCTION

Monoclonal antibodies have been used as a powerful tool in the
analysis of differentiation of the T lymphocytic lineage (25,26) and
in the identification of subclasses of lymphocytic leukemia cells
(4,13,22). More recently the possibility of inducing suppression of
tumor growth in vivo with monoclonal antibodies has also been
demonstrated (1,11).

Although an increasingly large number of monoclonal antibodies
directed against lymphoid cells has been described (17,22,25,26), only
a few directed against myeloid and myelomonocytic cells are presently
available. Two monoclonal antibodies, OKM1 and Mac 1, that react with
granulocytes, monocytes and natural killer cells have been reported
(5,29, 32), as well as several monoclonal antibodies that react specifically with human monocytes (31). But there is no information
available thus far to indicate the stage of differentiation of the
myeloid and monocytic lineages at which the antigens recognized by
antibodies are expressed. There are indications that such monoclonal
antibodies do not react, or react weakly, with myeloid leukemic cells
(5,31).

We have described two monoclonal antibodies (B13.4 and B9.8) specific for mature myelomonocytic cells and with myelomonocytic leukemia
cells (24). More recently we have examined the lineage and differentiation stage specificity of some other monoclonal antibodies directed
against mature and immature bone marrow cells. Some of these antibodies have been found to be reactive with surface antigens expressed on
myeloid leukemia and erythroleukemia cells either in culture or
freshly obtained from patients.

MATERIAL AND METHODS

1. Patients and sample preparation:

All patients in this study were evaluated at the Division of
Oncology, Children's Hospital of Philadelphia. The diagnosis of acute
lymphoblastic, myeloid or undifferentiated leukemia or chronic myelogenous leukemia was made by clinical, morphologic and cytochemical
criteria. Approximately 0.5 ml of heparinized bone marrow was
collected from untreated leukemic patients, from treated leukemic
patients in remission or relapse, and from patients with solid tumors
during evaluation for metastases. Consent was obtained for use of
each specimen in research.

Red cells and the majority of the granulocytes were separated from
the mononuclear cells in the samples using a Ficoll Hypaque (d =
1.078) density gradient centrifugation (3). All neoplastic samples
used in this study had at least 80% leukemic cells.

2. Cell lines:

HL60 (8) KG1 (15), ML3 (21) and K562(S) (7) cells were grown in
Breitman's synthetic medium (18) or in RPMI medium containing 15%
fetal bovine serum. All lymphoid lines were grown in RPMI containing
15% fetal bovine serum. HL60 cells were induced to differentiate in

culture into macrophage-like cells by treatment with TPA as previously described (19,27,28).

3. Production of monoclonal antibodies:

Monoclonal antibodies (16) were obtained as previously described (30). Balb/c mice were immunized with 2×10^7 peripheral blood cell subpopulations (granulocytes, monocytes) or with the myeloid leukemia cell line HL60. Spleen cells (10^8) obtained from the immunized animals were fused with 2×10^7 P3-x63-Ag8 or P3-x63-Ag8-6.5.3 mouse myeloma cells using 40% polyethylene glycol 1000 (30). Hybrids were selected in HAT medium. Positive clones were identified in radioimmunoassay 2 weeks after fusion: 5×10^5 target cells identical to those used for immunization were incubated with supernatant from growing hybrids. A second labeled antibody (lactoperoxidase ^{125}-labeled goat F(ab')$_2$ anti-mouse IgG/M) (Cappel Laboratories) was added after 3 washes and bound radioactivity in the pellet determined.

4. Testing of specific monoclonal antibodies:

Specificity of the antibodies for a given cellular lineage was determined by 1) a second radioimmunoassay against purified lymphocytes, granulocytes, monocytes and erythrocytes, 2) multi-parameter analysis of the peripheral blood cell population using a Cytofluorograf System 50HH (Ortho Instruments, Westwood, Mass.) equipped with a Lexcel Model 95-4 Argon Ion Laser (at 488 nm) and connected to a Data General MP200 Microprocessor Computer system, or 3) by sorting experiments. The hybrids producing monoclonal antibodies that reacted with only one or two lineages were cloned by limiting dilution. Positive colonies were expanded into mass cultures. Supernatants from the clones, concentrated 20 times by 50% (NH$_4$)$_2$SO$_4$ precipitation, were used thereafter. Immunoglobulin isotype was determined by immunodiffusion in Ouchterlony plates using goat anti-mouse Ig class antibodies (Meloy).

5. Indirect immunofluorescence:

$2-5 \times 10^5$ target cells were treated with 10 μl of the specific antibody at a chosen dilution, incubated at room temperature for 30 min and washed 3 times. The cells were then incubated with 20 μl of fluorescein-conjugated goat F(ab')$_2$ anti-mouse Ig (heavy and light chain) (Cappel) for 30 min at 4°C, and the percentage of fluorescent cells determined (18).

6. Analysis and sorting of bone marrow cells reactive to monoclonal antibodies:

Approximately 2×10^6 bone marrow cells, separated by Ficoll Hypaque gradient centrifugation (d = 1.078) were suspended in phosphate-buffered saline and were incubated with each antibody and stained by indirect immunofluorescence as described above. A control bone marrow cell suspension was treated only with fluorescein-conjugated second antibody. The level of background fluorescence was determined in the Cytofluorograf System 50HH using the control bone marrow, and a 1% and 5% positive cell baseline value was established.

The samples to be tested were then analyzed and sorted at a rate of 3,000 cells/sec with an 85% efficiency. Both positive and negative cell populations were collected, cytocentrifuged on slides, stained with May Grundwald-Giemsa and examined.

7. Other Reagents:

A monocytic-specific monoclonal antibody (63D3) described by Ugolini et al (31) was purchased from BRL.

RESULTS

In this study we have used monoclonal antibodies that are specific for myeloid cells, for monocytes and for both. We have also studied one antibody specifically reactive with immature erythroid cells.

The cell type specificity of the monoclonal antibodies was documented using peripheral blood leukocytes and the Cytofluorograf System 50HH cell sorter. Peripheral blood buffy coat was incubated with different antibodies and the cell population was analyzed using three parameters: forward light scatter, right angle light scatter and green fluorescence (Fig. 1). The lymphocytic, monocytic and granulocytic clusters were identified as described by Hoffman et al (12), and the percentage of cells within each cluster reacting with the antibodies tested was determined. Antibodies reacting specifically with monocytes, granulocytes or both populations are listed in Table I. The same Table also indicates the type of cells used for immunization, the type of immune response and the isotype of each monoclonal antibody.

TABLE I

Characteristics of monoclonal antibodies

Monoclonal antibody	Immunizing cells	Type of immune response	Mouse myeloma partner	Ig Isotype	Cellular Specificity
R1B19	HL60	secondary	P3-x63-Ag8-6.5.3	IgM	myelocytic
B34.2	granulocytes	secondary	P3-x63-Ag8-6.5.3	IgM	myelocytic
L11.1	HL60	primary	P3-x63-Ag8-6.5.3	IgM	myelocytic
B40.1	granulocytes	secondary	P3-x63-Ag8-6.5.3	IgM	myelocytic
B44.1	monocytes	secondary	P3-x63-Ag8-6.5.3	IgM	monocytic
B13.4	mononuclear peripheral blood cells	primary	P3-x63-Ag8	IgM	myelomono-cytic
B9.8	mononuclear peripheral blood cells	primary	P3-x63-Ag8	IgM	myelomono-cytic
L5.1	HL60	secondary	P3-x63-Ag8-6.5.3	IgG2a	immature erythroid

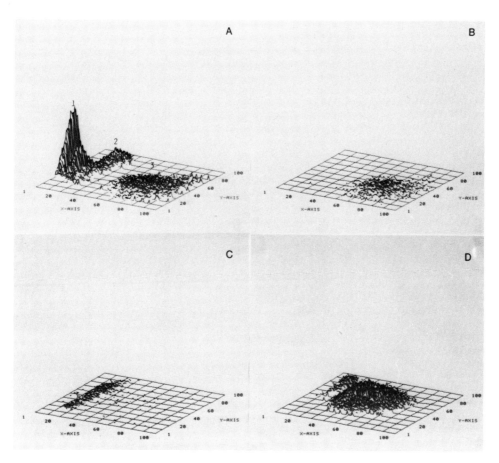

FIG. 1. Multiparameter analysis of normal peripheral blood
buffy coat. x axis, right angle light scatter; y axis, forward light scatter; z axis, number of cells.
A) Control untreated buffy coat cells. 1, lymphocytes; 2,
monocytes; 3, granulocytes.
B) Cells reacting with myeloid-specific antibody R1B19.
C) Cells reacting with monocytic-specific antibody B40.1.
D) Cells reacting with myelomonocytic-specific antibody
B13.4.
Peripheral blood buffy coat cells (10^6) were prepared as
described by Hoffman and co-workers (12) and incubated with
the indicated monoclonal antibodies. The washed cells were
incubated with FITC-conjugated F(ab')$_2$ goat anti-mouse
(IgG/M) immunoglobulin. Background fluorescence staining was
obtained by incubating cells with P3 cells supernatant and
developing with IgG/M-FITC.

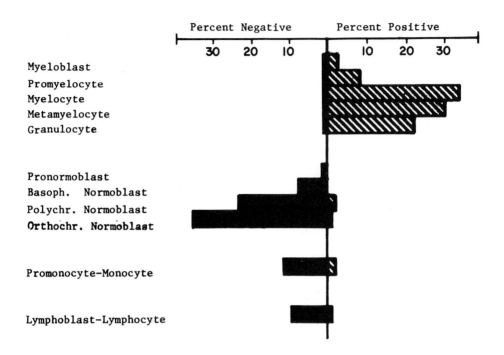

FIG. 2. Sorting analysis of bone marrow cells after incubation with a myeloid-specific antibody. Bone marrow cells
were incubated with R1B19 and developed with IgG/M-FITC.
On the right side of the panel are the cells positive with
the antibody expressed as percentages of the positively
sorted population. On the left side are the non-reactive
cells expressed as a percentage of the negatively sorted
population. Values represent pooled results from 3 separate
bone marrow sortings. Sorting efficiency was 85% The total
positive cells sorted were 31.5% of the total population.

In order to determine specificity for lineage and for differentiation stage, the antibodies listed in Table I were tested on bone
marrow elements. The positive and the negative cell populations were
sorted, collected by cytocentrifugation on slides and identified
morphologically after May Grundwald staining. Four granulocyte-
specific antibodies (R1B19, L11.1, B34.2, B40.1) reacted with every
morphologically recognizable immature, intermediate and mature myeloid
element. The cellular specificity of R1B19 is shown in Fig. 2.
Essentially the same pattern was observed with the other three antibodies of this group.

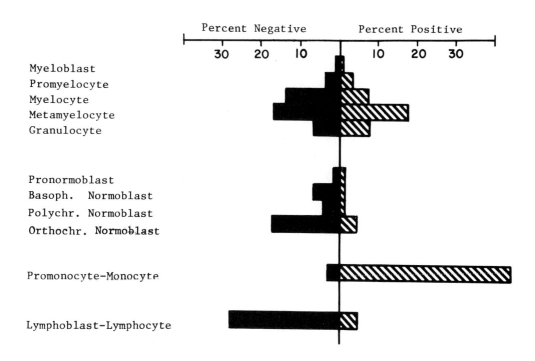

FIG. 3. Sorting analysis of bone marrow cells after incubation with monocytic-specific antibody (B44.1). See legend of Fig. 2 for experimental conditions. The total positive cells sorted were 8.6% of the total population.

The only monocyte-specific monoclonal antibody (B44.1) that we have tested so far reacted with monocytes, promyelocytes and a fraction of the bone marrow myelocytes and metamyelocytes (Fig. 3).

Two antibodies (B13.14 and B9.8) reacted with granulocytes and monocytes from the peripheral blood and with late and intermediate cells of the myeloid lineage (monocytes, metamyelocytes, a fraction of myelocytes).

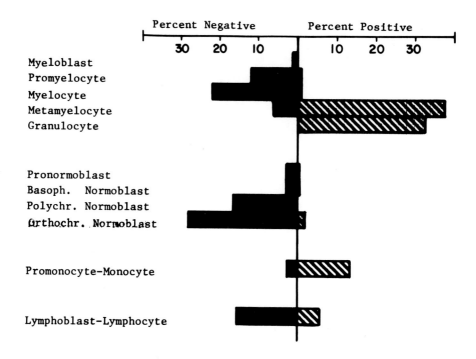

FIG. 4. Sorting analysis of bone marrow cells after incubation with myelomonocytic-specific antibody (B13.4). See
legend of Fig. 2 for experimental details. The total positive cells sorted were 20.3% of the total population.

Fig. 4 shows the reactivity of B13.4 with marrow cells. L5.1 antibody
was generated by immunizing Balb/c mice with HL60 human promyelocytic
leukemic cells and selected because of its negative reactivity with
peripheral blood white cells and weak positivity with HL60 cells.
When tested against normal marrow cells, only the cluster containing
immature erythroid cells was found to be positive (Fig. 5).

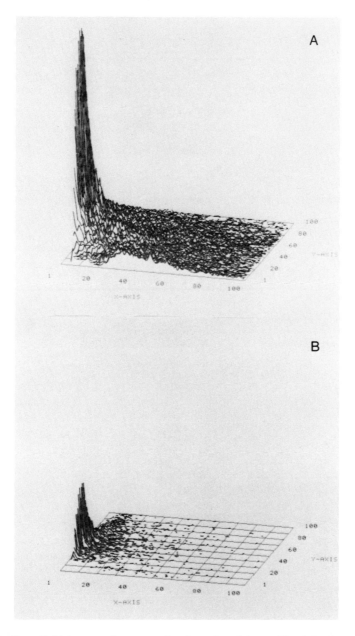

FIG. 5. Multiparameter analysis of anti-erythroblast-specific monoclonal antibody (L5.1). x axis, right angle light scattering; y axis, forward light scattering; z axis, number of cells. A) Bone marrow (Ficoll cut); B) Population of cells from A reacting with L5.1 antibody.

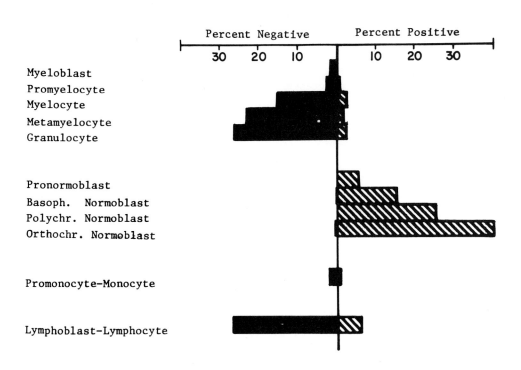

FIG. 6. Positive (right side of panel) and negative (left side of panel) cells morphologically identified after sorting of bone marrow cells treated with antibody L5.1. For experimental details see legend of Fig. 2. The total positive cells sorted were 22.9% of the total population.

Sorting analysis of bone marrow cells (Fig. 6) indicated that L5.1 antibody reacts with proerythroblasts, basophilic, polychromatic and orthochromatic erythroblasts but does not react with mature erythrocytes.

Reactivity of leukemic cells with monoclonal antibodies:
Some of the monoclonal antibodies described here were tested
against marrow and peripheral blood samples obtained from leukemic
patients and in which leukemic cell replacement was at least 80%.
Table II lists the clinical diagnosis and the reactivity of these
antibodies with the leukemic cells.

B13.4 reacted only with myelomonocytic leukemias but not with
other types of myeloblastic leukemia. R1B19, B34.2 and B40.1 reacted
with acute myeloblastic leukemias. All anti-myeloid reagents reacted
with chronic myeloid leukemia cells. None of the myeloid-specific
antibodies have so far been found to react with clearly documented
cases of T or B lymphoblastic leukemias.

TABLE II

Reactivity of a panel of monoclonal antibodies with leukemia cells

Type of Leukemia	Monoclonal Antibody					
	R1B19	B34.2	B40.1	B13.4	B9.8	L5.1
Acute myeloblastic	1/1	1/1	1/1	0/1	0/5	NT
Acute promyelocytic	1/1	1/1	1/1	0/1	0/2	NT
Acute myelomonocytic	1/1	1/1	1/1	1/1	NT	NT
Acute monocytic	1/1	1/1	1/1	NT	NT	0/1
Chronic myelocytic	1/1	5/5	4/4	2/2	2/2	NT
T ALL	0/2	0/4	0/4	0/3	0/2	NT
B and Null ALL	0/2	0/18	0/16	0/10	0/18	0/1
Non-classified	NT	1/4	1/4	0/2	0/4	NT

The number of cases positive out of the total number of cases tested with
each antibody is reported.
The monoclonal antibodies were tested by indirect immunofluorescence at dilutions previously determined by titration to saturate all binding sites on positive cells.
Leukemic cells were at least 70% of total population in all cases tested.
Positivity indicates that at least 50% of the cells reacted with a given
monoclonal antibody.

NT - not tested.

Reactivity of monoclonal antibodies against established cell
lines:
When the monoclonal antibodies were tested against different
myeloid and erythroid cell lines, the pattern of reactivity was quite
typical (Table III). The K562(S) reacted with the L5.1 but also with
monoclonal antibodies directed against immature myeloid markers
(R1B19, B34.2, L11.1, B40.1).

Myeloid leukemic cell lines (HL60, ML3, KG1) reacted with all the
antibodies recognizing immature myeloid leukemic cell markers.
However HL60 cells also reacted with the anti-erythroid L5.1. The
percentage of cells positive with this antibody fluctuated with

TABLE III

Reactivity of monoclonal antibodies with leukemic cell lines

Cell Line	Monoclonal Antibodies					
	R1B19	B34.2	L11.1	B13.4	B40.1	L5.1
HL60	100	100	100	0	75	25
ML3	100	100	100	0	95	0
KG1	2	25	10	0	30	6
K562(S)	35	55	55	0	35	55

*All monoclonal antibodies were added at dilutions previously deter-
mined by titration to saturate all binding sites on positive cells.
The values indicate percent of positive cells by indirect
immunofluorescence.

culture conditions. Sorted positive cells were promyelocytes. Eight
B lymphoid cell lines and five T lymphoid cell lines were found to be
negative by radioimmunoassay with all the antibodies tested.

Expression of differentiation antigens in leukemic cells induced
to differentiate:
It was of interest to determine whether surface antigen expression
was modified after treatment of human promyelocytic leukemia (HL60)
cells with TPA, an agent which causes HL60 cells to differentiate into
macrophage-like cells (19,27,28). A monocyte-specific antibody
(B44.1), a myelomonocytic-specific antibody (B13.4), a myeloid-
specific antibody that is non-reactive with monocytes (R1B19), and the
anti-erythroblast antibody (L5.1) were tested on TPA-treated HL60
cells. A monocytic-specific antibody (63D3) developed by Ugolini et
al (31) was also tested. A time sequence of changes of such surface
markers after TPA treatment is reported in Table IV. The
myelomonocytic-specific antibody reacted with TPA-treated HL60, but
monocytic-specific antibodies did not react with HL60 cells at any
time after TPA treatment. The antibody R1B19, reacting specifically
with myeloid cells and HL60 cells prior to treatment, also reacted
with TPA treated-cells. Positivity of HL60 cells to the erythroblast-
specific antibody, L5.1, disappeared after TPA treatment.

TABLE IV

Appearance of Surface Antigens Following Treatment of HL60 cells with TPA

Days after TPA treatment[1]	Monoclonal Antibodies				
	R1B19	B13.4	B44.1	L5.1	63D3[2]
day 0	100	0	0	25	0
day 1	100	0	0	NT	0
day 2	100	100	2	0	0
day 3	100	80	0	NT	0
day 4	100	80	0	NT	0

All monoclonal antibodies were added at dilutions previously determined by titration to saturate all binding sites on positive cells. Values represent percent of positive cells by indirect immunofluorescence.

[1] TPA (12-O-tetradecanoyl-phorbol-13-acetate) was added to the cultures at the final concentration of 1.6×10^{-8} M.

[2] 63D3 is a monoclonal antibody against monocytes described by Ugolini et al (11).

DISCUSSION

We have presented here a preliminary characterization of several monoclonal antibodies reacting with normal and leukemic cells of the myeloid, monocytic and erythroid lineages. Granulocytic-specific and erythroid-specific monoclonal antibodies have not been described until now, though Ugolini et al (31) have reported a monocyte-specific antibody. The myelomonocytic antibodies described here (B9.8 and B13.4) differ from OKM1, which is reactive with granulocytes, monocytes and natural killer cells, in that they do not react with any peripheral blood subpopulation of lymphocytes. It is not presently clear whether the different antibodies within each given class recognize the same surface determinants. Competition experiments as well as biochemical characterization of the surface antigens recognized by such antibodies are currently in progress. Preliminary results indicate that the two myelomonocytic antibodies react with two distinct antigenic determinants.

The presence of markers of both erythroid and myeloid lineages in vitro on K562(S) cells and the fact that an anti-erythroid antibody reacts with HL60 cells suggests the possibility that some leukemic cell lines in culture are bipotent or multipotent. Our data confirm the finding of Drew et al (9), who have shown, using conventional antisera, that the erythroleukemic cell line K562 expresses specific human granulocytic antigens. It remains to be determined whether such bipotent or multipotent leukemic cells occur in some types of leukemias in vivo. The increased availability of monoclonal reagents in panel form should answer such questions.

The appearance of only some mature surface markers in vitro during the process of differentiation induced by the phorbol diester TPA indicates that the program of macrophagic differentiation in HL60 promyelocytic leukemia cells is incompletely expressed.

The reactivity of monocytic-specific antibodies with a fraction of myeloid immature cells could be interpreted in two ways. Either the surface markers detected by such antibodies are also expressed on a small subpopulation of myeloid cells, or a subpopulation of myelocytes and metamyelocytes are the natural precursors of monocytes and macrophages. The antibodies described here could be valuable for several reasons. An adequate number of monoclonal antibodies could be used in panel form for more accurate differential diagnosis of lymphoblastic and myeloblastic leukemias and in the positive identification of some undifferentiated leukemias. Such distinctions are important because of the drastically different prognosis and therapeutic approach of the two types of leukemias (23). Secondly, it is possible that those antibodies reacting with myeloid leukemia cells might have some future therapeutic value in vivo; they could be used individually or, even better, in association to reduce the number of leukemic cells present in the organism, either by reacting directly with the target cells or indirectly, as carriers for toxic agents like subunits of ricin or diphtheria toxin (10). The fact that all the myeloid lineage leukemic cells as well as normal cells could be selectively depleted by such treatment should not represent a major obstacle, provided that multipotent stem cells could recolonize such lineages. Studies on the effect of such antibodies on progenitor and stem cells in adequate colony assays and long term cultures will indicate how far back in the process of differentiation the surface antigens detected are expressed on the surface of the cells. More information about the reactivity of such antibodies against non-hematopoietic cells will also be needed since the pattern of reactivity with other cell types in the organism is known presently for only a few of these antibodies. It is possible that the IgM monoclonal antibodies will not be effective in vivo (2), and thus the coupling of the antibodies to toxic agents or other chemotherapeutic agents should then be considered to obtain more efficient target cell killing in vivo.

In conclusion, the availability of these and other antibodies directed against myeloid monocytic and erythroid cell precursors will allow us to understand better the differentiative disorders of non-lymphocytic leukemias.

ACKNOWLEDGEMENTS

This work was supported by grants CA-10815, CA-11796, CA-14489, CA-20833, CA-21069, CA-21124 and CA-25875 from the National Cancer Institute and from the W.W. Smith Memorial Fund. Beverly Lange is a clinical fellow of the American Cancer Society.

We thank Dr. J. Minowada for the gift of ML3 cells and Drs. H.P. Koeffler and D. Golde for the gift of KG1 cells.

We thank Marina Hoffman for editing and Ann McNab for typing the manuscript.

REFERENCES

1. Bernstein, I.D., Nowinski, R.C., Tam, M.R., McMaster, B., Houston, L.L. and Clerk, F.A. (1980): In: Monoclonal Antibodies, edited by R.H. Kenneth, T.J. McKearn, K.B. Bechtol, pp. 275-291. Plenum, New York.
2. Bernstein, I.D., Tam, M.R. and Nowinski, R.C. (1980): Science, 207: 68-71.
3. Boyum, A. (1968): Scand. J. Clin. Lab. Invest., 21(Suppl. 97): 77-89.
4. Bradstock, K.F., Janossy, G., Pizzolo, G., Hoffbromd, A.V., McMichael, A., Pilch, J.R., Milstein, C., Beverley, P. and Bollum, F.J. (1980): J. Nat. Cancer Inst., 65: 33-39.
5. Breard, J., Reinherz, E.L., Kung, P.C., Goldstein, G. and Schlossman, S.F. (1980): J. Immunol., 124: 1943-1948.
6. Breitman, T.R., Collins, S.J. and Keene, B.R. (1980): Exp. Cell Res., 126: 494-497.
7. Cioe, L., McNab, A., Hubbell, H.R., Meo, P., Curtis, P. and Rovera, G. (1981): Cancer Res., 41: 237-244.
8. Collins, S.J., Gallo, R.C. and Gallagher, R.E. (1977): Nature, 270: 347-349.
9. Drew, S.I., Terasaki, P.I., Bellmy, R.J., Bergh, O.J., Minowada, J. and Klein, E. (1977): Blood, 49: 715-718.
10. Gilliland, D.G., Steplewski, Z., Collier, R.J., Mitchell, K.F., Chang, T.H. and Koprowski, H. (1980): Proc. Nat. Acad. Sci., 17: 4539-4543.
11. Herlyn, D.M., Steplewski, Z., Herlyn, M.F. and Koprowski, H. (1980): Cancer Res., 40: 717-721.
12. Hoffman, R.A., Kung, P.C., Hansen, W.P. and Goldstein, G. (1980): Proc. Nat. Acad. Sci. USA, 77: 4914-4917.
13. Janossy, G., Bollum, F.J., Bradstock, K.F. and Ashley, J. (1980): Blood, 56: 430-441.
14. Kekwick, R.A. (1940): Biochem. J., 34: 1248-1257.
15. Koeffler, H.P. and Golde, D.W. (1980): Blood, 56: 344-350.
16. Koehler. G. and Milstein, C. (1975): Nature, 256: 495-497.
17. Ledbetter, J.A., Evans, R.L., Lipinski, M., Cunningham Rundles, C., Good, R.A. and Herzemberg, L.A. (1981): J. Exp. Med., 153: 310-323.
18. Loor, F., Forni, L. and Pernis, B. (1972): Eur. J. Immunol., 2: 203-212.
19. Lotem and Sachs. (1979): Proc. Nat. Acad. Sci. USA, 76: 5158-5162.
20. McMichael, A.M., Pilch, J.R., Galfre, G., Mason, D.Y., Fabre, J.W. and Milstein, C. (1979): Eur. J. Immunol., 9: 205-210.
21. Minowada, personal communication
22. Nadler, L.M., Ritz, J., Hardy, R., Pesando, J.M., Schlossman, S.F. and Stashenko, P. (1981): J. Clin. Invest., 67: 134-140.
23. Necheles, T.F. (1979): The Acute Leukemias: Clinical Monographs in Hematology., edited by T.F. Necheles. Stratton Interc. Med. Book Corp.
24. Perussia, B., Lebman, D., Ip, S.H., Rovera, G. and Trinchieri, G. (1981): submitted for publication.
25. Reinherz, E.L. and Schlossman, S.F. (1980): Cell, 19: 821-827.
26. Reinherz, E.L. and Schlossman, S.F. (1980): New Engl. J. Med., 203: 370-372.

27. Rovera, G., O'Brien, T. and Diamond, L. (1979): Science, 204: 868-870.
28. Rovera, G., Santoli, D. and Damsky, C. (1979): Proc. Nat. Acad. Sci. USA, 76: 2779-2783.
29. Springer, T., Galfre, G., Secher, D.S. and Milstein, C. (1979): Europ. J. Immunol., 9: 301-306.
30. Tonkonogy, S., Trinchieri, G., Perussia, B. and Nabholz, M. (1980): Human Immunol., 1: 111-120.
31. Ugolini, V., Nunez, G., Smith, R.G., Stastny, P. and Capra, J.D. (1980): Proc. Nat. Acad. Sci. USA, 77: 6764-6768.
32. Zarling, J.M. and Kung, P.C. (1980): Nature, 288: 394-396.

Expression of Differentiated Functions in Cancer Cells, edited by R. F. Revoltella et al., Raven Press, New York © 1982.

Structural and Functional Markers During Induced Differentiation in Human Leukemia Cell Lines

*†Leif C. Andersson, **Martti A. Siimes, †Eero Lehtonen, and ‡Carl G. Gahmberg

*Transplantation Laboratory, Departments of †Pathology, **Pediatrics, and ‡Biochemistry, University of Helsinki, SF-00290 Helsinki 29, Finland*

The cells of the hematopoietic system undergo continuous renewal. Originating from a common pluripotent stem cell the functionally specialized blood and lymphoid tissue cells emerge through differentiation along discrete pathways. The proliferation and maturation in the different hematopoietic lineages are normally strictly regulated by still incompletely known homeostatic mechanisms.

Malignant transformation in the hematopoietic system does not always imply a complete loss of the basic feature of the hematopoietic cell, namely its differentiation capacity. E.g., in the Philadelphia chromosome positive chronic granulocytic leukemia the karyotypic marker can be followed to a stem cell level. This indicates that the oncogenic transformation has occurred at an early progenitor stage. The malignant cells continuously differentiate during the chronic phase of the disease. Eventually the differentition stops and immature blast cells accumulate resulting in blast crisis. Leukemias and lymphomas are currently classified according to the phenotype of the majority of the accumulating cells. Information about the earliest malignantly transformed cell is rarely obtained.

Maturation arrest of malignant cells at a level before the loss of the proliferative capacity is a prerequisite for successful establishment of hematopoietic cell lines. Such cell lines originating from human leukemias and lymphomas have provided useful models for detailed studies on cytobiological mechanisms acting during normal and malignant hematopoiesis. As first demonstrated in the murine system with the Friend leukemia cells (6), malignant hematopoietic blasts can be induced to further functional differentiation under tissue culture conditions. Recently several hematopoietic human cell lines have been described which upon cultivation in the presence of different compounds are inducible to morphological and functional differentiation.

We have recently been investigating cell lines which represent main lineages of the hematopoietic system. Some of our findings are briefly summarized here.

The K562, a human erythroleukemic cell line was originally established by Lozzio & Lozzio from the pleural effusion of a patient with chronic granulocytic leukemia in terminal blast crisis. This cell line was considered to represent an early progenitor of the granulocytic series (12). However, the real phenotype of this cell line was under dispute. The K562 cell line was not originally cloned and the possibility exists that there are several sublines available with slightly different phenotypic characteristics.

Our K562 cell line was obtained from professor G. Klein, Stockholm. When analyzing the surface glycoprotein profiles of a large panel of human hematopoietic cell lines, we observed that the K562 cell line showed a surface glycoprotein profile which was distinctly different from that obtained with cells of the granulocytic series of either benign or malignant origin (3). We also found that a heteroantiserum raised against K562 cells and extensively adsorbed to nonreactivity against granulocytes and myeloblasts still showed strong reactivity with the erythroid lineage of normal bone marrow (3). Subsequently we observed that the K562 line showed a strong surface expression of glycophorin A which is the main sialoglycoprotein of the normal red cell membrane. This protein has been shown to constitute a selective marker for the erythroid lineage in normal hematopoiesis (8). Finally, a low but constant basal synthesis of fetal hemoglobin (2) was demonstrated in K562 cells. These findings have been confirmed by other investigators (13).

Since these findings strongly indicated the K562 cell line to be an early representative of the erythroid lineage we tried to induce further differentiation in vitro with compounds previously reported to be active in the murine Friend leukemia system. Our K562 cells did not respond to dimethyl sulphoxide (DMSO). Instead, sodium butyrate at concentrations of 1-2 mmol induced enhanced hemoglobin synthesis, benzidine positivity and formation of spherical, hemoglobin-containing particles in culture (2). We have recently found that diazepam at concentrations of 50-60 ug/ml and retinoic acid at concentrations of 10^{-7}-10^{-8}M also are efficient inducers of differentiation in the K562 cells (Fig. la). Rutherford et al. first reported that hemin is also an inducer of maturation in K562 cells (13). The addition of hemin increases synthesis of embryonic and fetal hemoglobin.

During the sequence of induced differentiation in K562 cells there is a decrease in the surface expression of glycophorin A and a switch in the mobility of a major surface glycoprotein, GP105. The latter may be due to changes in the carbohydrate portion of the glycoprotein and not caused by induction of synthesis of new surface proteins (1).

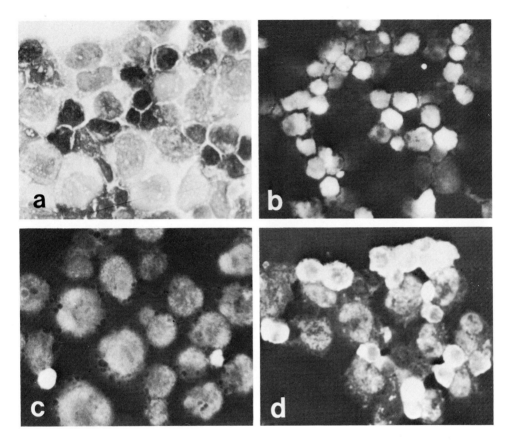

Figure 1.   a) Accumulation of normoblast-like, condensed
cells in a culture of K562 treated with retinoid acid (RA)
10^{-7} M for five days.   MGC staining.
b) RA-induced K562 cells stained with FITC-conjugated
rabbit anti-fetal hemoglobin antiserum.
c) Non-induced K562 cells stained with FITC-conjugated
anti-spectrin antiserum.
d) RA-induced K562 stained with FITC-conjugated rabbit
anti-spectrin antibodies.

The K562 cell line provides a tool for studies on biosynthesis of previously well-characterized erythroid
components.   We have recently isolated the messenger RNA
fraction from K562 cells, which codes for the glycophorin A
molecule, and studied the synthesis of glycophorin A in a
cell-free system (10).   In the absence of membranes a
precursor form of glycophorin A was synthesized.   This was
identified by antiserum.   The molecular weight of the
carbohydrate-free precursor was 19 500.   This exceeds the

molecular weight of the glycophorin A apoprotein with approximately 5000 which may correspond to a signal sequence of about 45 amino acid residues. In the presence of membranes from dog pancreas the synthesized glycophorin A precursor was both N and O glycosylated. The oligosaccharide side-chains of the in vitro synthesized glycophorin remained incompleted and corresponded to the glycosylated precursor form of glycophorin A which we have previously isolated from intact K562 cells (11). The glycophorin A molecule which carries both N and O glycosidic side-chains constitutes an interesting model for further in vitro studies on the principles for the assembly of different carbohydrate structures of mammalian surface glycoproteins.

We have recently studied the distribution of another erythroid component, spectrin, in uninduced and induced K562 cells by direct immunofluorescence with rabbit antispectrin antiserum. In uninduced K562 cells the antispectrin antiserum stains the nuclear areas and a weak net-like configuration is seen in the cytoplasm (Fig. 1c). During sodium butyrate or retinoic acid induction there is an increase in the spectrin staining in the cytoplasm. The spectrin accumulates close to the outer surface and especially in the normoblast-like, fetal hemoglobin containing condensed cells (Fig. 1d).

CHANGES IN THE SURFACE GLYCOPROTEIN PATTERN OF THE PROMYELOCYTIC LEUKEMIA LINE HL-60 DURING INDUCED MORPHOLOGICAL AND FUNCTIONAL DIFFERENTIATION

The HL-60 promyelocytic leukemia line was established by Collins et al. (4). This cell line can be induced to terminal granulocytic differentiation by cultivation in the presence of DMSO (5). The HL-60 cells acquire phagocytotic and chemotactic capacities during differentiation. We followed the changes in the surface glycoprotein pattern during the sequence of induced differentiation of the HL-60 cells. The uninduced cells had a major surface glycoprotein with an apparent molecular weight of 160000 (GP160). During morphological and functional differentiation this band disappeared and a new band with a lower molecular weight of 130000 (GP130) occurred. The expression of the GP130 coincided with the acquisition of mitotic and chemotactic capacities. The molecular weight of this protein on the induced cells corresponds to the major labeled band of normal granulocytes. We observed an inversed relationship between the presence of GP160 and GP130 which suggests a product/precursor relationship. This was further confirmed by the finding that both GP160 and GP130 could be precipitated with the same rabbit heteroantiserum which apparently reacted with common determinants (9). The changed electrophoretic mobility might therefore be due to alterations in the carbohydrate moieties of the glycoprotein occurring during the differentiation of the cells. A possible functional involvement of the GP130 was obtained through the observation that this protein is poorly visualized after surface labeling of granulocytes from patients with monosomy-7 (7). Granulocytes from such patients have a normal random mobility but do not respond to chemotactic stimuli (14). This indicates that GP130 might be involved in the chemotactic response and that the expression and/or glycosylation of this particular protein is related to chromosome 7.

JOK-1, A HAIRY CELL LEUKEMIA LINE INDUCIBLE TO DIFFERENTIATION

During the past few years the derivation of the cell accumulating in bone marrow and spleen in hairy cell leukemia or malignant reticuloendotheliosis has been extensively discussed. Mitotic figures are rarely seen in biopsy material. The accumulating cells might therefore represent an end stage of a differentiation process. In most instances the hairy cells have been found to carry monoclonally distributed immunoglobulins on their surface indicating a relationship to the B lymphocytic lineage.

We have recently established a continuously growing cell line from the blood of a patient with hairy cell leukemia (1). This cell line, called JOK-1, grows in suspension cultures and shows a surface glycoprotein profile rather similar to that obtained from cells freshly isolated from patients with hairy cell leukemia. The cells also form colonies in soft agar, have an abnormal hyperdiploid karyotype and are phenotypically different from EBV-infected lymphoblastoid cell lines established from the same patient. Scanning electron microscopy has revealed that the JOK-1 cell line has rather smooth outer surface. After cultivation for 2-3 days in the presence of 2 mmol sodium butyrate or TPA 10^{-7} M, the JOK-1 cells form larger aggregates and the surface is covered by slender "hairy" projections (Fig. 2). Concomitantly cells acquire increased tartrate-resistant phosphatase activity which is considered to be a typical marker for the hairy cell leukemia. During this sequence of maturation slight changes in the surface glycoprotein profile have also been observed. "New" bands with apparent molecular weights of 57000, 46000 and 37000 appeared (1). An increased alpha-naphthyl-acetate esterase activity could also be recorded during induced differentiation.

These findings indicate that the JOK-1 cell line apparently respresents a precursor form of the mature hairy cells. The phenotype of the JOK-1 is compatible with that of an early representative of the B lymphocytic lineage.

CONCLUDING REMARKS

The continuous hematopoietic human cell lines described here exemplify the panel of currently available inducible lymphoma and leukemia lines. Such cell lines give additional information about the biological behaviour of hemato-

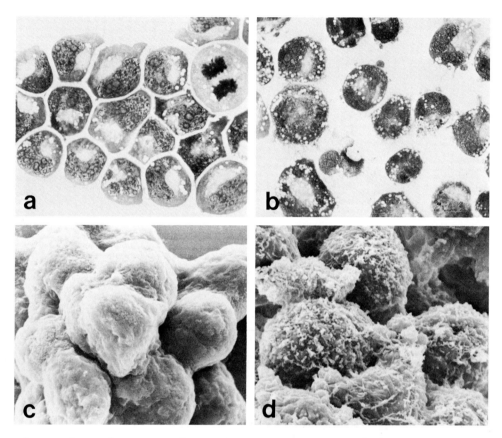

Figure 2. a) Smear of JOK-1 cells. MGG-staining.
b) Smear of JOK-1 cells cultivated in the presence of 2 mM
Na-butyrate for three days.
c) Scanning electron microscopy photographs of non-induced
JOK-1 cells and
d) butyrate-induced JOK-1 cells.

poetic malignancies. They show that the leukemia or
lymphoma cells are not definitely "frozen" at a certain
stage of differentiation but have merely lost their
responsiveness to physiological stimuli which guide the
maturation of the corresponding normal cell lines. Recent
observations indicate that malignant hematopoietic cells
freshly isolated from both patients and cell lines established from lymphomas and leukemias can be induced to
further and sometimes terminal differentiation in vitro
with a variety of compounds. This opens interesting
approaches for the future treatment of hematopoietic
malignancies.

Changes in surface glycoprotein profile observed during induced differentiation of various normal and malignant hematopoetic cells are usually characterized by differences in the quantitative expression and/or electrophoretic mobility of certain surface proteins. Such changes are apparently due to alterations of the glycosylation of preexisting molecules and does not necessarily imply neosynthesis of surface proteins. It is tempting to assume that many of the surface structures recently recognized by monoclonal antibodies as differentiation antigens are in fact alterations in the carbohydrate structures of preexisting molecules. This would also imply that the genetic regulations of the differentiation-associated surface antigens might be expressed through activation and inactivation of specific carbohydrate transferases or hydrolases.

REFERENCES

1. Andersson, L.C., and Gahmberg, C.G. Proc. 3rd Annual Bristol-Myers Symposium on Cancer Res., 1980, in press.
2. Andersson, L.C., Jokinen, M., and Gahmberg, C.G. (1979): Nature 278:364.
3. Andersson, L.C., Nilsson, K., and Gahmberg, C.G. (1979): Int. J. Cancer 23:143.
4. Collins, S.J., Callo, R.C., and Gallagher, R.E. (1977): Nature 270:347.
5. Collins, S.J., Ruscetti, F.W., Gallagher, R.E., and Callo, R.C. (1978): Proc. Natl. Acad. Sci. U.S.A. 75:2458.
6. Friend, C., Scher, W., Holland, J.G., and Soto, T. (1971): Proc. Natl. Acad. Sci. U.S.A. 68:378.
7. Gahmberg, C.G., Andersson, L.C., Ruutu, P., Timonen, T., Hänninen, A., Vuopio, P., and de la Chapelle, A. (1979) Blood 54:401.
8. Gahmberg, C.G., Jokinen, M., and Andersson, L.C. (1978): Blood 52:379.
9. Gahmberg, C.G., Nilsson, K., and Andersson, L.C. (1979): Proc. Natl. Acad. Sci. 76:4987.
10. Jokinen, M., Ulmanen, I., Andersson, L.C., Kääriäinen, L., and Gahmberg, C.G. (1981): Eur. J. Biochem. 114:393.
11. Jokinen, M., Gahmberg, C.G., and Andersson, L.C. (1979): Nature 279:604.
12. Lozzio, C.B., and Lozzio, B.B. (1975): Blood 45:321.
13. Rutherford, T.R., Clegg, J.B., and Weatherall, D.J. (1979): Nature 280:164.
14. Ruutu, P., Ruutu, T., Vuopio, P., Kosunen, T., and de la Chapelle, A. (1977): Nature 265:146.

Expression of Differentiated Functions in Cancer Cells, edited by R. F. Revoltella et al., Raven Press, New York © 1982.

Induction of Differentiation in the Human Diploid Multipotential Cell Line CM-S

R. P. Revoltella, E. Vigneti, R. H. Butler, E. Gresick,
*G. Lambertenghi-Deliliers, **M. D. Cappellini, †P. Musiani,
†M. Piantelli, and ‡G. Monaco

*Laboratorio di Biologia Cellulare, C.N.R., Roma; *Prima Cattedra e **Terza Cattedra di Clinica Medica, Università degli Studi di Milano, Milano; †Istituto di Anatomia Patologia dell'Università Cattolica del Sacro Cuore, Roma; ‡Istituto di Anatomia Comparata, Università degli Studi di Roma, Roma, Italy*

Within the past few years, various autonomous haematopoietic cell lines have been established that retain distinctive markers of primitive haematopoietic cells and are capable of spontaneous or inducible further maturation and differentiation in vitro, depending upon the specific microenvironment the cells inhabit (8,10,19,7,3,4,13,1,14,11). The majority of these cell lines, however, show chromosome alterations, usually aneuploidy, and are frequently tumorigenic in syngeneic or athymic mice hosts. Although these lines have provided useful models for studying some cell differentiated functions as well as some of the regulatory factors acting during haematopoiesis, these lines probably do not fulfil the genetically programmed functional state of "normal" haematopoietic stem cells, due to their malignant origin.

We report that we have now isolated an autonomous haematopoietic diploid cell line, CM-S, where the cells retain, so far, a stable euploid karyotype, do not spontaneously grow in agar or in athymic mice, are multipotential (carry distinctive markers of early precursors of the monocytic, granulocytic and erythroid series) and, in the presence of appropriate inducing compounds added to their microenvironment, can further differentiate in liquid culture, at least along the monocyte-macrophagic and erythroid lineages.

The present report will review, in part, the results of our preliminary studies on CM-S cells and the patterns of differentiation observed
when CM-S cells are grown in vitro in the presence of various inducing
agents.

CM-S cells.

CM-S was established as an autonomous cell line approximately 14 months ago, from a bone marrow sample obtained from a 3 year-old male patient
affected by congenital hypoplastic (Diamond-Blackfan) anemia (5,6,9),
an uncommon non-neoplastic childhood defect in erythropoiesis. CM-S grow
in suspension culture in tightly closed flasks at 37°C , in Dulbecco's
modified Eagle's medium supplemented with 20% fetal calf serum, 10% try-
pticase soy broth and antibiotics. When the cells are seeded at a concentration of 1.0-1.5 x10^6 cells per ml, they reach a saturation density of
5-6 x10^6 cells per ml in 4-5 days , with a doubling time of approximately
48 hours. Instead, when they are seeded at lower concentrations, their
growth capacity is delayed and below about 0.1-0.3 x10^6 cells per ml they
do not replicate.

Untreated CM-S : morphologic and functional characteristics.

CM-S cells grow in suspension, but tend to aggregate and form clumps.
By May-Gründwald-Giemsa (see Fig.1), the majority of the cells (70 to 90
%) are undifferentiated, large, mononuclear cells. Rarely (0.1 to 10%)
giant, polynuclear cells are seen. The remaining cells are small, mononuclear cells displaying morphologic characteristics of more differentiated
haematopoietic cells. The cells, in general, show an eccentric indented
nucleus with fine, dispersed chromatin and one to several nucleoli; the
abundant cytoplasm of the larger cells often contains some azurophilic
granules. The cells often show a perinuclear halo. Transmission electron
microscopy (Plate 1, c) showed that CM-S cells have indented nuclei,
frequent mitochondria, a relatively abundant endoplasmic reticulum profi-

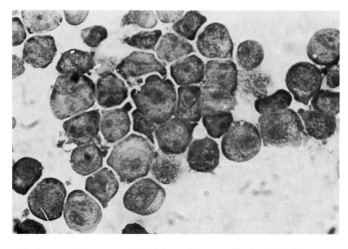

Fig. 1. Morphology of CM-S cell line (May-Gründwald-Giemsa stain,x1,600)

le, free ribosomes and a well developed Golgi apparatus. The cytoplasm of the larger cells often contains vacuoles and rare lysosomal bodies.

Under normal culture conditions, CM-S cells express some enzyme markers and functional properties characteristic of granulocytic, monocytic and erythroid cells. No evidence of lymphoid cells was detected ,by combined cytochemical and immunological analyses. Table 1 summarizes these properties.

TABLE 1.   PROPERTIES OF THE CM-S CELL LINE

Properties/Reagents	Percent Positive Cells[1]			
	Untreated	TPA $(10^{-6}M)$	Dexamethasone $(25\,\mu g$ per ml$)$	PHA-CM $(.05$ ml 1:10 per ml$)$
Enzyme cytochemical staining:				
Granulocytic markers:				
Sudan black	10	0	0	0
Specific esterase (AS-D-chloroacetate)	30	20	2-10	0
Myeloperoxidase	20	0	0	0
Monocyte-macrophage markers:				
Acid phosphatase	40	80	15	0
Cytochrome oxidase	100	100	10	10
α-Naphthol-acetate esterase				
NaF -	100	100	5-15	10
" + (1.5 mg/ml)	10	10	0	0
α-Naphthyl-acetate esterase	80	100	20	10
Erythroid markers:				
Glycophorin-A	90	60	100	100
Spectrin	2-5	0	50	80
Hemoglobin (Hbγ)	0	0	1-5	80
Lymphoid markers:				
Ig (all classes):				
intracellular,surface,release	0	0	0	0
Sheep erythrocyte-receptors	0	0	0	0
β-Glucuronidase	0	0	0	0
Functional properties:				
Receptors F_c	1-5	60-80	20	20
C3	1-5	60-80	15-30	20
Adherence	no	yes	no	no
Phagocytosis	1-5	80	20	20

[1] After 4 days in culture.

CM-S express membrane histocompatibility (HLA.ABC and HLA.DR) antigens(15). (Table3)In collaboration with Dr.Gianni Rovera, The Wistar Institute of Anatomy and Biology of Philadelphia, we have also tested CM-S cells with a panel of monoclonal antibodies directed against different surface-differentiation antigens specifically associated with granulocytic, monocytic and erythroid cell precursors. The results of these preliminary screenings, reported in Table 2, confirmed that unstimulated CM-S cells are rather heterogeneous, comprising cells at different levels of maturation along different haematopoietic pathways.

TABLE 2 . IMMUNOLOGICAL MARKERS ON CM-S CELLS DETECTED
BY MONOCLONAL ANTIBODIES.

Monoclonal antibodies[1]	Lineage Specificity	Positive Cells[2] %
Anti-HLA.DR:H-5-12 (polyvalent)	–	83.5
Granulocytic:		
R1B19	Total	6.4
DS1-1	Total	4.6
S5-22	Early	1.9
L-12-1	Middle-Late	8.0
S5-28	Late	3.9
Monocytic:		
S-5-25	Total	10.6
H-14-1	Total	24.6
Erythroid:		
S-4-6	Total	37.4

[1] See Ref.17 and :Perussia et al. (This volume).
[2] As determined by immunofluorescence, using ORTHO-Cytofluorograph system H50 and ORTHO-Cytofluorograph ICP-22A.

Stimulation of monocyte-macrophage differentiation.

When CM-S cells are incubated with some potent tumor-promoting phorbol diesters such as 12-0-tetradecanoyl-phorbol-13-acetate (TPA), the cells rapidly differentiate, acquiring several of the morphologic and functional characteristics of monocyte-macrophages (15). The morphology of the cells dramatically changes within a few hours of exposure to TPA: cells rapidly become adherent to the culture plate and show prominent spreading and flattening (see Plate 1, a and b). By transmission electron microscopy (Plate 1, d) , cells treated for 2 days with TPA show an apparently increased relative cell size; nuclei show deep indentations and prominent polymorphism; nucleoli are usually in good evidence: in

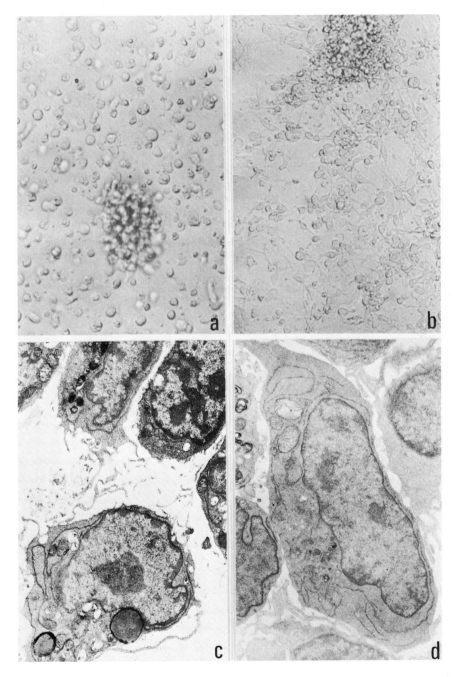

Plate 1. Morphology observed on CM-S cells before and after incubation with TPA (10^{-7} M) : a and c) untreated CM-S; b and d) after 2 days of exposure to TPA. a and b) Nomarski ; c and d) transmission electron microscopy (×6750) .

the cytoplasm ,mitochondria appear larger, swollen and possibly increase in number, as compared to those of the controls. The endoplasmic reticulum profile appears elongated around the nucleus and, frequently, lysosomal bodies are in clear evidence.

Most TPA-treated cells express Fc-and C_3-receptors, phagocytize inert particles or bacilli and show active immuno-phagocytosis (15). Cytochemical analyses showed that, after 3-4 days of culture in the presence of TPA, most of the cells express enzyme markers abundant in monocyte-macrophages. Table 1 summarizes these properties.

These cells show a significantly decreased expression of membrane histocompatibility antigens (Table 3).

TPA affects CM-S proliferation : terminal cell differentiation is accompanied by an almost complete arrest of cell division.

These effects were related to the concentration and structure of the phorbol diester and were not related to toxicity. Other non-tumor-promoting phorbols (such as phorbol-12,13-diacetate, PDA) were not effective.

TABLE 3 . EFFECT OF DIFFERENT INDUCING AGENTS ON
HISTOCOMPATIBILITY ANTIGEN EXPRESSION BY CM-S.

Addition to culture[1]	Antigens[2]				Total No. of cells
	(HLA.ABC)(HLADR)		(HLA.ABC)(HLA.DR)		$(\times 10^6 / \text{ml})$
	(cell lysate)		(culture supernate)		
	$(\text{I.U.}_{50} / 10^6 \text{cells})$				
CM-S ---	2780	1630	5128	3146	4.2
CM-S + TPA (10^{-9}M)	1810	1030	3140	1664	3.6
" + " (10^{-7}M)	1450	580	2850	1518	2.4
" + " (10^{-6}M)	1200	320	2120	1005	1.6
" + DPA (10^{-6}M)	2628	1414	4880	3020	4.1
CM-S + Dexamethasone (25 ug/ml)	820	660	2510	2080	4.0
CM-S + PHA-CM (.05 ml 1:10/ml)	373	80	1340	440	4.2
CM-S + Con-A-CM (.05 ml 1:10/ml)	2520	1378	4620	2850	4.1
CM-S + PHA (5 ug/ml)	2810	1430	4850	2320	3.2
CM-S + Con-A (4 ug/ml)	2620	1375	4620	2583	3.5

[1] CM-S were seeded at a concentration of 1.25×10^6 cells/ml and cultured for 4 days with or without inducers. The results are the mean of three separate experiments run in triplicates.Cell viability was approximately 70% in all cultures. [2] As measured by radioimmunoassay (20,15).

Stimulation of erythroid differentiation.

Congenital hypoplastic anemia (CHA) is characterized by an absolute
reticulocytopenia and a paucity of bone marrow erythroid cells more mature than pro-erythroblasts. Glucocorticoid therapy often improves marrow
erythroid cellularity and remission of anemia in CHA patients. It has
been found that steroids also improve the erythropoietin response of CHA-
erythroid precursors, by the in vitro plasma clot method (16). We investigated the effects of dexamethasone on CM-S. Time course kinetic studies with varying concentrations of dexamethasone revealed that this steroid does not affect the rate of proliferation of CM-S. However, the mo-
dal size of the proliferating cells markedly decreases in a time and dose dependent fashion (18). Concomitantly, the resulting predominant cell
population acquires morphologic characteristics and specific immunological markers of erythroid precursors.(Fig. 3 and Table 1).

In searching for other compounds capable of promoting differentiation of CM-S, we tried conditioned media (CM) from lectin-stimulated human peripheral blood mononuclear cells (PBL) . Conditioned medium from
PBL stimulated for 6 days in culture with phytohemagglutinin (PHA-CM),
proved to stimulate CM-S differentiation resulting within 4-5 days in a
predominant erythroid cell population developing spectrin and fetal hemoglobin (Hbγ)-positive cells .(Fig. 4). As seen with dexamethasone,
the number of cells progressively increases in the presence of PHA-CM
while the resulting cell population shows an increasing percentage of
erythroid cells and a decreasing percentage of cells with myeloid markers (Table 1). Expression of histocompatibility antigens also decreases,
in a time dependent fashion.(Table 3).

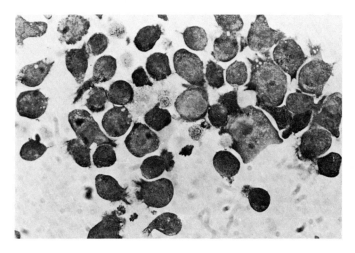

Fig.3 . Morphology of CM-S induced to erythroid differentiation after 3
        days of exposure to dexamethasone (25 ug/ml). Precursor erythroid
        cells predominate in culture (May-Grünwald-Giemsa stain,x1,600).

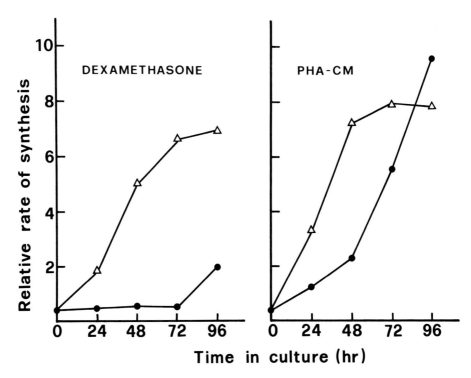

Fig. 4. Synthesis of spectrin (△) and Hbγ (●) during treatment of CM-S with dexamethasone (25 ,ug/ml) and PHA-CM (0.05 ml 1:10 dilution/ml). The rates of synthesis of these antigens were quantitatively measured by inhibition-solid-phase-radioimmunoassay (18) and plotted in arbitrary units, related to the rate of synthesis measured in untreated cells (From:Revoltella et al.,1981).

Conditioned media from unstimulated PBL or from PBL incubated with different lectins (e.g. concanavalin-A and pokeweed mitogen), as well as a variety of different chemical compounds (e.g. dimethylsulfoxide,butyric acid, hexamethylenbisacetamide,etc.) which can induce differentiation of certain myeloid and erythroid leukemia cells (8,4), were all uneffective in promoting CM-S differentiation (18).

Production of cell growth factors.
    Preliminary experiments indicated that serum-free conditioned medium of 4 day-old unstimulated CM-S cultures (CM-S-CM) is capable of enhancing colony proliferation of the myeloid leukemia HL-60 cell line and also of the erythroid K-562 cell line, in semi solid or viscous medium. In addition, CM-S-CM stimulates, under the same culture conditions, proliferation and differentiation of myeloid precursors (e.g. CFU-C) and early (but apparently not late) erythroid precursors (e.g. BFU-E) from human normal bone marrow cells. CM-S also elaborate constitutively as

well as upon induction with TPA or lypopolysaccharides high titers of an interleukin-I (apparent 13,000 MW, by Sephadex G100 chromatography) which induces human and mouse thymocytes to proliferate in the in vitro assay described by Lachman et al. (12) . CM-S cells do not elaborate T-cell growthfactor (interleukin-II)-like activity ,as assessedby the method of Bonnard et al. (2).

Concluding remarks.

The findings here reported favour the conclusion that CM-S is a multipotential cell line, comprising a replicating population of early haematopoietic progenitor cells capable, in the presence of suitable inducing compounds of differentiating to various stages at least along the monocytic-macrophagic and erythroid lineages.

Experiments performed on the line at different cell passages (from the 10th passage to the more recent 70th passage) gave very repetitive and comparable results. This stability of CM-S could be due to its euploid karyotype. Moreover, our combined morphologic, cytoenzymatic and immunologic data indicate that differentiation of CM-S occurs in a clonal-like fashion, as if the effective inducing compound (TPA, dexamethasone, PHA-CM) promotes a selective cell amplification and/or differentiation process, leading to a resulting predominant population of cells committed along a single pathway. Attempts to clone CM-S cells are in progress in order to clarify the potential capacity of differentiation of the CM-S precursor cells. CM-S should thus provide a convenient cell system for studying the mechanism of action of these differentiation-promoting substances.

CM-S cells contain the genetic determinants for several membrane and cytoplasmic markers of blood cell differentiation: the products seem to become coordinately expressed in a time dependent fashion, during induced cell differentiation. Since CM-S can provide unlimited quantities of cells in liquid culture, biochemical and immunologic studies of early markers of haematopoietic differentiation should be facilitated using this cell line.

Finally, the CM-S line constitutively elaborates several cell growth factors. It is possible that the cell line proliferates in culture in response to its own growth factors. The line could therefore be used both as a source for isolation and chemical characterization of these factors as well as a model for the study of their synthesis and action.

Acknowledgments.

The authors wish to thank Dr.P.Cornaglia-Ferraris,Istituto G.Gaslini of Genova for providing human bone marrow specimens. Dr.E.Gresick was on a leave of absence from the Department of Anatomy,The Mount Sinai School of Medicine of New York.
Reprint requests to:Roberto P.Revoltella,M.D.,Ph.D.,Laboratory of Cell Biology,C.N.R.,Via Romagnosi 18A,00196 Roma,Italy.

References.

1. Andersson,L.,Jokinen,M. and Gahmberg,C.G.(1979):Nature 278:364-365
2. Bonnard,G.D.,Yasaka,K. and Maca,R.D.(1980):Cell.Immunol.51:390-401
3. Collins,S.J.,Gallo,R.C. and Gallagher,R.E. (1977):Nature 270:347-349
4. Collins,S.J.,Ruscetti,F.W.,Gallagher,R.E. and Gallo,R.C.(1978):Proc.
   Natl.Acad.Sci.USA 75:2458-2462
5. Diamond,L.K.and Blackfan,K.O. (1938):Am.J.Dis.Child.56:464-474
6. Diamond,L.K.,Allen,M. and MaGill,F.B.(1961)Am.J.Dis.Child.102:149-158
7. Fibach,E. and Sachs L.(1975) :J.Cell Physiol. 86:221-228
8. Friend,C.,Scher,W.,Holland,J.G. and Sato,T.(1971) :Proc.Natl.Acad.Sci.
   USA 68:378-382
9. Hoffman,R.,Zanjani,E.D.,Vila,J.,Zalusky,R.,Lutton,J.D.and Wasserman,L.
   R(1976):J.Clin.Invest. 61:489-498
10.Ichikawa,Y.(1970):J.Cell.Physiol.76:175-181
11.Koren,H.S.,Anderson,S.J. and Larrick,J.W.(1979):Nature 279:328-331
12.Lachman,L.B.,Hacker,M.P. and Handschumaker,R.E.(1977):J.Immunol.119:
   2019-2023
13.Lozzio,C.B. and Lozzio,B.B.(1975):Blood 45:321-334
14.Lozzio,C.B.,Lozzio,B.B.,Bamberger,E.G. and Feliu,A.S.(1981):Fed.Proc-
   eedings 40:754(Abstract)
15.Monaco,G.,Vigneti,E.,Lancieri,M.,Cornaglia-Ferraris,P.,Lambertenghi-
   Deliliers,G. and Revoltella,R.(1981):Submitted for publication
16.Nathan,D.G.,Clarke,B.J.,Hillman,D.G.,Alter,B.P. and Housman,D.E.(1979)
   :J.Clin.Invest.61:489-498
17.Perussia,B.,Trinchieri,G.,Lebman,D.,Jankiewicz,J.,Lange,B. and Rovera
   G.(1981):Blood :In press.
18.Revoltella,R.P.,Vigneti,E.,Crcsick,E.,Lambertenghi-Deliliers,G.,Anna-
   loro,C. and Cappellini,M.D.(1981):Submitted for publication
19.Sachs,L.(1978):Nature 274:535-539
20.Tosi,R.,Tanigaki,N.,Centis,D.,Rossi,P.L.,Alfano,G.,Ferrara,G.B. and
   Pressman,D.(1980):Transplantation 29:302-305

Expression of Differentiated Functions in Cancer Cells, edited by R. F. Revoltella et al., Raven Press, New York © 1982.

Induction of Terminal Differentiation of HL-60 and Fresh Leukemic Cells by Retinoic Acid

Theodore R. Breitman

Laboratory of Tumor Cell Biology, National Cancer Institute, Bethesda, Maryland 20205

For many years now, acute myeloid leukemia has been looked upon as a disease which at least in part involves a block in differentiation (20). In its simplest terms, it is possible that some leukemia cells do not mature because they either have a decreased ability to respond to differentiative factors or because the production of specific differentiative factors is suppressed.

The development of tissue culture cell lines has made possible studies on the regulation and control of differentiation of specific cell types and the effect on these cells of known mediators and modulators. The most widely characterized leukemic cell lines have been those derived from the mouse: Friend erythroleukemia cells and Ml myeloid leukemia cells (18,31). Differentiation of one or both of these cell lines is induced by a wide variety of compounds including dimethyl sulfoxide, hemin, ouabain, prostaglandin (PG) E, butyric acid and other short-chain fatty acids, purines particularly hypoxanthine, 6-thioguanine, and 6-mercaptopurine, corticosteroids including dexamethasone and standard chemotherapeutic agents such as actimomycin D (2,15,18,25,30,31,37,42,43,46,53-55,61,65,66).

The HL-60 cell line, developed from a patient with acute promyelocytic leukemia (8), also serves as a useful, more recent model of differentiation. These cells proliferate continuously in suspension culture and consist predominantly of promyelocytes. HL-60 is induced to terminally differentiate to morphologically mature granulocytes by exposure to a wide variety of compounds including butyric acid, hypoxanthine, actinomycin D, dimethyl sulfoxide and hexamethylene bisacetamide(7,9). Moreover, these induced HL-60 cells have many of the functional characteristics of normal human peripheral blood granulocytes, including phagocytosis, lysosomal enzyme release, complement receptors, chemotaxis, hexose monophosphate shunt activity, and the ability to reduce nitroblue tetrazolium (NBT) (9,10,49). These cells lack leukocyte alkaline phosphatase (19), and while differentiating HL-60 cells do not develop secondary (specific) granules (17) and the specific protein markers for secondary granules, lactoferrin (17,49) and B-12 binding protein (17) they still provide a unique system for studies on human myeloid differentiation <u>in vitro</u>.

INDUCTION OF DIFFERENTIATION OF HL-60 BY RETINOIC ACID

Retinoids (vitamin A and its natural and synthetic analogs) influence the normal differentiation of epithelium. Retinoid deficiency in rats leads to premalignant lesions in a wide variety of epithelial tissue that are reversed by the administration of retinoids(69). Certain of these compounds inhibit the growth of transformed cells (41,47) and induce differentiation of mouse embryonal carcinoma cells in vitro (60).

Until recently, terminal differentiation of HL-60 could be induced only either by non-physiological compounds, e.g., dimethyl sulfoxide or by physiological chemicals at markedly greater than physiological concentrations, e.g., hypoxanthine. We have now found that all-trans-β-retinoic acid (RA) is the most potent inducer of granulocytic differentiation of HL-60 (5). This compound induces differentiation at concentrations 1/1000th to 1/1,000,000th the concentration of other inducers (Fig. 1), induces relatively more extensive morphological differentiation than other inducers, and probably more importantly induces at concentrations that are physiological (14).

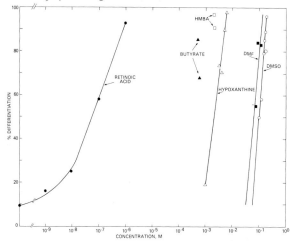

FIG. 1. Terminal differentiation of HL-60 cells induced by various compounds. Differentiation was measured at Day 5 of incubation and is expressed as the percent of cells capable of reducing nitroblue tetrazolium (NBT).

Differentiation of HL-60 in the presence of RA is concentration and time dependent with the sequential appearance of maturing granulocytes easily measured (Fig. 2). The data in Fig. 2 also show that in 1 μM RA and after 8 days, 70% of the cell population has matured to banded and segmented neutrophils.

To determine how long an exposure to RA was required for HL-60 cells to differentiate, cells were incubated with 1 μM RA for various time intervals, washed, and then resuspended in fresh growth medium without RA (Fig. 3). Continuous exposure to RA was necessary for optimal differentiation. However, cultures exposed to RA for 12 to 24 hr. exhibit an increase in differentiation after a delay of approximately two days. This differentiation continues to increase in the absence of RA to day 7 and then declines (Fig. 3) as undifferentiated cells repopulate the cultures (Fig. 4). These undifferentiated cells can be fully induced to

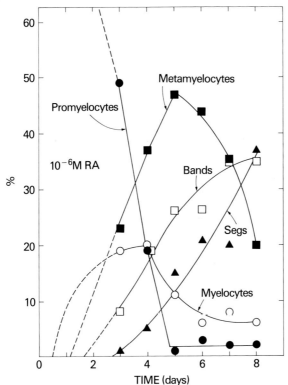

FIG. 2   Morphological   maturation   of   HL-60   cells   induced   by   1 μM RA.

mature by a second challange with RA (Fig. 3).

In the continuous presence of 1 μM RA, alterations in growth were apparent by day 3 and growth ceased by day 4 (Fig. 4). These cells no longer proliferated even when resuspended in growth medium without added RA. Thus, as expected, morphologically and functionally mature HL-60 cells induced by RA have also lost the capacity for further proliferation. The growth patterns of the cultures treated with RA for 12 and 24 hr. (Fig. 4) were a reflection of the extent of differentiation (Fig. 3).

Induction of HL-60 Differentiation by Other Retinoids

A total of 13 retinoids have been tested for their relative activities on induction of granulocytic differentiation of HL-60 as assayed by NBT reduction (Table 1). These results indicate that the most effective retinoid inducers of HL-60 differentiation, RA and 13-cis-RA, possess a carboxylic acid function at the C-15 terminal carbon. This activity is retained in spite of alterations in the ring as in the 4-hydroxy and 4-keto substituted derivatives and α-RA. Substitutions at the C-15 position result in markedly decreased activity. These activity-structure relationships emphasize the specificity of the RA effect on induction of HL-60 and makes more likely the possibility that this phenomenon, observed <u>in vitro</u>, is an expression of a true physiological process.

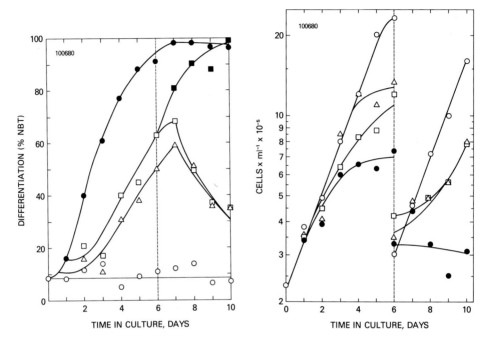

FIG. 3 (left).   Differentiation of HL-60 cells after various exposure times to RA.   Cells (2×10^5 per ml) were incubated in the absence (O) or in the presence of 1 μM RA continuously (●) or for 12 (Δ) or 24 (□) hr before being washed and resuspended in growth medium without RA.   At day 6, the cells from each culture were harvested, washed, and resuspended in fresh medium without RA.   Cells from the culture previously treated with RA for 24 hr were also retreated with RA (■).

FIG. 4 (right).   Growth of HL-60 cells after various exposure times to RA.   The conditions and symbols are the same as in the legend to Fig. 3.   Cell counts were performed on a Coulter cell counter.

TABLE 1. Effect of Retinoids on Differentiation of HL-60 Cells

Retinoid	Concentration (M)	Differentiation (% NBT)	Retinoid Concentration (M) for	
			50% NBT	25% NBT
Control	0	5	–	–
β-Retinoic Acid	10^{-6}	96	1×10^{-8}	2×10^{-9}
	10^{-7}	78		
	10^{-8}	46		
	10^{-9}	16		
	10^{-10}	5		
13-cis- Retinoic Acid	10^{-6}	96	1×10^{-8}	2×10^{-9}
	10^{-7}	85		
	10^{-8}	53		
	10^{-9}	15		
4-keto- Retinoic Acid	10^{-6}	93	9×10^{-8}	1.8×10^{-8}
	10^{-7}	55		
	10^{-8}	16		
	10^{-9}	5		
4-hydroxy- Retinoic Acid	10^{-6}	87	9×10^{-8}	1.8×10^{-8}
	10^{-7}	42		
	10^{-8}	13		
	10^{-9}	5		
α-Retinoic Acid	10^{-6}	67	3×10^{-7}	3×10^{-8}
	10^{-7}	35		
	10^{-8}	24		
	10^{-9}	9		
N-(4-carboxyphenyl)- Retinamide	10^{-6}	25	–	1×10^{-6}
	10^{-7}	13		
	10^{-8}	5		
	10^{-9}	6		
Retinal	10^{-6}	22	–	1×10^{-6}
	10^{-7}	9		
	10^{-8}	5		
	10^{-9}	6		

HL-60 cells were incubated with the indicated concentrations of retinoid for five days. The following retinoids produced less than 25% NBT reduction at a concentration of 1 μM: N-(4-hydroxyphenyl)-retinamide; N-ethyl-retinamide; retinylidene dimedone; retinol; retinyl acetate; N-(2-hydroxyethyl)-retinamide.

Studies on the Mechanism of Action of RA

The mechanism by which RA enhances differentiation of HL-60 cells or affects other cells is unknown. Mechanisms such as exerting an effect in the nucleus after binding to a highly specific cytoplasmic receptor (cellular RA-binding protein) (6), and promoting glycosylation of membrane glycoproteins (13), have been considered. It is also unknown whether the mechanism of induction by RA is the same as that of polar compounds such as dimethyl sulfoxide; in preliminary experiments the effects of combinations of RA and dimethyl sulfoxide were synergistic, suggesting that these two inducers act by different pathways.

The report of Levine and Ohuchi (39) that in MDCK cells RA enhances the deacylation of cellular lipids with a consequent increase in prostaglandin (PG) production suggested possible early biochemical steps for RA induction of HL-60 differentiation. PGE induces erythyroid differentiation in Friend murine erythroleukemia cells (61) and induces lysozyme activity, but not other functional or morphological markers of mature macrophages, in the murine myeloid leukemia cell line, M1 (28,29). This phase of our study was initiated to investigate the possible involvement of PG's in terminal differentiation of HL-60. All experiments in this section were conducted in a serum-free medium (3).

If a primary action of RA was to enhance the synthesis of PG's then it would be expected that inhibitors of PG synthesis would inhibit RA-induced differentiation of HL-60 and that PG's added alone without RA would be potent inducers. Indomethacin and aspirin, inhibitors of the PG synthetic enzyme, cyclooxygenase, had no inhibitory effect on RA-induced differentiation of HL-60 (Table 2). The concentration of aspirin and the lowest indomethacin concentration used here (2.8 µM) are at least 5-fold greater than concentrations reported to suppress completely PG synthesis in a wide variety of cell types and cell lines

TABLE 2. Effects of Aspirin and Indomethacin on RA-Induced Differentiation of HL-60 Cells

Condition	Differentiation, Day 4 (% NBT)
Control	8±3
RA, 0.1 µM	68±8
1 µM	95±2
Aspirin, 0.56 mM	7
plus RA, 1 µM	95
Indomethacin, 2.8 µM	10±3
plus RA, 0.1 µM	76
plus RA, 1 µM	90
Indomethacin, 14 µM	9
plus RA, 0.1 µM	88
Indomethacin, 28 µM	10
plus RA, 0.1 µM	94

including rat neutrophils (59), murine macrophages and human monocytes (35), MDCK cells, HeLa cells and human fibroblasts (12). However, addition of PGE to HL-60 cultures promoted differentiation in a concentration dependent manner (Table 3). Compared to RA at least 60-fold greater concentrations of PGE were required to promote differentiation to the same extent (data not shown). The most striking finding is that PGE_2 and PGE_1 are very effective inducers in combination with RA. That this combination is synergistic and not additive is indicated in Table 3 and is demonstrated clearly by an isobologram. RA is present in normal human plasma at 10 nM (14) and PGE is routinely found in human peripheral blood at 0.1 nM and can increase to 400 nM in localized areas of trauma, inflammation or infection (1). Thus, it is possible that the effects on differentiation with 10 nM RA and various concentrations of PGE (Table 3) reflect *in vitro* what can occur *in vivo* where concentrations of RA can be expected to be fairly steady and concentrations of PGE vary widely.

TABLE 3. Modulation of PGE of RA-Induced Differentiation of HL-60

RA(M)	PGE_2(M)	Net Differentiation,* Day 4 (% NBT)	Expected if Additive
10^{-8}		17	
10^{-7}		60	
	10^{-8}	7	
	10^{-7}	13	
	10^{-6}	22	
10^{-8}	10^{-8}	52	24
10^{-8}	10^{-7}	64	30
10^{-8}	10^{-6}	70	39

*Observed differentiation minus spontaneous differentiation of 8%.

The other PG's, either alone or in combination with RA, were much less active than PGE in inducing differentiation of HL-60 (Table 4) indicating a great degree of biological specificity by HL-60 in distinguishing between these structurally similar compounds This specificity is related to substitutions in the cyclopentane ring as there are no significant differences in biological activity between the PG-1's and PG-2's in each class.

PGE acts on many cell types by binding to a specific receptor, activating membrane adenylate cyclase and increasing intracellular levels of cAMP (22,26,34). The finding that exogenous dbcAMP also induces differentiation of HL-60 is consistent with this mode of action of PGE (Table 5). The addition of theophylline, an inhibitor of cAMP phosphodiesterase, results in a relatively small increase in the extent of HL-60 differentiation when added alone or in combination with RA or dbcAMP (Table 5). The combination of dbcAMP with RA or PGE_2 results in increases in differentiation that appear to be synergistic with RA and additive with PGE_2 (Table 5). However, a definitive judgement on these effects must await studies on intracellular cAMP concentrations. Preliminary results have indicated that PGE increases the intracellular cAMP concentration of HL-60 approximately 5-fold.

TABLE 4. Differentiation of HL-60 Cells by Combinations of RA, PGF, PGB, and PGA

| | | Differentiation, Day 4 (% NBT) | | | |
| | | PG Concentration, μM | | | |
PG	RA, 10 nM	0	1	3	10
None	–	8			
	+	25			
$F_{1\alpha}$	–		4	7	11
	+		24	25	53
$F_{2\alpha}$	–		12	16	25
	+		26	27	47
B_1	–		12	20	33
	+		26	37	82
B_2	–		9	11	23
	+		34	52	76
A_1	–		19	25	
	+		62	68	
A_2	–		18	25	
	+		53	70	

TABLE 5. Modulation of RA-Induced HL-60 Differentiation by cAMP

Condition	Differentiation, Day 4 (% NBT)
Control	8±3
RA, 10 nM	25±6
PGE_2, 10 nM	18
dbcAMP,	
10 μM	12
100 μM	33±5
dbcAMP, 100 μM	
plus 10 nM RA	92±7
plus PGE_2, 10 nM	54
theophylline, 100 μM	17
plus 10 nM RA	35
plus 100 μM dbcAMP	59

The data presented above indicate that PGE_1 and PGE_2 are potent modulators of RA-induced differentiation of HL-60 cells. The possibility that RA induction is mediated by endogenous synthesis of PG is doubtful because potent PG synthetase inhibitors do not decrease the extent of RA-induced differentiation (Table 2). These results indicate that HL-60 does not synthesize PG's and support the findings of Moore (48) that PGE is not produced by HL-60 either constitutively or after stimulation with endotoxin. The possibility that HL-60 does not have a characteristic of normal granulocytes is unlikely because of the findings of Kurland and Bockman (35) who could not detect PG production in highly purified human granulocytes. These authors conclude that reports in the literature of PGE synthesis in human granulocytes is most likely due to contamination with low numbers of monocytes which synthesize large amounts of PGE.

It is possible that the effects of RA and PGE on HL-60 cells may be explained on the basis of a cAMP-dependent protein kinase activity. The phosphorylation of specific proteins has been implicated as playing a central role in a large number of biological processes (24). In murine melanoma cells, RA increases cyclic AMP-dependent protein kinase activity (45) with no change in intracellular cAMP levels (40,45). Thus, in HL-60, RA may induce or increase the synthesis of a specific protein kinase in a concentration dependent manner. The activity of this enzyme would, however, be dependent on the intracellular level of cAMP, which in vitro is increased by adding PGE or dbcAMP. An enhancement in protein kinase activity to a critical level for differentiation can be obtained by either increasing the amount of enzyme protein (which we propose for RA alone) or activating more of the constitutive enzyme (which we propose for PGE or dbcAMP alone). Combinations of RA and PGE (or dbcAMP) yielding equal increases in protein kinase activity would be expected to produce similar increases in differentiation of HL-60 . This interrelationship between protein kinase synthesis and activation may explain the synergy observed between RA and PGE. Effects of PG's and cAMP on differentiation have been observed with other tissue culture cell lines. Friend erythroleukemia cells synthesize PG's (58) and are induced to synthesize hemoglobin by addition of PGE (58,61). These cells have been reported to have increased (21) or no increased (57) intracellular levels of cAMP during induction of differentiation by dimethyl sulfoxide and to be induced by agents that increase intracellular cAMP (21). Exogenous cAMP has no effect on Friend erythroleukemia differentiation either alone (21,57,61) or in combination with dimethyl sulfoxide (57). Differentiation of MDCK cells is induced by exogenous dbcAMP and PGE, and by compounds known to increase intracellular levels of cAMP (38). In the murine myeloid leukemia cell line, M_1, dexamethasone, and other glucocorticoid hormones, induce differentiation into forms morphologically identifiable as granulocytes and macrophages. These morphological changes are accompanied by functional characteristics of macrophages/granulocytes such as phagocytosis, locomotion, and lysozyme activity (29). Dexamethasone induces the synthesis of PGE in M_1 cells and this synthesis as well as the other differentiation associated properties is inhibited by indomethacin (29). This inhibition is counteracted by exogenous PGE. PGE or cAMP alone induce lysozyme activity but not the other functional and morphological markers of mature cells (28,29). In the M_1 system, RA induces lysosomal activity and markedly inhibits dexamethasone-promoted differentiation (63). The results with dexamethasone are an example of the difficulty of developing a mechanism for induction of differentiation of various cell systems that take into account the contradictory effects of PG's and cAMP. Dexamethasone inhibits both PG synthesis and dimethyl sulfoxide induced differentiation of Friend erythroleukemia cells (58). In contrast, it induces both PGE synthesis and differentiation of M_1 cells and has no effect on differentiation of HL-60 cells (7) even though these cells have glucocorticoid receptors (33) and dexamethasone inhibits the expression of Fc receptors (11).

The results we have obtained on HL-60 cells in vitro may reflect events occurring during normal granulocytic differentiation in vivo. It is well known that PGE and cAMP are potent inhibitors of both normal bone marrow granulocyte/macrophage colony forming units and of myeloid leukemia cell lines in semi-solid medium (32,36,62,68). However, these studies do not provide a clear distinction between decreased colony numbers resulting from terminal differentiation or from cytotoxicity. In the microenvironment of the developing granulocyte the interplay between RA, derived ultimately from the diet, and PGE and colony stimulating activity derived from monocytes may be one of the important controls of granulocytic maturation.

RA-Induced Differentiation of Fresh Human Promyelocytic Leukemia Cells in Primary Culture

The finding that RA is a potent inducer of HL-60 terminal differentiation prompted an investigation to determine whether fresh leukemic cells shared this response. In a recent report (4) we incubated fresh human myeloid leukemia cells in short-term suspension cultures in the presence of RA. Twenty-one leukemic patients were studied. The diagnosis was acute myelocytic leukemia in thirteen patients, acute myelomonocytic leukemia in two patients, acute promyelocytic leukemia in two patients, chronic myelocytic leukemia in blastic phase in three patients, and chronic myelomonocytic leukemia in accelerated phase in one patient. Differentiation of the leukemic cells from two of the twenty-one patients was induced by RA. The only inducible specimens were from the two patients with acute promyelocytic leukemia both of whose cells incubated in the absence of RA did not morphologically differentiate and did not reduce NBT.

None of the other patients' cells showed any significant granulocytic differentiation induced by RA. In no specimen did RA significantly affect viability or the total cell counts. In several of the cultures, especially those diagnosed as myelomonocytic leukemia, cells morphologically resembling monocytes/macrophages developed after a few days in suspension culture. These cells were NBT positive, also a functional characteristic of monocytes and macrophages (70). Similar spontaneous differentiation of fresh leukemic cells in short-term culture has been described (50). However, RA had essentially no effect on this spontaneous differentiation.

Since this initial report we have received peripheral blood and/or marrow from two additional acute promyelocytic patients. The cells from both of these patients responded to RA in vitro (Fig. 5 and Table 6). When the cells from patient P.V. were originally tested there was a marked response to RA alone (Fig. 5). This patient's cells, that had incubated for 5 days in medium, responded markedly in the next 3 days to RA alone. This patient was treated with conventional chemotherapy but returned 6 weeks later with a partial relapse. Another specimen was received and tested in vitro. These cells responded to RA alone and possibly to a combination of RA and PGE_2 (Table 6). Cells from another acute promyelocytic patient (M.S.) also exhibited RA-induced differentiation.

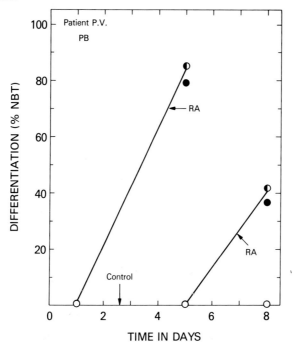

FIG. 5 Terminal differentiation of fresh leukemic cells isolated from the peripheral blood of a patient with acute promyelocytic leukemia. Cells (2 x10^5/ml) were incubated in the presence of 0.1 µM (●) and 1.0 µM (◑) RA or no RA (O).

TABLE 6. Induction of Differentiation of Fresh Acute Promyelocytic Leukemia Cells by RA

Patient	Treatment	Differentiation (% NBT) Day 4
P.V.	Control	3.5
	RA, 1 µM	80
	0.1 µM	66
	RA, 0.1 µM plus PGE$_2$, 10 nM	77
M.S.	Control	2.5
	RA, 1 µM	41
	0.1 µM	37

Like HL-60, the four specimens induced by RA were acute promyelocytic leukemias, suggesting that to respond to this compound it is necessary that leukemic cells be at the promyelocytic stage of differentiation.

Specific cytologic alterations (64,67) as well as a common karyotypic abnormality (56), also distinguish acute promyelocytic leukemia from other acute leukemias. In our experience less differentiated leukemic specimens do not show a response to RA.

In the four acute promyelocytic leukemias granulocytic differentiation occurred in RA treated cultures without an increase in cell number or a significant loss of cell viability. This would suggest that in these short term cultures cell division is not required for differentiation, a finding that has been confirmed with HL-60 (see below).

Studies of leukemic cells in soft agar (51) in diffusion chambers (27), and in suspension culture (16,50), suggest at least partial retention of granulocytic or monocytic/macrophage differentiation by at least some of the cells. The therapeutic role of agents which induce differentiation in human leukemia remains in question whether used alone or in combination with conventional chemotherapy, but any factor mediating differentiation of leukemic cells might be expected to favorably affect the progression of the disease. Moreover, 13-cis-RA, which is as active as RA in inducing HL-60 (5), has been used systemically to treat certain skin disorders and is well-tolerated (52). The utility of RA in this regard remains conjectural and from our results would apparently be limited to patients with acute promyelocytic leukemia, accounting for 13% of acute nonlymphocytic leukemias (23).

Evidence That RA-Induced Differentiation of HL-60 Does Not Require Cell Growth

When it seemed possible that RA might have clinical utility it became of interest to examine in vitro the effects on RA-induced differentiation of cell-growth inhibiting chemotherapeutic agents. It was also felt that such studies might yield further insight into the mechanism of RA-induction and more generally into granulocytic terminal differentiation.

Two chemotherapeutic agents were studied: hydroxyurea (HU) and arabinosylcytosine (araC). Both of these agents inhibit cell growth by specifically inhibiting DNA synthesis. The experimental design was to grow HL-60 with various concentrations of drug, with and without RA. The concentration of HU that inhibited growth by 50% was 100 μM for cultures growing either with or without 1 μM RA (Fig. 6). RA, as expected, decreased growth alone and increasing concentrations of HU decreased the cell number still further. However, HU inhibition of cell growth had no effect on the extent of RA-induced HL-60 differentiation (Fig. 7). HU alone had little, if any effect on the extent of HL-60 differentiation.

A similar study was conducted with various concentrations of araC and 0.3 μM RA (Figs. 8 and 9) and the extent of RA induction of HL-60 was not markedly reduced by araC. From a clinical point of view it is of interest that plasma levels of approximately 200 nM araC are obtained when it is used as a sole agent. Thus, the effects in vitro shown here may have direct clinical application. In addition araC alone had a small inductive effect on HL-60 (Fig. 9).

These results with two clinically employed anticancer agents indicate that neither drug interferes with the differentiative action of RA and that RA does not interfere with their growth inhibitory activity. Thus, RA can probably be considered for combination therapy in a program aimed at both inhibiting the proliferation and inducing terminal differentiation of immature leukemia cells.

Other experimental evidence indicating that growth of HL-60 is not a requisite for differentiation is: (a) omission of either insulin alone, transferrin alone, or insulin and transferrin from defined medium has essentially no effect on RA-induced differentiation, and (b) as shown above, fresh leukemia cells in primary culture differentiate either spontaneously or can be induced under non-growth conditions.

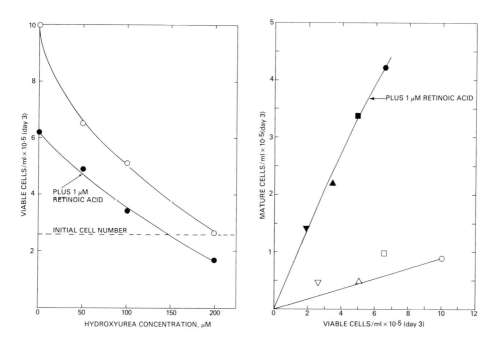

FIG. 6 (left). Inhibition of growth of HL-60 cells by hydroxyurea in the presence (●) or absence (○) of 1 μM RA.

FIG. 7 (right). RA-induced terminal differentiation of HL-60 cells in the presence of various concentrations of hydroxyurea. Solid symbols, with 1 μM RA; open symbols, no RA. Hydroxyurea concentrations were: none, (●,○); 50 μM, (■,□); 100 μM, (▲,△); 200 μM, (▼,▽). Mature cells were calculated by the formula:

$$\text{mature cells/ml} = \frac{\%\ NBT\ positive\ cells \times viable\ cells/ml}{100}$$

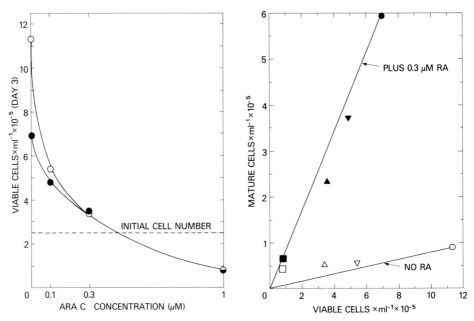

FIG. 8 (left). Inhibition of growth of HL-60 cells by ara C in the presence (●) or absence (0) of 0.3 µM RA.

FIG. 9 (right). RA-induced terminal differentiation of HL-60 cells in the presence of various concentrations of ara C. Ara C concentrations were: none, (●,0); 0.1 µM, (▼,▽); 0.3 µM, (▲,△); 1 µM, (■,□). Mature cells were calculated as in legend to Fig. 7.

ACKNOWLEDGEMENTS

I thank Beverly R. Keene for excellent technical assistance, Dr. R. C. Gallo for continued support, and Anna Mazzuca for expert secretarial assistance.

REFERENCES

1. Berenbaum, M.C., Cope, W.A., and Bundick, R.V. (1976): <u>Clin.Exp. Immunol.</u>, 26:534–541.
2. Bernstein, A., Hunt, D.M., Crickley, V., and Mak, T.W. (1976): <u>Cell</u>, 9:375–381.
3. Breitman, T.R., Collins, S.J., and Keene, B.R. (1980): <u>Exp. Cell Res.</u>, 126:494–498.
4. Breitman, T.R., Collins, S.J., and Keene, B.R. (1981): <u>Blood,</u> (in press).
5. Breitman, T.R., Selonick, S.E., and Collins, S.J. (1980): <u>Proc. Nat. Acad. Sci., U.S.A.,</u> 77:2936–2940.
6. Chytil, F. and Ong, D.E. (1979): <u>Fed. Proc. Fed. Am. Soc. Exp.Biol.,</u> 38:2510–2514.

7. Collins, S.J., Bodner, A., Ting, R., and Gallo, R.C. (1980): Int. J. Cancer, 25:213-218.
8. Collins, S.J., Gallo, R.C., and Gallagher, R.E. (1977): Nature (Lond.), 270:347-349.
9. Collins, S.J., Ruscetti, F.W., Gallagher, R.E., and Gallo, R.C. (1978): Proc. Nat. Acad. Sci., U.S.A., 75:2458-2462.
10. Collins, S.J., Ruscetti, F.W., Gallagher, R.E., and Gallo, R.C. (1979): J. Exp. Med., 149:969-974.
11. Crabtree, G.R., Munck, A., and Smith, K.A. (1979): Nature (Lond.), 279:338-339.
12. Crutchley, D.J., Conanan, L.B., and Maynard, J.R. (1980): Cancer Res., 40:849-852.
13. DeLuca, L.M., Bhat, P.V., Wiodzimierz, S., and Adamo, S. (1979): Fed. Proc. Fed. Am. Soc. Exp. Biol., 38:2535-2539.
14. DeRuyter, M.G., Lambert, W.E., and DeLeenheer, A.P. (1979): Anal. Biochem., 98:402-409.
15. Ebert, P.S., Wars, I., and Buell, D.N. (1976): Cancer Res., 36:1809-1813.
16. Elias, L., and Greenberg, P. (1977): Blood, 50:263-274.
17. Fontana, J.A., Wright, D.G., Schiffman, E., Corcoran, B.A., and Deisseroth, A.B. (1980): Proc. Nat. Acad. Sci. (Wash), 77:3664-3668.
18. Friend, C., Scher, W., Holland, J.G., and Sato, T. (1971): Proc. Nat. Acad. Sci. (Wash), 68:378-382.
19. Gallagher, R., Collins, S., Trujillo, J., McCredie, K., Ahearn, M., Tsai, S., Metzgar, R., Aulakh, G., Ting, R., Ruscetti, F., and Gallo, R.C. (1979): Blood, 54:713-733.
20. Gallo, R.C. (1973): In: Modern Trends in Human Leukemia, edited by R. Neth, R.C. Gallo, S. Spiegelman, and F. Stohlman, Jr., pp. 227-237. J.F. Lehmanns, Munich, West Germany.
21. Gazitt, Y., Reuben, R.C., Deitch, A.D., Marks, P.A., and Rifkind, R.A. (1978): Cancer Res., 38:3779-3783.
22. Gilman, A.G., and Nirenberg, M. (1971): Nature, 234:356-358.
23. Goldman, J.M. (1974): Br. Med. J., 1:380-382.
24. Greengard, P. (1978): Science, 199:146-152.
25. Gusella, J.F., and Housman, D. (1976): Cell, 8:263-269.
26. Hittelman, K.J., and Butcher, R.W. (1973): In: The Prostaglandins, edited by M.F. Cuthbert, pp. 151-165, J.B. Lippincott, Philadelphia.
27. Hoelzer, D., Kurrle, E., Schmucker, H., and Harriss, E.B. (1977): Blood, 49:729-744.
28. Honma, Y., Kasukabe, T., and Hozumi, M. (1978): Biochem. Biophys. Res. Commun., 82:1246-1250.
29. Honma, Y., Kasukabe, T., and Hozumi, M. (1979): Cancer Res., 39:2190-2194.
30. Honma, Y., Kasukabe, T., Okabe, J., and Hozumi, M. (1977): Gann, 68:241-246.
31. Ichikawa, Y. (1969): J. Cell Physiol., 74:223-234.
32. Koeffler, H.P., and Golde, D.W. (1980): Cancer Res., 40:1858-1862.
33. Koeffler, H.P., Golde, D.W., and Lippman, M.E. (1980): Cancer Res., 40:563-566.
34. Kuehl, F.A., Jr., and Humes, J.L. (1972): Proc. Nat. Acad. Sci., U.S.A., 69:480-484.
35. Kurland, J.I., and Bockman, R. (1978): J. Exp. Med., 147:952-957.
36. Kurland, J.I., Hadden, J.W., and Moore, M.A.S. (1978): Cancer Res., 37:4534-4538.

37. Leder, A., and Leder, P. (1975): Cell, 5:319–322.
38. Lever, J.E. (1979): Proc. Nat. Acad. Sci., U.S.A., 76:1323–1327.
39. Levine, L., and Ohuchi, K. (1978): Nature, 276:274–275.
40. Lotan, R., Giotta, G., Nork, E., and Nicolson, G.L. (1978): J. Natl. Cancer Inst., 60:1035–1041.
41. Lotan, R., and Nicolson, G.L. (1977): J. Natl. Cancer Inst., 59:1717–1722.
42. Lotem, J., and Sachs, L. (1974): Proc. Nat. Acad. Sci., U.S.A., 71:3507–3511.
43. Lotem, J., and Sachs, L. (1975): Int. J. Cancer, 15:731–740.
44. Lotem, J., and Sachs, L. (1980): Int. J. Cancer, 25:561–564.
45. Ludwig, K.W., Lowey, B., and Niles, R.M. (1980): J. Biol. Chem., 255:5999–6002.
46. Maeda, S., and Sachs, L. (1978): J. Cell Physiol., 94:181–186.
47. Meyskens, F.L., Jr., and Salmon, S.E. (1979): Cancer Res., 39:4055–4057.
48. Moore, M.A.S. (1979): In: Clinics in Haematology, edited by L.G. Laijtha, pp. 287–309. W.B. Saunders Co. Ltd., London.
49. Newburger, P.E., Chovaniec, M.E., Greenberger, J.S., and Cohen, H.J. (1979): J. Cell Biol., 82:315–322.
50. Palu, G., Powles, R., Selby, P., Summersgill, B.M., and Alexander, P. (1979): Br. J. Cancer, 40:719–730.
51. Paran, M., Sachs, L., Barak, Y., and Resnitzky, P. (1970): Proc. Nat. Acad. Sci., U.S.A., 67:1542–1549.
52. Peck, G.L., Olsen, T.G., Yoder, F.W., Strauss, J.S., Downing, D.T., Pandya, M., Butkus, D., and Arnaud-Battandier, J. (1979): N. Eng. J. Med., 300:329–333.
53. Preisler, H.P., and Lyman, G. (1975): Cell Differentiation, 4:179–185.
54. Reuben, R.C., Wife, R.L., Breslow, R., Rifkind, R.A., and Marks, P.A. (1976): Proc. Nat. Acad. Sci., U.S.A., 73:862–866.
55. Ross, J., and Sautner, D. (1976): Cell, 8:513–520.
56. Rowley, J.D., Golomb, H.M., Vardiman, J., Fukuhara, S., Dougherty, C., and Potter, D. (1977): Int. J. Cancer, 20:869–872.
57. Rubin, C.S. (1978): J. Cell. Physiol., 94:57–68.
58. Santoro, M.G., Benedetto, A., and Jaffe, B.M. (1980): In: In Vivo and in vitro Erythropoiesis: The Friend System, edited by G.B. Rossi, pp. 553–562. Elsevier/North-Holland Biomedical Press, Amsterdam.
59. Siegel, M.I., McConnell, R.T., Porter, N.A., Selph, J.L., Truax, J.F., Vinegar, R., and Cuatrecasas, P. (1980): Biochem. Biophys. Res. Commun., 92:688–695.
60. Strickland, S., and Mahdavi, V. (1978): Cell, 15:393–403.
61. Tabuse, Y., Furusawa, M., Eisen, H., and Shibata, K. (1977): Exp. Cell Res., 108:41–45.
62. Taetle, R., and Koessler, A. (1980): Cancer Res., 40:1223–1229.
63. Takenaga, K., Hozumi, M., and Sakagami, Y. (1980): Cancer Res., 40:914–919.
64. Tan, H.K., Wages, B., and Gralnick, H.R. (1972): Blood, 39:628–636.
65. Tanaka, M., Levy, J., Terada, M., Breslow, R., Rifkind, R.A., and Marks, P.A. (1975): Proc. Nat. Acad. Sci., (Wash), 72:1003–1006.
66. Terada, M., Epner, E., Nudel, U., Salmon, J., Fibach, E., Rifkind, R.A., and Marks, P.A. (1978): Proc. Nat. Acad. Sci. (Wash), 75:2795–2799.

67. Valdiviesco, M., Rodriguez, V., Orewinko, B., Bodey, G.P.. Ahearn, M.J., McCredie, K.B., and Freireich, E.J. (1975): <u>Med. Ped. Oncol.</u>, 1:37.
68. Williams, N. (1979): <u>Blood,</u> 53:1089-1094.
69. Wolbach, S.B., and Howe, P.R. (1925): <u>J. Exp. Med.</u>, 42:753-777.
70. Zakhireh, B., and Root, R.K. (1979): <u>Blood,</u> 54:429-439.

Expression of Differentiated Functions in Cancer Cells, edited by R. F. Revoltella et al., Raven Press, New York © 1982.

Control of Gene Expression in Friend Erythroleukemia Cells Induced to Differentiate

E. A. Stringer and C. Friend

Center for Experimental Cell Biology, Mollie B. Roth Laboratory, Mount Sinai School of Medicine, CUNY, New York, New York 10029

Continuous lines of murine erythroleukemia (FL) cells, which originate either from the spleen cells of mice infected with Friend leukemia virus (FLV) or from hematopoietic cells transformed in vitro with the virus, are being widely used to study the molecular control of erythrodifferentiation. The cells can be induced to differentiate and to synthesize hemoglobin by treatment with dimethyl sulfoxide (DMSO) or one of a variety of unrelated compounds. Although the mechanism of action of these agents is not well understood, differentiation in the treated cells is characterized by morphological changes similar to those seen in the normal erythropoietic transition from proerythroblasts to orthochromophilic erythroblasts. The morphological changes are accompanied by a decrease in the proliferative capacity of the cells and by the expression of late erythroid events, such as an increase in iron uptake and heme synthesis, the accumulation of hemoglobin and the appearance of erythrocyte-specific membrane antigens. The ease with which the transition to a program of terminal differentiation can be made is enabling us to study the mechanisms involved in the "switching" to the developmental program. The literature describing studies on induced FL cells is extensive and progress in the field has been well documented in a number of reviews (5,6,8,10).

The observations that heme is involved in differentiation of FL cells have raised the possibility that modulation of translational controls in the commitment of FL cells to differentiate may be similar to that found in rabbit reticulocyte protein synthesizing systems. In rabbit reticulocytes, hemin blocks the formation of a translational inhibitor by preventing the conversion of an inactive proinhibitor to an active inhibitor. This inhibitor, the hemin-controlled repressor (HCR), also known as the heme-regulated inhibitor (HRI), possesses a protein kinase activity which can specifically phosphorylate the initiation factor, eIF-2, and inhibit the initiation of new protein chains. We were led to study the translational control in induced FL cells by the report that uninduced cells possessed a translational inhibitor with similar specificity (13), but which differed from HCR of rabbit reticulocytes in that it did not respond to the presence of hemin (2).

In the present communication, we have confirmed Cimadevilla's observations (2) that the translation of the globin mRNA in rabbit reticulocytes is greatly diminished in the presence of uninduced lysates of FL cells, while translation of mRNA from the uninduced lysates is unaffected, and have further shown that uninduced FL cell lysates similarly affect protein synthesis in induced FL cell lysates. When lysates of uninduced and induced FL cells are mixed, there is a reduction in the total amount of amino acid incorporated.

We also show that addition of hemin or HCR to lysates of FL cells induced to differentiate with either hexamethylbisacetamide (HMBA) or aminonucleoside of puromycin (AMS) does not affect the rate of protein synthesis. The induced FL cells, although they are actively synthesizing hemoglobin and exhibiting other features characteristic of terminal erythroid differentiation, are as refractory to heme and its associated translational inhibitor, HCR, as are the uninduced FL cells.

MATERIALS AND METHODS

Establishment, growth conditions and characterization of the subclone 5-86 of the prototype FL cell line 745A have been previously described (6). Cells were seeded at a concentration of 1×10^5 cells/ml and were maintained in a basal medium/Eagle (GIBCO, Grand Island, N.Y.), supplemented with 10% fetal calf serum (Reheis Chem. Co., Kankankee, Ill.), penicillin and streptomycin. The cultures were kept at a constant temperature of 37°C in an atmosphere of 5% CO_2 in air.

Aminonucleoside of puromycin (Sigma Chem. Co., St. Louis, Mo.) and HMBA (kind gifts from Drs. Roberta Reuben and Yair Gazitt) were added to cultures at concentrations of 10 μg/ml and 5 mM respectively at the time of seeding. The cultures were scored for benzidine-positive (B+) cells by the wet benzidine method of Orkin et al (12).

Preparation of Lysates

Rabbit reticulocyte lysates were prepared by the method of Ranu and London (16). The same method was used to prepare lysates of FL cells harvested 4-5 days after initiation of the cultures with and without inducers except that total lysis of the cells was accomplished by additional mechanical disruption in a Dounce hemogenizer. Lysates were stored in small aliquots in liquid nitrogen.

Purification of the Hemin-Controlled Repressor (HCR)

The reversible form of the hemin-controlled repressor was purified according to the method of Trachsel et al (18). The ability of HCR to inhibit protein synthesis in the presence of optimal levels of hemin was used as a measure of its activity (16).

Assay of Protein Synthesis in Cell-free Lysates

Immediately upon thawing, the lysates were made 50 μg/ml in creatine phosphokinase and 5 mM in creatine phosphate. Amino acid incorporation was measured using a modification of the procedure of Ranu and London (16). The details are included in the legend to Fig. 1. Radioactivity was measured by liquid scintillation in 10 ml toluene counting fluid containing 4 g 2,5-diphenyloxazole (POP) and 40 mg 1,4 bis [2(5-phenyloxazolyl)]-benzene (POPOP) per liter of toluene.

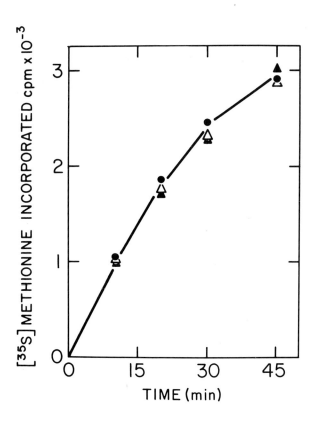

FIG. 1. Effect of HMBA and AMS on Amino Acid Incorporation in
Rabbit Reticulocyte Lysates. The reaction volume of 80 μl contained a mixture of 20 mM Tris-HCl (pH 7.5), 80 mM potassium
acetate, 0.5 mM magnesium acetate, unlabelled amino acid at concentrations related to their frequency in rabbit globin, (^{35}S)-
methionine (4,000 cpm/pm), 10 μg creatine phosphokinase, 5 mM
creatine phosphate and 15 μM hemin. Reaction mixtures were incubated at 30°C for 45 min and, during the course of the incubation, 8 μl aliquots were removed at 15 min intervals and treated
according to the method of Kramer (9). The aliquots were diluted
in 1.0 ml of a solution of 0.5 M NaOH and 1.5% H_2O_2, incubated
at 37 C for 10 min, then made 5% in TCA and incubated at 90°C for
a further 10 min. Following cooling in ice for 10 min, the precipitate formed was collected on nitrocellulose filters (0.45 μm
pore size, type HAWP, Millipore Corp., Bedford, Mass.) and washed
with three 5 ml volumes of 5% TCA. The dried filters were counted
in a scintillation counter as outlined in Methods. ●-●-● complete system (30 μl rabbit reticulocyte lysate); Δ-Δ-Δ complete
system plus 5 mM HMBA; ▲-▲-▲ complete system plus 10 μg/ml AMS.

RESULTS

The Effect of Addition of Hemin and HCR to Uninduced and Induced FL Cell Lysates

Since it had been reported that neither hemin nor HCR had any effect on protein synthesis in lysates of uninduced FL cells (2,3), it was of interest for us to investigate whether lysates from cells induced to differentiate exhibited the same characteristics. Two potent inducers which differ in their ability to stimulate ornithine decarboxylase (ODC) in FL cells (7) were selected for these studies: HMBA stimulates ODC activity and AMS does not. In order to ensure that the inducers do not inhibit protein synthesis by inactivating components of the translation system or by activating HCR, we first tested the inducers at the concentrations used to stimulate FL cell differentiation, adding them separately to the in vitro amino acid incorporating system from rabbit reticulocytes.

As Fig. 1 clearly demonstrates, the addition of either 5 mM HMBA or 10 µg/ml AMS to the rabbit reticulocyte lysate system had no effect on the rate of protein synthesis. Amino acid incorporation was virtually linear for 45 min during the course of the incubation with or without the inducer. Hemin was present at a final concentration of 15 µM to prevent activation of HCR.

The typical response to the addition of hemin of the rabbit reticulocyte lysates used in these experiments is shown in Fig. 2A. In the absence of added hemin, HCR becomes activated and amino acid incorporation ceases after 10 min. The addition of exogenous hemin to give a final concentration of 15 µM prevents activation of the repressor, and amino acid incorporation remains linear during the 45 min incubation period. Lysates from uninduced FL cells do not exhibit biphasic kinetics in the absence of added hemin (Fig. 2B). Amino acid incorporation is continuous throughout the course of the incubation. Addition of hemin in concentrations which prevent activation of HCR in rabbit reticulocyte lysates has no effect. Similarly, lysates from FL cells induced to differentiate by treatment with HMBA incorporate amino acids into polypeptides whether or not hemin is present (Fig. 2C). Lysates from FL cells induced to differentiate by AMS show identical results (data not shown).

In view of these results, we next investigated the effect of adding highly purified preparations of HCR from rabbit reticulocytes to lysates of induced and uninduced FL cells, since the effect of hemin on rabbit reticulocyte lysates is mediated through HCR.

The amount of HCR (0.01 µg) added in all cases was sufficient to give marked inhibition of amino acid incorporation in rabbit reticulocyte lysates whether or not hemin was added. Addition of HCR to the rabbit reticulocyte lysate amino acid incorporating system drastically reduced the rate of synthesis to a level close to that observed in the absence of hemin (Fig. 2A). When similar amounts of HCR were added to lysates from uninduced FL cells (Fig. 2B), no change in the rate of amino acid incorporation was observed, confirming the observations of Cimadevilla et al that uninduced FL cell lysates are refractory to HCR (3). The effect of the addition of HCR to lysates of FL cells induced to differentiate by HMBA is shown in Fig. 2C. The rate of amino acid incorporation was not altered. The addition of 0.01 µg of HCR to the induced cells had no effect during the course of the incubation. Identical results were obtained with lysates from FL cells induced to differentiate by AMS (data not shown). The addition or omission of hemin had no effect.

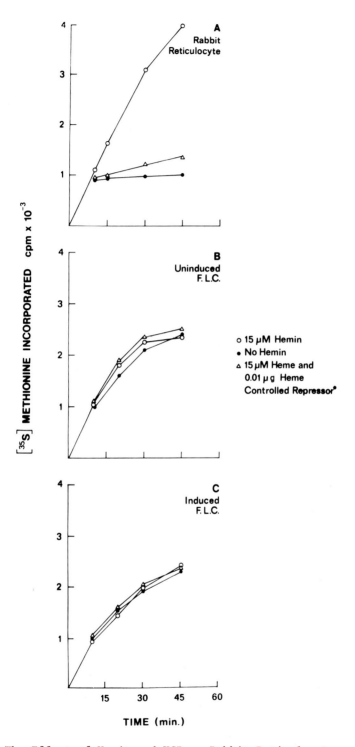

FIG. 2. The Effect of Hemin and HCR on Rabbit Reticulocytes, uninduced and Induced FL Cell Lysates. Reaction mixtures and incubation conditions were the same as those outlined in Fig. 1.

The Effect of Mixing Uninduced FL Cell Lysates with Rabbit Reticulocyte
Lysates or Lysates from Induced FL Cells

Reports that uninduced FL cells contain an inhibitor which prevents
protein synthesis in rabbit reticulocyte lysates (13) and our evidence
that induced FL cells, although actively synthesizing hemoglobin, are
not under the control of HCR (Fig. 2C) led us to examine the effect of
adding lysates of uninduced FL cells to induced FL cell lysates.

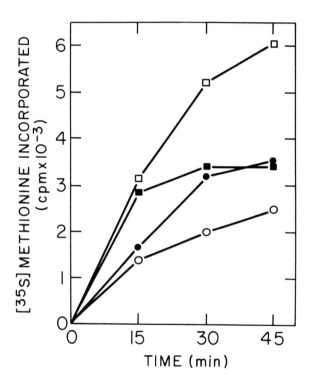

FIG. 3.   The Effect of Mixing Uninduced FL Cell Lysates
With Rabbit Reticulocyte Lysates.   Reaction mixtures and
incubation conditions were the same as those outlined in
Fig. 1.   ●-●-● rabbit reticulocyte lysate; o-o-o uninduced
FL cell lysates; ■-■-■ rabbit reticulocyte lysate plus
uninduced FL cell lysate; □-□-□ theoretical value of
rabbit reticulocyte lysate plus uninduced FL cell lysate.

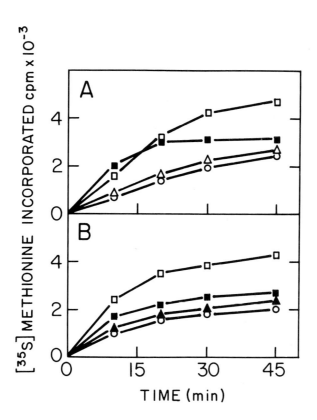

FIG. 4. The Effect of Mixing Uninduced FL Cell Lysate with HMBA- and AMS-induced FL Cell Lysates. Reaction mixtures and incubation conditions were the same as those in Fig. 1. o-o-o uninduced FL cell lysate; Δ-Δ-Δ HMBA-induced FL cell lysate; ▲-▲-▲ AMS-induced FL cell lysate; ■-■-■ uninduced FL cell lysate plus induced FL cell lysate; □-□-□ theoretical value of uninduced FL cell lysate plus induced FL cell lysate.

As has been reported by Cimadevilla and Hardesty (2), the addition of uninduced FL cell lysates to rabbit reticulocyte lysates resulted in a decrease in the total amount of amino acid incorporation observed (Fig. 3). Analysis of the products of translation shows that synthesis of rabbit globin is reduced up to 90%, while synthesis of uninduced FL cell proteins is unaffected (data not shown).

Similar results are obtained when uninduced FL cell lysates are mixed with lysates from FL cells induced to differentiate by either HMBA or AMS (Fig. 4A and 4B, respectively). The total amino acid incorporation observed is much less than that expected from the sum of the values from the individual lysates. These data suggest that the inhibitor in the lysates from uninduced FL cells is curtailing, in the lysates of differentiated FL cells and reticulocytes, the synthesis of the proteins which have specialized functions relating to differentiation.

DISCUSSION

The results presented in this paper confirm earlier observations of Cimadevilla and Hardesty (2,3) that: 1] protein synthesis in uninduced FL cell lysates is not stimulated by hemin at concentrations which are necessary to maintain linear incorporation of amino acids in rabbit reticulocyte lysates for periods up to 1 hr (Fig. 2), and 2] purified preparations of the reversible form of HCR from rabbit reticulocytes have no effect on amino acid incorporation in lysates from uninduced FL cells, while effectively inhibiting synthesis in rabbit reticulocyte lysates with the characteristic kinetics of inhibition observed by many workers (for review, see Ochoa and deHaro, ref. #11).

As is well known, the cells grown in the presence of inducers exhibit changes characteristic of erythroid differentiation and synthesize appreciable amounts of hemoglobin. The globins synthesized by FL cells induced to differentiate by DMSO are identical to the globins synthesized in DBA/2 mice, the strain from which the FL cell line was derived (5). Our data, however, demonstrate that the control of translation in induced FL cells is not the same as that found in reticulocytes which primarily synthesize globin. Lysates of FL cells treated with HMBA or AMS, at concentrations which induce differentiation but do not activate HCR or cause inactivation of the translation system (Fig. 1), were found to behave in a fashion similar to that of uninduced FL cell lysates. Neither hemin or HCR had an effect on the incorporation of amino acids into protein. Both hemin and HCR were added to lysates of induced FL cells in amounts which gave final concentrations that were in the range in which they were effective in the rabbit reticulocyte system (Fig. 2). These results clearly indicate that the control of translation of hemoglobin in induced FL cells is markedly different from that found in rabbit reticulocytes where the addition of hemin prevents the activation of HCR. This translational inhibitor possesses a protein kinase activity which specifically phosphorylates the initiation factor eIF-2. The phosphorylation of eIF-2 inhibits initiation of polypeptide synthesis in a manner that is still not completely understood. It most likely involves a conformational change of eIF-2 which prevents interaction with one or more additional protein factors for initiation complex formation (1,4,14,15,17). The possibility that FL cell lysates may modify or inactivate HCR or that FL cell lysates contain high levels of phosphatases capable of dephosphorylating eIF-2 is presently being investigated.

When uninduced FL cell lysates were mixed with rabbit reticulocyte lysates, the total amino acid incorporation observed was less than the sum of the values of the individual lysates (Fig. 3). When the products of translation were analyzed by polyacrylamide gel electrophoresis, the uninduced FL cell proteins were synthesized very efficiently, while synthesis of rabbit globin was inhibited. These results confirm those of Cimadevilla and Hardesty (2) and suggest uninduced FL cells possess a translational inhibitor which specifically prevents the translation of rabbit globin mRNA and only allows the synthesis of uninduced FL cell proteins to proceed. When uninduced lysates were mixed with lysates from induced cells, an inhibition of the total amino acid incorporation was observed (Fig. 4). Therefore, the inhibitor which is present in the lysates from uninduced FL cells not only curtails the synthesis of proteins from rabbit reticulocyte lysates but also proteins from induced FL cells.

Our preliminary findings indicate that, unlike reticulocyte lysates, protein synthesis in lysates of FL cells, whether or not they are induced, show no response to hemin nor to HRC. The fact that protein synthesis in FL cells appears to be operating under a control system different from that controlled by heme in reticulocytes suggests that alternative pathways to differentiation may be available in neoplastic cells.

Work is in progress to determine the nature of the inhibitor in FL cells and the nature of the products of translation.

REFERENCES

1. Amesz, H., Goumans, H., Haubrich-Morree, T., Voorma, H., and Benne, R. (1979): Eur. J. Biochem. 98:513-520.
2. Cimadevilla, J.M., and Hardesty, B. (1975): Biochem. Biophys. Res. Comm. 63:931-937.
3. Cimadevilla, J.M., Kramer, G., Pinphanichakarn, P., Konecki, D., and Hardesty, B. (1975): Arch. Biochem. Biophys. 171:145-153.
4. deHaro, C. and Ochoa, S. (1979): Proc. Nat. Acad. Sci. USA 76:1741-1745.
5. Friend, C. (1980): In: Differentiation and Neoplasia, edited by R. McKinnell et al, pp. 202-212. Springer Verlag, Heidelberg.
6. Friend, C. (In Press): In: Functionally Differentiated Cell Lines, edited by G. Sato. Alan R. Liss, New York.
7. Gazitt, Y., and Friend, C. (1980): Cancer Res. 40:1727-1732.
8. Harrison, P.R., Affara, N., Conkie, D., Rutherford, T., Sommerville, J., and Paul, J. (1976): In: Progress in Differentiation Research, edited by N. Muller-Berat, pp. 135-146. Elsevier/N. Holland, Amsterdam.
9. Kramer, G., Cimadevilla, J., and Hardesty, B. (1976): Proc. Nat. Acad. Sci. USA 73:3078-3082.
10. Marks, P.A., and Rifkind, R.A. (1978): Ann. Rev. Biochem. 47: 419-448.
11. Ochoa, S., and deHaro, C. (1979): Ann. Rev. Biochem. 48:549-580.
12. Orkin, S.H., Swan, D., and Leder, P. (1975): Proc. Nat. Acad. Sci. USA 72:98-102.
13. Pinphanichakarn, P., Kramer, G., and Hardesty, B. (1977): J. Biol. Chem. 252:2106-2112.
14. Ralston, R., Das, A., Grace, M., Das, H., and Gupta, N.K. (1979): Proc. Nat. Acad. Sci. USA 76:5490-5494.
15. Ranu, R.S. (1980) FEBS Letters 112:211-215
16. Ranu, R.S., and London, I.M. (1979): In: Methods in Enzymology, edited by K. Moldave and L. Grossman, Vol. LX pp. 459-482. Academic Press, New York.
17. Ranu, R., and London, I. (1979): Proc. Nat. Acad. Sci. USA 76:1079-1083.
18. Trachsel, H., Ranu, R.S., and London, I.M. (1979): In: Methods in Enzymology, edited by K. Moldave and L. Grossman, Vol. LX pp. 485-495. Academic Press, New York.

Expression of Differentiated Functions in Cancer Cells, edited by R. F. Revoltella et al., Raven Press, New York © 1982.

Murine Erythroleukemia Cell Differentiation: The Relation of Commitment to Terminal Cell Division, Globin mRNA Synthesis, and Cell Cycle Related Effects of Inducer

Paul A. Marks, Zi-xing Chen, Elliot Epner, Judy Banks, Roberto Gambari, and Richard A. Rifkind

Memorial Sloan-Kettering Cancer Center, New York, New York 10021

Over the past several years, evidence has accumulated from studies of several systems that in a cell lineage the transition to synthesis of proteins characteristic of the differentiated state requires cell division (1,2). It is not clear that this relationship between the cell division cycle, or more specifically, the S phase, and the programming of the cells to the synthesis of so-called differentiated proteins is characteristic of all developmental transitions (reviewed in 1-3). In our laboratory we have studied this question, employing the murine erythroleukemia cells (MELC) which are inducible to express a program of erythroid differentiation when cultured with one of several agents (for review, see 3). This program includes many biochemical functions characteristic of normal erythroid cells. Several lines of evidence have suggested that initiation of this program of differentiation by the action of inducers is cell cycle dependent. For example, Levy et al (4) and McClintock and Papaconstantinou (5) demonstrated that an inducer must be present through at least one S phase for MELC to differentiate along the erythroid line. Harrison (6) observed that MELC arrested in the cell cycle in the presence of inducer failed to differentiate. More recently, in our own laboratory, Gambari et al (7) provided evidence that inducer-mediated events during early S appeared to be critical to the expression of certain characteristics of MELC differentiation, including α and β globin mRNAs. Other studies suggested that the portion of MELC genes which replicate early in S may play a role in regulating cell growth as well as the expression of erythroid characteristics (7-9). More generally, DNA replication has been implicated in changes in gene expression in prokaryotes (10), eukaryotes (7-9, 11-17), bacteriophages (18), and animal viruses (19); the mechanisms that govern these changes are unknown.

In this paper, we will review the evidence on the
relationship between the induction of MELC to the commitment
of terminal cell division and the expression of differentiated characteristics, specifically, the accumulation of
newly synthesized α and β globin mRNA. In addition, we will
review the evidence suggesting that an action of the inducer
during the early S phase of the cell division cycle appears
to be critical to the subsequent expression of α and β
globin genes and that α and β globin gene sequences are
replicated in early S phase.

COMMITMENT TO TERMINAL CELL DIVISION

Commitment of MELC to terminal cell division and the
expression of erythroid-specific characteristics (defined as
the ability to continue to differentiate in the absence of
an inducer after initial exposure to inducer) is detectable
in non-synchronized cells between 12 and 16 hrs after onset
of culture, depending on the inducer added (Table 1).
Commitment can be assayed at the single cell level by culture in suspension of MELC with an inducer for various
periods of time, and then transfer of cells to a semisolid
cloning medium and scoring the colonies derived from single
cells for proliferation (colony size) and differentiation
(benzidine reactivity) (20,21). For example, by this
assay, commitment of MELC cultured with 5mM hexamethylene
bisacetamide (HMBA) can be detected as early as 16 hrs and
is essentially complete by 48 hrs (Table 1). Fully

TABLE 1. Globin mRNA accumulation and MELC commitment
after exposure to inducers[*]
(time of appearance)

Inducer		Globin		Commitment
		α	β	
		Hrs		Hrs
Me$_2$SO$_4$	Initial	16	24	16
	Max	96	96	>48
HMBA	Initial	12	24	12
	Max	72	72	48
BA	Initial	12	20	12
	Max	40	72	48
HEMIN	Initial	6	6	>48
	Max	24	24	>72

[*]These data are from Nudel et al (22).

differentiated colonies are small (fewer than 64 cells),
indicating that a committed cell is limited in proliferative capacity to about 5-6 cell divisions. The proportion
of cells that become committed to differentiation is
dependent upon the time and the concentration of inducer
exposure in the precloning suspension culture. The kinetics
of induction of commitment is not identical for all inducing
agents. MELC cultured with HMBA or butyrate (BA) accumulate
committed cells with similar kinetics, but achieve different
maxima (over 95% of the cells become committed with HMBA,
while only about 70% with BA). MELC cultured in the presence of hemin display a quite different pattern of commitment. Although an increase in newly synthesized globin
mRNA is detected as early as 6 hrs after onset of culture,
commitment to terminal cell division does not occur or
occurs only very late (after 72 hrs or more) and then only
in a relatively small proportion of the population (Table 1).
The observation that hemin could induce the expression of
α and β globin genes without commitment of the cells to
terminal cell division was among the evidence pointing to
the possibility that the events involved in the commitment
to terminal cell division were separable from those involved
in the expression of erythroid-specific genes, such as α and
β globin structural genes.

DEXAMETHASONE-MEDIATED INHIBITION OF CELL DIFFERENTIATION

Previous studies from several laboratories (23-27) have
demonstrated that dexamethasone is a potent inhibitor of
inducer-mediated terminal differentiation of MELC, including
suppression of terminal cell division and of accumulation of
globin mRNAs. Our laboratory (28) previously demonstrated
that tumor promoters, such as 12-0-tetradecanoyl-phorbol-
13-acetate (TPA), are also potent inhibitors of inducer-
mediated differentiation of MELC. It was found that TPA can
suppress the expression of characteristics of the committed
state, specifically, terminal cell division and hemoglobin
production, even when MELC are cultured with potent inducers
such as HMBA. Studies on the transfer of MELC from media
containing HMBA plus TPA, to media without either agent,
indicated that MELC retained, for a period, a "memory" of
the exposure to HMBA. The memory for HMBA induction to
commitment is expressed upon removal of the cells from
culture with HMBA plus TPA.
In present experiments, dexamethasone suppression of
expression of differentiated characteristics of MELC cultured with HMBA was studied to further define the nature
of commitment to terminal cell division and its temporal
relation to expression of α and β globin structural genes.
Dexamethasone inhibits accumulation of benzidine reactive
cells among MELC cultured with various inducers (Table 2).
Dexamethasone is a potent inhibitor of induction of MELC
cultured with Me_2SO, HMBA, actinomycin-D, or hemin, but not
butyric acid. The suppression of accumulation of benzidine

reactive cells in MELC cultured with HMBA and dexamethasone reflects an inhibition in accumulation of newly synthesized globin mRNA in the cytoplasm and an inhibition of accumulation of newly synthesized globin mRNA sequences in nuclear RNA (Table 3). These findings suggest that dexamethasone inhibits inducer-mediated increase in the rate of transcription or processing of globin mRNA in MELC cultured with HMBA.

TABLE 2.   Dexamethasone inhibition of accumulation of benzidine reactive cells in MELC cultured with various inducers

| | Benzidine Reactive Cells (%) * | |
| | Dexamethasone Added | |
Inducer	None	10^{-6}M
None	0.5	0.5
Me$_2$SO, 280mμ	80.7	3.0
HMBA, 5mM	100.0	4.3
Butyric acid, 1.2mM	86.4	77.6
Actinomycin-D, 1.5 ng/ml	90.7	7.2
Hemin, 75 μg/ml	56.1	12.7

*The accumulation of benzidine reactive cells was scored on day 5 of culture. Each value represents the average of at least 3 determinations. See Chen et al (29) for details of methods.

[The lack of inhibition of butyric acid induced accumulation of benzidine reactive cells in MELC is reflected in the lack of inhibition of accumulation of newly synthesized globin mRNA in MELC cultured with butyrate (data not shown).]

To examine the relationship between dexamethasone-mediated inhibition of HMBA-induced commitment, MELC were cultured with HMBA and, at intervals up to 72 hrs, aliquots of cells were transferred to semisolid cloning medium without or with 4×10^{-6}M dexamethasone, and without inducer (29). After a 30 hr exposure to HMBA, little or no commitment was apparent by cloning into media with dexamethasone, as compared with over 50% of the cells displaying commitment by cloning into media free of HMBA or dexamethasone. After 40 hrs in HMBA, 80% of the cells were committed, but only a little over 30% of the cells showed evidence of that commitment when cloned in media containing dexamethasone. After 50 hrs in HMBA, approximately 95% of the cells showed commitment cloned into media without or with dexamethasone. These studies suggest that the alterations induced by HMBA which lead to commitment to

TABLE 3. Dexamethasone inhibition of accumulation of newly synthesized globin mRNA in the nuclear and cytoplasmic fractions prepared from MELC cultured with 4mM HMBA without and with 10^{-6}M dexamethasone

Addition	^{3}H-Total RNA	
	Cytoplasm	Nucleus
	$\dfrac{cpm}{10^6 \; cells}$	
HMBA	74,000	468,000
HMBA plus dexamethasone	96,000	560,000

Addition	^{3}H-Globin mRNA*			
	Cytoplasm		Nucleus	
	$\dfrac{cpm}{10^6 \; cells}$	% of total cytoplasm ^{3}H-RNA	$\dfrac{cpm}{10^6 \; cells}$	% of total nuclear ^{3}H-RNA
HMBA	301	0.4	94	0.02
HMBA plus dexameth- asone	54	0.06	14	0.002

*See Chen et al (29) for details of methods to determine amount of total ^{3}H-RNA and of ^{3}H-globin mRNA. Cells were cultured for 65 hrs with HMBA or HMBA plus dexamethasone and then ^{3}H-uridine added and the culture continued for 30 min prior to harvesting of cells for preparation and assay of RNA. The experiment was repeated twice with similar results. In each experiment, cells cultured with HMBA were over 90% B+, and cells cultured with HMBA plus dexamethasone were less than 5% B+, as assayed 4 days after initiation of culture.

terminal cell division while initiated within 30 hrs,
require up to 48 hrs to become resistant to suppression by
dexamethasone (Figure 1).

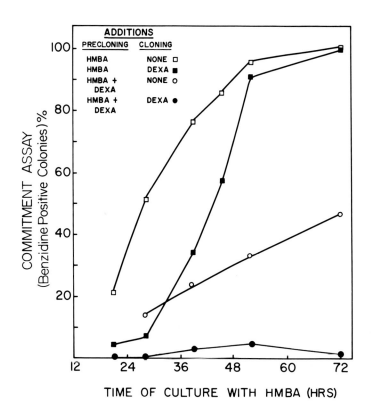

FIG. 1.   Effect of dexamethasone on commitment of MELC to
          erythroid differentiation. Cells cultured with 4mM
          HMBA and, at times indicated on the abscissa,
          aliquots of the suspension culture were transferred
          to semisolid cloning medium without dexamethasone
          (□———□) or with dexamethasone (■———■)
          to assay for commitment to terminal cell division
          (colony size) and hemoglobin synthesis (B+ colo-
          nies). Clones were scored on the fifth day after
          initiation of the cultures. In parallel experiments
          cells were cultured with 4mM HMBA plus 10^{-6}M
          dexamethasone and, at times indicated, aliquots of
          the suspension culture transferred to semisolid
          cloning medium without dexamethasone (o———o) and
          with 10^{-6}M dexamethasone (●———●). From Chen
          et al (29).

In a parallel series of experiments, cells were cultured in suspension culture with both HMBA and dexamethasone, and at intervals up to 72 hrs, aliquots were transferred to semisolid cloning medium without or with dexamethasone, and without inducer. Cells transferred after 30, 40, 50, and 72 hrs to media without dexamethasone showed progressively increasing proportions of colonies committed to terminal cell division. Cells transferred into media with dexamethasone showed little increase in committed colonies (Figure 1). These results suggest that MELC retain a memory of past exposure to HMBA even when such exposure is under conditions of culture where dexamethasone is suppressing the expression of differentiation.

To further examine the relationship of induced commitment to terminal cell division and expression of globin structural genes, the effect of hemin on dexamethasone suppression of HMBA induction was examined. MELC were cultured with HMBA alone, HMBA plus dexamethasone, and HMBA plus dexamethasone plus hemin (Table 4). Hemin reversed the dexamethasone suppression of HMBA-induced hemoglobin formation in MELC, but did not reverse the suppression of commitment to terminal cell division.

TABLE 4. Hemin reversal of dexamethasone inhibition of HMBA induction[+]

Addition	Cell Density* $(x10^6/ml)$	Commit- ment** (%)	Hb* $(\mu g/10^6 \text{ cells})$
None	1.82	1	0.71
HMBA (5mM)	2.12	94	6.70
HMBA + DEXA $(4x10^{-6}M)$	2.04	21	1.14
HMBA + DEXA + HEMIN (0.1mM)	1.78	12	5.40
HEMIN	2.00	3	4.71
HMBA + HEMIN	1.99	89	10.54
HEMIN + DEXA	1.97	6	4.02

* Assayed at 120 hrs after initiation of culture.
**Assayed at 72 hrs after initiation of culture.
[+] From Chen et al (29).

In a subsequent series of experiments, the accumulation and stability of newly synthesized α globin mRNA in MELC in culture with HMBA, or HMBA plus dexamethasone, or HMBA plus dexamethasone plus hemin, were examined (Table 5). These experiments demonstrated that dexamethasone inhibited the accumulation of newly synthesized globin mRNA in cells in culture with HMBA. The addition of hemin to cultures with HMBA plus dexamethasone resulted in a reversal of the dexamethasone effect, that is, the newly synthesized α globin mRNA accumulated at about the same level as in cells cultured with HMBA alone. The dexamethasone suppression of HMBA-induced globin mRNA appears to be primarily at the level of transcription or processing of the globin mRNA. Hemin reversal of the dexamethasone suppression appears to reflect an action at the level of transcription or mRNA processing early (25-38 hrs). At the late time (67-78 hrs), dexamethasone may also affect the stability of mRNA, possibly by affecting cell survival. This is suggested from the observation that when pulse chase experiments were performed, α globin mRNA appeared to be increased in stability in cells in culture with HMBA, dexamethasone plus hemin, as compared to cells in culture with HMBA alone, during the later times in culture.

TABLE 5. Accumulation and stability of newly synthesized α globin mRNA--at 27 hr and 67 hr in culture with HMBA; HMBA plus dexamethasone; HMBA and dexamethasone plus hemin; hemin.

Addition / Time in Culture (hrs)	HMBA	HMBA + DEXA	HMBA DEXA + HEMIN	HEMIN
	α globin mRNA (% of total cytoplasmic ^{3}H-RNA)			
27* Chase 38	.038	.016	.034	.036
	.031	.016	.034	.025
67** Chase 78	.148	.027	.053	.088
	.094	.022	.071	.033

Data from Chen et al (29).

* Cells in culture were labeled for 2 hrs with ^{3}H-uridine (from 25 to 27 hrs) and cells washed, resuspended, and cultured for 11 hrs with excess unlabeled uridine 27 to 38 hrs.

**As above--but cells labeled for 2 hrs from 65 to 67 hrs in culture and chased for 11 hrs from 67 to 78 hrs.

Eisen and his co-workers (30) recently described the protein, IP_{25}, which appeared on the chromatin of MELC early during induced differentiation in vitro. They suggested that this protein may play an important role in the control of proliferation and differentiation of MELC, as well as other cell types. We have examined the accumulation of IP_{25} in MELC cultured with HMBA, HMBA plus dexamethasone, HMBA plus dexamethasone plus hemin, and in the presence of hemin alone. Our observations confirm the report of Eisen et al (30) that IP_{25} accumulates in cells induced with HMBA. Dexamethasone does not inhibit the accumulation of IP_{25}. Hemin does not induce the appearance of IP_{25}. These results are consistent with the possibility that IP_{25} represents a change in chromatin protein which is associated with the action of the inducer leading to commitment to terminal cell division. The accumulation of IP_{25} per se, however, is not sufficient to cause terminal cell division (28), as suggested by findings with MELC in culture with HMBA and dexamethasone.

REPLICATION OF α AND β GLOBIN DNA SEQUENCES IN RELATION TO CELL CYCLE IN MELC

Previous studies in this laboratory as well as in others (4-19) suggest that the S phase in eukaryotic cells is temporally ordered with respect to replication of certain specific DNA sequences. For example, using BrdUrd density labeling to isolate newly synthesized DNA from synchronous cell populations and appropriate radioactive DNA probes, it was determined that ribosomal RNA genes replicate throughout S phase in HeLa and SV3T3 cells (11) and late in S phase in Chinese hamster cells (12). Replication of HeLa 5S RNA genes studied by similar techniques occurs primarily in early S phase (13). In our laboratory we studied the pattern of replication of α, β and rRNA genes in MELC. Synchronous populations of cells were obtained by centrifugal elutriation which separated cells into relatively discrete populations with respect to selected phases of the cell cycle (7,8,30). This technique avoids the use of cell cycle inhibiting agents to create synchrony, which alter cell metabolism and perturb the cell cycle. Newly synthesized DNA was isolated by incorporating BrdUrd into DNA and separating the BrdUrd-DNA from non-substituted DNA by centrifugation to equilibrium in neutral CsCl gradients to obtain double stranded DNA or in alkaline CsCl gradients to obtain single stranded BrdUrd-DNA. The results indicate that α and β globin gene sequences are predominantly located in regions of the genome that replicate early in S phase in logarithmatically growing MELC cells (Table 6 and Table 7). Ribosomal RNA genes are found to replicate in early, middle, and late S phase.

TABLE 6.   Hybridization of [^{32}P] α globin cDNA with BrdUrd-DNA (HL-DNA) and BrdUrd-free DNA (LL-DNA) prepared from cells predominantly in early, mid or late S of the cell cycle. HL-DNA and LL-DNA were separated on neutral CsCl gradients.

	^{32}P cpm/10μg*		
	HL-DNA	LL-DNA	Ratio HL/LL**
Early S	1607	645	2.5
Mid S	799	1338	.6
Late S	505	1265	.4

From Epner et al (31).

* 10μg of each DNA sample was immobilized on nitrocellulose filters, prehybridized, hybridized and washed.

**Ratio HL/LL is the ratio of $\dfrac{\text{cpm/10μg HL-DNA}}{\text{cpm/10μg LL/DNA}}$

TABLE 7.   Hybridization of [^{32}P] α globin cDNA, [^{32}P] β globin cDNA and [^{32}P] ribosomal RNA DNA with single stranded H-DNA (BrdUrd-DNA) prepared from cells predominantly in early, mid or late S phase of the cell cycle. BrdUrd-DNA was separated from non-substituted single stranded DNA (L-DNA) on alkaline (α,β) or neutral (ribosomal) CsCl gradients.

	α*	β*	Rib.*
Early S	100	100	100
Mid S	58	40	95
Late S	39	14	108

From Epner et al (31).

*Values represent the average of 3 determinations for β, 2 for α and 3 for ribosomal RNA DNA (Rib.). Cpm/μg DNA was normalized to 100 for early S phase values, for each experiment, and the results expressed as the average value. Actual cpm/μg DNA for early S phase were: α, 140 and 170; β, 255, 160 and 97 cpm/μg DNA; and ribosomal, 1034, 298 and 1476 cpm/μg.

Hybridization of cloned α and β globin cDNA to newly synthesized BrdUrd-DNA prepared from fractions of cells predominantly in middle or late S phase was observed at a level 15-25% of that for the BrdUrd-DNA isolated from cells predominantly in early S phase. One possible explanation for the low but distinct hybridization to mid and late S-DNA is contamination of middle and late S phase cell fractions by cells in early S phase. Also, BrdUrd-DNA could be contaminated with unsubstituted DNA, although this possibility should have been minimized under the denaturing conditions of the alkaline CsCl gradients. Alternatively, while both globin cDNA probes react primarily with the gene sequences active in mRNA transcription, namely, β major and β minor structural gene sequences with β cDNA probe and α_1 and α_2 structural gene sequences with α cDNA probe, there are DNA sequences in the region of these structural genes which hybridize with these probes and are apparently not translated (31,32). Under the present experimental conditions, over 95% of the hybridization of the cloned α and β cDNA probes was with DNA fragments corresponding in size to those containing globin structural sequences which are transcribed. These further results, taken together with previous studies in this laboratory which suggested that inducer-mediated events occurring during early S phase are critical to the subsequent expression of globin genes (8), provide a correlation between replication of the globin gene sequences and inducer effects leading to the expression of these sequences. It is possible that unique genes that are transcribed or have the potential of being transcribed, are preferentially replicated early in S phase. Non-transcribed heterochromatic regions, such as satellite DNA and inactive X chromosomes, replicate late in S phase (14-17).

ACKNOWLEDGMENTS

These studies were supported, in part, by grants CA-13696, CA-18314, and CA-08748 from the National Cancer Institute, and grant CH-68A from the American Cancer Society.

Roberto Gambari was a visiting fellow from the Istituto di Biologia Generale, Policlinico Umberto I, University of Rome, Italy.

REFERENCES

1. Rutter, W.K. et al (1973) Ann. Rev. Biochem. <u>42</u>:601-646.

2. Holtzer, H. et al (1972) Curr. Top. Dev. Biol. 7:229-256.

3. Marks, P.A. and Rifkind, R.A. (1978) Ann. Rev. Biochem. 47:419-448.

4. Levy, J. et al (1975) Proc. Natl. Acad. Sci. 72:28-32.

5. McClintock, P.R. and Papaconstantinou, J. (1974) Proc. Natl. Acad. Sci. 71:4551-4555.

6. Harrison, P.R. (1977) in International Review of Biochemistry of Cell Differentiation II, ed. Paul, J. (University Park, Baltimore, MD), 15:227-268.

7. Gambari, R. et al (1978) Proc. Natl.Acad. Sci. USA 75:3801-3804.

8. Gambari, R. et al (1979) Proc. Natl. Acad. Sci. USA 76:4511-4515.

9. Brown, E. and Schildkraut, C. (1979) J. Cell Physiol. 99:261-278.

10. Osley, M.A. et al (1977) Cell 12:393-400.

11. Balazs, I. et al (1973) Cold Spring Harbor Symposium, Quantitative Biology 38:239-245.

12. Stambrook, P.J. (1974) J. Mol. Biol. 82:303-313.

13. Ho, C. and Armentrout, R.W. (1978) Biochim. et Biophys. Acta 520:175-183.

14. Tobia, A.M. et al (1970) J. Mol. Biol. 54:499-515.

15. Tobia, A.M. et al (1971) Biochim. et Biophys. Acta 246:258-262.

16. Lima de Faria, A. and Jaworski, H. (1968) Nature (London) 217:138-142.

17. Pardue, M.L. and Gall, J.G. (1970) Science 168:1356-1358.

18. Riva, S. et al (1970) J. Mol. Biol. 54:85-102.

19. Thomas, G. and Mathews, M. (1980) Cell 22:523-533.

20. Fibach, E. et al (1977) Cancer Res. 37:440-444.

21. Gusella, J. et al (1976) Cell 9:221-229.

22. Nudel, U. et al (1977) Cell 12:463-469.

23. McClintock, P.R. et al (1977) J. of Cell Biology 75:351.

24. Tsiftsoglou, A.S. et al (1979) Cancer Res. 39:3849-3855.

25. Lo, S.C. et al (1978) Cell 15:447-453.

26. Scher, W. et al (1978) Proc. Natl. Sci. USA 75:3851-3855.

27. Santoro, N.G. et al (1978) BBRC 85:1510-1517.

28. Fibach, E. et al (1979) Proc. Natl. Acad. Sci. USA 76:1906-1910.

29. Chen, Z.X. et al (1981, in press).

30. Eisen, H. et al (1979) in In Vivo and In Vitro Erythropoiesis: The Friend System, ed. Rossi, G.B. 289-296.

31. Epner, E. et al (1981) Proc. Natl. Acad. Sci. USA (in press).

32. Nishioka, Y. et al (1980) Proc. Natl. Acad. Sci. USA 77:2806-2809.

33. Leder, P. et al (1980) Science 209:1336-1342.

Expression of Differentiated Functions in Cancer Cells, edited by R. F. Revoltella et al., Raven Press, New York © 1982.

The Expression of Non-Globin Genes During Red Blood Cell Differentiation

P. R. Harrison, N. Affara, C. Casimir, P. Goldfarb, and A. Lyons

Beatson Institute for Cancer Research, Glasgow G61 1BD, Scotland

How sets of structural genes which are usually located on different chromosomes come to be expressed selectively during the growth and differentiation of eukaryotic cells is a major biological question that is highly relevant to understanding the nature of the aberrant proliferation and differentiation of cancer cells.

The basic premise from which our own experimental approach stems is that the elucidation of the mechanisms by which sequential gene expression is coordinated during cell differentiation requires firstly a molecular analysis of the organisation, transcription and subsequent expression of such sets of unlinked specific structural genes; and then secondly, genetic definition of the (putative) regulatory genes involved. Cell differentiation in higher eukaryotes may well involve significantly different regulatory mechanisms to those operating in prokaryotes and lower eukaryotes; but on the basis of evidence from these simpler systems, a regulatory gene might be expected to act either on a particular structural gene to which it is covalently linked (i.e. act cis) or alternatively control a series of unlinked structural genes on different chromosomes (i.e. act trans), for example via a diffusible RNA or protein regulatory molecule. Structural information about several specific genes or gene clusters in higher eukaryotes is now becoming available (e.g. histones, vitellogenin, ovalbumin, globins, chorion proteins and the special case of immunoglobulins) and in a few cases evidence for cis-regulation exists (for the rosy and ocelliless loci in Drosophila controlling xanthine dehydrogenase and two chorion proteins respectively {1, 2} and also the human β -globin gene cluster {3, 4}. But molecular or genetic analysis of the regulation of unlinked structural gene sets in eukaryotes is rudimentary except in fungi, although other experimental systems are beginning to be studied such as ecdysone or heat shock-induced gene activation in Drosphila {5}, slime-mold development {6}, egg white protein synthesis and myogenesis.

We are therefore attempting to exploit murine erythropoiesis as an experimentally favourable model for elucidating the coordinate regulation of unlinked structural genes, in particular those coding for well-defined erythroid markers such as spectrin, glycophorin and the globins. As a first step in this approach, we have cloned certain non-globin messenger RNAs from erythroblasts and reticulocytes using recombinant DNA technology in order to provide specific probes for isolating and monitoring the activities of genes selectively expressed during red blood cell differentiation. We are currently characterising the proteins for which these non-globin recombinants code and studying the pattern of their expression during red blood cell maturation. In the course of these studies we have also identified a recombinant coding for a globin chain expressed specifically in foetal erythropoiesis and in Friend cells induced to undergo erythroid maturation in culture.

RESULTS

Reticulocytes and erythroblasts synthesise various proteins in addition to the globins required for establishing the specialised functions of the red blood cell and for maintaining its integrity in the peripheral circulation. Although globin mRNAs comprise greater than 90% of the total mRNA population in reticulocytes, a few other mRNAs are present as judged by protein synthesis studies of translation assays (Figure 1).

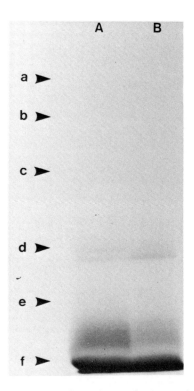

FIG.1. Translation of reticulocyte polyA-containing mRNAs. Total polyA- RNAs were isolated from peripheral blood of mice either 5d (A) or 3d (B) after induction of anaemia by acetyl phenyl hydrazine treatment. The buffy coat was removed from the blood sample prior to RNA extraction. PolyA-RNAs were then translated in the rabbit reticulocyte lysate system and the polypeptides synthesised analysed on polyacrylamide/SDS gels. The arrows at a, b, c, d, e, f mark the positions of markers at 94, 67, 43, 30, 20 and 14,000 daltons.

In contrast, erythroblasts contain a much more diverse range of mRNAs as estimated from the rate of hybridisation between complementary DNAs (cDNAs) and the total poly A-containing mRNA population from which they are transcribed (Figure 2).

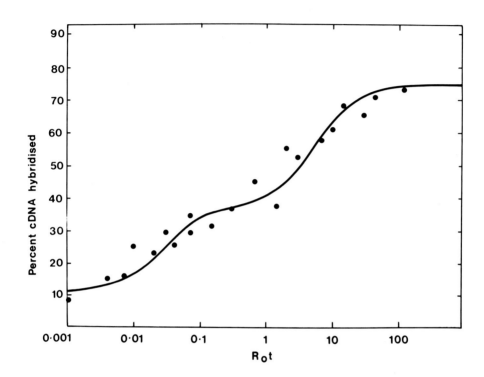

FIG.2. The complexity of foetal liver mRNAs. The total polyA-containing cytoplasmic RNAs from 14d foetal liver erythroblasts were transcribed into complementary DNAs (cDNAs) which were then hybridised back to excess template mRNA. Abscissa, Rot: RNA concentration X time (moles x sec/l). Hybridisation conditions were 0.3M NaCl, 70°. The Rot curve was then analysed into components by comuter programme using the globin mRNA/globin cDNA hybridisation as standard.

Computer analysis of such complex hybridisation reactions is consistent with there being a class about 15 abundant mRNAs representing about 40% of the total mRNA content together with about 5000 rarer mRNA sequences present at only a few copies per cell. The aim of our research has been to obtain probes for these non-globin but fairly abundant mRNAs present in reticulocytes and erythroblasts, especially those which are specific to red blood cells.

Cloning procedures

Our approach has been to clone double-stranded cDNAs transcribed from the total reticulocyte or foetal liver erythroblast polyA[+] mRNA population in plasmid vectors by creating appropriate cDNA libraries using the blunt-end ligation technique. Briefly, single-stranded cDNAs transcribed from the mRNA populations using reverse transcriptase were rendered double-stranded with DNA polymerase, treated with S1 nuclease to remove single-stranded regions including the hairpin loop and then treated with DNA polymerase again to render the termini absolutely flush-ended after the S1 treatment. Plasmid pAT153 was linearised with restriction enzyme BamH1 or Hind III, the sticky ends repaired with DNA polymerase and then treated with alkaline phosphatase to remove terminal phosphates so as to prevent recyclization of the plasmid vector alone. Double-stranded cDNA was then ligated to the phosphatase-treated pAT153 vector in equimolar amounts and the mixture used directly to transform E.Coli HB101 under Category II conditions. Transformants were isolated by selection for ampicillin-resistance, picked into master microtitre wells and transferred by transfer plate on to nitrocellulose filters for screening with ^{32}P-labelled foetal liver or reticulocyte cDNA by the Grunstein-Hogness procedure in order to identify recombinants positively. Recombinants were then grouped according to the relative extents of hybridisation with labelled cDNA from the appropriate mRNA used for cloning.

To determine which of the foetal liver recombinants coded for erythroid cell-specific mRNAs, replica filters were also hybridised to cDNA transcribed from primary fibroblast polyA-containing mRNAs. Thus foetal liver recombinants showing high hybridisation to fibroblast cDNA were eliminated from further screening. However, all reticulocyte cDNA recombinants were retained since reticulocytes contain a much more restricted mRNA population than erythroblasts and the identification which mRNAs remain after nuclear extrusion is an interesting biological question. Detailed results are given in ref.7.

Screening for non-globin recombinants

Recombinants coding for adult α -or β -globin mRNAs were next identified according to whether the hybridisation with reticulocyte cDNA was reduced by pre-hybridisation of the cDNA with excess α and β - globin cDNA recombinant plasmid DNAs (obtained from Dr. C. Weissmann, Zurich) (see ref. 7 for details). A novel alternative procedure is to use the sandwich transfer method to identify globin cDNA recombinants. In this technique rows of recombinants spotted from microtitre plates onto nitrocellulose filters were first hybridised with foetal liver or reticulocyte cDNA (Figure 3, left). The washed filter was then placed back-to-back with a replica filter containing rows of the same cDNA recombinants arranged at right angles, the cDNA hybridised melted briefly and then allowed to rehybridise. Both filters were then washed and autoradiographed so that transfer of cDNA from the recombinants on to the α or β globin cDNA recombinants could be detected (Figure 3, right). From this type of screening, recombinants coding for adult α , β globins were identified (e.g. AH3, AF3, AE4, and AE1) and eliminated from further screening. This technique is useful not only for identifying clones coding for α and β globins but also it indicates which code for the same or different sequences. Thus scrutiny of the pattern of cross-hybridisation between recombinants AH3, AF3, AE1 and AE4, for example, shows that the first three contain cDNAs transcribed from the same globin mRNA whereas AE4 contains a different globin cDNA.

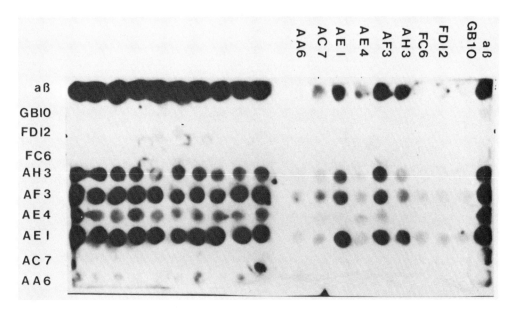

FIG.3. Screening of cDNA recombinants. Nine cDNA recombinants were spotted in rows onto a nitrocellulose filter (A, left) together with cloned ∝ and β globin cDNA recombinants, lysed and denatured, and then hybridised with ^{32}P-labelled foetal liver cDNA. After washing, filter A was then placed back-to-back with a second replica filter B arranged with the rows of recombinants at right angles to those on filter A. The filters were then briefly heated to melt any hybridised cDNA on filter A and then the cDNA allowed to rehybridise. The filters were then separated, washed and autoradiographed to detect transfer of cDNA from filter A (left) to filter B (right). Only if the recombinants placed back-to-back contain part of the same cDNA sequence should cDNA be transferred between recombinants on the two filters.

Putative non-globin cDNA recombinants identified in this way were grown up, plasmid DNA extracted, digested with restriction enzymes (eg. EcoR1 and HinF1) and then run on acrylamide on agarose gels. In this way the sizes of the cDNA inserts could be determined by comparison of the restriction patterns with that of pAT153 itself (results summarised in Table 1).

Identification of recombinants by translation assay

One uncertainty with the above screening procedures to eliminate globin cDNA recombinants is that a recombinant encoding a short region towards the 5'-end of an adult globin mRNA might fail to be identified since the available ∝ and β globin cDNA recombinants used for competition selection represent the 3'-region of the mRNA. To overcome this problem, DNA from putative non-globin cDNA recombinants was bound to DBM-filters, incubated with reticulocyte mRNA and then any hybridised mRNA eluted and translated in the wheat germ system. By analysing the translation products on acid-urea polyacrylamide gels, basic proteins such as the ∝ and β globins can be well resolved (Figure 4).

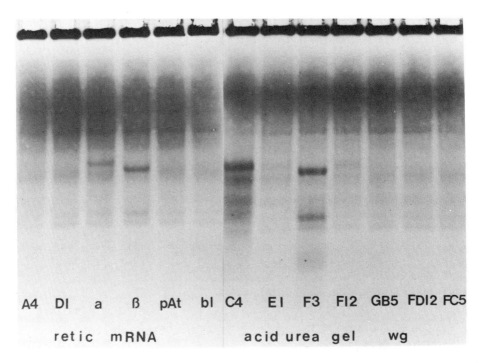

FIG.4. Identification of non-globin cDNA recombinants by translational assay. Plasmid pAT or foetal liver recombinant cDNAs were bound to discs of DBM-paper and then hybridised with reticulocyte mRNA. After washing, the bound mRNA was eluted, translated in the wheat germ system and analysed by electrophoresis on acid-urea gels. a,β:cloned ∝ or β globin cDNA recombinants; bl: polypeptides synthesised by lysate system alone.

These results show that under conditions where ∝ or β globin cDNA recombinants hybridise ∝ or β globin mRNAs specifically, some recombinants (such as A4, D1, FD12, FC5 and GB5) fail to hybridise either ∝ or β globin mRNA, whereas others (eg. C4, E1, F3 and F12) do. Interestingly even recombinants with short globin cDNA inserts (eg. F12 (107bp)) are detected by this translation assay although they remained undetected by the cDNA hybridisation experiments.

Attempts were then made to identify positively the proteins encoded by these non-globin cDNA recombinants by similar transation assays, except that the recombinant cDNAs were hybridised with the induced Friend cell total mRNA population, prior to translation of the bound mRNA in the reticulocyte lysate system and analysis of the translation products on SDS-polyacrylamide gels (Figure 5). It proved possible to identify some recombinants coding for fairly abundant induced Friend cell mRNAs in this way, for example, recombinants FA6 & FC5 seem to code

for protein(s) of molecular weight about 30,000 (possibly carbonic
anhydrase?) whereas recombinant A4 codes for a protein of molecular
weight 35,000.

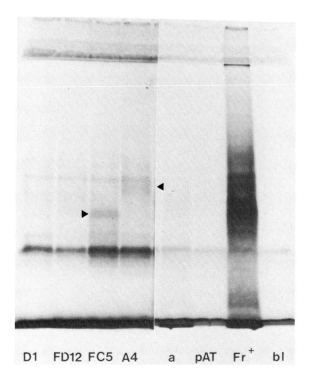

D1   FD12 FC5 A4   a   pAT Fr[+] bl

FIG.5. Characterisation of the proteins encoded by non-globin cDNA
recombinants by translational assay. Recombinants were analysed as
described in Fig.4, except that the hybridisation was to total induced
Friend cell polyA-containing RNA, the bound mRNAs were translated in the
rabbit reticulocyte lysate system and polypeptides synthesised were
analysed by electrophoresis on SDS/polyacrylamide gels.   Fr[+]:
translation products of total induced Friend cell polyA-containing mRNA.

The sizes of the mRNAs encoded by these non-globin cDNA recombinants
have also been investigated by electrophoresis of the induced Friend
cell mRNA population on formaldehyde/agarose gels followed by transfer
of the RNAs to nitrocellulose filters and hybridisation with the nick
translated recombinant cDNAs individually.   The sizes of the more
abundant mRNAs encoded by the non-globin cDNA recombinants are
summarised in Table 1.

The Tissue distribution of cloned non-globin mRNAs

To determine the stage of erythroid cell maturation at which the
mRNAs encoded by the non-globin cDNA recombinants are expressed, oligo
dT-primed cDNAs transcribed from the mRNA populations from various

TABLE 1: CHARACTERISTICS OF mRNAs ENCODED BY FOETAL LIVER AND RETICULOCYTE cDNA RECOMBINANTS

Recombinant	Insert size	size mRNA coded	size protein coded	mRNA abundance (% total)*		
				Uninduced FLC	Induced FLC	Reticulocyte
globin	370	9S	14,000	0.1	2.8	36
globin	530	9S	14,000	0.15	2.4	36
A. Foetal liver cDNA recombinants						
GB5	330 bp	9S	14,000 globin	0.05	3.0	0.8
FC5	287 bp	12S	30,000	0.07	0.3	0.1
FA6	250 bp	12S	30,000	0.1	0.4	0.1
D1	?	15S		0.05	0.15	2.0
A4	265 bp	13S	40,000	0.25	0.5	0.2
D6	194 bp	7-8S		0.25	0.44	0.2
G10	?			0.04	0.02	0.2
F4	140 bp			0.04	0.02	0.25
F5	10-12 bp			0.04	0.03	0.15
FD12	790 bp			0.05	0.14	0.1
GB10	?			0.02	0.05	0.1
B. Reticulocyte cDNA recombinants						
CC3	900			0.01	0.01	6
CC6	175			0.07	0.16	14
CC7	200			0.02	0.58	9.5
CC9	200			0.02	0.16	3.2

* Measured by titration of total cDNA with the recombinant DNA as described in Figure 6.

erythroid cell types were hybridised to each non-globin cDNA recombinant bound to nitrocellulose filters. The principle of the method is illustrated in Figure 6: under the conditions used, about 3% of the total induced Friend cell cDNA hybridised to ∝ or β globin cDNA recombinants, a figure in close agreement with values obtained by solution hybridisation experiments (8).

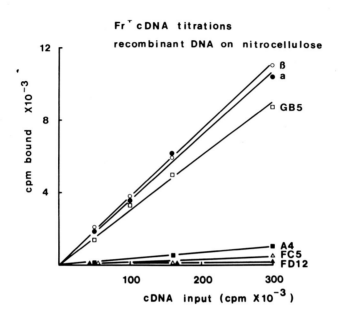

Fr⁺ cDNA titrations

recombinant DNA on nitrocellulose

FIG.6. Levels of mRNAs encoded by foetal liver cDNA recombinants in induced Friend cells. Increasing amounts of cDNA transcribed from induced Friend cell mRNA were hybridised with each recombinant DNA bound to nitrocellulose, the filters washed extensively and the amount of cDNA bound determined. Other details were as in Fig. 4.

Figure 6 also shows that the level of GB5 mRNA is high in induced Friend cells; whereas the levels of A4, FC5 and FD12 are much lower. Caution must be exercised in deducing the absolute levels of mRNAs encoded by the different recombinants from such experiments since the size and position of the cloned cDNA insert relative to the mRNA sequence could affect the level of hybridisation of 3'-primed cDNAs: clearly cloned cDNA inserts derived from the 5' end of the mRNA would be seriously underestimated in 3'-primed cDNA transcripts. However, such complications do not arise in comparing the relative amounts of the mRNA encoded by a single recombinant between various cDNA populations.

The results of many experiments of this kind are summarised in Table 1. One foetal liver cDNA recombinant (D1) encodes a mRNA expressed late in erythroid cell maturation; whereas others (e.g. A4, D6, FC5 and FA6) are expressed at a more pronounced level in mid erythroblasts (eg. induced Friend cells). The mRNAs encoded by five other recombinants are seemingly expressed at very low levels in all the erythroid cell types examined.

Most of the reticulocyte non-globin cDNA recombinants seem to code for mRNAs expressed at increased levels as the erythroblasts mature into reticulocytes (Table 1). Most of these mRNAs are also expressed at significant levels in other non-erythroid tissues such as fibroblasts and brain cells (up to 0.1-0.2%) of the total fibroblast mRNA in the case of a CC6 and 9 for example). This suggests that they contain cDNA transcripts of mRNAs coding for proteins (possibly enzymes) necessary for maintainance of cells in general.

Identity of the mRNA encoded by recombinant GB5

Interestingly, recombinant GB5 appears to contain a cDNA transcribed from a relatively abundant mRNA in induced Friend cells (Figure 6) coding for a small protein about the size of globin (not shown); yet the GB5 mRNA cannot be detected in adult reticulocyte mRNA (Figure 4). Since GB5 was cloned from the 13-15d foetal liver mRNA population, these results raise the possibility that GB5 might code for a foetal globin mRNA which fails to cross-hybridise with adult α or β globin cDNA recombinants under the hybridisation conditions used. To explore this possibility, yolk sac-derived nucleated erythrocytes from the 12d foetal-circulation were isolated and separated from any foetal liver-derived enucleated erythrocytes by centrifugal elutriation using the Beckman JE-6B rotor. Enucleated foetal erythrocytes from 15 day foetal peripheral blood were also separated from contaminating nucleated erythrocytes using the same technique. RNAs extracted from yolk sac-derived nucleated erythrocytes, foetal enucleated erythrocytes, adult reticulocytes and induced Friend cells were then hybridised to GB5 DNA, the bound RNA translated in the wheat germ system and the translation products analysed by elctrophoresis on acid-urea gels. These experiments (see ref. 7 for details) showed that pGF5 codes for a β -like globin mRNA present in foetal liver erythroblasts, foetal erythrocytes and in induced Friend cells whereas it is absent in yolk-sac derived nucleated erythrocytes and adult reticulocytes. Recently, the entire 330 bp cDNA insert in pGF5 has been sequenced (ref. 7) and shown to differ from the adult β major and β minor mRNA sequences although it is virtually identical to the ey_3 globin gene sequence over the limited conserved region which has been published. However the amino acid sequence encoded by GB5 cDNA is substantially different from the embryonic globin chains ey_2 and ez.

For convenience the present state of our information concerning the nature of the mRNAs encoded by our cDNA recombinants is summarised in Table 1.

DISCUSSION

Our results have shown it to be possible to isolate recombinants from a total erythroblast or reticulocyte cDNA library which contain cloned cDNAs transcribed from non-globin mRNAs expressed at various stages of erythroblast maturation. In the case of recombinants coding for fairly abundant mRNAs, the sizes of the corresponding mRNAs and proteins encoded have been determined. Thus two recombinants FA6 & FC5 code for (probably the same) protein of M.W. about 30,000 daltons. We are currently attempting to determine whether these two recombinants code for carbonic anhydrase by immune precipitation of the translated protein and by direct sequencing of the cDNA inserts. The nature of the proteins encoded by A4 and other recombinants is being analysed by fractionating the translation products by the two dimensional isoelectrofocussing/PAGE technique.

Our future plans are to isolate genomic DNA fragments coding for the mRNAs encoded by our cDNA recombinants by screening mouse genomic DNA libraries and then to search for structural similarities in the DNA sequences surrounding the set of structural genes expressed during red blood cell differentiation. This may enable us to elucidate how these genes are recognised as those to be expressed specifically during red blood cell maturation. In order to study the molecular mechanisms involved in the selective expression of these genes, we plan to determine the chromatin organisation and pattern of transcription and processing of the non-globin genes in various cell lines derived from haemopoietic cell precursors or more distantly-related cell types.

EXPERIMENTAL PROCEDURES

All procedures were performed as described previously (7).

ACKNOWLEDGEMENTS

We acknowledge financial support from the Medical Research Council and the Cancer Research Campaign. We are grateful to Dr. J. Paul for useful discussions and in particular the suggestion of the sandwich transfer technique.

REFERENCES

1. Chovnick, A., Gelbart, W. and McCarron, M. (1977): Cell, 11: 1-10.
2. Spradling, A.C., Waring, G.L. and Mahowald, A.P. (1979): Cell, 16: 609-616.
3. Fritsch, E.F.,Lawn, R.M. and Maniatis, J. (1979): Nature, 279: 598-603.
4. Van der Ploeg, L.A.T., Konings, A., Ooyt,M., Roos, D., Bernini, L. and Flavell, R.A. (1980): Nature, 283: 637-642.
5. Asburner, M. and Bonner, J.J. (1979): Cell, 17: 241-254.
6. Kimmel, A.R. and Firtel, R.A. (1979): Cell, 16: 787-796.
7. Affara, N., Vass, K., Goldfarb, P., Lyons, A. and Harrison, P.R. Nucleic Acids Research, submitted.
8. Affara, N. and Daubas, P. (1979): Dev. Biol, 72: 110.

Expression of Differentiated Functions in Cancer Cells, edited by R. F. Revoltella et al., Raven Press, New York © 1982.

The Erythropoietic Component of Friend Virus Erythroleukemias: Role of Erythropoietic Hormone(s) and SFFV Genome

*†C. Peschle, **G. Colletta, †A. Covelli, † R. Ciccariello, †G. Migliaccio, and *G. B. Rossi

*Istituto Superiore di Sanità, Rome; †Istituto Patologia Medica, **Chair of Viral Oncology, Istituto Patologia Generale, IInd Faculty of Medicine and Surgery, University of Naples, Naples, Italy

Abbreviations

Friend Leukemia Virus, FLV; polycythemic and anemic, FLV-P and FLV-A. Friend Murine Leukemia Virus, F-MuLV; polycythemic and anemic, F-MuLVp and F-MuLV$_A$. Spleen Focus-Forming Virus, SFFV; polycythemic and anemic, SFFVp and SFFV$_A$. Colony-forming unit(s), CFU; spleen CFU, CFU-S, erythroid CFU, CFU-E; granulo-macrophage CFU, CFU-GM. Burst-forming unit(s), erythroid, BFU-E. Erythropoietin, Ep. Burst-promoting factor(s), BPF. Colony-stimulating factor(s), CSF. Spleen conditioned medium (lectin-stimulated or not), SCM. Fetal calf serum, FCS.

PRELIMINARY REMARKS

FLV-induced erythroleukemias show a kinetic pattern characterized by: (a) amplification of the splenic pool of BFU-E and CFU-E (17);(b) enhanced cycling of BFU-E (17); (c) Ep-independent growth of splenic CFU-E from FLV-P- but not FLV-A-infected mice (16,17) (heretofore FLV-P or FLV-A mice). In line with (c), erythropoiesis is effective in FLV-P animals, thus leading to polycythemia, but is abortive in FLV-A mice, hence causing anemia (6).

These results relate to recent advances on mechanisms regulating normal erythropoiesis (cfr. 18). In vitro, differentiation of normal BFU-E (8,25) and CFU-E (1) is largely controlled by BPF and Ep respectively; BPF also modulates the cycling activity of BFU-E (25). In vivo, Ep levels regulate the erythropoietic rate (cfr 18). The in vivo role of BPF, although

311

still under scrutiny, is conceivably similar to that played in culture (cfr. 18). Additionally, the T-lymphocyte-macrophage complex is apparently involved in production of BPF (21, see also 18)and perhaps Ep (19). These studies shed light on possible mechanism(s) underlying the kinetics of erythroid progenitors in FLV leukemias. Since FLV infection causes enhanced cycling of BFU-E, the possibility may be considered that BPF is elevated in FLV leukemias. On the other hand, Ep-independent growth of splenic CFU-E from FLV-P mice suggests that: (a) Ep-like activity is released in culture (by macrophages?), or (b) transformed CFU-E are capable to differentiate independently of physiologic hormonal control. Hypothetically, transformed CFU-E might respond to the low levels of Ep present in plated FCS: this possibility, however, is excluded by the Ep-independent growth of these progenitors in FCS-free cultures (20).

These considerations should be seen in the perspective of recent molecular studies on the FLV complex (11,12,14,15). Indeed, cloning of FLV components has allowed to establish the following: (a) both strains of FLV (i.e., FLV-P, FLV-A) contain a helper-independent Murine Leukemogenic Virus (F-MuLV$_P$ and F-MuLV$_A$, which are either identical or intimately cross-related). (b) FLV-P also consists of the defective Spleen Focus Forming Virus (SFFVp), which is by definition biologically active. (c) FLV-A also includes SFFV$_A$, i.e. SFFVp-related sequences exerting   an erratic biologic action (possibly caused by faulty glycosilation of its marker gp$_{52}$, E.M. Scolnick, personal communication).

SFFVp is apparently linked to the erythropoietic component of FLV-P leukemia. SFFVp pseudotypes, derived (12) or not (4,13) from plasmid purified DNA, were rescued by a number of unrelated helper viruses, including F-MuLVp. All pseudotypes induced Ep-independent growth of splenic CFU-E (4,13) and erythroblastosis + polycythemia (12), whereas the type of leukemia was always dependent upon the given helper virus (4,12,13). Furthermore, Ep-independent growth of CFU-E in different mouse strains is directly correlated with their susceptibility to SFFVp (17). It may be conceded therefore that, in keeping with C. Friend's appraisal (6), the SFFVp genome does not cause per se any bona fide leukemic event, but exerts an Ep-like action on erythropoiesis.

Recent observations at molecular and cellular level therefore suggest that expression of SFFVp and enhanced activity of erythropoietic hormone(s) underlie the erythroid component of FLV-P leukemia. In this regard, enhanced cycling of BFU-E in FLV mice may be hypothetically mediated via elevated BPF activity, in turn mediated via SFFV expression. Circumstancial support to a linkage between BFU-E cycling and SFFV expression is provided by observations showing that the gene locus (Fv-2) controlling BFU-E proliferation also regulates susceptibility to SFFVp (22).

EXPERIMENTAL APPROACH

The present studies have been devised to probe (a) the role of erythropoietic hormone(s) (BPF, Ep) in the erythroid component of FLV leukemias and (b) the presence of SFFVp-related sequences in erythroid or GM-colonies from leukemic and normal mice. The first aspect was assessed in culture under stringent conditions, i.e., in presence of O (C. Peschle, unpublished observations) or 4% FCS (9). The second one has been assayed by hybridization studies (3) on cytoplasmic RNA's extracted from pools of erythroid bursts or GM-colonies, which were picked up from standard methylcellulose cultures (17); each pool contained as little as $\sim$1-2x10^6 nucleated cells. The colonies derived from marrow or spleen of FLV-infected and normal mice. The probes were conventional cDNA's against whole FLV-P or SFFVp-specific sequences (3).

RESULTS AND DISCUSSION

Detailed results are being published elsewhere. In this paper, we concisely show some representative data. We then discuss the possible role of erythropoietic hormones and SFFV$_p$, and finally propose a model for the pathophysiology of FLV leukemias.

Studies on Erythropoietic Hormones

In FLV-P mice infected from 10-12 days, the cloning of splenic BFU-E and CFU-E is fully BPF- and Ep-independent respectively (Table 1). The "hormone independence", however, is either total or only partial if evaluated at different times after infection (Fig. 1, and data not shown). In striking contrast, growth of GM-colonies always requires CSF addition (Table 1 and results not presented here).

Erythroid progenitors from marrow of FLV-P mice show a less clearcut hormone independence, while CFU-GM remain fully dependent of CSF addition (Table 1 and unpublished data).

TABLE 1. Cloning of hemopoietic progenitors from spleen or marrow of normal, FLV-P and FLV-A mice in 4% FCS-free cultures.[a]

Progenitors	Plated Hormones[b]	Uninfected mice Spleen[c]	Marrow[d]	FLV-P mice Spleen[c]	Marrow[d]	FLV-A mice Spleen[c]	Marrow[d]
BFU-E	BPF, Ep	12	21	14	23	10	19
	Ep	0	0	13	4	5	0
CFU-E	Ep	312	162	1200	174	960	120
	none	36	24	1140	72	252	24
CFU-GM	CSF	50	151	40	156	47	126
	none	0	0	0	0	0	0

a) A representative experiment from normal or 10-12-day infected DBA/2 mice (female, 18-22 g) is shown here (2-3 mice and 2 plates/group).

b) BPF and CSF: ConA-stimulated SCM, prepared as in (25) (each plate contained 20% SCM, i.e. plateau levels of both factors). Ep: Step III sheep Ep (Connaugth Medical Research Laboratories, Toronto) containing <1 ng endotoxin/IU (1.5 IU/plate).

c) Colonies/1.5x10^5 nucleated cells/plate.

d) Colonies/5x10^4 nucleated cells/plate.

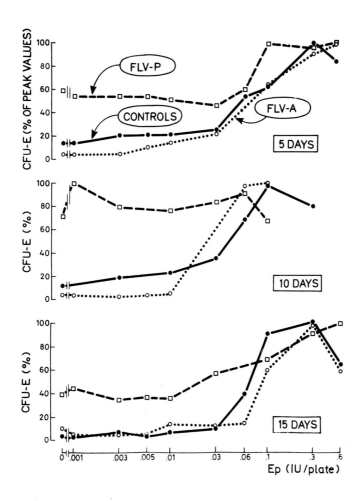

Fig. 1 Ep dose/response curves of CFU-E from spleen of control (—), FLV-P (--) or FLV-A (··) mice (see Table 1) at 5,10, or 15 days after infection. The assay was carried out in FCS-free cultures (9) stimulated by human uri̱nary Ep, semi-purified as described (17). Mean values from at least 2 experiments are presented. Data are expressed as % of peak levels.

These data suggest that (a) erythroid progenitors from FLV-P spleen differentiate independently of physiologic hormone stimuli,or (b) they respond to enhanced activity of erythropoietic hormones released in culture. As an initial attempt to discriminate between these two hypotheses, we have prepared (25) medium conditioned by FLV-P splenocytes in the absence of Concanavalin A stimulus (ConA⁻ SCM). This SCM, tested in FCS-free cultures of normal splenocytes, exerted a discrete but significant BPF- and Ep-like effect (i.e., induced growth of BFU-E and CFU-E respectively) (data not shown). CSF-like activity was not observed, thus in line with the hormone dependence of CFU-GM from FLV-P spleen. These observations, although in need of confirmation, indicate that FLV-P splenocytes release in vitro BPF- and Ep-like activity. This may in turn suggest FLV infection of the T-lymphocyte-macrophage complex, which would be thereby stimulated to release BPF and possibly Ep-like factor(s) in absence of lectin stimulus (indeed, early infection by FLV-P of splenic macrophages has been documented (24)). Accordingly, the discrete magnitude of BPF- and Ep-like activity in ConA⁻ SCM might be referred to the dramatic decrease of the relative lymphocyte content in FLV-P spleen at 7-14 day after infection (<20% lymphocytes in the whole splenic population, as compared to ∿80-90% in control organ).

In FLV-A mice, the "hormone independence" of erythroid progenitors is less clearcut in spleen, and absent in marrow (Table 1). In line with this erratic pattern, ConA⁻ SCM from FLV-A animals exerts a more variable BPF- and Ep-like activity, as compared to that from FLV-P mice (data not shown).

Expression of FLV Sequences in Erythroid and GM-colonies

Cytoplasmic viral RNA's has been evaluated (a) in pooled bursts and GM-colonies from spleen or marrow of FLV-infected or normal mice, and (b) in corresponding whole spleen or marrow cell populations. It seemed necessary to insure that the assay of viral sequences in colonies was not biased by spread of FLV infection to uninfected, non-contiguous cells during the culture period. In this regard, addition of anti-gp$_{70}$ serum in FLV-P dishes did not significantly modify the pattern of RNA's hybridization against the FLV-P probe, as compared to that observed in control FLV-P plates (data not shown). These experiments seemingly exclude the in vitro spread of FLV infection from infected cells to uninfected, non-contiguous ones.

Results available so far can be summarized as follows: (a)

TABLE 2. FLV-P specific sequences in normal and 15-20-day FLV-P-infected mice.[a]

Source of cytoplasmic RNA[b]	Levels of FLV-P-specific sequences[c]	
	Crt 1/2[d]	% viral RNA
Normal spleen cells	600	0.0023
Infected spleen cells	25	0.056
Infected spleen bursts	120	0.0116
Infected spleen CFU-GM colonies	75	0.018
Normal marrow cells	2000	0.0007
Infected marrow cells	300	0.0046
Infected marrow bursts	140	0.010
Infected marrow CFU-GM colonies	160	0.0087

a) Mean values from 2-4 experiments are shown here. Mice as in Table 1.

b) Cytoplasmic RNA was extracted as previously described (3).

c) The level of viral specific sequences in cytoplasmic RNA was determined by hybridization of the extracted RNA with radioactive cDNA probe against whole FLV-P specific sequen ces, as previously described (3).

d) Crt value (expressed as moles x liter^{-1} x sec^{-1}) required to reach 50% of final hybridization value.

the levels of both FLV-P- (Table 2) and SFFVp-specific (data
not shown) RNA's are comparable in pooled BFU-E- and CFU-GM-
derived colonies from both spleen and marrow of FLV-P mice.
(b) In whole spleen, both RNA species are more abundant than
in whole marrow (Table 1 and results not presented here). A
similar difference has been demonstrated in FLV-A mice (not
shown). Both FLV-P- (Table 1) and SFFVp-specific (not present
ed here) sequences are detected in bursts and GM-colonies
from spleen of FLV-P mice. Comparable or slightly lower leve
ls are present in corresponding colonies from FLV-P marrow
(Table 1 and data not shown). (c) In normal animals, these
viral sequences have been detected at low levels in whole mar
row and spleen (Table 1 and results not presented), in keeping with data of (2). Furthermore, they were barely and occa
sionally detected in GM-colonies, but not in bursts from either organ (not shown).

   Data in (a) reflect on previous studies on "target cell(s)"
in FLV-leukemias. In this regard, Tambourin and Wendling
(23) suggested that an erythroid progenitor functions as tar
get of FLV-P. Furthermore,   normal marrow cells, infected
in vitro by FLV-P, showed significant burst formation in absence of added Ep (7). The number of bursts was increased
when cell fractions from normal spleen, enriched for "late"
BFU-E and CFU-E,were similarly infected (10). In both cases
(7,10), however, macrophages and/or lymphocytes coseeded with
erythroid progenitors might have mediated burst formation,
via elevated BPF-like activity. The molecular data hereby re
ported suggest that FLV-P sequences are equally expressed in
both erythroid, granulocytic and macrophage lineage (in this
last regard, $\sim$90% pure G- and M-colonies showed virtually i-
dentical hybridization patterns, data not shown). Since virus
spread in culture was excluded by anti-gp_{70} serum addition,
it may be postulated that FLV-P infects in vivo a progenitor
of both erythroid and GM-lineage (i.e., a cell closely-relat
ed to CFU-S). Furthermore, these data militate against the
possibility that in FLV leukemia the "primary" phenomenon is
represented by infection and transformation of a distal erythroid progenitor, while enhanced cycling and BPF-independen
ce of BFU-E would constitute "secondary" aspects (i.e., not
directly caused by virus infection).

   Results in (b) are in keeping with studies described in
previous section: they indicate that the spleen is the selec
tive organ for both virus replication and expression of the
erythroid component of FLV leukemias.

   (c) Presence of SFFVp-specific sequences in normal marrow
and spleen (but not in thymus and lymphonodes) has been pre-

viously shown (2), and is confirmed here. Furthermore, we have detected these sequences at low levels in GM-colonies but not in bursts: it is thus apparent that they are selectively restricted to particular hemopoietic lineages.

CONCLUDING REMARKS: A TENTATIVE MODEL FOR FLV LEUKEMIAS

Admittedly, further studies shall be necessary to confirm and extend results discussed in previous sections. The data available so far, however, fit neatly together to suggest a model for the physiopathology of FLV leukemias.

We suggest that the erythropoietic component in FLV-P leukemia is at least in part mediated via enhanced activity of erythropoietic factor(s) in splenic microenvironment. These include BPF- and Ep-like factor(s). The enhanced activity may be mediated via (a) elevation of hormone(s) production over normal levels, and/or (b) enhancement of the response of transformed progenitors to discrete levels of erythropoietic hormone(s) released under normal conditions. It must be emphasized that enhanced pressure for erythropoietic differentiation is not associated with a stimulus for GM-proliferation. On the basis of the previous discussion, the enhanced levels of BPF- and possibly Ep-like activity may be tied to expression of $SFFV_p$.

In FLV-A leukemia a similar, although less prominent rise of erythropoietic hormone(s) activity may take place in spleen. This borderline pattern is possibly related to the erratic biologic activity of $SFFV_A$, as shown by erythropoietic spleen foci formation. Both phenomena are in keeping with the ineffective type of erythropoiesis in FLV-A mice.

We also suggest that the rise of erythropoietic hormone-like activity in spleen is possibly mediated via early infection of the T-lymphocyte-macrophage complex by FLV-P, and perhaps FLV-A. This may trigger release of either BPF (and possibly Ep in FLV-P mice) or BPF- and Ep-like factor(s). Two aspects may be tied to this hypothesis. (a) The enhanced activity of erythropoietic factor(s), although demonstrated in spleen cultures, is only slight or absent when plating marrow from FLV-P or FLV-A mice respectively. This difference is in keeping with prevalent expression of leukemia in spleen; furthermore, it may be referred to presence of a more abundant population of T-lymphocytes-macrophages in spleen than in marrow. (b) The hormone-independence of splenic erythroid progenitors from FLV-P and even more FLV-A animals is gradually dampened in the course of the leukemia.

This may be related to progressive decrease of the relative number of T-lymphocytes and/or macrophages in spleen, caused by massive expansion of erythropoietic cells.

It may be postulated that $SFFV_P$, and perhaps $SFFV_A$, mediate the erythropoietic component of FLV-P and FLV-A leukemia respectively. Conversely, the leukemogenic transformation would be mediated by $F-MuLV_P$ and $F-MuLV_A$. In this regard, two aspects deserve further comment: (a) the relationship between enhanced activity of erythropoietic hormone(s) and leukemogenesis; (b) the target cell(s) of F-MuLV (i.e., the transformed progenitor(s) giving rise to the leukemic progeny).

In regard to (a), it is tempting to suggest that enhanced BPF-like activity and leukemogenesis are not only temporally related, but also linked by a cause/effect relationship. In this regard, BPF is known to modulate cycling of normal BFU-E, and presumably CFU-S (25). The cycling BFU-E (and possibly the closely-related CFU-S) is considered a suitable target for FLV infection and transformation (22). Thus, a hypothetical sequence of events in FLV leukemia may be as follows: (I) rise of BPF-like activity, particularly in spleen, thus forcing BFU-E and CFU-S into cycling; (II) infection and leukemic transformation of cycling BFU-E and/or CFU-S by FLV; (III) development of a leukemia with preferential erythropoietic expression, due to sustained production of BPF-like (and possibly Ep-like) activity.

In line with this model, the equivalent expression of viral RNA's in bursts and GM-colonies suggests that the target for FLV transformation is a progenitor of both lineages, i.e. the CFU-S or a closely-related element. Alternatively, FLV erythroleukemia might not be of clonal origin, thus at variance with other models such as chronic meyelocytic leukemia in humans (5). If this alternative hypothesis is accepted, FLV leukemias might be mediated via a multi-target mechanism, whereby prevalent erythropoietic expression would be anyway mediated via enhanced activity of erythropoietic factor(s), particularly in spleen.

ACKNOWLEDGEMENTS

Supported by Grants from: Volkswagen Foundation, Hannover (°); EURATOM, Bruxelles (No. BIO-C-353-I) (°); CNR, Rome (Progetto Finalizzato "Controllo della crescita neoplastica" No.80.01615.96° and 80.01943.96^; Progetto Finalizzato "Virus", No.79.00435.84+). We wish to express our appreciation for the excellent technical help of Mr. P. Ciaglia and secretarial asistance of Ms. G. Di Lauro.

REFERENCES

1. Axelrad, A.A., McLeod, D.L., Shreeve, M.M., and Heath, D.S. (1974): In: Hemopoiesis in Culture, edited by W.A. Robinson, pp. 226-334. GPO, Washington.

2. Bernstein, A., Gamble, C., Penrose, D., and Mak, T.W. (1979): Proc. Natl. Acad. Sci. USA, 76:4455-4459.

3. Bilello, J.A., Colletta, G., Warnecke, G., Koch, G., Frisby, D., Pragnell, I.B., and Ostertag, W. (1980): Virology, 107:331-344.

4. Fagg, B., Vehmeyer, K., Ostertag, W., Jasmin, C., and Klein, B. (1980): In: In vivo and in vitro Erythropoiesis: the Friend System, edited by G.B. Rossi, pp. 163-172. Elsevier/North-Holland, Amsterdam.

5. Fialkow, P.J. (1979): Ann.Rev. Med., 30:135-143.

6. Friend, C., Scher, W., Tsuei, D., Haddad, J., Holland, J.G., Szrajer, N., and Haubenstock, M. (1979): In: Oncogenic Viruses and Host Cell Genes, edited by Y. Ikawa, pp. 279-301. Academic Press, New York.

7. Hankins, W.D., Kost, T.A., Koury, M.J., and Krantz, S.B. (1978): Nature, 276:506-508.

8. Iscove, N.N. (1978): In: Hemopoietic Cell Differentiation, edited by D.W. Golde, M.J. Cline, D. Metcalf and C.F. Fox, pp. 37-52. Academic Press, New York.

9. Iscove, N.N., Guilbert, L.J., and Weyman, C. (1980): Exp. Cell. Res., 126:121-126.

10. Kost, T.A., Koury, M.J., and Krantz, S.B. (1981): Virology, 108:309-317.

11. Linemeyer, D.L., Ruscetti,S.K., Menke, J.G., and Scolnick, E.M. (1980): J. Virol., 35:710-721.

12. Linemeyer, D.L., Ruscetti, S.K., Scolnick, E.M., Evans, L.H., and Duesberg, P.H. (1981): Proc. Natl. Acad. Sci. USA, 78:1401-1405.

13. McDonald, M.E., Johnson, G.R., and Bernstein, A. (1981): Virology, 110:231-236.

14. Oliff, A.I., Hager, G.L., Chang, E.M., Scolnick, E.M., Chan, H.W., and Lowy, D.R. (1980): J. Virol., 33:475-486.

15. Oliff, A.I., Linemeyer, D.L., Ruscetti, S.K., Lowe, R., Lowy, D.R., and Scolnick, E.M. (1980): J. Virol., 35:924-936.

16. Opitz, U., Seidel, H.J., and Bertoncello, I. (1978): J. Cell. Physiol., 96:95-104.

17. Peschle, C., Migliaccio, G., Lettieri, F., Migliaccio, A.R., Ceccarelli, R., Barba, P., Titti, F., and Rossi, G.B. (1980): Proc. Natl. Acad. Sci. USA, 77:2054-2058.

18. Peschle, C. (1980): Ann. Rev. Med., 31:303-314. Peschle, C. (in press): In: BIMR Pediatrics-Volume I Ha-

ematology and Oncology,edited by M.L.N. Willoughby and
S.E. Siegel. Butterworth, London.

19. Rich, I.N., Heit, W., and Kubanek, B. (1980): Exp. Hemat., 8 (Suppl. no.8): 307-310.

20. Rossi, G.B., and Peschle, C. (1980): In: In vivo and in vitro Erythropoiesis: the Friend System, edited by G.B. Rossi, pp. 139-149. Elsevier/North-Holland, Amsterdam.

21. Schreier, M.H., and Iscove, N.N. (1980): Nature, 287: 228-230.

22. Suzuki, S., and Axelrad, A.A. (1980): Cell, 19:225-236.

23. Tambourin, P.E., and Wendling, F. (1975): Nature, 256: 320-322.

24. Toniolo, A., Matteucci, D., Pistillo, M.P., Gori, Z., and Bendinelli, M. (1980): J. Gen. Virol., 49:203-208.

25. Wagemaker, G. (1980): In: In vivo and in vitro Erythropoiesis: the Friend System, edited by G.B. Rossi, pp. 87-95. Elsevier/North-Holland, Amsterdam.

Expression of Differentiated Functions in Cancer Cells, edited by R. F. Revoltella et al., Raven Press, New York © 1982.

Integration and Expression of Polyoma Virus Genomes in Transformed Rat Cells

Claudio Basilico, Robert G. Fenton, and Giuliano Della Valle

Department of Pathology, New York University School of Medicine, New York, New York 10016

Polyoma is a small DNA tumor virus which exhibits two types of interaction with susceptible cells. A productive or lytic interaction in which the virus multiplies and - kills the infected cells, and a transforming interaction, in which a fraction of the infected cells become phenotypically "transformed" and tumorigenic, without substantial virus production or cell death. The type of interaction depends mainly on the species of the infected cells. Permissive cells, such as mouse, although transformable, give rise almost exclusively to a lytic interaction, while in non-permissive cells, such as rat and hamster, transformation is easily detected(1). About 50% of the total coding capacity of polyoma DNA (5.3 kb) is dedicated to the synthesis of proteins which are involved in transformation. These are three early proteins (also called T antigens), and it has been conclusively shown that polyoma transformation requires the integration of the viral genome into the DNA of the host cells,and the expression of the early viral genes. Integration is a necessary, although not sufficient condition for the expression of viral genes in transformed cells, as it ensures the regulated transmission of these DNA sequences to the cells' progeny.

To learn more about the interaction between polyoma virus and the genome of animal cells, we have studied the process of integration of polyoma viral DNA into the genome of transformed rat cells, the stability of such an association, and the mode of transcription of integrated viral genomes. The results of some of the experiments will be discussed in this manuscript.

INTEGRATION

Polyoma DNA encodes three early proteins small (20k), middle (56 k), and large (100 k) T antigen (Fig.1). While middle T antigen is probably the viral gene-product mainly responsible for conferring to cells a transformed phenotype(2-6), it has long been known that large T-Ag plays a role at least in the establishment of transformation(7-9). Polyoma temperature sensitive mutants of the A complementation group (producing a thermolabile large T-Ag) are greatly impaired in the ability to induce transformation at non-permissive temperature; however, the

phenotype of the cells remains transformed when ts-a
transformed cells are shifted from 33⁰ to 39.5⁰(7-11).
These findings suggested the possibility that large T-Ag
regulated or promoted the integration of polyoma DNA into
the genome of the infected cells, and for this purpose we
undertook experiments aimed at. elucidating the role of this
protein in transformation.

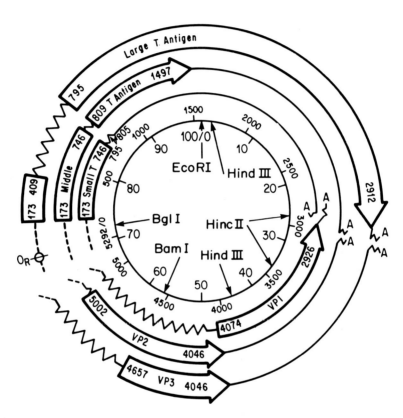

Fig.1: Physical and functional map of polyoma virus DNA
(A2 strain). The physical map is divided in map units
starting clockwise from 0 at the EcoRl site) or nucleotide
number (starting clockwise from 0 at the origin of replication). The mRNAs for the three T antigens and the late
proteins VP1, VP2, VP3 are shown with their coding regions
([   ] ⟩, 3' non-coding regions (————) and intervening
sequences (∿∿∿). The numbers within the coding regions
represent initiation and termination codons and splice
junctions. Note that the mRNAs for the three T antigens
start with the same reading frame and are then shifted to
three different frames by the splicing out of different
intervening sequences. Adapted from (1).

Table 1

Transforming Ability of Polyoma ts-a Mutant DNA and of Wild Type Restriction Enzyme Fragments*

DNA or DNA Fragment	Transformation° at 39°	Transformation° at 33°	Transformation° at 37°
wt Form I	100	100	100
ts-a Form I#	4.8	100	ND
BamHI cleaved wt•	ND	ND	16.7
EcoRI cleaved wt•	ND	ND	1.4
wt HincII-1 fragment (m.u. 36-26)	ND	ND	25
wt HindIII-1 (m.u. 45-2)	ND	ND	1.3
wt HindIII-2 (m.u. 2-45)	ND	ND	<0.01

*These results are the average of several independent experiments. Rat F2408 cells were transfected with polyoma DNA or DNA fragments (1µg/100 mm plate) in the presence of carrier rat cell DNA as described. 24-36 hours later the cells were trypsinized and plated in agar medium at 1x10^5 cells/plate (5).

°Transformation was measured from the frequency of cells forming colonies in agar medium at 20-25 days after plating, and is expressed in percent of wild type values. Absolute transformation frequencies produced by wt DNA ranged between 3 and 8x10^{-3}.

#Ts-a DNA (or virions) always transform even at 33° at lower frequency than wt DNA. These values are the ratios 39°/33° normalized for wt DNA.

•DNAs were cleaved with the indicated restriction enzyme and then treated with S1 nuclease to produce deletions at the site of cleavage (5).

Two types of experiments were performed. In one, the
ability of ts-a polyoma DNA to transform cells at 33° or
39° was compared with that of wt DNA. In another, the
transforming ability of viral DNA molecules or fragments
specifically cleaved as to encode information for only
small and middle, but not large T-Ag (Fig.1) was compared
to that of intact polyoma DNA. All experiments gave
concording results(5). Polyoma DNA molecules deleted
within the late region gave frequencies of transformation
only slightly lower than those obtained by intact viral
DNA. Molecules not encoding small and middle T-Ag did not
produce any detectable transformation. Polyoma DNA
fragments containing sequences capable of encoding small
and middle T-Ags but not large T-Ag transformed at a
frequency 10-20 fold lower than molecules encoding intact
early regions. Similarly, transfection with ts-a DNA at
39° produced some transformed colonies, but at a
frequency about 20 fold lower than that obtained at
33°(Table I). Taken together, these results confirm the
hypothesis that large T-Ag increases the efficiency of
transformation, but is not absolutely required for either
its initiation or maintenance. Cells transformed by
molecules lacking large T-coding regions were fully
transformed in vitro and tumorigenic in animals.

Table 2

Tandem and Single Copy Integration* in Rat Cells Transformed by Different Forms of Polyoma Virus DNA

Transforming DNA	Clones With Single Copy# Integrations	Clones With Tandem Integrations
ts-a at 39°	18/20	2/20
EcoRl cleaved wt	7/8	1/8
BamHl cleaved wt	2/7	5/7
wt or ts-a at 33°	0/9	9/9

*Determined by restriction enzyme analysis and "Southern"
blot hybridization with ^{32}P-labeled polyoma DNA of high
m.w. DNA extracted from the transformed lines(5).

#Or less than one copy.

To determine how large T-Ag enhanced the efficiency of transformation, we studied the integration pattern of cells transformed in the presence or absence of large T-Ag function. The results of these experiments are shown in Table 2. As previously shown (12-14), polyoma integration in cells transformed under conditions permissive for all viral functions generally consists of a head to tail tandem arrangement of integrated viral DNA molecules. In contrast, cells transformed in the absence of large T-function (whether ts-a DNA at 39° or wt DNA molecules specifically cleaved to inactivate large T coding sequences) almost invariably display multiple or unique insertions of viral DNA molecules in less than a single copy arrangement(5).

These and other results strongly suggest that the role of large T antigen in promoting transformation consists of allowing tandem insertion, this type of integration being the most efficient one for transformation.

TRANSCRIPTION OF INTEGRATED POLYOMA GENOMES

Once the polyoma genome is integrated into the host DNA, transformation is maintained by the transcription and translation of specific viral genes. It therefore became important to define the modalities of viral transcription in transformed cells, and to determine whether they differ from those manifested during productive infection. In this work, we followed the pioneering work of Kamen et al.(15,16) describing transcription of the polyoma genome in the lytic cycle. However, we exploited particularly the properties of polyoma ts-a transformed cells, which at 39° have totally stable integration and do not produce free viral DNA(14,17). The presence of free viral genomes would have made it difficult to study the transcription of integrated molecules.

Transcription of Cells Containing Intact Early Regions, Whether in Single Copy or Tandemly Arranged The modalities of transcription of these DNA sequences can be summarized as follows: Transcription invariably starts from viral promoters; no evidence of host initiated transcription can be detected. Transcription is limited to the early region of polyoma DNA. Studies of polyadenylated cytoplasmic mRNAs reveal the presence of three types of RNAs, indistinguishable in their 3' and 5' ends and splice junctions from those detected early in lytic infection and coding for small, middle and large T-Ag (Fig.1) . No evidence of stable transcripts hybridizing to polyoma late sequences can be found (18).

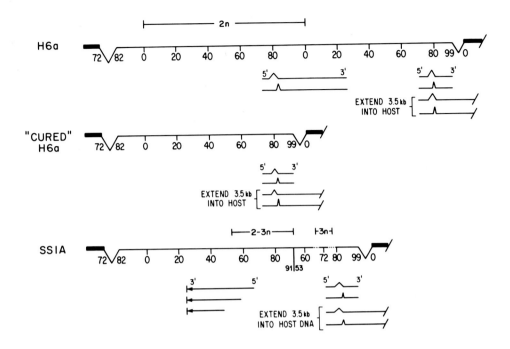

Fig.2: Schematic representation of the structure of viral
DNA insertions and viral RNAs produced in the polyoma
transformed rat cell lines H6A and its derivatives SS1A and
one of the "cured" H6A revertants(13,14). Heavy lines
represent host sequences flanking proviral DNA. Numbers
above the proviral insertion (thin lines) are viral DNA map
units. The approximate positions of the host/viral DNA
junctions are also shown. "2n", "3n" indicate that the
bracketed DNA sequences are repeated twice or three times.
Cytoplasmic mRNAs are diagrammed below the map of the viral
DNA insertion, and their polarity and splices are indicated.
The RNAs for small and middle T-antigens are not distinguished in the diagram, but are both represented by the RNAs
with the short early splice near 86 m.u. Only the body
sequences of late RNAs produced in SS1A are shown, since the
exact size of their splices is not known.

**Transcription from Cells Containing Truncated or Otherwise
Deleted Viral Early Regions** Deletion of the major early
region poly(A) attachment site at 25.8 m.u. on the polyoma
map results in the generation of readthrough transcripts and
increased utilization of an alternative poly(A) addition
signal at 99 m.u.(15). This can be produced by the joining
of viral sequences upstream from 25 m.u. to host DNA, or by
deletions which remove this region from the viral genome.

In the first case transcripts extend variable distances into host DNA and are polyadenylated at a host site (Fig.2). When defective viral DNA molecules are tandemly arrayed, multimeric viral transcripts are produced, and these are homologous both to early and anti-late viral sequences(18). It is not clear whether these long transcripts encode any novel protein, or whether they can only encode small, middle and truncated large T-Ags. Transcripts terminating at 99 m.u. contain sufficient information to code for small and middle T-Ags.

In conclusion, when transcription of integrated polyoma genomes is compared to that occurring in the lytic cycle,the new transcripts observed seem in general to result from alterations of the 3' viral DNA sequences due to the process of integration. The 5' ends of these novel viral mRNAs are generally indistinguishable from those observed early in lytic infection(15,18). These data strongly suggest that viral gene expression depends on the presence of promoter regions of viral origin.

Specificity of Transcription of Integrated Viral DNA   As mentioned above, late region transcripts are not detected in polyoma or SV40 transformed cells, under conditions in which no free viral DNA is made (1). In our present study of at least 12 independent transformed cell lines, and of several cell lines derived from them, we could never detect the presence of stable cytoplasmic polyadenylated late mRNAs, i.e., RNAs hybridizing to the coding (L) strand of the polyoma late region (rather than to the antilate strand). The problem of why late transcripts are not made from integrated viral DNA molecules is important since it may provide important clues to eukaryotic gene expression. We wish to report here that we have detected late transcription from integrated DNA in one polyoma transformed line.

The transformed line SS1A was isolated as a subclone of a ts-a polyoma transformed line designated H6A, which contains a single insertion of integrated viral DNA consisting of full length molecules arranged in a head to tail tandem repeat(14). The SS1A cell line has undergone excision of full length molecules and as such does not produce a functional large T-Ag. In addition, this line has acquired a new arrangement of head to tail tandem repeats of a 38% segment as well as of a 10% segment of the viral genome, both containing the Py origin of replication and the promoter regions(19). A map of this integrated arrangement is shown in Fig.2. SS1A produce transcripts corresponding to the truncated early region on the right side of insertion, that are also present in the parental line H6A and its cured derivatives. Most important, SS1A cells do not produce free viral DNA, as expected from their inability to produce large T-Ag(17), but transcribe viral late regions. The late mRNAs are produced in low amounts, and

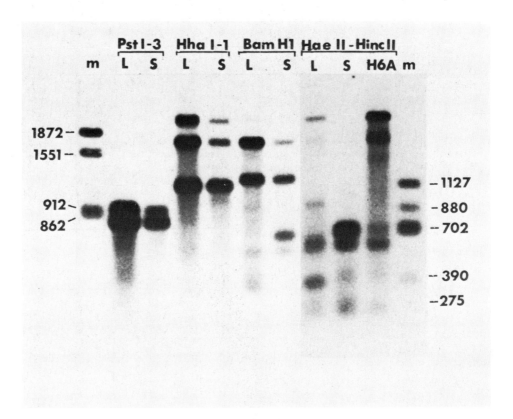

Fig.3: Alkaline S1 analysis of viral RNAs produced by the
SS1A cell line(S) and late in the polyoma virus lytic
cycle (L). Briefly 0.5 µg of poly(A)+ cytoplasmic late
lytic RNA (isolated from 3T3 mouse cells 36h post infection
with 10 pfu/cell of wt virus) or 10µg of poly(A)+ cytoplasmic SS1A RNA were hybridized to an excess of the
unlabeled Py DNA fragments indicated. Following hybridization, duplexes were treated with S1 nuclease and the
products electrophoresed on denaturing alkaline agarose
gels. Protected DNA segments were visualized by blot-
transfer onto nitrocellulose and hybridized with ^{32}P-
labeled Py DNA as described(18). Markers(m) are Py DNA
cleaved with PstI (left) or MspI (right). Sizes in
nucleotides are shown. The PstI-3 fragment spans m.u.
33-50, and the HhaI-1 fragment m.u. 27-72. Therefore, they
represent almost uniquely viral late sequences (see Fig.1).
Bam H1 is polyoma DNA linearized by BamH1 cleavage (m.u.58)
and the HaeII-HincII fragment spans m.u. 72-26, and
therefore contains only early sequences. RNAs produced by
the H6A cell line did not protect any sequence of the PstI-
3 and HhaI-1 fragments.

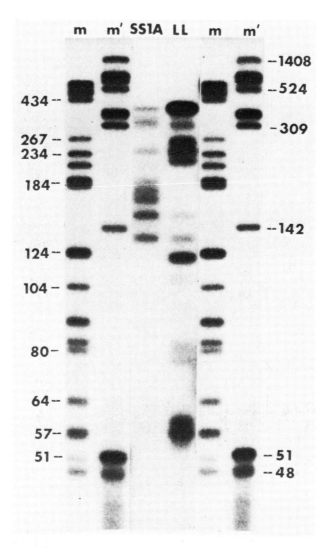

Fig.4: Identification of heterogeneous 5' ends of late lytic or SS1A RNA by a modification of the Berk and Sharp techniques(25). 0.5 µg of poly(A)+ cytoplasmic late lytic RNA or 20 µg of SS1A RNA were hybridized to excess of the BclI-EcoRl Py restriction fragment (m.u. 65-0) ^{32}P-end labeled at the BclI 5' end. Thus, radioactivity is exclusively in the L-strand, i.e. homologous to late mRNAs. Following hybridization, RNA:DNA duplexes were digested to completion with S1 endonuclease, hybrids denatured by heating at 90°C in 50% formamide, and electrophoresed on 1mm thick 8 m urea, 8% polyacrylamide gels. The gel was dried and bands visualized by autoradiography. "m" is ^{32}P-end labeled pBR 322 cleaved with HaeIII and run as marker. m' is end labeled polyoma DNA cut with Hinf I. Bands observed in experimental lanes represent protected DNA fragments extending from the BclI site (65 m.u.) to the 5' ends of the viral mRNAs.

consist of 3' exons indistinguishable from those of the
three late mRNAs previously described (20) (Fig.3). With
regard to the origin of 5' exons, more precise mapping
indicates that L-strand DNA sequences known to be
transcribed in late leader sequences are present in SS1A
mRNA, but the precise size of these fragments is not always
identical to the late 5' exons (Fig.4). This last point is,
however, difficult to evaluate because, as shown previously
(21), late lytic Py mRNAs have 5'ends which are extremely
complex and heterogeneous (fig.4).

The occurrence of late transcription in the SS1A cell
line seems clearly due to the amplification of integrated
viral DNA in the origin and promoter regions (Fig.2). This
interpretation is supported not only by the fact that this
is the only polyoma transformed cell lines described so far
to perform late transcription, but also by the transcription
patterns of the parental H6A line, and its cured
derivatives. In the latter cell lines, excision of
integrated viral DNA molecules has occurred like in SS1A,
but no amplification of the DNA segments containing the
origin of replication has taken place (Fig.2). Neither H6A
or its cured derivatives transcribe any viral late
sequences. While the molecular mechanism of late
transcription in SS1A is not clear at this moment, several
hypothesis can be advanced and will be reviewed in the
Discussion.

DISCUSSION

Integration of Polyoma Viral DNA   The results in this
paper show that polyoma virus DNA can integrate into the
genome of transformed cells, in tandem or single copy
arrangement. The efficiency of transformation is greatly
dependent on the presence of a functional large T antigen
which is, however, not necessary for the expression of the
transformed phenotype. Restriction enzyme analysis of a
number of transformed lines showed a strong correlation
between the presence of a functional large T antigen and the
integration pattern of viral genomes in "head to tail"
tandem repeats. Cells transformed in the absence of a
functional large T antigen almost invariably contained one
or more single copy insertions(5).

Polyoma large T-Ag is known to be necessary for the
initiation of viral DNA replication(1), and if the main role
of polyoma large T in the establishment of transformation is
allowing the formation of tandem head to tail integration,
this integrated arrangement may result from a replication
process. The model best supported by our results postulates
that polymers of viral DNA arranged in "head to tail"
tandems are the precursors of the integrated form. Such
polymers could be produced by replication of the viral DNA
by mechanisms that allow DNA synthesis without separation of
the newly formed DNA molecules. A rolling circle mechanism

of viral DNA synthesis would meet many of the requirements of this hypothesis. The rolling circle is both a replicative intermediate and an oligomer containing viral genomes in "head to tail" sequence. Such structure could integrate by a double crossing-over event, leading to insertions of multiple viral genomes. Models including a double crossing-over event would predict the deletion of the host DNA between the two cross-over sites. The rolling circle is not the normal replicative form of Py DNA(22), but viral DNA molecules replicating in such manner have been observed(23). Alternatively, a model such as that suggested by Harshey and Bukhari (24) for integration of transposable elements, which also postulates a rolling circle replication leading to the formation of tandem insertions, would also be applicable to our data. An important diffference between these two models however is that the latter does not predict deletions of host DNA. Clearly, further experiments may help differentiating between these two hypothesis.

Together with previously published results on excision and amplification of integrated polyoma genomes(14,19), these data firmly establish that large T antigen is the major polyoma gene product involved in processes of replication and integrative recombination. While the recombination-promoting role may be indirect, a protein which binds to DNA and initiates replication may have to fulfill functions (such as helix destabilization, unwinding, etc.) which are also required in the process of recombination. This latter property of large T-Ag molecules may be important in promoting excision and amplification.

Expression of Integrated Polyoma Genomes   The data presented show that the regulation of transcription of integrated polyoma genomes depends mainly on viral controlling elements. No evidence of transcription initiating from host DNA has been detected, and the mRNAs produced from integrated intact early regions are indistinguishable from those seen early in the infectious cycle. When deletions of 3'early region sequences including the most used polyadenylation signal at 25.8 m.u. occur, novel viral transcripts are produced. These consist of fused transcripts of viral and host DNA, or of long polymeric viral transcripts including RNA homologous to "antilate" sequences(18).In addition the poly(A) addition site at 99 m..u. is used much more frequently. It is possible that sequences around 26 m.u. signal transcription and when these are deleted, transcription continues into host or viral sequences normally not transcribed. Alternatively, endonucleolytic cleavage and polyadenylation of mRNA percursors may be very efficiently directed by these sequences.

A further demonstration that viral controls are operating also on integrated polyoma molecules comes from the study of the extent of early transcription in ts-a transformed cells at 39° and 33°. In the lytic cycle large T-Ag autoregulates its own production presumably by binding near the origin of replication and inhibiting early transcription(1). Thus, polyoma ts-a infected cells produce approximately 6-10 fold more early RNAs at 39°, where large T-Ag is non-functional, than at 33°. This type of regulation is present also in ts-a transformed cells, which also overproduce early mRNAs at 39° (Fenton and Basilico, in preparation). This clearly shows that transcription of integrated polyoma DNA is still sensitive to its normal controlling elements.

As discussed in Results, one unique finding of our studies was the discovery of a polyoma transformed cell line producing late viral mRNAs. These cytoplasmic RNAs are similar to those produced late in lytic infection, and contain heterogeneous late sequences in their 5' ends. The unusual structure of integrated viral DNA sequences in the SS1A cell line strongly suggest that late transcription results from the presence of repeats of the origin-promoter region of polyoma DNA. One of the repeats could be inverted, and thus late transcription could be under the control of an early promoter. Other possibilities are alterations in the repeated sequences, undetectable by Southern blots, or conformation effects, which would render late promoterss more accessible to RNA polymerase. Molecular cloning of the viral insertion in SS1A cells, followed by DNA sequencing and other viral studies should indicate which, if any, of these hypotheses is the correct one.

ACKNOWLEDGEMENT

This investigation was supported by U.S. PHS grants CA16239, CA 11893 and CA 26070 from the Nat. Cancer Institute.

REFERENCES

1. The Molecular Biology of Tumor Viruses Part 2 (1980). J. Tooze ed. Cold Spring Harbor Laboratory.

2. Israel, M.A., Simmons, D.T., Mourihan, S.L., Rowe, W.P. and Martin, M.A. (1979). Proc. Natl. Acad. Sci. USA 76:3713-3716.

3. Novak, U., Dilworth, S.M. and Griffin, B.E. (1980). Proc. Natl. Acad. Sci. USA 77:3278-3282.

4. Hassell, J.A., Topp, W.C. Rifkin, D.B. and Moreau, P.E. (1980). Proc. Natl Acad. Sci. USA 77:3978-3982.

5. Della Valle, G., Fenton, R. and Basilico, C. (1981). Cell 23:347-355.

6. Treisman, R., Novak, U., Favaloro, J. and Kamen, R. (1981). Nature, in press.

7. Fried, M. (1965). Proc. Natl. Acad. Sci. USA 53:486-491.

8. DiMayorca, G., Callender, J., Marin, G. and Giordano, R. (1969). Virology 38:126-133.

9. Eckart, W. (1969). Virology 38:120-125.

10. Seif, R. and Cuzin, F. (1977). J. Virol 24:722-728.

11. Fluck, M.M. and Benjamin, T.L. (1979). Virology 96:205-228.

12. Birg, F., Dulbecco, R., Fried, M. and Kamen, R. (1979). J. Virol. 29:633-648.

13. Basilico, C., Gattoni, S., Zouzias, D. and Della Valle, G. (1979). Cell 17:645-659.

14. Basilico, C., Zouzias, D., Della Valle, G., Gattoni, S., Colantuoni, V., Fenton, R. and Dailey, L. (1979). Cold Spring Harbor Symp. Quant. Biol. 44:611-619.

15. Kamen, R., Favaloro, J., Parker, J., Treisman, R., Lania, L., Fried, M. and Mellor, M. (1979). Cold Spring Harbor Symp. Quant. Biol. 44:63-75.

16. Favaloro, J., Treisman, R. and Kamen, R. (1980). Methods in Enzymology 65:718-749.

17. Zouzias, D., Prasad, I. and Basilico, C. (1977). J. Virol 24:142-150.

18. Fenton, R.G. and Basilico, C. (1981). J. Virol, in press.

19. Colantuoni, V., Dailey, L. and Basilico, C. (1980). Proc. Natl. Acad. Sci. USA 77:3850-3854.

20. Kamen, R. Favaloro, J. and Parker, M. (1980). J. Virol. 33:637-651.

21. Treisman, R. (1980). Nucleic Acid Res. 8:4867-4888.

22. Hirt, B. (1969). J. Mol. Biol. 40:141-144.

23. Bjursell, G. (1978). J. Virol. 26:136-142.

24. Harshey, R.M. and Bukhari, A.I. (1981). Proc. Natl. Acad. Sci. USA 78:1090-1094.

25. Berk, A.J. and Sharp, P.A., (1977). Cell 12:721-732.

Expression of Differentiated Functions in Cancer Cells, edited by R. F. Revoltella et al., Raven Press, New York © 1982.

Expression of the Polyoma Virus Middle-T Protein is Sufficient to Establish and to Maintain the Transformed State

R. H. Treisman, A. Cowie, U. Novak, J. Favaloro, and R. Kamen

Transcription Laboratory, Imperial Cancer Research Fund, London WC2A 3PX, England

The early region of polyoma virus DNA encodes at least three polypeptides, the large-T, middle-T, and small-T proteins (24,21,20,37; see ref. 43 for a review). Conclusive evaluation of the individual roles of the three proteins in virally induced oncogenic transformation has been difficult because the DNA sequences (11,40) which encode them overlap extensively (Figure 1). It is known that expression of the large-T protein is insufficient to transform cells (29,3), and that the 3'-terminal half of the early region, which encodes only C-terminal sequences of large-T protein, is not required to maintain (26,30) or to establish (22,34,19,2) the transformed state. Attention has therefore focused on the 5'-terminal half of the early region, which encodes the small-T and middle-T proteins as well as the N-terminal portion of the large-T protein. Since all previously reported mutations within this region of the genome affect at least two of the three T-proteins (3,39,15,31,14), rigorous assignment of the resulting phenotype to a change in any individual gene product has not been possible. We now report the construction of an altered polyoma virus early region which encodes exclusively the middle-T protein, and describe the mode and consequences of the expression of this DNA when it is introduced into cultured rat cells.

CONSTRUCTION OF A VIRAL EARLY REGION ENCODING ONLY THE MIDDLE-T PROTEIN

We constructed a modified viral early region capable of encoding exclusively the middle-T protein by specific deletion of the middle-T protein intervening sequence (see Figures 1 and 2). Using a recombinant plasmid containing full length wild type viral DNA (p53.A6.6) we achieved this by replacing a small genomic restriction fragment spanning the small-T and middle-T protein intervening sequences with the corresponding shorter fragment from a cloned partial cDNA copy (44) or the middle-T protein mRNA (Figure 2). From our knowledge of the structures of the Py early region mRNAs (44; Figure 1) we predicted that the plasmid produced, pPyMT1, would encode only middle-T protein. The polyoma virus early region mRNAs are generated by the differential splicing of a common precursor. This involves the ligation of two splice donors (at nucleotides 409 and 746) to two splice acceptors (at nucleotides 795 and 809) in three of the four possible combinations (Figure 1). The mature mRNA for middle-T protein (spliced from 746 to 809) lacks the acceptor (at 795) used in large-T and small-T mRNAs. Moreover, since the highly conserved consensus sequences at splice donor sites lie largely within the intervening sequences (5,38), the splice donor at nucleotide 746 in the middle-T mRNA should also be inactive. The only potential splicing signal remaining in this mRNA would be the donor (at nucleotide 409) used in the large-T mRNA splice. The primary transcript of the viral early region in pPyMT1

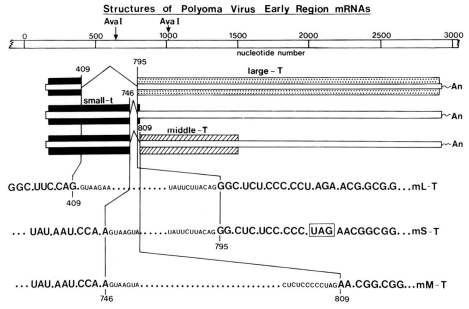

FIG. 1: The spliced structures of the principal Py early region mRNAs. At the top of the figure we show a linearized map of the Py early region, with conventional nucleotide numbers (37) indicated. The three differentially spliced principal mRNAs (44) are aligned with this map. The coding regions of the mRNAs are boxed; solid boxes, dotted boxes and hatched boxes refer to reading frames (as defined in ref.40) 1, 2 and 3 respectively. The nucleotide sequences across the splice joints are shown in the bottom half of the figure (44).

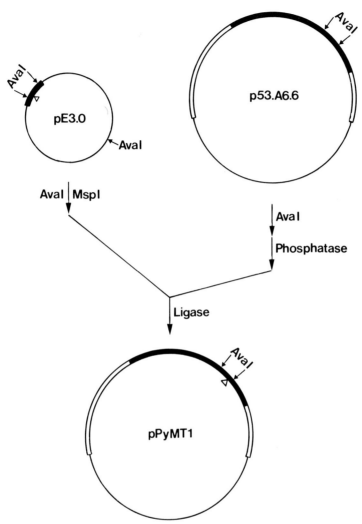

FIG. 2: Construction of a modified polyoma virus early region able to
encode only the middle-T protein. Plasmid pE3.0 (44) consists of a
partial cDNA copy of the middle-T protein mRNA (solid bar) inserted at
the PstI site of plasmid pAT153 (45). The absence of the intervening
sequence is indicated by V. Plasmid p53.A6.6 consists of a complete
wild type Py genome inserted via the unique BamHI site into a derivative
of pAT153 in which the plasmid AvaI site had been removed. The Py early
region is shown as a solid bar, and other Py sequences as open bars.
Plasmid pE3.0 was digested with AvaI+MspI. Plasmid p53.A6.6 digested
with AvaI was treated with calf intestine alkaline phosphatase (47).
Equimolar amounts of the two plasmid digests were ligated at 25μg/ml
p53.A6.6. Following transfection into E. coli HB101, ampicillin resistant colonies were picked and plasmid DNAs prepared (4). Recombinants
were analysed for the substitution of the Py genomic AvaI fragment by
the pE3.0 cDNA AvaI fragment using restriction endonucleases AvaI, AvaII,
HinfI and MspI. One recombinant with the appropriate restriction map,
pPyMT1, was chosen and large quantities of its DNA were prepared (4).

TABLE 1.   Transformation of F2408 rat fibroblasts by pPyMT1 DNA and control plasmid DNA.

	plasmid	µg	number of foci	foci per µg viral DNA	ratio pPyMT1/p53.A6.6
ExpI	pPyMT1	0	0	–	
		0.1	59	1000	0.40
		1.0	137	232	
	p53.A6.6	0	0		
		0.1	149	2530	
		1.0	409	693	
ExpII[a]	pPyMT1	0.05	100)	3930	0.45
		0.05	132)		
	p53.A6.6	0.05	248)	8810	
		0.05	275)		
ExpIII	pPyMT1	0	0	–	
		0.2	15	127	0.20
		1	82	139	0.28
		5	181	61	
	p53.A6.6	0	0	–	
		0.2	76	644	
		1	294	498	
		5	>500	–	
ExpIV	pPyMT1	0	0	–	
		0.1	77	1305	0.20
		1.0	324	549	
		5.0	361	122	
	p53.A6.6	0	0	–	
		0.1	375	6360	
		1.0	>500	–	
		5.0	>500	–	

Subconfluent monolayers of cells (90mm cultures) were transfected with the indicated quantities of plasmid DNAs. Dense foci were counted 14-21 days later.

a. In this experiment, the cells were trypsinized and divided among four dishes 24 hours after transfection.

(cf sequence in Figure 1) could therefore not be spliced to generate mRNAs encoding normal large- or small-T proteins, but it would encode the middle-T protein. A novel splice could perhaps join the large-T mRNA donor to an otherwise unused acceptor, but we considered this possibility to be improbable, and indeed found that such splices did not occur.

TRANSFORMATION OF RAT CELLS WITH pPyMT1

We tested the biological activity of the viral genome in

pPyMT1 by transfecting Fisher rat cells (F2408 cell line;
10), using the calcium phosphate technique (46), and quanti-
tating dense foci overgrowing the normal monolayer which
appeared after 2-3 weeks of incubation in the presence of
5% fetal calf serum. We used as a control the plasmid
p53.A6.6, the parent of pPyMT1, which contains a normal
polyoma virus genome (Figure 2). In repeated assays, the
transformation efficiency of pPyMT1 was 20-45% that of the
control plasmid when non-saturating amounts of DNA were
used (Table 1). No foci appeared when cells were transfected with carrier DNA alone, or with the plasmid vector
and carrier DNA. Twenty foci induced by pPyMT1 and six
induced by p53.A6.6 were picked and grown into cell lines
for further analysis without recloning.

All of the transformed cell lines were initially screened
for the presence of viral T-antigens by indirect immunofluorescence using a serum from a Py tumour-bearing rat.
Of the six control cell lines transformed by the unmodified
parental plasmid, five showed the strong nuclear fluorescence pattern characteristic of the polyoma virus large-T
antigen. None of the twenty cell lines derived from
pPyMT1 transfections displayed such fluorescence, although
many of them showed a weak specific immunofluorescence
which appeared to be distributed throughout the cell.

PROPERTIES OF RAT CELL LINES TRANSFORMED BY pPyMT1

Eight pPyMT1 and two control lines were selected at
random for more detailed study. The properties measured
were saturation density, ability to form foci when grown
with untransformed rat cells and the ability to grow in
semi-solid medium. All ten cell lines displayed, by these
criteria, the usual range of phenotypes characteristic of
polyoma virus transformed rat cells. Those transformed by
pPyMT1 could not be distinguished from the control cell
lines. The cell lines also had the morphological characteristics of transformed cells when examined by phase contrast
microscopy at high cell densities. Most significantly, all
cell lines tested produced tumours in vivo. Fisher rats
were injected subcutaneously with cells from lines 1.6,
1.7, 2.4, 2.8, 4.1 and 4.6. Within three weeks after injection of 4×10^5 cells, tumours were detected with all six
cell lines; pPyMT1 transformed lines 1.6 and 2.4, moreover,
produced tumours within the same time period when only
4×10^4 cells were injected. We conclude that the lines derived from pPyMT1-induced foci are transformed by all of
the parameters tested. We reserve judgement, however, on
whether differences between these cell lines and those
transformed by genomic viral DNA might be demonstrable by
measurement of other parameters of the transformed state.
In particular, we have noted that many, but not all, of
the pPyMT1-transformants grew poorly on plastic when
seeded at very low cell densities in 5% fetal calf serum.

TABLE 2. Properties of pPyMT1 and control plasmid transformed cell lines.

cell line	efficiency of focus formation,%[*]	efficiency of growth in agar,%[+]	saturation density[§] cells/cm^{2}x10^{-6}
pPyMT1			
1.2	0.4, 2.2	4.4, 10	>0.99
1.6	2.7, 3.2	6.2, 96	>1.4
1.7	3.7, 93	5.4, 60	>1.0
1.8	1.0, 5.0	3.3, 1.2	>1.1
2.4	2.3, 1.6	0.8, 1.6	>1.3
2.6	1.0, 2.4	0.8, 0.9	>1.1
2.8	1.4, 12.8	2.5, 0.9	>0.97
2.9	1.4, 4.4	2.5, 0.9	>0.83
p53.A6.6			
4.1	3.0, 4.7	1.7, >0.02	>0.70
4.6	1.7, 4.8	1.6, 20	>1.20
F2408 rat cells	none	<0.01	0.28

[*] Transformed cells ($5x10^2$ and $5x10^3$) were plated in separate experiments with either $2x10^5$ (first number) or $2x10^4$ (second number) F2408 rat cells on 50mm dishes. Foci were counted after 14 days of growth in DMEM containing 5% fetal calf serum.

[+] Transformed cells ($5x10^2$ and $5x10^3$) were grown in DMEM, 5% fetal calf serum, 0.3% (w/v) agar. Microscopically visible colonies were counted after 14 days. Results of two independent assays are listed, done after extensive passage of the cell lines in culture (first number) or shortly after the original foci had become established as cell lines (second number).

[§] Cells ($5x10^5$) were plated on 50mm dishes and grown in DMEM/5% fetal calf serum, with medium changes every 24 hours after the third day. The control F2408 cultures reached the indicated density at day four and increased no further. All transformed lines continued to divide until the cells came away from the plastic, and thus the numbers listed are minima.

VIRAL PROTEINS SYNTHESISED BY pPyMT1 TRANSFORMED CELL LINES

The prediction that the viral early region in plasmid pPyMT1 would encode only the middle-T protein was confirmed by analysis of the viral proteins synthesised by the transformed cell lines. A randomly selected set of cell lines transformed by p53.A6.6 or pPyMT1 were labelled with ^{35}S-methionine and the proteins precipitable by polyoma virus anti-T serum were fractionated on SDS-polyacrylamide gels (Figure 3). In each pPyMT1 cell line tested, the

only specifically immunoprecipitated protein detected co-
migrated with the normal viral middle-T protein synthesised
in mouse or rat cells infected with polyoma virus. This
polypeptide was also immunoprecipitated by a monoclonal
antibody directed against Py middle-T protein (S. Dilworth,
personal communication). The amount of middle-T protein
produced was within the usual range obtained with Py transformed rat cells. No large-T, truncated large-T, or
small-T proteins were found. These conclusions were
strengthened by analysis of the viral mRNA present in the
cell lines, as discussed below. Two control lines transformed by the control plasmid p53.A6.6 were similarly
analysed. Both synthesised middle-T protein and small-T
protein. One also produced a full length large-T polypeptide (line 4.1), while the other (line 4.6, which was
T-antigen negative by immunofluorescence) synthesised

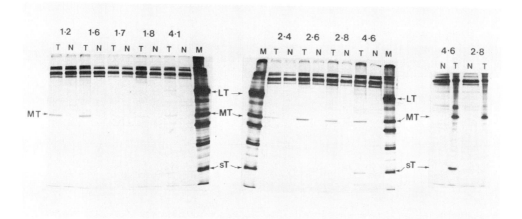

FIG. 3: Viral proteins synthesized by rat cells transformed by modified
plasmid pPyMT1 (cell lines 1.2, 1.6, 1.7, 1.8, 2.4, 2.6, 2.8 and 2.9) or
by control plasmid p53.A6.6 (cell line 4.1 and 4.6). Cultures grown in
50mm plates were labelled with ^{35}S-methionine (0.3mCi per plate) for
3 hours. Proteins were extracted and precipitated with Py anti-T protein serum (lanes T, immune serum; lanes N, non-immune serum) as
described previously (24); they were then fractionated on 10% SDS-
polyacrylamide gels, using the viral proteins precipitated from Py-
infected mouse cells (lanes M) as markers. A background band, migrating
just below the small-T protein, appears in all lanes in the first two
panels. The further experiment shown in the small panel on the right
clearly established, however, that cell line 4.6 (p53.A6.6 transformed)
synthesized the small-T protein, whereas cell line 2.8 (pPyMT1 transformed) did not.

instead a shorter polypeptide which was probably a truncated large-T molecule like those frequently found in other polyoma virus transformed rat cell lines (26,30).

VIRAL mRNAs SYNTHESISED BY pPyMT1 TRANSFORMED CELL LINES

We investigated the structure of the viral mRNAs in several transformed lines for two reasons. Firstly, we wanted unambiguous evidence demonstrating that the pPyMT1 transcripts were not spliced to produce mRNAs which could encode viral proteins other than middle-T. Secondly, we were interested to know how the transformed cell lines generated stable cytoplasmic mRNA encoding middle-T protein from the modified genome in pPyMT1. Previous reports (17, 18,16) had suggested that RNA splicing is an obligatory step in the expression of genes which normally contain intervening sequences. We therefore thought it possible that the transformed cell lines always contained viral genomes integrated such that the early region and a host intervening sequence could be co-transcribed. However, because several genes in higher eucaryotes are known to express unspliced transcripts as stable cytoplasmic mRNAs (12,1,32), a direct mode of expression could not be discounted.

The S1-gel mapping experiments shown in Figure 4 (see figure legend for precedural and interpretative details) clearly examined, the principal mRNAs had 5'-termini mapping in the same position (ca nucleotide 150; 73 mu) as those of productively infected cells or other cell lines transformed by genomic viral DNA (30,7), and that these mRNAs were colinear with the pPyMT1 DNA sequence throughout the region which encodes the middle-T protein. This demonstrated that none of the usual splicing events occurred. Three of the transformed lines also produced variable amounts of a transcript beginning somewhere in vector or host DNA sequence 5' to the early region, which was also unspliced. In other experiments not presented here, we used a 3'-labelled single-stranded DNA probe to detect specifically splices originating from the donor used in the large-T mRNA (see Figure 1): control cell lines, but none of the pPyMT1-induced cell lines, showed utilisation of this splicing donor. Therefore, the only known early region viral polypeptide which could be made from the mRNAs in pPyMT1 transformed cell lines is the middle-T protein.

The data shown in Figure 4 also established that, at least in the case of two pPyMT1 lines mapped in detail (line 2.4 and 2.8), viral mRNAs were produced which were colinear with the modified viral DNA sequence for the entire extent of the early region and had polyadenylated 3'-ends mapping within viral sequence at the normal position. This strongly suggested, for reasons which shall be discussed below, that RNA splicing was not involved in the biogenesis of these messengers. Maps of the viral mRNAs produced by pPyMT1 transformed lines and by one p53.A6.6 line (4.6) are shown in Figure 6. The third pPyMT1 line

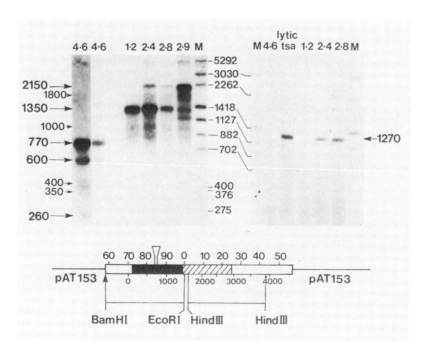

FIG. 4. Characterisation of the viral mRNA in pPYMT1 transformed cell lines (1.2, 2.4, 2.8, and 2.9) and in a p53.A6.6 transformed cell line (4.6) by alkaline agarose gel electrophoresis of nuclease S1-resistant DNA-RNA hybrids. Experimental procedures were previously decribed in detail (9).

The diagram below the autoradiographs illustrates the structure of the Py DNA insert in the plasmids, with the middle-T protein coding region shaded, the remainder of the early region hatched, and the restriction fragments used in the S1-mapping experiments indicated. The position of the deletion in pPyMT1 is also shown. Left panel: S1-resistant DNA from 100μg of total cytoplasmic RNA from the indicated cell lines, hybridised to the unlabelled homologous DNA fragments extending from a BamHI to an EcoRI (58.0-100 mu; nt 4632-1565; see diagram beneath) site in plasmids pPyMT1 or p53.A6.6. After electrophoresis, the S1-resistant DNA products were transferred to nitrocellulose and visualised by annealling to nick-translated viral DNA. The lane on the left is from a longer exposure of the same gel (on this exposure, the indicated 350 nucleotide product was visible with the pPyMT1 transformants). Lane M shows Py restriction fragments run as size markers. The calculated lengths of S1-resistant products are indicated to the left. Larger numbers refer to principal products. Smaller numbers refer to products resulting from S1 cleavage within DNA-RNA hybrids at 93 mu, a phenomenon always found in S1 mapping of Py early region mRNAs which is probably a methodological artefact (44). Product assignments are: line 4.6 - the 600 and 260 nucleotide products represent the alternative 5'-colinear RNA segments, as shown in Figures 1 and 6; the 770 nucleotide product represents the 3'-colinear RNA segments, extending from the splice acceptors at nt 795 and 809 to the end of the restriction fragment at nt 1565; the minor 400 and 350 nucleotide products derive from the 770 by S1 cleavage at 93 mu (ca nt 1200). In lines 1.2, 2.4 and 2.8, the 2150 nucleotide product represents a continuous transcript extending from the BamI site to the EcoRI of pPyMT1 DNA; the 1800 nucleotide product is the result of cleavage of the 2150 at 93 mu; the major 1350 nucleotide product represents a continuous transcript extending from the normal 5'-end position of Py early region mRNAs (nt 150; ref. 7) to the EcoRI site in pPyMT1 DNA; the minor 1000 and 350 nucleotide products represent cleavage of the 1350 at 93 mu. Line 2.9 – pattern too complex for analysis. Right panel: Polyadenylated cytoplasmic mRNA from the indicated transformed cell lines, or from mouse cells productively infected with Py thermolabile mutant tsa (44), annealled to the unlabelled Py HindIII fragment illustrated in the diagram below. The transfer was annealled to a ^{32}P-labelled probe (9) which detects only transcripts of the E–DNA strand, and therefore the 1270 nucleotide product maps the 3'-colinear segments of early region mRNAs extending from the HindIII site (1.8 mu; nt 1650) to the previously determined polyadenylation site at 25.8 mu (ca nt 2930). No bands were detected with RNA from cell lines 4.6 and 1.2 because the 3'-ends of viral sequence in these mRNAs lie before (1.2) or shortly after (4.6) the HindIII site.

---

examined in detail, 1.2, had mRNAs with 3'-ends of colinear viral sequence which mapped within that portion of the early region which, in genomic DNA, uniquely encodes the C-terminal part of large-T protein. This has often been found in other Py transformed rodent cell lines, and indeed is also the case with the one control line analysed here (line 4.6, see Figure 5). It usually indicates the position of a virus-host integration junction (26,30). Since such integration events remove the principal viral polyadenylation site, cell lines like 1.2 and 4.6 have often been found to produce relatively large amounts of mRNA terminating at the alternative viral polyadenylation site, which occurs at 99 mu (26,44), as illustrated in Figure 5. One of the pPyMT1 cell lines (2.8; see Figure 5) also produced a continuous transcript of the L DNA strand of the late region, extending from a 5'-end at an undetermined point in the flanking vector or host DNA sequence to a polyadenylated 3'-end mapping at the same position as that of late region mRNAs produced in lytically infected cells.

The middle-T mRNAs synthesised by the pPyMT1 transformed cell lines, 2.4 and 2.8, are identical in structure to the middle-T mRNAs produced during productive infection (Figure 5). The mRNAs in the transformed lines, however, have not been spliced between their 5'-ends and polyadenylated 3'-termini. This strongly suggests that RNA splicing does not occur during the biogenesis of these messengers. We cannot at this time rigorously exclude the alternative possibility that the mRNAs derive from longer precursors which had been spliced and then subsequently processed to generate the 5'- or 3'-ends of the mature species. We consider processing at the 5'-end to be unlikely, because the ends detected are indistinguishable from those generated by normal use of the viral early promoter (7); it is firmly established in several other systems (6,13) that mRNA 5'-ends correspond to transcriptional initiation points.

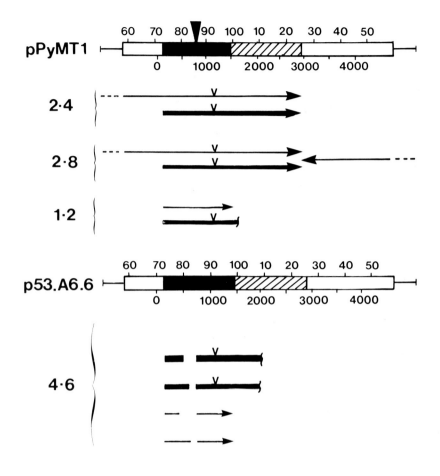

FIG. 5: Structures of Py mRNAs in pPyMT1 and p53.A6.6 transformed rat
cell lines, as deduced from S1-gel mapping studies not presented here.
The mRNAs are aligned below line diagrams of the viral DNA inserts in
the plasmids used, but it should be noted that we have not determined
the structures of the viral DNA actually present in the transformed cell
lines. The middle-T protein coding regions are shaded, and the rest of
the early regions are hatched. mRNAs are represented by thick and thin
lines to suggest their relative abundancies. The 5'-ends of read-through
transcripts have not been mapped and are therefore indicated by dotted
lines. Arrow heads are polyadenylation sites. The S1-sensitive site
at 93 mu is indicated by V. The 3'-ends of viral sequence indicated by
ʃ probably represent the positions of virus/host joints, as frequently
found in other Py transformed cell lines (26). The four cell lines all
contained detectable amounts of mRNAs ending at the 99 mu alternative
polyadenylation site (26,44), but these are only illustrated for lines
1.2 and 4.6 where they comprised significant proportions of the viral
messenger. Note that in cell line 4.6 there must be mRNAs with the two
different small splices (see Figure 1) because this line produces both
small and middle-T proteins, but these cannot be distinguished by agarose gel analysis.

Similarly, we believe that cleavage and 3'-polyadenylation
after downstream splicing is equally improbable because
polyadenylation has been shown to precede splicing during
processing of Ad2 and SV40 RNAs (33,28).   The efficiency
with which the transformed lines produce cytoplasmic mRNAs
may however be slightly impaired by the absence of splicing
since we have noted above that the transformation efficiency of pPyMT1 DNA is 2-3 fold lower than that of the
parental plasmid DNA.   The level of expression obtained
from integrated Py DNA has been shown to vary considerable
among transformed cell lines, although each appears to use
the viral early promoter (26).   This difference in level
is probably a chromosomal position effect; similar observations have been made in the case of avian sarcoma virus
transformed mammalian cell lines (35).   Thus, we may have
selected among the pPyMT1 transformants a sub-set of
integrated genomes which are transcribed at a particularly
high level to compensate for a defect in subsequent processing.   Alternatively, the reduced transformation
efficiency of pPyMT1 may have little to do with RNA

synthesis and instead reflect the absence of the small-T
protein (see below).   To address this question, we have
begun experiments comparing nuclear RNA with cytoplasmic RNA
in the pPyMT1 transformed cell lines.   We are also studying
the expression of pPyMT1 DNA shortly after transfection into
rat cells: preliminary results indicate that the amount of
viral cytoplasmic RNA synthesised from the modified genome
is similar to that produced by unmodified DNA at 60 hours
after DNA transfection, but better quantitation is required
to resolve the issue.

The production of stable, unspliced, cytoplasmic middle-T
mRNA from the modified genome in pPyMT1 does not necessarily
conflict with the results of previous studies (17,18,16).
The conclusion that RNA splicing is obligatory could not be
generalised from the few instances examined in these earlier
experiments.   Moreover, if instead of proposing that splicing in itself is essential, one hypothesises that there is
an RNA sequence, often but not always located within introns,
which has a positive function in RNA maturation, all of the
available data could be accommodated.   Given the pattern of
differential splicing evolved by polyoma virus to produce
three mRNAs from one precursor, it would not be surprising
if such a sequence occurred somewhere outside the 63 nucleotides comprising the middle-T protein intervening sequence.
This hypothesis would also better explain the expression of
genes such as those for the adenovirus protein IX (1) and
interferons (32) which lack introns, or the abundant production of unspliced late SV40 19S mRNA (12) in certain
situations.   The effect of deletion mutations which interfere with the splicing of the SV40 small-T protein mRNA has
also been investigated (27), the general result being that
unspliced mRNAs were usually not expressed.   It is possible,
however, that most of the deletions caused preferential
splicing of the precursor to yield large-T, rather than un-

spliced, mRNAs. Indeed, one (dl 884) of the deletions removing the small-T mRNA splice donor appeared to synthesise a truncated small-T protein, perhaps by translation of an unspliced messenger (27).

THE ROLES OF THE POLYOMA VIRUS EARLY PROTEINS IN TRANSFORMATION

Our results strongly suggest that expression of the polyoma virus middle-T protein is sufficient to establish and maintain a transformed state. What of the other two viral early proteins? Viable deletion mutants (the hr-t mutants) have been isolated (3) which synthesise normal large-T protein but no detectable small or middle-T proteins (37). These mutants do not transform cells (29,3). Moreover, the integration of such DNA into the rat cell genome can result in cell lines which express the large-T protein but are phenotypically normal (29). Deletion mutants lacking DNA which encodes the C-terminus of the middle-T protein, but which encode normal small-T protein, are severely impaired in transforming activity (U. Novak and B.E. Griffin, submitted for publication), as are certain internal deletions mapping within the middle-T/large-T overlap region (15,31,14) and a point mutant which causes premature termination of only the middle-T protein (D. Templeton and W. Eckhart, manuscript in preparation). These observations are consistent with our demonstration of the critical role of middle-T protein in transformation; they also suggest that expression of the small-T protein alone cannot transform cells. It is therefore now clear that of the three early proteins, only individual expression of the middle-T can induce the dramatic changes in cell regulation identified as viral transformation. We found, however, that pPyMT1 DNA has a slightly reduced transformation efficiency, which may reflect either an impairment in middle-T gene expression or the absence of an additional gene product. It will be interesting to construct plasmids containing two modified early regions which independently encode middle-T and one of the other T-proteins and to determine whether any of these have a fully restored transformation potential. Further, we have not as yet systematically studied in the pPyMT1 transformed lines all relevant parameters of the transformed state. If the middle-T transformed lines prove to be different in some selectable property, it will be possible to assess the roles of the other T-proteins by super-transfection with the appropriate cDNA recombinants.
Our results are in prima facie disagreement with the recent work of Cuzin and collaborators (Rassoulzadegan, M., Gaudray, P., Canning, M., Trejo-Avila, L. and Cuzin, F., submitted for publication) which suggested an involvement of the amino-terminal portion of the large-T protein in the maintenance of the transformed state. It is conceivable that the disagreement reflects differences in the way in which the transformants were obtained, although preliminary results indicate that pPyMT1 DNA does transform FR3T3 rat

cells under the conditions used by these workers (F. Cuzin, personal communication). We anticipate that collaborative experiments now in progress between our two laboratories using the plasmid DNA described here will resolve this issue.

The mechanism whereby middle-T protein causes transformation is unknown. Of the three polyoma virus T-proteins, a unique property of the middle-T is its association with the plasma membrane (39,23), although efforts to detect it on the cell surface have been unsuccessful (25). Several groups have also found a protein kinase activity probably associated with the Py middle-T protein which results, in vitro, in the phosphorylation of a tyrosine residue in the middle-T protein itself (41,42,36). We tested four pPyMT1-transformed cell lines (1.2, 2.4, 2.6 and 2.8) and one p53.A6.6-transformed cell line (4,6) for this kinase activity: they were all positive, demonstrating that no viral protein other than middle-T is required. However, it is not proven that the kinase is an activity of the middle-T protein rather than that of a bound host enzyme. Introduction of the modified viral early region from pPyMT1 into a bacterial expression vector in order to obtain large amounts

of the middle-T protein is therefore of high priority. The middle-T protein produced in this heterologous system could be used to directly assess whether it is a tyrosine-specific protein kinase, and to assay other potential functions.

REFERENCES

1. Alestrom, P., Akusjarvi, G., Perricaudet, M., Mathews, M.B., Klessig, D.F. and Pettersson, U. (1980) Cell 19: 671-681.
2. Bastin, M., Bourgaux-Ramoisy, D. and Bourgaux, P. (1980) J. Gen. Virol. 50: 179-184.
3. Benjamin, T. (1979) Proc. Natl. Acad. Sci. USA 67: 394-398.
4. Birnboim, H.C. and Doly, J. (1979) Nucl. Acids Res. 7: 1513-1523.
5. Breathnach, R., Benoist, C., O'Hare, K., Gannon, F. and Chambon, P. (1978) Proc. Natl. Acad. Sci. USA 75: 4853-4857.
6. Contreras, R. and Fiers, W. (1981) Nucl. Acids Res. 9: 215-236.
7. Cowie, A., Jat, P. and Kamen, R., in preparation.
8. Eckhart, W., Hutchinson, M.A. and Hunter, T. (1979) Cell 18: 925-933.
9. Favaloro, J., Treisman, R. and Kamen, R. (1980) Meths. Enzymol. 65: 718-748.
10. Freeman, A.E., Gilden, R.B., Vernon, M.L., Wolford, R.G., Hugunin, P.E. and Huebner, R.J. (1973) Proc. Natl. Acad. Sci. USA 70: 2415-2419.
11. Friedmann, T., Esty, A., LaPorte, P. and Deininger, P. (1979) Cell 17: 715-724.

12. Ghosh, P.K., Reddy, V.B., Swinscoe, J., Lebowitz, P. and Weissman, S.M. (1978) J. Mol. Biol. 126: 813-846.
13. Gidoni, D., Kahana, C., Canaani, D. and Groner, Y. (1981) Proc. Natl. Acad. Sci. USA 78: 2174-2178.
14. Griffin, B.E. and Maddock, C. (1979) J. Virol. 31: 645-656.
15. Griffin, B.E., Ito, Y., Spurr, N., Dilworth, S., Smolar, N., Pollack, R., Smith, K. and Rifkin, D. (1980) Cold Spring Harbor Symp. Quant. Biol. 44: 271-284.
16. Gruss, P., Lai, C.-J., Dhar, R. and Khoury, G. (1979) Proc. Natl. Acad. Sci. USA 76: 4317-4321.
17. Gruss, P. and Khoury, G. (1980) Nature 286: 634-637.
18. Hamer, D.H. and Leder, P. (1979) Cell 17: 737-747.
19. Hassell, J.A., Topp, W.C., Rifkin, D.B. and Moreau, P.E. (1980) Proc. Natl. Acad. Sci. USA 77: 3978-3982.
20. Hunter, T., Hutchinson, M.A. and Eckhart, W. (1978) Proc. Natl. Acad. Sci. USA 75: 5917-5921.
21. Hutchinson, M.A., Hunter, T. and Eckhart, W. (1978) Cell 15: 65-77.
22. Israel, M.A., Simmons, D.T., Hourihan, S.L., Rowe, W.P. and Martin, M.A. (1979) Proc. Natl. Acad. Sci. USA 76: 3713-3716.
23. Ito, Y., Brocklehurst, J.R. and Dulbecco, R. (1977) Proc. Natl. Acad. Sci. USA 74: 4666-4670.
24. Ito, Y., Spurr, N. and Dulbecco, R. (1977) Proc. Natl. Acad. Sci. USA 74: 1259-1263.
25. Ito, Y. and Spurr, N. (1980) Cold Spring Harbor Symp. Quant. Biol. 44: 149-157.
26. Kamen, R., Favaloro, J., Parker, J., Treisman, R., Lania, L., Fried, M. and Mellor, A. (1980) Cold Spring Harbor Symp. Quant. Biol. 44: 63-75.
27. Khoury, G., Gruss, P., Dhar, R. and Lai, C.-J. (1979) Cell 18: 85-92.
28. Lai, C.-J., Dhar, R. and Khoury, G. (1978) Cell 14: 971-982.
29. Lania, L., Griffiths, M., Cooke, B., Ito, Y. and Fried, M. (1979) Cell 18: 793-802.
30. Lania, L., Hayday, A., Bjursell, G., Gandini-Attardi, D. and Fried, M. (1980) Cold Spring Harbor Symp. Quant. Biol. 44: 597-603.
31. Magnusson, G. and Berg, P. (1979) J. Virol. 32: 523-529.
32. Nagata, S., Mantei, N. and Weissmann, C. (1980) Nature 287: 401-408.
33. Nevins, J.R. and Darnell, J.E. (1978) Cell 15: 1477-1494.
34. Novak, U., Dilworth, S.M. and Griffin, B.E. (1980) Proc. Natl. Acad. Sci. USA 77: 3278-3282.
35. Quintrell, N., Hughes, S.H., Varmus, H.E. and Bishop, J.M. (1980) J. Mol. Biol. 143: 363-393.
36. Schaffhausen, B.S. and Benjamin, T.L. (1979) Cell 18: 935-946.
37. Schaffhausen, B.S., Silver, J.E. and Benjamin, T. (1978) Proc. Natl. Acad. Sci. USA 75: 79-83.
38. Seif, I., Khoury, G. and Dhar, R. (1979) Nucl. Acids Res. 6: 3387-3398.
39. Silver, J., Schaffhausen, B. and Benjamin, T. (1978) Cell 15: 485-496.

40. Soeda, E., Arrand, J.R., Smolar, N., Walsh, J.E. and
    Griffin, B.E. (1980) Nature 283: 445-453.
41. Smith, A.E., Smith, R., Griffin, B.E. and Fried, M.
    (1979) Cell 18: 915-924.
42. Smith, A.E., Fried, M., Ito, Y., Spurr, N. and Smith,R.
    (1980) Cold Spring Harbor Symp. Quant. Biol. 44: 141-147.
43. Tooze, J. (ed.) The Molecular Biology of Tumor Viruses
    II. DNA Tumour Viruses (Cold Spring Harbor Laboratory,
    New York, 1980).
44. Treisman, R.H., Cowie, A., Favaloro, J.M., Jat, P. and
    Kamen, R. (1981) J. Mol. Appl. Gen. 1: 83-92.
45. Twigg, A.J. and Sherratt, D. (1980) Nature 283: 216-218.
46. Van der Eb, A.J. and Graham, F.L. (1980) Meths. Enzymol.
    65: 826-838.
47. Weaver, R.F. and Weissmann, C. (1979) Nucl. Acids Res.
    6: 1175-1193.

Expression of Differentiated Functions in Cancer Cells, edited by R. F. Revoltella et al., Raven Press, New York © 1982.

Biological and Biochemical Studies of Polyoma Virus Transformation

Thomas L. Benjamin

Department of Pathology, Harvard Medical School, Boston, Massachusetts 02115

Malignant transformation of cells by polyoma virus results from the continual expression of a single viral gene, designated "hr-t". The normal function of the hr-t gene is to alter the physiological state of the host in a manner which facilitates productive viral infection. The action of the hr-t gene is pleiotropic and results in the induction of a transformed cellular phenotype that is manifested transiently during productive infection or abortive transformation but permanently when the viral genome is integrated in stably transformed cells. Hr-t mutants are defective in their growth in mice, and in most cultured cell lines. They are unable to induce tumors or any of the morphological, structural or growth-related changes which accompany cell transformation by the wild type virus.

The 22K small T antigen and the 56K middle T antigen are proteins encoded in the early region of viral DNA and constitute the dual products of the hr-t gene. Hr-t mutants are localized in a narrow segment of the early region that specifies an amino acid sequence shared by these two overlapping proteins. Current efforts to link structural (mutational) changes with functional changes in these proteins center around the 56K middle T antigen and its associated protein kinase activity. Assayed in vitro, this activity leads to phosphorylation of the 56K protein itself, predominantly at a specific tyrosine residue in the C-terminal portion of the molecule. The middle T protein is anchored in the plasma membrane by a hydrophobic tail close to the C-terminus. Membrane association appears to be essential for transformation as well as for the associated kinase activity. In vivo, the 56K protein undergoes multiple phosphorylations involving serine or threonine residues which appear to affect its in vitro kinase activity. The altered middle T antigens of hr-t mutants show no protein kinase activity in vitro; they also fail to undergo at least some of the in vivo phosphorylations found in the wild type middle T antigens. These kinase reactions, originating in the plasma membrane but potentially affecting pathways into the cytoplasm and nucleus, currently provide the most plausible biochemical mechanism underlying the pleiotropic effects of the hr-t gene.

353

I.   Introduction

     The long range goal of research on tumor viruses is to elucidate
the steps and mechanism of malignant cell transformation. Viruses of
two distinct biological groups have been intensively studied as model
systems in pursuing these goals. These are the small DNA-containing
tumor viruses of the papova group including polyoma and SV-40, and the
RNA-containing retraviruses of which the best studied example is the
Rous sarcoma virus. While papova viruses and retraviruses differ pro-
foundly from one another in their structure and life cycle, their
actions in inducing malignant transformation of their respective host
cells show dramatic similarities. In each virus system, two distinct
viral genes are essential for the transformation process. The first of
these is an "initiation" function whose action results in the integration of all or part of the viral genome into host DNA. Once the genome
has been stably integrated, the initiation function is no longer required
for the cell to remain transformed. The action of the second viral gene
results in the multiple phenotypic alterations of the cell associated
with malignant transformation. The latter viral functions affecting the
"maintenance" of the transformed state are carried out by the src gene
in the case of Rous sarcoma virus and by the hr-t gene in the case of
polyoma virus. The single genes in each virus system affecting the maintenance of transformation act in a pleiotropic way affecting morphological, structural and growth-related changes of the transformed cell.
The pleiotropic effects of the hr-t gene plays a role in the polyoma
growth cycle, both in cultured cells and in the animal. This is in contrast to the situation with retraviruses in which the src gene appears
to be non-essential in the life cycle of the virus.

     Genetic and biochemical studies of these two virus systems have led
to identification of the products of the transforming genes. An important clue concerning the biochemical mode of action of the src gene
came with the discovery of a protein kinase activity associated with
the src gene product (1,2). A similar protein kinase activity with
specificity for tyrosine (3) is seen associated with the polyoma
virus middle T antigen, which is one of the products of the hr-t gene.
The protein kinase activities specified by the src and hr-t genes appear
to reside at least in part on the cytoplasmic side of the plasma membrane of transformed cells. Non-transforming mutants in the src and
hr-t genes fail to show the protein kinase activity. The initial step
in the maintenance pathway for transformation thus appears to involve
protein phosphorylating events occurring at or near the plasma membrane.
In this article, I will review the history of the isolation and the
general biological properties of hr-t mutants and discuss more recent
findings concerning phosphorylation events associated with the polyoma
middle T antigen. A more extensive review on the hr-t gene will appear
elsewhere (4).

II. The Isolation and Preliminary Characterization of Hr-t Mutants

     The hr-t gene was uncovered in the course of attempts to understand
polyoma virus-cell interactions along lines suggested by temperate bacteriophage. Nucleic acid hybridization experiments indicated clearly
that at least a portion of the polyoma virus genome persists in transformed cells and continues to be expressed. However, radiobiological
and other experiments suggested a function for the expressed gene(s)
which was not expected of a prophage. Specifically, viral genes expressed in polyoma transformed cells appeared to promote virus growth
rather than to repress it in the manner of a temperate bacteriophage

repressor. The realization that viral genes expressed by the integrated virus in a transformed cell also played a role in the productive infectious cycle of the virus led to the notion of screening for a "polyoma transformed cell-dependent" host range phenotype. Polyoma transformed mouse 3T3 cells were therefore utilized as the permissive host and normal 3T3 cells as the non-permissive host in the screenings for host range mutants. It was expected that such mutants, selected for deficiencies which could be complemented by the integrated virus in transformed cells, would themselves be unable to induce transformation (5).

A total of nineteen mutants were isolated according to this selection. When tested for transformation of normal rat or hamster embryo fibroblasts, all were found to be defective, thus confirming the prediction that the deficiency selected for involved a function that was required for cell transformation as well as for virus growth (5, 6). Complementation analysis with these nineteen host range mutants showed that all nineteen fell into a single complementation class (6). The designation "hr-t" was given to this class indicating the dual nature of the defect affecting both the host range for growth and cell transformation.

a) The HR-T gene acts on the cell to induce a permissive state.

Subsequent studies on the host range character of hr-t mutants revealed several classes of cells that were capable of serving as permissive hosts for replication of the mutants without themselves being transformed by polyoma virus (7,8). Among such non-polyoma transformed permissive cells were mouse embryo fibroblasts in primary passage and normal mouse 3T3 cells infected by and producing any one of several different murine leukemia viruses. The finding of cell types such as these, free of polyoma information but which nevertheless could complement the growth of hr-t mutants, gave rise to the hypothesis of indirect complementation. The hr-t gene, according to this hypothesis, acts as a pleiotropic regulatory gene bringing about a profound alteration in the physiological state of the host which is essential for efficient virus growth (6). While the hr-t gene normally acts to induce the cellular permissive state, the latter can also be expressed constitutively by the cell as shown by the permissivity of normal mouse embryonic fibroblasts. The precise role of the cellular permissive factor(s) in the virus growth cycle is not clear, although they appear to act at a late stage in the virus growth cycle. When hr-t mutants infect a non-permissive host such as normal 3T3 cells, viral DNA and viral capsid proteins are made in essentially normal amounts, although the yield of infectious virus particles is only a few percent of that of a wild type viral infection. Thus, the hr-t block in virus growth - and hence the role of the cellular permissive factor(s) - appears to be concerned in some way with virus maturation or assembly.

The indirect complementation hypothesis assumes that the loss of transforming ability arises concomitantly in hr-t mutants with the inability to induce the expression of the cellular permissive state. It should thus be possible to isolate hr-t mutants using normal mouse embryo fibroblasts in place of polyoma transformed 3T3 cells as the permissive hosts (6). Results confirming this prediction have recently been obtained. Five host range mutants were isolated using primary mouse embryo fibroblasts as the permissive host. All five of these mutants are negative for transformation and indistinguishable from "polyoma transformed cell dependent" hr-t mutants by complementation and other physiological tests (9).

III.   Role of the Hr-t Gene in Cellular Alterations
     In line with the putative role of the hr-t gene in inducing the
cellular permissive state for viral replication, a number of discrete
alterations of cellular components and processes are seen to occur following infection by wild type virus and which fail to occur in the same
manner following hr-t mutant infections. Alteration of the cell surface
leading to agglutination by lectins is one such example ([10]). Within
24 hours after infection by wild type virus, normal 3T3 cells become
readily agglutinable by conconavalin A or wheat germ agglutinin. Cells
infected by hr-t mutants on the other hand remain non-agglutinable over
this time period and even for longer times. The hr-t gene is also required to induce morphological and cytoskeletal changes following infections of rat fibroblasts ([11]). Dramatic changes in cell shape accompanied by decreased cell-substrative adhesion and extensive cell-cell
underlapping occur in a majority of cells infected by wild type virus
24-36 hours post-infection. These changes are also accompanied by the
disappearance of stress fibers, corresponding to a loss of the bundle
arrangement of the actin-containing microfilaments. None of these
changes are seen to occur following infection of cells by hr-t mutants
(11).

     The hr-t gene also plays a role in activation of the cell cycle in
resting fibroblasts. Infection by wild type virus results in a continuous recruitment of cells from the G-1 phase of the cycle into S-phase
and subsequently into G-2 and M, persisting throughout several cell generations. In contrast, hr-t mutant infections lead to the induction of
only a single cycle of DNA synthesis and cell division(11).The mitogenic
effect of hr-t mutants is therefore restricted in a quantitative sense,
compared to that of the wild type virus. The activation of multiple cycles of growth in the case of wild type virus is accompanied by a loss
of growth control. This is demonstrated by the ability of wild type virus infected fibroblasts to grow in soft agar ([12]). This loss of anchorage dependence of growth is not seen following infection by hr-t virus mutants ([13]).

     A final example of hr-t gene-related modifications of cellular com-
ponents is provided by the study of histones found in purified virus
particles. The cellular histones isolated from purified wild type polyoma virions show extensive acetylation of the two arginine-rich species
H3 and H4. The same histone species isolated from hr-t mutant particles
show a normal, i.e., "low", level of acetylation ([14]). The significance of histone hyperacetylation in terms of the action of the hr-t viral gene is not clear. The activity may reflect a viral induced stimulation of cellular gene expression perhaps related to the mechanism
whereby the hr-t gene induces expression of cellular permissive and
transformation related functions (6,15). The absence of high levels of
histone acetylation in hr-t mutant viral chromatin may also be related
in some manner to the apparent maturation defect of the mutants. The
ensemble of these results on hr-t gene-induced cellular alterations, affecting nuclear, cytoplasmic and cell surface structures, emphasize the
pleiotropic nature of the action of this viral gene, and raises the
challenge to uncover the underlying biochemical mechanism.
IV.   The Middle T Antigen Associated Protein Kinase Activity
     Incubation of polyoma T antigen immune precipitates with γ-P^{32} la-
beled ATP leads to the incorporation of radioactive phosphate into the
middle T antigen species (3,16,17). This incorporation occurs predominantly if not exclusively on tyrosine residues ([3]). The activity is
present in all wild type and tsA mutant virus infected or transformed

cells, as well as in cells infected by different viable deletion mutants
with altered middle T antigens, provided that the latter retain a wild
type transforming capacity. Hr-t mutants, however, are defective
in this kinase reaction. Phenotypically normal revertants of polyoma transformed cells fail to express the middle T antigen and its associated kinase activity (18). These results point to the essential
role of this enzymatic activity in the transformation process.

Cell fractionation experiments have shown that the middle T antigen
species is associated with membrane fractions of the cell (19,20). When
monolayers of transformed cells are lightly treated with a non-ionic detergent such as Triton X-100 and incubated directly with ATP, and the T
antigens subsequently extracted and immune-precipitated, radioactive
phosphate is again incorporated into the middle T antigen (21). This
incorporation is also on tyrosine, indicating that the kinase reaction
demonstrable in immune precipitates also occurs in situ. The kinase-ac-
tive fraction of middle T molecules appears to be largely non-extracta-
ble in Triton-containing buffer and remains preferentially associated
with the residual cell framework (21).

Examination of the primary sequence of the middle T antigen shows a
polypeptide chain of 421 amino acids with a hydrophobic sequence of 22
residues close to the C-terminal end. The sequence is similar to those
found in several trans-membrane proteins and presumably constitutes the
membrane anchoring site of the middle T antigen. In order to demonstrate that this sequence is indeed the membrane anchor and to investigate the importance of association of the middle T protein with membranes, we have constructed a mutant of middle T which lacks the hydrophobic tail (22). This mutant has been made by introducing a chain-
terminating codon just upstream of the hydrophobic tail. This "tail-
less" middle T antigen containing most of the body of the middle T protein (384 out of 421 amino acids) is no longer recovered in membrane
fractions but rather in the cytosol. The truncated middle T antigen
produced by this mutant, when immuno-precipitated from cell extracts,
fails to show kinase activity. In addition, this mutant is unable to
transform cells. These results underline the importance of membrane localization of middle T antigen via its hydrophobic tail for both biological and biochemical activity (22).

A closer examination of the products of the in vitro kinase reaction separated on SDS-acrylamide gels reveals two species of middle T
antigen which are active in incorporating phosphate (18,21). The more
rapidly migrating species corresponds to the 56K middle T antigen detectable by S[35]-methionine metabolic labeling. The second species migrates
slightly more slowly with an apparent molecular weight of 58K. This 58K
species is closely related to the 56K species as shown by analysis of
partial proteolytic digestion fragments (18,21). The apparent difference
between the 58K and 56K species resides in the C terminal portion of the
molecule as indicated by comparisons of partial proteolytic digestion
fragments from various viable deletion mutants affected in this region
of the protein (18,21). The 58K species comprises roughly 50% of the in[35]
vitro labeled product, but corresponds to only trace amounts of an S[35]-
methionine labeled species, indicating that it is roughly ten times more
active as a phosphate acceptor in the in vitro reaction than the 56K.
The tyrosine serving as the acceptor site in the in vitro kinase reaction has been mapped to a specific residue in the C-terminal portion of
the molecule, and lies just downstream of an extraordinary cluster of
six glutamic acids. Both the 56K and 58K species appear to utilize this

same tyrosine residue as the phosphate acceptor (18,21).

V.   Phosphorylations of Middle T Antigens In Vivo

Both 56K and 58K middle T antigen species are readily detected by labeling infected or transformed cells with P^{32}-orthophosphate(16,18,21,23). In contrast to the in vitro kinase reaction however, the phosphate linkages of in vivo labeled middle T antigens appears to be primarily to serine or threonine residues (23). Furthermore, comparisons of proteolytic digestion products of in vivo labeled 56K and 58K proteins shows that these two species are phosphorylated at different sites. The region of the molecule showing the difference in in vivo phosphorylations corresponds to the same region which contributes to the apparent molecular weight difference seen by mapping of the in vitro labeled material.

Hr-t mutants show incorporation of phosphate in vivo into their altered middle T species, despite the fact that these species are negative in the in vitro kinase reaction. Interestingly, the hr-t mutant (NG-59) shows only a single species corresponding to the 56K form by labeling with P^{32}-orthophosphate in vivo (16,18).The results on in vivo phosphorylation show that the polyoma middle T antigen species of wild type virus are substrates for cellular kinases, and suggest furthermore that phosphorylation(s) of middle T antigen by cellular enzymes may in fact activate the middle T protein as revealed in the in vitro kinase reaction. Hr-t mutants are at least partially defective in the presumptive activation by the in vivo kinase reactions, and are completely defective in the in vitro kinase reaction.

VI.   Summary and Conclusions

The hr-t gene of polyoma virus acts as a pleiotropic regulator affecting the cell in a manner which leads it to express permissive factors that promote effective virus growth. Action of this same gene leads to multiple cellular alterations giving rise to the transformed phenotype. The hr-t viral gene codes for two products, the 22K small T antigen and the 56K middle T antigen. The latter species has come under intensive study in recent years stimulated by the finding of a protein kinase activity associated with the species in immune precipitates. This activity may reflect an intrinsic enzymatic activity (autophosphorylation), or alternatively may be due to a cellular kinase which recognizes and coprecipitates with the middle T proteins. While this question cannot presently be resolved, it is clear that retention of the in vitro kinase activity is critical for cell transformation. Middle T protein appears to be acted upon by cellular protein kinase(s). Association of the middle T protein with membrane fractions of the cell appears to be necessary for the acquisition of the in vitro kinase activity as well as for biological activity in transformation. The phosphorylation reactions associated with the middle T antigen appear to provide a plausible mechanism for the initial steps in transformation by polyoma virus._ _

Acknowledgement - The work in this laboratory has been supported by grants from the National Cancer Institute and the American Cancer Society.

References

1.   Collett, M. and Erikson, R. (1978) PNAS 75: 2021.
2.   Levinson, A.D., Oppermann, H., Levintow, L., Varmus, H.E. and Bishop, J.M. (1978) Cell 15: 561.
3.   Eckhart, W., Hutchinson, M.A. and Hunter, T. (1979) Cell 18: 925.
4.   Benjamin, T.L. (submitted 1981) BBA Reviews on Cancer.
5.   Benjamin, T.L. (1970) PNAS 67: 394.

6. Staneloni, R.J., Fluck, M.M., and Benjamin, T.L. (1977) Virology 77: 598.

7. Benjamin, T.L. and Goldman, E. (1974) 39th Cold Spring Harbor Symp. on Quantitative Biology, p. 41.

8. Goldman, E. and Benjamin, T.L. (1975) Virology 66: 372.

9. Feunteun, J. and Benjamin, T.L. (manuscript in preparation).

10. Benjamin, T.L. and Burger, M.M. (1970) PNAS 67: 929.

11. Schlegel, R. and Benjamin, T.L. (1978) Cell 14: 587.

12. Stoker, M. (1968) Nature 218: 234.

13. Fluck, M.M. and Benjamin, T.L. (1979) Virology 96: 205.

14. Schaffhausen, B.S. and Benjamin, T.L. (1976) PNAS 73: 213.

15. Benjamin, T.L. (1976) Cancer Research 36: 4289.

16. Schaffhausen, B.S. and Benjamin, T.L. (1979) Cell 18: 935.

17. Smith, A., Smith, R., Griffin, B. and Fried, M. (1979) Cell 18: 915.

18. Schaffhausen, B.S. and Benjamin, T.L. (1981) J. Virology, in press.

19. Ito, Y., Brocklehurst, J.R., and Dulbecco, R. (1977) PNAS 74: 4666.

20. Silver, J., Schaffhausen, B. and Benjamin, T.L. (1978) Cell 15: 485.

21. Schaffhausen, B.S. and Benjamin, T.L. (1981) 8th Cold Spring Harbor Conference on Cell Proliferation, in press.

22. Carmichael, G.G., Dorsky, D.I., Schaffhausen, B.S., Olliver, D. and Benjamin, T.L. (manuscript in preparation).

23. Schaffhausen, B.S., Silver, J. and Benjamin, T.L. (1978) PNAS 75: 79.

Expression of Differentiated Functions in Cancer Cells, edited by R. F. Revoltella et al., Raven Press, New York © 1982.

Herpes Simplex Virus Host Cell Interactions Related to Cancer of the Human Cervix

J. H. Subak-Sharpe, R. P. Eglin, H. C. Kitchener, J. B. Clements, J. C. M. Macnab, and N. M. Wilkie

Institute of Virology, University of Glasgow, Glasgow G11 5JR, Scotland

Two types of herpes simplex virus (HSV) are recognised to exist in the human population (Nahmias and Roizman, 1973). HSV type 1 (HSV-1) is universally endemic in human populations producing disease ranging from relatively mild skin lesions around the lips and mouth to fatal encephalitis. HSV type 2 (HSV-2) is usually found infecting the genital regions of males and females, but may also produce lesions in other parts of the lower body.

After primary infection the virus characteristically remains latent in neurological tissue and in a proportion of infected individuals it can reactivate, leading to peripheral lesions. During the latent phase infectious virus is not present nor is it demonstrable by homogenising or otherwise disrupting tissue samples. However, when intact latently infected tissue samples are explanted and incubated the virus reactivates and infectious virus is produced. Latent HSV-1 has been shown to reside in the sensory dorsal root (trigeminal) ganglia of naturally infected humans (Bastian et al., 1972). Baringer (1974) reactivated and isolated HSV-2 from sacral ganglia of humans.

In the various animal model systems which have been developed, e.g. mice (Stevens and Cook, 1971), guinea pigs (Scriba, 1975) and rabbits (Stevens et al., 1972), the virus similarly resides in the ganglia.

Tobin et al. (1978) were able to reactivate HSV-2 from Frankenhauser's plexus in latently infected mice subsequent to vaginal infection with HSV-2. HSV-1 has been successfully reactivated following explantation of human ganglia, not only from the trigeminal ganglia but also from superior cervical, vagus and thoracic ganglia (Warren et al., 1978; Lonsdale et al., 1979; Price et al,, 1975).

Cytological (Niab, Nahmias and Josey, 1966) and sero-epidemiological surveys (Rawls, Tomkins and Melnick, 1969; Adam et al., 1973; Skinner,

Whitney and Hartley, 1977) have provided evidence suggesting an association of HSV-2 with cervical anaplasia. More recently, the later stages of cervical intraepithelial neoplasia (CIN) were found to exhibit increasingly significant correlation with prior HSV-2 infection (Thomas and Rawls, 1978).

Other experimental approaches have also led to the direct detection of HSV-coded material in cervical neoplasia. Immunofluorescence tests using general anti-HSV sera have given positive results in some cases (Nahmias, Del Buono and Ibrahim, 1975) but failed to do so in others (Pasca et al., 1975). Dreesman et al. (1980) reported positive results in immunoperoxidase tests on biopsies of both CIN and squamous cell carcinoma using specific antisera to HSV-2 coded ICSP.

Using in situ hybridisation of radiolabelled HSV-2 DNA to RNA transcripts in tissue sections McDougall, Calloway and Fenoglio (1980) obtained quantitative evidence for the presence of HSV-specific RNA in a series of CIN but not in squamous cell carcinoma biopsies (0/5). By quantitative analysis of in situ hybridisation Eglin et al. (1981) detected HSV-specific RNA in 72% CIN (31/43) and 60% squamous cell carcinoma (21/35) as against 2% of non-neoplastic cervical biopsies (1/56). However, unlike McDougall et al. (1980), Eglin et al. (1981) found all three stages of CIN to give similar results and moreover they detected transcripts in all four clinical stages of squamous cell carcinoma of the cervix. McDougall (pers. comm., Atlanta, 1980) has now also observed HSV-specific RNA in 2 out of 7 squamous cell carcinomas. We now report further confirmation and extension of the use of the in situ hybridisation technique by extending the investigation to matched paired punch biopsies of squamous cell carcinoma and by employing cloned fragments of the HSV-2 genome. The cloned fragments were used to detect the regions of the HSV-2 genome transcribed in the neoplastic cervical cells of different individuals. In addition, we report the reactivation of infectious HSV from explanted uterosacral ligament tissue.

METHODS AND MATERIALS

Biopsy Samples

From the same patient, matched paired punch biopsies from neoplastic and non-neoplastic regions (10 patients with CIN and 5 patients with early stage squamous cell carcinoma) were obtained and immediately snap frozen in liquid nitrogen. In each case the diagnosis was confirmed histologically by Dr. R. Denham of the Western Infirmary, Glasgow. Single biopsies were also collected from 10 squamous cell carcinoma patients at clinical stages 1 - 3. In no case could infectious HSV be isolated from ectocervical swabs or cell-free tissue extracts of any of these patients using the methods described previously (Eglin et al., 1981).

Preparation of Tissue Samples and in situ Hybridisation

Serial 7 micron sections of the tissue biopsies were prepared at
-30°C and fixed as described by Eglin et al. (1981). The virus DNA
probes (HSV-2, adenovirus-2 and bacteriophage lambda) were prepared
from whole virus as previously described and were radiolabelled with
^{125}I to a specific activity of approximately 5 x 10^7ct/min/ ug. Cloned
fragments of HSV-2 DNA were similarly labelled. In situ hybridisation
was performed as previously described (Eglin et al., 1981) and the
grains present in 10 standard fields (each 3.6 x 10^{-2}mm^2) were counted
using an Optomax Video Image Analyser.

Culture of Uterosacral Ligaments

Uterosacral ligaments were collected at hysterectomy, one was snap
frozen in liquid nitrogen and the other was cultured in vitro at 37°C
in 5 ml. Glasgow-modified Eagle's medium supplemented with 10% calf
serum. Supernatant was checked for presence of infectious virus every
48 hours for 14 days when the ligament tissue was minced, sonicated
and plated onto monolayers of BHK C13 indicator cells. Any virus producing a cytopathic effect in the indicator cells was harvested, stored
at -70°C and typed by restriction enzyme analysis of its DNA using the
method of Lonsdale et al. (1980).

Production of Cloned Fragments of HSV-2 DNA

The HSV-2 Hind III and Bam HI fragments used had been litigated into
the Hind III and Bam HI sites respectively of plasmid vector pAT 153
(Twigg and Sherratt, 1980) and transfected into the host bacterium
E. coli K12 HB101. The Hind III and Bam HI clones were provided by
our colleagues, A.J. Davison and A. Easton, who had mapped them at
the co-ordinates on the HSV-2 genome shown in Table 1. The Hind III DNA
fragments from clones pGz2 and pGz11 was recut with EcoR1 and the fragments produced were separated by electrophoresis on 1% agarose gels,
the individual HSV-2 DNA bands were cut out and the DNA fragments isolated by hydroxylapatite chromatography.

RESULTS

Matched Paired Biopsies from Squamous Cell Carcinoma and non-Neoplastic Biopsies

Eglin et al. (1981) analysed matched paired punch biopsies from
the neoplastic and benign regions of 29 cervices and reported that
HSV-specific RNA transcripts were detected only in the neoplastic cells
of a cervix with CIN. We have extended this approach to investigate a
small series of squamous cell carcinoma cases where it was possible to
identify some non-neoplastic region of the cervix. Table 2 shows the

TABLE 1

Clones of HSV-2 DNA

	RESTRICTION ENZYME FRAGMENTS	MAP UNITS
pGz 26	HIND III a	0.52 - 0.72
pGz 11	HIND III b	0.07 - 0.27
pGz 25	HIND III e	0.40 - 0.52
pGz 10	HIND III h	0.29 - 0.40
pGz 23	HIND III 1	0.88 - 0.93
pGz 12	HIND III k and 1	0.84 - 0.87; 0.93 - 0.99
pGz 32	HIND III n	0.27 - 0.29
pGz 1	Bam H1 f	0.74 - 0.78; 0.05 - 0.06
pGz 65	Bam HI g	0.81 - 0.85; 0.98 - 1.00; 0.00 - 0.02
pGz 64	Bam H1 p	0.78 - 0.81; 0.02 - 0.05
pGz 26a	pG1 1 recut with EcoR1	0.52 - 0.64
pGz 26b	pG1 1 recut with EcoR1	0.64 - 0.65
pGz 26c	pG1 1 recut with EcoR1	0.65 - 0.72
pGz 11a	pG1 2 recut with EcoR1	0.07 - 0.11
pGz 11b	pG1 2 recut with EcoR1	0.11 - 0.21
pGz 11c	pG1 2 recut with EcoR1	0.21 - 0.27

TABLE 2

Background-corrected grain counts for matched paired biopsies from squamous cell carcinoma patients after in situ hybridisation

	HSV-2				Ad 2		M.lys	
	Ca	N-N	Ca	N-N	Ca	N-N	Ca	N-N
	446	28	88	58	79	86	37	35
	236	97	20	31	61	11	52	28
	424	170	24	16	19	69	6	80
	196	134	43	83	87	85	43	28
	154	79	21	28	76	63	88	27
mean	291	102	39	43	64	63	45	40
SEM	54	21	12	19	11	12	12	9
p for t test	0.005 < 0.01		> 0.05		> 0.05		> 0.05	

Ca   squamous cell carcinoma biopsy

N-N   non-neoplastic matched biopsy   Ad 2   adenovirus type 2 DNA probe

HSV-2   Herpes simplex virus type 2 DNA probe   M.lys   Micrococcus leisodeiticus DNA probe

bacteriophage lambda DNA probe

background-corrected grain counts of squamous cell carcinoma and non-neoplastic samples for the 5 cases we have examined using HSV-2, adenovirus type 2, lambda and <u>Micrococcus lysodeikticus</u> DNAs as probes. In all five cases the neoplastic region produced higher grain counts with the HSV-2 DNA probes than any other combination. For 4 out of 5 of the cases this is equal to at least twice the value found in the non-neoplastic matched region or with any of the other probes. This is a small number of cases but it confirms and extends the findings previously made with 29 matched punch biopsies from CIN cases. We have had some difficulty in obtaining squamous cell carcinoma cases where a clearly non-neoplastic region of the cervix could be identified.

Reactivation of HSV from Explanted Utersacral Ligaments

HSV was isolated in BHK cells following reactivation from explanted uterosacral ligaments cultured for 14 days. The DNA of the viruses isolated was typed by restriction enzyme analysis with the results shown in Table 3. Two points should be noted, first the much higher number (5 out of 10 attempts) of successful reactivations from the uterosacral ligaments of squamous cell carcinoma patients and second, that in one of the five cases the virus isolated was HSV type 1. No virus was isolated from explants of cervical epithelium of these patients, or from swabs of ectocervix. When 5 additional uterosacral ligaments were sonicated and individually plated onto indicator cells on the day of collection no virus was recovered.

Our success in isolating virus from explanted uterosacral ligaments caused us to look for typical nerve cells in these structures. Portions of uterosacral ligaments approximately 3 cm long and proximal to the uterus were obtained at hysterectomies. Serial 20 micron sections have disclosed the presence of a typical small ganglion through eight successive sections in one of three such ligaments examined so far (Fig. 1).

Detection of HSV-Specific RNA Transcripts Using Cloned Segments of the HSV-2 Genome as Probes

The genome of HSV-2 comprises a long unique sequence (U_L15.5kbp) each flanked by inverted repeated regions (TR_L/IR_L10 kbp; TR_S/IR_S6 kbp) joined at IR_L-IR_S(Fig. 2). Approximately equal amounts of the four genome arrangements, arrising from all possible combinations of inversions of the two unique regions, are normally found in DNA preparations. As a result, certain cloned fragments contain sequences that identify more than one region of the genome, i.e. clones pGz 1, 12, 64 and 65.

The differences in mean grain counts (background-corrected) between CIN and matched non-neoplastic cervical epithelium, or squamous cell carcinoma and non-neoplastic cervical epithelium controls were analysed

TABLE 3

Isolation of HSV following reaction from uterosacral ligaments

Pathology of Cervix	No. of Isolates		No. of Uterosacral ligaments screened
	HSV-1	HSV-2	
C.I.N.	0	0	2
Squamous cell carcinoma	1	4	10
Non-neoplastic	0	1	11

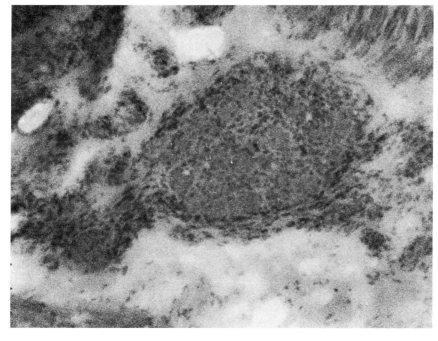

FIGURE 1

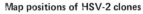

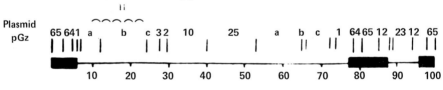

Map positions of HSV-2 clones

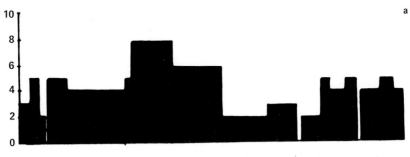

Matched paired C.I.N.

C.I.N. versus mean non-neoplastic cervical epithelium

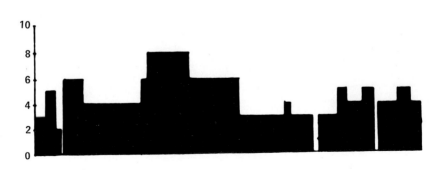

Squamous cell carcinoma versus mean non-neoplastic cervical epithelium

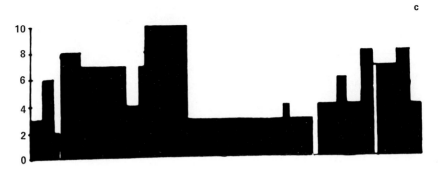

FIGURE 2

statistically for each nucleic acid probe used and are shown in Table 4. In the case of the non-neoplastic samples the actual background-corrected count is given in the table; while the values shown for the neoplastic biopsies are the differences between the matched CIN and non-neoplastic background corrected means or squamous cell carcinoma and non-neoplastic background corrected means. Statistically significant elevated grain counts were obtained for the CIN group after in situ hybridisation with clones pGz 11a, 32, 10 and 25 which cover map units 0.07 - 0.11 and 0.27 - 0.52 of the HSV-2 genome. The squamous cell carcinoma group showed significantly higher grain counts after in situ hybridisation with clones pGz 11a, 11b, 32, 10 and 12 which cover map units 0.07 - 0.21, 0.27 - 0.40, 0.84 - 0.87 and 0.93 - 0.99; but since pGz 65 did not hybridise significantly to the squamous cell carcinoma group, the significantly transcribed region should be considered to lie within limits 0.07 - 0.21, 0.27 - 0.40, 0.85 - 0.87 and 0.93 - 0.98.

It is reassuring, that the hybridisations against whole HSV-2 DNA in both cases give statistically significant elevated grain counts, while the lambda DNA or no DNA controls disclose no differences (Table 4).

Due to the difficulty in obtaining matched non-neoplastic cervical epithelial tissue for each squamous cell carcinoma biopsy, we have had to use the mean non-neoplastic results to evaluate the squamous cell carcinoma grain counts. To show that this can be justified, the CIN mean grain count differences have been plotted both as individually matched results (Fig. 2a) and as individual cases compared with the mean values for the non-neoplastic biopsies (Fig. 2b). As can be seen from the comparison of Fig. 2a and 2b, the plots were reassuringly similar.

For each neoplastic tissue group the number of individual samples which contain significantly detectable amounts of HSV-specific RNA varied across the genome (Fig. 2a, b, c). Both in CIN and squamous cell carcinoma at least two neoplastic samples showed significant graining (outside the 5% confidence limit for the non-neoplastic sample) with every clone used. No single biopsy gave significant graining when hybridised with each cloned probe. For the region map units 29 - 40, 8 out of 10 CIN cases and 10 out of 10 squamous cell carcinoma cases disclosed significantly elevated grain counts.

It is clear that RNA transcripts able to hybridise against different regions of the HSV-2 genome occur with very different frequencies in the tissue samples from different individual cases; at the same time the general frequency distribution seems to be rather similar in the CIN and squamous cell carcinoma cases.

TABLE 4

Background-corrected mean grain counts + SEM per standard area for tissue sections after in situ hybridisation with cloned fragments of HSV-2 DNA. There are 10 different biopsies in each tissue group.

CLONE (pGz)	11a	11b	11c	32	10	25	26a	261b	26c	1	64	65	23	12	HSV-2		No Probe DNA
Map co-ordinates	7-11	11-21	21-27	27-29	29-40	40-52	52-64	64-65	65-72	74-78 5-6	78-81 2-5	81-85 0-2 98-100	88-93	93-99 84-87	0-100		
$\bar{x}$	189	175	211	145	209	269	292	154	161	165	136	157	114	153	117	57	41
Nn																	
SEM	±20	±31	±34	±30	±30	±28	±29	±14	±18	±18	±28	±28	±28	±23	±22	±8	±7
$\bar{x}$CIN−$\bar{x}$Nn	67	0	15	44	138	143	41	40	27	35	64	20	56	53	210	10	−5
p for t test	.05-.01	.05-.01		.05-.01	.05-.01	.05-.01									<.001		
$\bar{x}$SCC−$\bar{x}$Nn	94	78	20	112	179	20		9	−14	4	86	21	96	111	134	1	−9
p for t test	.05-.01	.05-.01		.05-.01	<.001										<.001		

CIN   cervical intraepithelial neoplasia

SCC   squamous cell carcinoma

Nn   non-neoplastic cervical epithelium

DISCUSSION

In our previous studies (Eglin et al., 1981) we obtained internally consistent data from 43 CIN cases - 11 CIN I, 16 CIN II, 16 CIN III- suggesting a strong association (72%) between the detectable presence of transcripts able to hybridise against HSV-2 DNA and CIN. This association was further confirmed by data from 29 matched paired CIN biopsies. In 35 cases of squamous cell carcinoma (SCC) a strong association (60%) could similarly be discerned. Again the data were internally consistent when broken down into 5 SCC 1, 18 SCC 2, 10 SCC 3, 2 SCC 4. We have confirmed and extended these findings by the 5 matched paired cases of squamous cell carcinoma reported in Table 2. It is unfortunately very difficult to obtain matched paired cases for squamous cell carcinoma because at that stage very few clearly non-neoplastic regions of cervical epithelium remain. In fact, closer examination of the data of Table 2 discloses that in three of the five cases there is evidence of some elevation of grain counts following in situ hybridisation of HSV-2 DNA to the matched non-neoplastic cervical epithelium; this suggests the possible presence in the non-neoplastic sample of a small number of visually undetected cancer cells. When checked against the adenovirus type 2 DNA and lambda DNA probes, neither the squamous cell carcinoma nor the non-neoplastic sections showed any evidence of specific hybridisation.

The observations and conclusions concerning the association between HSV-2 and squamous cell carcinoma of the cervix are supported by our preliminary findings with explanted pieces of uterosacral ligaments: in 5 out of 10 cases of squamous cell carcinoma explantation resulted in reactivation and subsequent isolation of infectious HSV. It is of considerable interest that in one case this was HSV-1 and in four cases HSV-2, identified by restriction enzyme analysis performed on the isolated DNAs. As on previous occasions when comparing restriction enzyme fragment profiles from fresh isolates, each isolate could be distinguished. HSV was isolated from only one of eleven uterosacral ligament explants from non-neoplastic cervix controls. Again this could be identified as HSV-2. We failed to isolate infectious HSV from the uterosacral ligaments of two CIN patients. Clearly a more extensive series of uterosacral ligament explants is desirable so as to obtain a better assessment of the prevailing situation. A ganglion-like structure has been identified in one of three uterosacral ligament pieces which have been sectioned. It should perhaps be stressed that we only obtained a 3 cm long cut piece of uterosacral ligament with the hysterectomy specimen. It is tempting to speculate that the reactivated HSV isolated from the explanted uterosacral ligaments was present latent in ganglion-like structures. However, more extensive data are needed before this inference can be accepted.

The cloned fragments of HSV-2 DNA which we have used cover 96% of the HSV-2 genome and it is of interest that transcripts hybridising to all of them were found in at least 2 out of 10 CIN and 2 out of 10 squamous cell carcinoma cases. No two individual neoplastic biopsies produced identical patterns of significant graining with all probes.

Our limited data indicate that some regions, e.g. map co-ordinates 0.29 - 0.40, are transcribed in the great majority if not all cases, whereas others, e.g. map co-ordinates 0.52 - 0.64 are only detected as transcribed in fewer than a third of the examined cases. In general, the distribution of transcripts does not seem to differ between CIN and squamous cell carcinoma, except possibly in the region map co-ordinates 0.40 - 0.52 which seems more frequently transcribed in CIN. Additional data are needed before firm conclusions concerning the comparative distribution of transcripts in CIN and squamous cell carcinoma can be made. It should, however, be noted that the HSV-2 morphological transforming region, map co-ordinates 0.58 - 0.62 (Reyes et al., 1979) 0.51 - 0.62 (Cameron and Macnab, 1980), is clearly not transcribed in such amounts as to be regularly detectable by the used method of in situ hybridisation.

There appears to be some discrepancy between the preliminary results not given in detail but quoted by McDougall et al., 1980, who found hybridisation only at map co-ordinates 0.07 - 0.32 and the results reported here.

Other workers have reported immunological studies which indicate that certain HSV-2 specific antigens are frequently expressed in cancer of the cervix cells. In particular, the report by Rawls et al., 1980, identified two polypeptides of molecular weight 38,000 and 118,000 which map at co-ordinates 0.56 - 0.61 and at 0.35 respectively. Dreesman et al., 1980 report the consistent presence of the polypeptide ICSP 11/12 which maps left of co-ordinate 0.40 (K. Powell, pers. comm.).

The here reported frequent in situ hybridisation to transcripts involving morphological transforming region 1 (map co-ordinates 0.29 - 0.40) in comparison with much rarer positive hybridisation with transcripts from morphological transforming region 2 (map co-ordinates 0.58 - 0.62) may reflect differences in the level of transcription or in stability of transcripts from these regions. These and other possible explanations will have to be further investigated. It is noteworthy that transcripts hybridising to the short terminal repeat which codes for the 175K immediate early polypeptide are frequently observed. The 175K polypeptide has been implicated as essential for the switch from immediate early transcription (Preston, 1979) and its continuous function is known to be necessary for the production of early and late mRNAs (Watson and Clements, 1980).

ACKNOWLEDGEMENTS

We wish to thank Dr. J.W. Cordiner of the Department of Midwifery and Mr. J. Monaghan of the Department of Gynaecological Oncology, Queen Elizabeth Hospital, Gateshead for the provision of tissue biopsies; Dr. R. Denham of the Department of Pathology for histopathological diagnosis; and Professor W.F. Lee of the Department of Ophthalmology for kindly allowing us to make use of his Optomax Video Image Analyser. We also thank Professor C.R. Whitfield of the Department of Midwifery for his continued support and interest. It is also a pleasure to acknowledge the excellent technical assistance provided by Mr. D.P. McNab and Mr. R.C. Stevenson. This work was supported by Grant number SP 1341/1 from the Cancer Research Campaign.

REFERENCES

Adam, E., Kaufman, R.H., Melnick, J.L., Levy, A.H. and Rawls, W.E. (1973). Am. J. Epidemiol., 98, 77–83.

Baringer, J.R. (1974). N. Engl. J. Med., 291, 828 – 830.

Bastian, F.O., Rabson, A.S., Yee, C.L. and Tralka, T. (1972). Science, 178, 305 – 307.

Cameron, I.R. and Macnab, J.M.C. (1980). In: The Human Herpesviruses p. 634. Eds. A.J. Nahmias, W.R. Dowdle and R.F. Schinazi. Elsevier, New York.

Dreesman, G.R., Burek, J., Adam, E., Kaufman, R.H., Melnick, J.L., Powell, K.L. and Purifoy, D.J. (1980). Nature (London), 283, 591 – 593.

Eglin, R.P., Sharp, F., MacLean, A.B., Macnab, J.C.M., Clements, J.B. and Wilkie, N.M. (1981). Cancer Research, 41, in press.

Lonsdale, D.M., Brown, S.M., Subak-Sharpe, J.H., Warren, K.G. and Koprowski, H. (1979). J. gen. Virol., 43, 151 – 171.

Lonsdale, D.M., Brown, S.M., Lang, J., Subak-Sharpe, J.H., Koprowski, H. and Warren, K.G. (1980). Annals. N.Y. Acad. Sci., 354, 291 – 308.

McDougall, J.K., Galloway, D.A. and Fenoglio, C.M. (1980). Int. J. Cancer, 25, 1 – 9.

Nahmias, A.J., Del Buono, I. and Ibrahim, I. (1975). In: Oncogenesis and Herpesviruses II, p. 309 – 311. Eds. G. de The, M.A. Epstein and H. zur Hausen. I.A.R.C., Lyon, France.

Nahmias, A.J. and Roizman, B. (1973). N. Engl. J. Med., 289, 667 – 671.

Niab, Z.M., Nahmias, A.J. and Jozey, W.E. (1966). Cancer, 19, 1026 – 1031.

Pasca, A.S., Kummerlander, L., Pejtsik, B. and Pali, L. (1975). J. Natl. Cancer Inst., 55, 775 - 781.

Preston C.M. (1979). J. Virol., 29, 275 - 284.

Price, R.W., Katz, B.J. and Notkins, A.L. (1975). Nature (London), 257, 686 - 687.

Rawls, W.E., Clarke, A., Smith, K.O., Docherty, J.J., Gilman, S.C. and Graham, S. (1980). In: Viruses in Naturally occurring Cancers, p. 117 - 133. Eds. M. Essen, E. Todaro and H. zur Hausen. Cold Spring Harbor Laboratories, New York.

Rawls, W.E., Tomkins, W.A.F. and Melnick, J.L. (1969). Am. J. Epidemiol., 89, 547 - 552.

Reyes, G.R., La Femina, R., Hayward, S.D. and Hayward, G.S. (1979). Cold Spring Harbor Symp. Quant. Biol., 44, 629 - 641.

Scriba, M. (1975). Infect. Immun., 12, 162 - 168.

Skinner, G.R.B., Whitney, J.E. and Hartley, C. (1977). Arch. Virol., 54, 211 - 221.

Stevens, J.G. and Cook, M.L. (1971). Science, 173, 843 - 846.

Stevens, J.G., Nesburn, A.B. and Cook, M.L. (1972). Nature (London), New Biol., 235, 216 - 217.

Thomas, D.B. and Rawls, W.E. (1978). Cancer, 42, 2716 - 2725.

Tobin, S.M., Wilson, W.D., Fish, E.N. and Papsin, F.R. (1978). Obstet. and Gynaecol., 51, 707 - 712.

Twigg, A.J. and Sherratt, D.J. (1980). Nature (London), 283, 216 - 218.

Warren, K.G., Brown, S.M., Wroblewska, Z., Gilden, D., Koprowski, H. and Subak-Sharpe, J.H. (1978). N. Engl. J. Med., 298, 1068 - 1069.

Watson, R.J. and Clements, J.B. (1980). Nature (London), 285, 329 - 331.

Expression of Differentiated Functions in Cancer Cells, edited by R. F. Revoltella et al., Raven Press, New York © 1982.

Transcription of Virus-Specific Sequences in Moloney Sarcoma Virus Infected Cells

Dino Dina

Department of Genetics, Albert Einstein College of Medicine, Bronx, New York 10461

Origin of the Transforming Sequences of Retroviruses

Several different mammalian and avian retroviruses induce acute leukemias and sarcomas in susceptible animals (1). Most of these viruses also induce neoplastic transformation of target cells in culture (1). With the exception of avian sarcoma virus (ASV) all transforming retroviruses are replication-defective and need a competent helper virus to be propagated (1). Biochemical and genetic analysis of their genomes has led to the conclusion that they all carry specific sequences which code for a transforming protein. The transforming genes of different oncogenic viruses vary with respect to their length and position on the viral genome, and show little if any sequence homology. Normal uninfected cell DNA has been shown to contain sequences sharing extensive homology with the viral transforming sequences (5,9,10,11,13,15,17,18,19,21).

The expression of viral oncogenes is thought to be controlled by viral sequences present on the long terminal repeat (LTR) present at either end of the proviral DNA. The structure of mRNA molecules coding for the transforming gene product has been found to vary in different viruses and is usually dependent on the position occupied by the tranforming gene on the viral DNA. In Harvey and Kirsten Sarcoma viruses the "onc" sequences are located next to the LTR and are apparently translated directly from the viral genomic RNA into p21, the polypeptide they encode. Differently, a number of acute leukemia and sarcoma viruses code for a fusion protein carrying covalently linked gag-onc sequences. These fusion proteins are also translated from genome size viral mRNA molecules. Finally, a third category of acute leukemia and sarcoma viruses expresses onc sequences which are located distally from the LTR by means of subgenomic-length spliced mRNAs containing a leader sequence which overlaps with the 5' terminus of the genomic viral RNA and is covalently linked to the onc sequences. Moloney murine sarcoma virus (MSV), a replication defective virus capable of transforming fibroblasts and myoblasts in vitro, appears to belong to this third group of viruses. The transforming (v-mos) gene of MSV is located near the 3' terminus of the viral RNA and its nucleotide sequence has been recently determined (16,22 and E. Benz, J. Hurwitz and D. Dina, unpublished observations). These sequence data support the notion that a polypeptide of MW 30-40 K may be encoded by this portion of the MSV genome. In this study we report the results of sequencing experiments and the mapping of virus-specific mRNAs. Our data strongly suggest that the transforming activity of the v-mos gene may be encoded by the 3' proximal 900 nucleotides of this region. This information is present on a spliced mRNA of about 2,000 nucleotides in length containing sequences from the 5' terminus of the MSV genome (U$_5$ region) linked to v-mos and sequences from the 3' terminus (U$_3$ region). The implications of these findings are discussed.

MATERIALS AND METHODS

Cells and viruses

The origin and culture conditions for NIH 3T3 (5), NRK (14) and thymus-bone marrow cells infected with Moloney sarcoma virus 124 (TBMSV 124) (14) and Balb 3T3 (5) have all been described. Moloney MSV 124 and Moloney MuLV Cl 1 have also been described earlier (5). Cloning of individual transformed cells was performed early after infection with virus by plating in DME-methylcellulose. Individual colonies were picked and grown up in microtiter wells two to three weeks after plating.

Analysis of intracellular virus specific mRNAs.

The procedures for the preparation of cell polysomal RNA, total RNA and DNA have been described elsewhere (5). After extraction the polyA+ RNA was selected by oligo dT cellulose chromatography and fractionated on methylmercury hydroxide denaturing agarose gels. After electrophoresis the gels were blotted directly onto nitrocellulose filters (20) and the blots were processed for hybridization. Details of hybridization to individual probes are given in the figure legends.

Preparation of labeled DNA reagents

All v-mos fragments were prepared by cleavage of a recombinant plasmid, p101 and its subclones with appropriate restriction enzymes. Representative v-mos probes were obtained by cleavage of p101 with Xba + Hind III (see Fig. 2b). The v-mos fragment, 1160 bp, is the shortest of those generated by these enzymes and was shown to be free of contaminating DNA after polyacrylamide gel purification. Mos-1 probes were derived from the largest Pst I-Pst I v-mos fragment as described elsewhere (Gattoni et al., in press).

U5 and U3 probes were derived from plasmid p600 (2). The recombinant plasmid was cleaved with Pst I + Sac I + Kpn I. U$_3$ sequences are present on a fragment ~ 400 bp long while U$_5$ sequences are on a ~ 100 bp fragment. All fragments were routinely purified on 5% polyacrylamide gels, electroeluted and labeled with reverse transcriptase and calf thymus DNA primers.

RESULTS

Selection of MSV infected cell clones and their characterization

Recent experiments performed in our laboratory supported the notion that the synthesis of active v-mos mRNA(s) was dependent on a splicing event joining 5' leader sequences to the v-mos region of the genome. However, subgenomic length virus specific mRNA with a variety of structures may be generated either by splicing or by deletions of the proviral DNA template. It seemed therefore important to isolate a series of MSV infected cell clones and characterize the integrated MSV proviruses to detect the presence of abnormal deleted or rearranged genomes. Balb 3T3 cells were infected with freshly harvested (3 hr) MSV (MLV) virus. One day after infection the cells were plated in methylcellulose to select for transformed clones and to prevent superinfection by newly synthesized MSV (MLV) virions. A number of large colonies were picked and grown in microtiter wells. Cells were expanded and their DNA was analyzed for the presence of integrated MSV proviruses. Since uninfected cells contain a large number of endogenous sequences which cross hybridize to the whole MSV genome a v-mos DNA fragment was utilized in this analysis. This fragment recognized a unique c-mos DNA locus which is present in uninfected cells from all vertebrate species so far examined (10,13,21,15). After cleavage with SacI, which releases a 5.4 kb fragment carrying 90% of the MSV genome, two major bands were observed in most clones: a 7.0 kb band representing the cellular c-mos sequences and the 5.4 kb viral genomic sequences completely separated from adjacent cellular sequences (Fig. 1). As shown in the 3B8 lane, the presence of extra bands of a length different from the 5.4 kb unit readily reveals the existence of abnormal MSV genomes. With the exception of clone 3B8 which was not used for transcriptional studies, all other clones were estimated to carry 1-5 integral copies of MSV and no smaller deleted genomes. The faint band at 2 kb is a c-mos cross-hybridizing cellular sequence found also in uninfected 3T3 cells (13). All clones obtained in these experiments contained multiple integrated genomes, a feature which cannot be readily explained.

Structure of spliced v-mos RNAs

As mentioned in the introduction, the transforming gene of Moloney MSV has been mapped rather accurately by a combination of biochemical and genetic techniques (3,4). Moreover, nucleotide sequencing data (16,22) have located the area in which the mos sequences are positioned between the Xba I and Hind III restriction sites (see Fig. 2b).

Genetic information downstream from the gag sequences can be expressed either in the form of a polyprotein or as a separate protein translated from a spliced mRNA. Alternatively it can be translated from transcripts originating at specific promoter sites adjacent to the transforming gene (C. Van Beveren, pers. comm.). The leader sequences of several retroviral mRNAs have been characterized by molecular hybridization, nucleotide seuqencing (J.M. Bishop and W.S. Hayward,

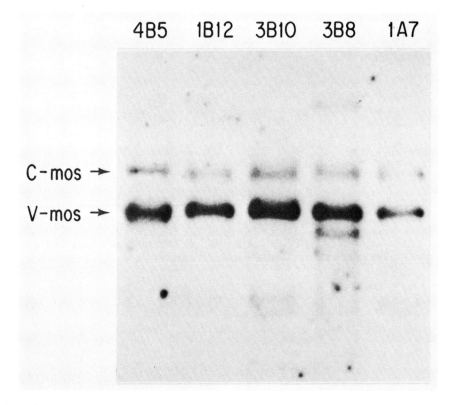

FIG. 1: Characterization of integrated MSV genomes.

DNA was prepared from a series of MSV infected Balb 3T3 cell clones termed 1A7, 3B8, 3B10, 1B12 and 3B5. Each DNA sample (20 μg) was digested with restriction endonuclease Sac I and electrophoresed on a 1% agarose gel. The DNA was transferred onto a nitrocellulose filter and the blot was hybridized to ^{32}P labelled mos-1 DNA. Bands identified as the endogenous cellular mos sequences (c-mos) and the MSV proviral DNA sequences (v-mos) are marked.

personal communication) and electron microscopy (8) and have been shown to be a few hundred nucleotides long. We have demonstrated that MSV-infected producer and non-producer cells synthesize a spliced subgenomic RNA species containing v-mos information (6). The notion that the MSV transforming gene is expressed through the synthesis of a spliced mRNA is in agreement with the fact that MSV RNA does not code for a transformation related polyprotein translated directly from genomic vRNA like other sarcoma viruses (1). Interestingly, we found that similar v-mos subgenomic spliced mRNAs were efficiently packaged into MSV virions, together with larger proportions of heterogenous

vRNAs. The presence of these mRNAs in the 70S complex of mature MSV
virions is possibly due to the fact that they carry a leader sequence
containing genetic information important in the packaging of the viral
RNAs.

Fig. 2a shows schematically the basic structure of a putative
v-mos RNA suggested by previous hybridization (6) and electron
microscope (8) mapping experiments. The dotted line represents the
fact that the exact splice junction sites of the v-mos mRNA(s) could
not be derived from the published information. Fig. 2b shows an
expanded map of the v-mos region and the 3' terminus of MSV. According
to published nucleotide sequences of this area three putative AUG start
codons may be present on a v-mos mRNA and direct the synthesis of
polypeptides terminating either before the Hind III site (22) or beyond
the the Hind III site (16). These data indicate that all three ATGs
are followed by an open reading frame through the entire v-mos region.
According to our sequencing data in clone p101 (Benz, Hurwitz and Dina,
unpublished observations) ATG #1 is in the second reading frame and
leads to early termination. ATG #2 and #3 are instead in the third
reading frame which does code for the same putative polypeptide
described by van Beveren et al (22). The only difference between
polypeptides starting at any of the 3 ATGs is obviously in the size of
the synthesized proteins. A polypeptide starting at ATG#2 would be 31
amino acids shorter than one starting at ATG#1 while a polypeptide
starting at ATG#3 would be missing 97 amino acids.

Analysis of intracellular mos-specific mRNAs

To confirm and extend earlier results obtained with cytoplasmic
poly(A)+ RNA from producer and non-producer MSV infected fibroblasts
(6) we prepared polysomal polyA+ mRNA from MSV-infected line 1B12. The
RNA was run on denaturing agarose gels, blotted and hyridized to
various labeled DNAs. Since hybridization patterns obtained with
MSV-infected cell RNA have been consistently very poor, we first tested
our RNA preparations for possible degradation. One lane of the blot,
containing 1B12 polysomal RNA was hybridized to a labelled cDNA clone
representing an abundant "house-keeping" mRNA normally expressed in
rodent fibroblasts. The translation product of this mRNA is unknown,
but its size has been found to be 20S in all cells examined (L.
Garfinkel and B. Nadal-Ginard, unpublished observations). Since we had
indications that the size of the v-mos mRNA should be similar this
seemed like an appropriate control for possible degradations occurring
either in the MSV transformed cells or during extraction. As shown in
Fig. 3 a unique 20S RNA band with no apparent degradation products is
visualized by the recombinant DNA probe. When a parallel (last lane,
labeled "C") nitrocellulose strip was hybridized to labelled mos-1 DNA,
three major species were visualized: a 30S RNA, (presumably the MSV
genome) a 28S RNA of unknown function and a 20S RNA, analogous to the
previously described v-mos mRNA (Fig. 3). The same RNA species were
observed with the 5' probe confirming earlier results obtained with
total cytoplasmic RNAs (6). Analogous patterns were obtained with all
the MSV infected mouse cell lines tested (not shown, see Fig. 1 for DNA
restriction patterns).

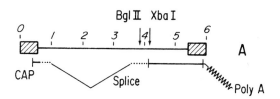

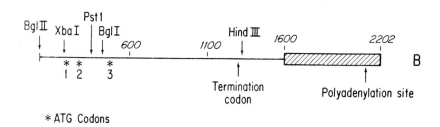

FIG. 2: A schematic representation of the spliced v-mos mRNA(s).

A. The upper line represents the MSV DNA template with LTRs (hatched regions). the v-mos mRNA 5' terminus is represented by the CAP. The dotted lines represent the undetermined portions of spliced leader and mRNA sequences.

B. Expanded map of the v-mos region and 3' terminus of MSV. The three putative AUG start codons potentially present on the v-mos mRNA(s) are shown on the map. Their position is based on the available nucleotide sequence information. It should be noted that while in the two published sequences all three ATGs are followed by an open reading frame through the whole v-mos region, in the p101 sequence ATG #1 is in the second readig frame and leads to early termination. ATG #2 and #3 are in the third reading frame which codes for nearly the same putative polypeptide described by Van Beveren et al (22). The only difference is obviously in the size of the polypeptides which would be about 30 amino acids smaller if started at ATG #2 and 97 amino acids smaller if started at ATG #3.

Characterization of total polyA+ MSV specific RNA.

Messenger RNA present on the cell polyribosomes is presumed to be active in protein synthesis and should therefore contain virus-specific mRNA species coding for the transforming gene product. To verify whether all virus-specific mRNAs synthesized in the cell were actually represented in the polyribosomal fraction, we conducted gel

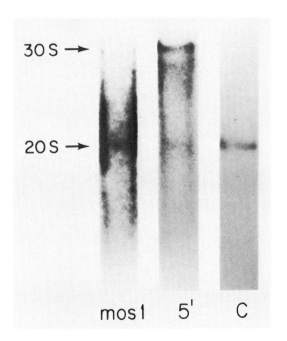

FIG. 3: Mapping of polysomal RNA from MSV infected cells.

    RNA was extracted from a crude polysomal pellet obtained from cell
clone 1B12. The polyA+ fraction was run on agarose gels and blotted
onto nitrocellulose filters. Two parallel filters were hybridized to
pMSV-5 and pmos-1. A third filter was hybridized to a control plasmid
carrying a cDNA sequence from an unidentified house-keeping gene.

fractionation/hybridization experiments with total cellular polyA+ RNA
from the same set of cells used to prepare virus-specific polysomal
mRNA. As shown in Fig. 4 the pattern obtained with total MSV infected
cell RNA is much more complicated than that displayed by polysomal
mRNA. By using a mos-1 probe (first lane), 5 distinct polyA containing
RNAs were detected. Their approximate size was calculated to be 5,400
nucleotides for the 30S species, 4,800 nucleotides for the 28S species,
3,000 nucleotides for the 24S species, 2,500 nucleotides for the 22S
species and 2,100 nucleotides for the 20S species. Hybridization to
p-MSV 5 DNA, which represents the 5' terminus of the vRNA and should
detect only subgenomic length RNAs which are spliced, revealed all the
major RNA molecules except for the 22S RNA. Therefore the only spliced
mRNA transcribed exclusively from the v-mos region is the 20S molecule.
To map the 5' end of this RNA more closely, the same RNA blot was
hybridized to a DNA fragment (Xba-PstI, Fig. 2b) which contains ATG #1
and #2. The 20S mRNA was not detected by this probe, while all other

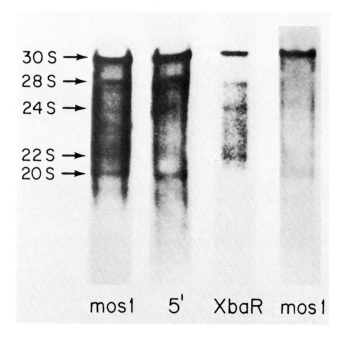

FIG. 4: Mapping of total virus-specific cellular RNAs in MSV
          infected cells.

PolyA+ RNA was prepared from cell lines containing multiple intact
MSV genomes. The RNA was run on a 1.5% agarose gel containing 10 mM
methylmercury hydroxide in parallel lanes. After blotting onto
nitrocellulose, individual lanes were hybridized to pMSV-5, pmos-1 and
Xba-Pst1 lableled DNA fragments (Fig. 2b). After autoradiography the
filter from the Xba-Pst I hybridization experiment was washed for 30
minutes at 80°C in 50% formamide, checked for residual radioactivity
and rehybridized to labeled pmos-1 DNA. The resulting autoradiogram is
shown to the right of the Xba-Pst I lane.

larger RNAs hybridized efficiently. To confirm this result, the same
blot was washed and rehybridized to a mos-1 probe which again detected
all the RNA species, including the 20S. In a recent experiment, not
shown in Fig. 2, we have hybridized a similar blot to a probe spanning
the Xba I to Bgl I region (Fig. 2b). This probe detected the 20S RNA,
indicating that the splice junction between the 5' leader and the v-mos
region must occur somewhere to the right of the PstI site. These data
clearly exclude the possibility that ATG #1 and #2 could be the
initiation codons for a v-mos gene product translated from the spliced
20S mRNA.

Further characterization of transcripts by electron
microscopy of RNA.DNA hybrids

The existence of spliced mRNA molecules in the cytoplasm of MSV
infected cells and the size of such mRNA was further investigated by
electron microscopic techniques.   In these experiments mRNA molecules
are annealed to single stranded DNA molecules synthesized in the
presence of actinomycin D (7) which are complementary to the entire MSV
RNA genome.   This cDNA represents the whole viral genome except that
the strong stop sequence (R + U5) is circularly permuted and located at
its 5' terminus.

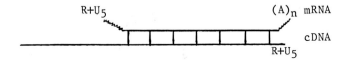

Hybrids obtained with spliced RNA should have the structure shown
above.   When the 5' terminus of the mRNA hybridizes to the 5' terminus
of the cDNA, structures as those shown in Fig. 5a and 5b will be seen.
Measurement of a large series of panhandles obtained both with viral
RNA and mRNA indicates that two main species of spliced RNA can be
detected.   One covers about 1/2 of the genome and presumably
corresponds to the mRNA described by Donoghue et al (8) while the other
accounts for about 1/3 of the genome and should correspond to the 20S
molecules consistently detected by gel electrophoresis.   Since these
molecules could only be generated by molecular splicing of larger
transcripts, it is obvious that alternate processing pathways for vRNA
must exist.   Additional panhandle species possibly representing other
minor components observed by gel electrophoresis, including the 28S RNA
molecules, were also observed in small numbers.

DISCUSSION

The existence of nucleotide sequences on the Moloney MSV genome
which are involved in the initiation and maintenance of malignant
transformation has been established by experiments involving cross
hybridization, DNA transfection and genetics.   Nucleotide sequencing
data show that the cell derived v-mos insert has the capacity to code
for a 40K polypeptide initiating at ATG #1 of Fig 2b.   This polypeptide
is presumed to be the product of the v-mos transforming gene (22).
According to our own v-mos sequence, derived from a biologically active
MSV recombinant DNA clone (p101), the first ATG in the sequence is not
followed by an open reading frame and may not be used to initiate a
v-mos polypeptide.   The second and third ATG are instead possible
initiator codons, since they are followed by a large open reading frame
allowing the synthesis of a 30-35K polypeptide.   To establish which
part of the v-mos sequence is actually used to code for the
transforming gene product we have mapped the v-mos mRNAs present in MSV
infected cells.   Only one major v-mos mRNA species of about 2,000

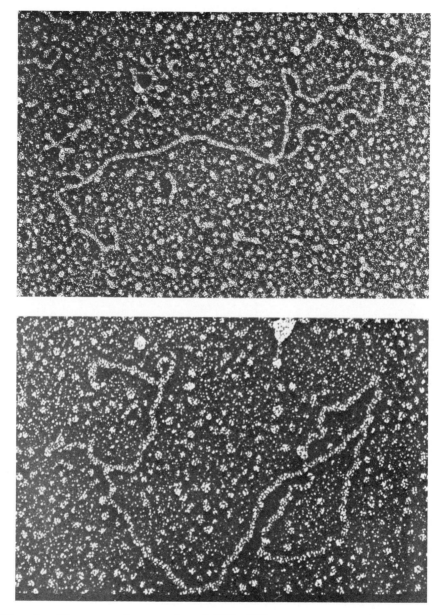

Fig. 5: Electron micrographs of MSV mRNA·MSV cDNA hybrids.

nucleotides in length has been detected on active polyribosomes. This mRNA has been mapped by hybridization to labeled cloned MSV DNA fragments and has been shown to carry only two thirds of the mos region, including ATG#3 but not ATG#1 and #2. This indicates that this part of the gene may be the one essential for the synthesis of the v-mos gene product. This result is particularly intriguing in view of recent reports about the extensive homology existing between the -COOH portions of three non-homologous transforming gene products , v-mos, v-src, and v-fes. According to these results, the portion of v-mos gene represented on the 20S RNA is the one which codes for the region of v-mos protein showing the highest level of similarity to pp60 src (22) and the putative polypeptide encoded by v-fes (C. Scherr, pers. comm.). These extensive similarities between the gene prodducts of different oncogenic retroviruses contradict the earlier notion, supported by cross-hybridization experiments, that all these oncogenes were quite different. Since recognizable similarities exist only among the polypeptides and no detectable homology is seen at the level of nucleotide sequence this constitutes a remarkable example of conservation of protein sequence with extensive drift in coding sequence.

ACKNOWLEDGEMENTS

We thank J. Pyati for her skillful technical assisitance and Drs. E. Benz and J. Hurwitz for their assistance in obtaining the nucleotide sequence of v-mos. This work was supported by NCI grant CA24223 and NSF grant PCM 7907594. D.D is the recipient of an ACS Junior Research Faculty Award.

REFERENCES

1. Recent experimental evidence on the structure of viral oncogenes is collected in: Cold Spring Harbor Symposia on Quantitative Biology, Viral Oncogenes, Volumne XLIV, 1979.

2. Benz, E.W., Wydro, R.M., Nadal-Ginard, B. and Dina, D. (1980): Nature

3. Canaani, E., Robbins, K.C. and Aaronson, S.A. (1979): Nature, 282: 378-383.

4. Dina, D. (1978): Proc. Natl. Acad. Sci. U.S.A., 75: 2694-2698.

5. Dina, D. and Penhoet, E.E. (1978): J. Virology, 27: 768-775.

6. Dina, D. and Nadal-Ginard, B. (1979): Cold Spring Harbor Symposia on Quantiative Biology, 44: 901-905.

7. Dina, D. and Benz, E.W., Jr. (1980): J. Virol., 33: 377-389.

8. Donoghue, D.J., Sharp, P.A. and Weinberg, R.A. (1979): <u>Cell,</u> 17:

9. Ellis, R.W., DeFeo, D., Maryak, J.M., Young, H.A., Shih, T.Y., Change, E.H., Lowy, D.R. and Scolnick, E.M. (1980): <u>J. Virol.,</u> 36: 408-420.

10. Frankel, A.E. and Fischinger, P.J. (1976): <u>Proc. Natl. Acad. Sci. U.S.A.,</u> 73: 3705-3709.

11. Goff, S.G., Gilboa, E., Witte, O.N., and D. Baltimore (1980): <u>Cell,</u> 22: 777-785.

12. Graiser, M., Soeller, W. and Dina, D. (1980): In: <u>Animal Viral Genetics.</u> ICN-UCLA Symposia on Molecular and Cell Biology, Vol. <u>XVIII,</u> eds. Fields, B. and Jaenish, R. (Academic Press). 18.

13. Jones, M., Bosselman, R.A., vande Horn, F.A., Bern, A., Fan, H. and Verma, I.M. (1980): <u>Proc. Natl. Acad. Sci. U.S.A.,</u> 77: 2651-2655.

14. Maisel, J., Dina, D. and Duesberg, P. (1977): <u>Virology,</u> 76: 295-312.

15. Oskarsson, M., McClements, W.L., Blair, D.G., Maizel, J.V. and Vande Woude, G.F. (1980): <u>Science,</u> 207: 1222-1224.

16. Reddy, E.P., Smith, M.J., Cananni, Robbins, K.C., Trocknick, S.R., Zains, and Aaronson, S.A. (1980): <u>Proc. Natl. Acad. Sci. U.S.A.,</u> 5234-5238.

17. Sheiness, D. and Bishop. J.M. (1979): <u>J. Virol.,</u> 31: 514-521.

18. Stehelin, D., Varmus, H.E., Bishop. J.M. and Bogt, P.K. (1976): <u>Nature,</u> 260: 170-173.

19. Stehelin, D., Saule, S., Roussel, M., Sergeant, A., Lagrou, C., Rommens, C. and Raes, M.B. (1979): <u>Cold Spring Harbor Symp. Quant. Biol.,</u> 44: 1215-1223.

20. Thomas, P.S. (1980): <u>Proc. Natl. Acad. Sci. U.S.A.,</u> 77: 5201-5205.

21. Tronick, S.R., Robbin, K.C., Canaani, E. Devarc, S.K., Anderson, P.R. and Aaronson, S.A. (1979): <u>Proc. Natl. Acad. Sci. U.S.A.</u> 76: 6314-6318.

22. Van Beveren, C., Galleshaw, J.A., Jones, M., Berns, A.J.M., Doolittle, R.F., Donaoghue, D.J. and Verma, I.M. (1981): <u>Nature,</u> 289: 258-262.

Expression of Differentiated Functions in Cancer Cells, edited by R. F. Revoltella et al., Raven Press, New York © 1982.

Preliminary Studies on BSB: A Virus Complex That Causes Erythroleukemia in C57BL Mice

Natalie M. Teich and Janice Rowe

Imperial Cancer Research Fund, Lincoln's Inn Fields, London WC2A 3PX, England

SUMMARY

BSB is a virus complex that causes erythroleukemia and polycythemia in C57BL strain mice. This situation contrasts dramatically to that observed with either the anemia or polycythemia variants of the Friend erythroleukemia virus complex (FV-A and FV-P, respectively). FV-A and FV-P cause erythroleukemia in adult mice of most mouse strains; however, adult mice of the C57BL strain are totally resistant to the changes in erythropoiesis and rapid tumor development, due mainly to the presence of the homozygous recessive allele $Fv-2^{rr}$. Because BSB induces a predominantly identical disease spectrum, independent of the $Fv-2$ gene effects, a comparative analysis of BSB to FV was initiated.

We have investigated the leukemogenicity of BSB virus in C57BL, (C57BL x DBA)F_1, and congenic (B10.D2) mice and have confirmed the results of Steeves et al. (30) that the host range of disease parallels FV-P with no $Fv-2^{rr}$ restriction.

We have also undertaken to separate the various components of the BSB virus complex by biological cloning techniques. The complexity of the BSB stock is greater than that observed with any other multi-component retrovirus complex. Because BSB does not induce foci of transformed cells in fibroblast cultures, the various infected cell clones have been classified into two main categories: virus producers and virus nonproducers. The evidence so far indicates that there are several distinct replication competent viruses which fall into numerous phenotypic classes based on the numbers and molecular weights of virus envelope (env) gene proteins synthesized in infected cells. In addition, we have identified at least three distinct nonproducer clone classes; it is not yet clear if these represent defective variants of the replication competent viruses or unique entities per se in the original BSB stock.

Neither the uncloned BSB stock nor any derivatives synthesize gp55, the env gene related glycoprotein considered the hallmark of the oncogenic component, spleen focus forming virus (SFFV), of FV stocks. In addition, a slight polycythemia rather than anemia is detected after infection of BALB/c neonatal mice, suggesting that the original Friend helper virus is no longer present. However, some of the clones synthesize env gene related proteins of 43,000 and 50,000 daltons (p43 and p50) and it is intriguing to speculate that these proteins could represent recombinant proteins important in the oncogenic activity, as is the case for the gp55 of SFFV. Preliminary analysis of the different clones for viral proteins and oncogenicity is described.

INTRODUCTION

In mice, RNA tumor viruses (retroviruses) cause a diverse spectrum of neoplasms including leukemias, sarcomas and carcinomas. Studies of murine viral-induced erythroleukemias began with the initial finding by Friend (7) that passage of an ascites tumor through mice eventually resulted in a new tumor type, originally identified as a reticulum cell sarcoma. Many of the later virus-induced tumors, however, were characterized as erythroleukemias. Virus recovered from these tumors caused anemia, hepatosplenomegaly and erythroleukemia in adult mice after a very short latency period. Further in vivo passage of the virus resulted in polycythemia rather than anemia (1, 21). The virus stocks became known as the anemia and polycythemia variant strains (FV-A and FV-P, respectively). It is now known that both FV-A and FV-P stocks contain at least two virus entities: a replication competent helper virus (Fr-MLV) and a replication defective virus which causes foci of erythroid cells in spleens of infected mice (the spleen focus forming virus, SFFV). As far as can be discerned by molecular analysis, the helper viruses in the two variant populations are essentially identical; this virus causes anemia and erythroblastosis in neonatally infected animals of certain mouse strains (e.g., NIH Swiss and BALB/c) (24, 32). On the other hand, the SFFV components, although somewhat related, are not identical biologically or molecularly and are therefore named SFFV-A and SFFV-P to distinguish them. Pseudotypes of these defective components with other helper viruses, prepared by biological or molecular cloning techniques, induce the full "Friend disease" spectrum in adult mice (6, 20); thus, classical Friend erythroleukemia is due to SFFV and not the helper viruses.

Friend disease in adult mice is influenced by a number of genetic loci, including Fv-1, Fv-2, H-2, Sl, W, f, Rgv-3, and Fv-4. However, most important to the issue described in this paper is the Fv-2 locus. This locus has two alleles, Fv-2^S and Fv-2^r, which determine susceptibility or resistance to Friend disease, respectively (18, 23). The resistance allele is recessive; thus Fv-2^{rs} mice (as, for example, in F$_1$ hybrid mice) are sensitive to disease, albeit with a somewhat decreased frequency and severity. The C57BL strain and a few other related mice contain the resistance allele in a homozygous state and adult mice are absolutely resistant to Friend virus disease. However, neonatal C57BL mice and adult C57BL mice experimentally made anemic (e.g., with phenylhydrazine treatment) become sensitive to some of the virus induced manifestations of Friend disease. The mechanism of action of Fv-2 is unknown, although it has no apparent effects on the replication of Fr-MLV.

One further important difference between SFFV-A and SFFV-P involves the nature of the induced erythropoietic defects. In SFFV-P infected mice, the erythroid progenitor cells, called CFU-E, differentiate in the absence of their normal physiological regulator, erythropoietin (Epo) (22). However, measurements of CFU-E from SFFV-A infected mice show that Epo dependence is maintained (6, 20).

At the molecular level, SFFV-A and SFFV-P are related but not identical. Their genomes contain deletions and/or defects affecting all three replicative genes of the virus: gag, pol and env. The gag gene encodes the structural proteins of the virion; pol encodes the RNA-dependent DNA polymerase (reverse transcriptase); and env encodes the envelope proteins (in the case of murine retroviruses, these are a 70,000 dalton glycoprotein, gp70, and a 15,000 dalton nonglycosylated protein, p15E). Nonproducer cells containing SFFV-A or SFFV-P genomes do not synthesize any of the mature pol or env proteins, although they may synthesize differing numbers and levels of gag polypeptides (2, 33). On the other hand, there is one protein specifically encoded by SFFV, a 55,000 dalton glycoprotein (gp55) (4, 26, 29), in all SFFV producer and nonproducer cell clones and by a molecularly cloned DNA copy of the SFFV genome (19). This env related protein is apparently the result of a recombinational event between the Fr-MLV helper virus env gene and the env gene of an endogenous xenotropic virus (34).

Thus, in discussing Friend disease in relation to expression and regulation of the Friend virus components, one encompasses the following salient features: (a) absolute control regulated by the Fv-2 locus; (b) anemia and polycythemia in adult mice attributable to SFFV-A and SFFV-P, respectively; (c) Epo independence vs. Epo dependence of CFU-E maturation in SFFV-P and SFFV-A, respectively, (d) expression of the SFFV encoded gp55, and (e) helper virus induced anemia in certain mouse strains.

BSB virus induces polycythemia, hepatosplenomegaly and erythroleukemia in many strains of mice, most importantly including C57BL. It was derived by Steeves and his colleagues (30) from numerous blind passages of an FV-P stock through Swiss and C57BL mice, eventually yielding a potent erythroleukemogenic virus for C57BL mice. Thus, it is independent of the restrictive actions of the $Fv-2^r$ locus. We considered that study of this virus in comparison to FV-A and FV-P might shed some light on the role of different viral genes in erythroleukemia induction and the way in which they interact with cellular genetic loci. To this end, we have cloned the virus in rat cells by low multiplicity infection and micromanipulative single cell cloning. The preliminary results indicate that there are a minimum of three distinct replication competent viruses and several potential replication defective viruses within the original BSB virus stock. In no case is the synthesis of SFFV gp55 detected; on the other hand, 43,000 and 50,000 dalton proteins precipitable with anti-env sera have been observed. A number of these producer and nonproducer clones containing the different BSB elements are described below.

MATERIALS AND METHODS

Cells and Viruses

NIH/3T3 mouse cells (12), 208F, a thioguanine resistant variant of Fischer strain Rat-1 cells (25), and mink cells (American Type Culture Collection, CCL64) were grown in Dulbecco's modified Eagle's medium (DMEM) supplemented with 10% heat-inactivated calf serum.

The polycythemia strain of Friend virus was chronically produced in the Friend erythroleukemia cell line F4N (15), kindly provided by W. Ostertag. A Graffi virus induced myeloid leukemia was kindly provided by B. Micheel. The original stocks of NB-tropic Moloney MLV and amphotropic MLV were kindly provided by J. Hartley. The original stock of BSB virus was kindly provided by R. Steeves.

Several assays were used to titrate infectious virus: the XC plaque assay (28), the reverse transcriptase assay (31), the spleen focus assay (1), and the fibroblast focus assay (8).

Mice

Newborn and adult mice of the C57BL/Icrf, B10.D2, DBA/2, (C57BL x DBA/2)F$_1$ (BDF$_1$) and BALB/c strains were bred in the ICRF specific pathogen free Animal Unit. We gratefully acknowledge the technical assistance of Ron Raymond of the Animal Unit.

Antisera and Gel Electrophoresis

Sera prepared against disrupted Rauscher murine leukemia virus, Rauscher virus gp70 and Rauscher virus p30 were kindly provided by the Office of Program

Resources and Logistics (National Cancer Institute, Bethesda, Maryland).

Cells were incubated for 1 hr at 37°C in the presence of 200 μCi/ml ^{35}S-methionine (600-1000 Ci/mM; Amersham) in DMEM lacking methionine. Cytoplasmic extracts were incubated with antiserum and precipitated with Staphylococcus aureus protein A (13). Sodium dodecyl sulfate polyacrylamide gel electrophoresis (SDS-PAGE) and fluorography were performed as described by others (3, 16, 36).

RESULTS

Analysis of Original BSB Virus Stock

The pathogenicity of the original BSB stock was assessed in several strains of newborn and adult mice, including DBA/2, B10.D2, BALB/c, BDF$_1$ and C57BL mice. In each case, 80-100% of the animals showed pathological conditions within 1-3 months. These symptoms included polycythemia (with hematocrits of up to 92% in adult mice), hepatic enlargement, splenomegaly (up to 4.5 grams), and mortality. As has already been reported by Steeves et al. (30), the number of spleen foci observed in BSB infected mice is extremely low, particularly in comparison to FV. Therefore, the probability of isolating the SFFV-like component by biological cloning in vitro presents a logistical problem.

The second step in the analysis of the BSB stock included a focus assay on mouse and rat fibroblasts; no foci were detected, even with the undiluted preparation. This finding rules out the possibility that BSB complex contains a classical murine sarcoma virus component capable of morphological transformation of fibroblasts. Unfortunately, it eliminates one of the major selective screening techniques used for isolating many replication defective virus components.

A new virus stock was prepared by infection of mouse NIH/3T3 cells. A high level of chronic virus production was attained. To determine the complexity of virus components within the system, preliminary characterization of virus related proteins in cell extracts was performed by SDS-PAGE. As shown in Figure 1, the number of proteins precipitated by specific viral antisera was markedly greater than those observed in NIH/3T3 cells infected with the Graffi strain of MLV or in Friend erythroleukemia cells chronically producing Fr-MLV and SFFV-P.

Based on this analysis and other gels, we have tentatively identified at least 6 high molecular weight env related proteins; these have been designated p86, p83 (which often is seen to migrate as a doublet), p70, p68, p50 and p43. Assuming that the BSB virus complex is analogous to other murine retroviruses, p86 and p83 most likely represent two distinct forms of the glycosylated env precursor polyprotein, gPr85^{env}, whereas p70 and p68 would be considered analogues of the mature structural envelope glycoprotein, gp70. Although the possibility arose that these could represent alternative forms of related proteins, for example due to differences in the extent of glycosylation, this possibility is ruled out by the segregation patterns, described below, following low multiplicity infection and selection of single cell clones. It should also be noted that there is no evidence for the synthesis of SFFV specific gp55. On the other hand, the two lower molecular weight env related proteins, p50 and p43, have not been described in analyses of other murine retroviruses. Breakdown products of MLV env proteins have been reported on occasion (14), but the data presented below suggest that these proteins are apparently unique to BSB and may represent products of a viral oncogene sequence. These findings emphasized the need to separate the multiple viral elements.

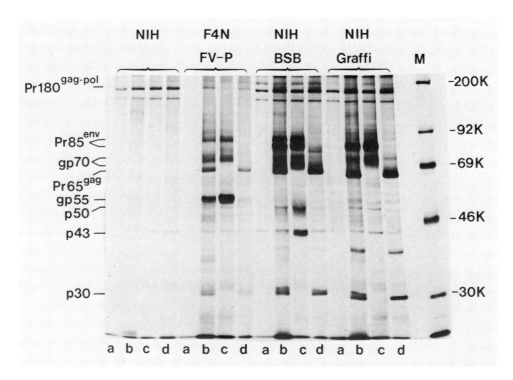

FIG. 1. Analysis of Virus Specific Proteins. Uninfected NIH/3T3 cells, F4N Friend erythroleukemia cells productively infected with FV-P, and NIH/3T3 cells productively infected with uncloned BSB or Graffi virus stocks were extracted, immunoprecipitated, and analyzed by SDS-PAGE. Antisera used for immuno-precipitation were: (a) normal goat serum, (b) goat anti-whole virus serum, (c) goat anti-virus gp70 serum, and (d) goat anti-virus p30 serum. Track M contains radiolabeled protein standards; the molecular weights are given in kilodaltons.

Isolation of Producer and Nonproducer Cell Clones

To isolate the various BSB viral components separately, a single harvest from chronically infected NIH/3T3 cells was titrated, diluted to give an inoculum of 0.5-1.0 PFU/cell and used to infect 208F rat cells. At 18 hours post-infection, the cells were trypsinized and diluted; single cells were then isolated with micro-pipettes and transferred to microwell plates. More than 70 clones were isolated in this fashion. As we had noted that anti-gp70 serum detected numerous proteins identifiable by SDS-PAGE in cells infected with the original BSB stock, we used this serum to screen the clones for apparent segregation of virus specific proteins. Figure 2 shows an analysis of a number of these clones and illustrates several of the segregation patterns.

As is clearly seen in this analysis of ten individual clones, several patterns of segregation of the various env related proteins are evident. For example, three of the clones (numbers 16, 21 and 24) synthesize neither p50 nor p43, whereas the other seven show both of these proteins. The co-segregation of these two proteins has been a consistent finding in all clones we have tested thus far. This finding suggests that these two proteins are products of a single viral genome. Also evident in this figure is the segregation of the 4 higher molecular weight <u>env</u> proteins: p86 and p70 co-segregate independently of p50 and p43 (compare clones 16 and 19), and p83 and p68 co-segregate, also independently of p50 and p43 (compare clones 17 and 21).   Interestingly, these patterns do not necessarily reflect the replication status of the virus. For example, the <u>env</u> phenotype of clone 17, p83$^+$-p68$^+$-p50$^+$-p43$^+$, is identical to those of clones 25 and 26; however, clone 17 is replication defective whereas clones 25 and 26 are replication competent.   Also, clone 21 (p83$^+$-p68$^+$-p50$^-$-p43$^-$) is replication competent.   Characterization of numerous other clones led to an even more complex pattern in that additional new <u>env</u> related proteins were sometimes identified. On one hand, this phenomenon could be generated by the continued proliferation of cells that were originally infected by more than one virus particle, suggesting that the original multiplicity of infection was too high. This hypothesis is borne out, to some extent, by the fact that we also observed many cell clones which showed the same phenotype as the original BSB virus stock whereas relatively few clones with no viral <u>env</u> related proteins were isolated. This possibility must certainly be reckoned with, although putatively dually infected clones (rather than the original multiple component BSB stock) provide samples for further sub-cloning and aid in the preliminary screening for tumorigenic virus clones. On the other hand, it is also possible that the BSB viral components are highly mutable and unstable. So far, the continuous passage of some of the cell clones for at least four months has not led to a diversification in phenotype since the time of original classification.   Nevertheless, this characteristic will be assessed by further sub-cloning.

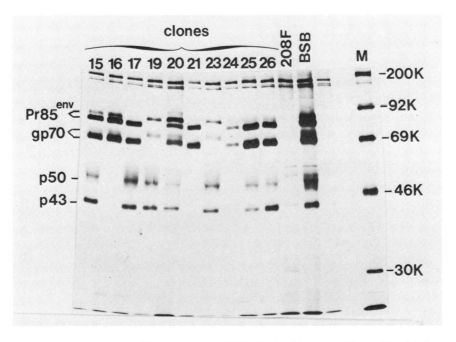

FIG. 2.   Analysis of BSB Infected 208F Cell Clones with gp70 Antiserum. Comparison by immunoprecipitation and SDS-PAGE analysis of uninfected 208F rat cells, 208F cells infected with the original BSB virus stock, and ten individual clones of 208F cells selected after infection at low multiplicity with BSB virus.

We also screened each clone for virus production by plaque and reverse transcriptase assays. From these analyses, replication competent viruses fell into eight "phenotypic" classes and replication defective viruses into three. These classes are summarized in Table 1.

TABLE 1. **Categories of BSB Virus Infected Cell Clones**

Virus Replication	Class	# Clones	env Related Proteins						New Proteins
			p86	p83	p70	p68	p50	p43	
Positive	Original	-	+	+	+	+	+	+	-
	I	5	+	+	+	+	-	-	-
	II	3	+	-	+	-	+	+	-
	III	1	+	-	+	-	+	+	p77, p63
	IV	3	-	+	-	+	+	+	-
	V	1	-	+	-	+	-	-	p52, p33
	VI	1	-	+	-	+	-	-	-
	VII	2	+	+	-	+	+	+	p76
	VIII	1	+	+	-	+		+	p40
Negative	IX	3	-	+	-	+	+	+	-
	X	1	-	+	-	+	-	-	-
	XI	1	-	-	-	-	+	+	p64, p62

It is quite clear from this type of analysis that there is always co-segregation of p50 and p43, of p83 with p68, and generally of p86 with p70. Furthermore, replication defective viruses of classes IX and X show env protein phenotypes that are shared by replication competent viruses (compare to classes IV and VI, respectively). The one exception is class XI, containing one cell clone only, in which the synthesis of the higher molecular weight proteins is not detected. It must also be mentioned that the cell clones containing replication defective viruses may be artefacts generated from replication competent viruses rather than important defective elements in the initial BSB virus complex.

Detection of a Dual-tropic Virus Component

In the last few years, murine retroviruses which grow in xenogeneic cells as well as in mouse cells have been isolated from the virally induced naturally occurring thymic lymphomas of high leukemia incidence mouse strains, such as AKR (10). The broad host range of infectivity is apparently due to a recombinant env gene arising from ecotropic (replication in murine cells predominantly) and xenotropic (replication in nonmurine cells) parental viruses (5, 17, 34). Such viruses have been called MCF (mink cell focus inducing) viruses because they cause cytopathic foci on mink cells. MCF isolates have also been obtained from spleen extracts of Friend and Rauscher virus infected mice (34, 35). Because of this property, we sought to determine whether the original BSB stock contained an MCF viral component.

Virus replication was readily detected in mink cell cultures infected with the original BSB stock. However, despite prolonged cultivation of cells infected with viruses of classes I, II, III and VI, no virus replication, as measured by reverse transcriptase activity, was attained in these cases. Thus, these 4 BSB virus classes represent ecotropic viruses only and the identification of the MCF component awaits further characterization.

Analysis of Replication Defects in Virus Nonproducer Clones

The previous analyses of the nonproducer nature of classes IX–XI were based on reverse transcriptase and infectivity studies. Also, the categorization into these classes was defined on the basis of the synthesis of env related proteins in the cells. To understand the replicative defects in further detail, some of these clones were analyzed by immunoprecipitation with antisera to whole virus or to gag related structural proteins. Figure 3 shows a comparison of clones infected with either a replication defective virus (clone 17) or a replication competent virus (clone 18) and an uncloned culture of 208F cells infected with the original BSB stock. As can be seen, all the proteins precipitated by anti-whole virus serum can be identified as being gag or env related. In BSB infected 208F uncloned cultures, two gag precursor polyproteins (Pr65^{gag}) are readily observed; this finding fits in well with the data suggesting multiple virus components in the original stock. The replication competent virus in clone 18 encodes fewer env related proteins, as discussed earlier, and only one gag precursor; such data support that notion that the individual components in the original BSB stock can be separated and phenotypically classified. Finally, clone 17 containing the replication defective virus lacks any detectable gag related proteins. This last finding suggests that the integrated virus contains a deletion or mutation in the gag gene which thus proscribes the formation of infectious progeny virions. However, there is no information provided to clarify whether the defective component pre-existed in the BSB stock before the cloning procedure or arose as a consequence of it. Clones representing all of the nonproducer classes have been analyzed in this fashion; none of them synthesize any gag related proteins.

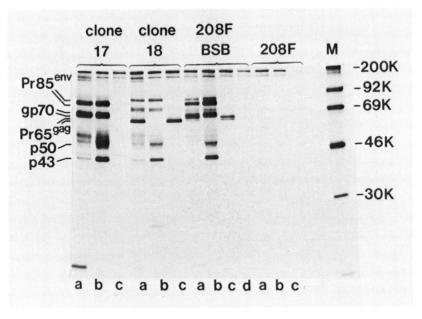

FIG. 3.　Analysis of BSB Stock and Subclones with Different Anti-viral Sera. 208F cells containing a replication defective virus (clone 17), a replication competent virus (clone 18), the original BSB stock and uninfected cells were immunoprecipitated before SDS-PAGE. Antisera used were: (a) anti-whole virus, (b) anti-gp70, (c) anti-p30, and (d) normal goat serum.

Rescue of Virus from Nonproducer Clones

To analyze the role of the replication defective viruses in the disease process, it is necessary to recover the viruses as infectious pseudotypes of helper retroviruses. Therefore, the nonproducer clones were superinfected with a variety of helper viruses, including the virus from BSB clone 18, Moloney MLV, and an amphotropic MLV (amphotropic viruses show a dual-tropic host range but are distinguishable from MCF viruses by the fact that there is no cross-interference with the env proteins of either ecotropic or xenotropic viruses) (9, 27). As is shown in Table 2, the BSB helper virus was unable to replicate in three clones representing the different nonproducer classes. This suggests that at least some of the env proteins synthesized in the nonproducer clones are expressed at the cell membrane and that their presence interferes with the adsorption and/or penetration of the helper BSB virus and thus must be closely related antigenically. Viruses from several other BSB producer clones representing other env phenotype classes were also tested and these too were unable to replicate. On the other hand, both Moloney MLV and amphotropic MLV are able to replicate in each of the nonproducer clones. Presumably, the BSB helper viruses share some unique antigenic specificities not found on Moloney or amphotropic MLV.

TABLE 2.   **Replication of Helper Viruses in BSB Nonproducer Clones**

Nonproducer BSB Class Infected	Replication[a] of		
	BSB Clone 18	Moloney MLV	Amphotropic MLV
Class IX	−	+	+
Class X	−	+	+
Class XI	−	+	+

[a]   Replication was determined by reverse transcriptase assay and SDS-PAGE.

The next stage, to determine whether the replication defective components have been rescued, is a more laborious process and is still in progress. At the present time, the only markers we have for the defective viruses are their env related proteins. Therefore, rescue can be measured only by using the super-natants from superinfected clones to infect new cells and to determine the env phenotype by SDS-PAGE. Such determinations are currently being made.

Analysis of Disease Potential of BSB and Virus Subclones

The most important criterion to define for the BSB virus complex is the virus(es) responsible for induction of the disease spectrum of polycythemia, hepatosplenomegaly, and erythroleukemia. By analogy to Friend virus complex, one might expect that a single virus component, like the replication defective SFFV in the case of FV, is responsible for the full pathological picture regardless of the helper virus used to permit replication of the defective component. Furthermore, the helper virus too might cause disease (e.g., the anemia and erythroblastosis in newborn mice induced by Fr-MLV). Alternatively, one replication competent virus of the BSB complex might suffice to induce the acute disease or a combination of particular virus entities might be required.

Because of the marked heterogeneity of the original BSB stock, it was necessary to confirm that an uncloned stock propagated continuously in NIH/3T3 cells was still capable of disease production to ensure that the oncogenic virus(es) was not lost by passage in vitro. Therefore, neonatal and adult mice of several strains were inoculated with a supernatant harvest from chronically infected cells after more than 10 passages. This virus harvest faithfully reproduced the full spectrum of BSB disease. Thus, we were confident that our in vitro propagated virus contained the disease producing entity.

Analysis of the in vivo effects of various BSB virus clones has only just begun and the data are yet meagre. To start, high titered virus harvests of some of the replication competent BSB clones were inoculated into newborn and adult mice of the DBA/2, BALB/c and C57BL strains. These three strains were chosen to delineate and compare the erythroleukemogenic diseases of BSB and FV: (a) DBA/2 mice are susceptible to both BSB and FV, (b) BALB/c mice are susceptible to both viruses and, in addition, are susceptible as neonates to Friend helper virus disease, and (c) C57BL mice are susceptible to BSB only.

At the time of writing, four replication competent clones have been inoculated into newborn and adult mice; in each case, the time since inoculation has been only 4-5 weeks. Thus, we are only just beginning to see the occurrence of the pathological symptoms typical of BSB disease. With the caveat that very few animals have yet been examined, it is interesting that clones representing classes II and III produce hepatosplenomegaly and polycythemia, whereas animals that received virus inocula representing classes I and VI show no disease at this time. Certainly it is still premature to conclude the lack of oncogenic potential in the latter two classes. However, it is informative that both of the disease producing clones contain the p50 and p43 env related proteins while the two disease negative clones lack these proteins. It is also interesting that class I viruses (disease negative) contain all of the four major high molecular weight env proteins (p86, p83, p70 and p68) whereas class II viruses (disease positive) lack p83 and p68. As both disease producing classes do not contain a dual-tropic MCF virus as described above, this finding indicates that MCF virus is not requisite to BSB disease. These very preliminary findings suggest the course of future tumorigenicity studies. Firstly, comparison of rescued pseudotypes of replication defective classes IX and X should determine the relevance of p50 and p43 in the disease process. Secondly, the last of the replication defective types, class XI, should emphasize the relative importance of the higher molecular weight env proteins associated with various replication competent clones. Thirdly, further subcloning of the replication competent disease inducing class II virus clones may perhaps lead to segregation of two env phenotypes: from $p86^+$-$p70^+$-$p50^+$-$p43^+$ to $p86^+$-$p70^+$-$p50^-$-$p43^-$ and $p86^-$-$p\overline{70}^-$-$p50^+$-$p43^+$ which should allow further evaluation of the etiological agents. Work is currently in progress along these lines.

CONCLUSIONS

The data reported in this paper represent the early movements in an as yet unfinished symphony. Because of the complex nature of the BSB virus system, definitive evidence to identify the oncogenic viral component(s) is still lacking. However, the system has been dissected to some extent compared to the original stock and it is hoped that future analyses will provide further elucidation.

Firstly, we have shown that continuous propagation of the uncloned stock in vitro does not lead to attenuation of pathogenic potential. This was an important point to assess because of the possibility that adventitious viruses in the stock could dominate and even replace the oncogenic agent. Furthermore, cell-free harvests from some of the cell clones derived following low multiplicity infection contain more simple phenotypic patterns of viral structural protein expression and yet still faithfully reproduce the BSB disease spectrum.

Preliminary analyses show that BSB virus complex shares some of the pathological potential of the polycythemia strain of Friend virus (FV-P) from which it was derived, but it also differs in several important aspects. The most important difference, which triggered our study, was the production of Friend disease in mice of the C57BL strain; in this regard, we have confirmed the initial report of Steeves et al. (30). On the other hand, two properties of FV-P are lacking: (a) no anemia is seen in neonatal BALB/c mice, as is observed following Friend helper virus (Fr-MLV) infection; in fact, a slight polycythemia was the prominent finding, and (b) no gp55 is observed in infected cells, whereas gp55 is the important hallmark of the SFFV component of FV which is responsible for Friend disease in adult mice. Thus, in the course of derivation of BSB, both Fr-MLV and SFFV have been lost, mutated, recombined or altered in some fashion.

Six major env gene related proteins were immunoprecipitated from cells infected with the original BSB stock: p86, p83, p70, p68, p50, and p43. It is most likely that these all represent glycoproteins, although we have not yet completed glucosamine labeling studies to conclude this with certainty. However, it is worth noting that Housman et al. (11) have shown changes in the apparent molecular weights of several viral proteins in BSB infected cells following glycosidase treatment, suggesting that a number of glycoproteins are present. At this stage, we interpret the two highest molecular weight proteins to represent two distinct env protein precursors ($gPr85^{env}$) and the next two bands to represent mature virion glycoproteins (gp70). Furthermore, from the segregation patterns, we would predict precursor-product relationships between p86 and p70 and between p83 and p68. The remaining two env proteins, p50 and p43, are apparently unique to BSB virus complex and co-segregate independently of any of the higher molecular weight proteins.

The overwhelming number of viral env gene proteins expressed in BSB infected cells emphasized the need for biological cloning. Following low multiplicity infection and micromanipulative cloning of BSB infected rat 208F cells, eleven env phenotypes were discerned; of these, 8 classes contained replication competent viruses and 3 classes were nonproducer cells.

The replication defective env phenotype classes do not synthesize any gag gene related proteins; this defect probably accounts, at least in part, for the absence of infectious virus production. We have not as yet analyzed these classes for disease potential because of the difficulty in deriving infectious pseudotypes following superinfection.

Of the replication competent virus classes, four have so far been analyzed in vivo. Class II and III viruses (env phenotype: $p86^+$-$p83^-$-$p70^+$-$p68^-$-$p50^+$-$p43^+$) induce disease, whereas class I ($p86^+$-$p83^+$-$p70^+$-$p68^+$-$p50^-$-$p43^-$) and class VI ($p86^-$-$p83^+$-$p70^-$-$p68^+$-$p50^-$$p43^-$) viruses do not. By subtractive analysis, it would appear that the $p50^+$-$p43^+$ phenotype was the most important for inducing the erythroid disease. This hypothesis will be assessed by investigating the in vivo effects of other replication competent and of rescued replication defective clones and further subcloning of disease inducing clones.

Although an MCF type of virus was detected in the original BSB stock, it has not yet been assigned to any of the env phenotypes. However, we have already shown that neither of the disease positive classes contains MCF virus. Thus, MCF virus in the inoculum is not responsible or necessary for induction of BSB disease; however, the possibility remains that such a virus, generated or induced in vivo, may be required in the disease process.

BSB disease in adult mice is very much like FV-P disease, engendering hepatosplenomegaly and polycythemia. In addition, marked stimulation of white blood cell production is also noted (30, and our own observations). In newborn BALB/c mice, we observe hepatosplenomegaly with a slight polycythemic response; this contrasts dramatically to the anemia observed in neonatal BALB/c mice infected with FV. Although distinct spleen foci of erythroid cells are evident following BSB infection, their titers are always several orders of magnitude lower compared to Friend virus stocks containing comparable levels of helper virus. Either BSB is less efficacious in inducing spleen foci or the levels of an SFFV-like component are in vast minority to those of other infectious components in the original stock or in subsequently derived clones. It will also be interesting to establish the levels and the erythropoietin dependence of the committed erythroid precursor cells, CFU-E, because of the disparity of effects induced by SFFV-A in comparison to SFFV-P.

It is hoped that answers to some of these unresolved questions will soon be forthcoming. Identification of discrete elements as the etiological agents in BSB disease will allow molecular cloning by recombinant DNA technology. Such reagents would provide knowledge on the origin of the distinct BSB components and their relationships to the various components associated with Friend virus disease. They would also provide information on the nature of the p50 and p43 env proteins, whether they represent truncated env gene products or new recombinant proteins, and whether they represent new oncogenic sequences. Finally, the initial stimulus in undertaking this analysis, that of understanding the interactions between the cellular Fv-2 gene and erythroleukemogenic viruses, will be investigated.

REFERENCES

1. Axelrad, A.A., and Steeves, R.A. (1964): Virology, 24:513-518.
2. Bernstein, A., Mak, T.W., and Stephenson, J.R. (1977): Cell, 12:287-294.
3. Bonner, W.M., and Laskey, R.A. (1974): Eur. J. Biochem., 46:83-88.
4. Dresler, S., Ruta, M., Murray, M.J., and Kabat, D. (1979): J. Virol., 30:564-575.
5. Elder, J.H., Gautsch, J.W., Jensen, F.C., Lerner, R.A., Hartley, J.W., and Rowe, W.P. (1977): Proc. Natl. Acad. Sci., 74:4676-4680.
6. Fagg, B., Vehmeyer, K., Ostertag, W., Jasmin, C., and Klein, B. (1980): In In Vivo and In Vitro Erythropoiesis: The Friend System, edited by G.B. Rossi, pp. 163-172. Elsevier/North-Holland Biomedical Press, Amsterdam.
7. Friend, C. (1957): J. Exp. Med., 105:307-318.
8. Hartley, J.W., and Rowe, W.P. (1966): Proc. Natl. Acad. Sci., 55:780-786.
9. Hartley, J.W., and Rowe, W.P. (1976): J. Virol., 19:19-25.
10. Hartley, J.W., Wolford, N.K., Old, L.J., and Rowe, W.P. (1977): Proc. Natl. Acad. Sci., 74:789-792.
11. Housman, D., Levenson, R., Vollach, V., Tsiftsoglou, A., Gusella, J., Parker, D., Kernen, J., Mitrani, A., Weeks, V., Witte, O., and Besmer, P. (1980): Cold Spr. Harb. Symp. Quant. Biol., 44:1177-1185.
12. Jainchill, J.F., Aaronson, S.A., and Todaro, G.J. (1969): J. Virol., 4:549-553.
13. Kessler, S.W. (1975): J. Immunol., 115:1617-1624.
14. Krantz, M.J., Strand, M., and August, J.T. (1977): J. Virol., 22:804-815.
15. Krieg, C.J., Ostertag, W., Clauss, U., Pragnell, I.B., Swetly, P., Roesler, G., and Weimann, B.J. (1978): Exp. Cell Res., 116:21-29.
16. Laemmli, U.K. (1970): Nature, 227:680-685.
17. Levy, J.A. (1973): Science, 182:1151-1153.
18. Lilly, F. (1970): J. Natl. Cancer Inst., 45:163-169.
19. Linemeyer, D.L., Ruscetti, S.K., Menke, J.G., and Scolnick, E.M. (1980): J. Virol., 35:710-721.
20. MacDonald, M.E., Reynolds, F.H., Jr., Van de Ven, W.J.M., Stephenson, J.R., Mak, T.W., and Bernstein, A. (1980): J. Exp. Med., 151:1477-1492.
21. Mirand, E.A. (1967): Science, 156:832-833.
22. Mirand, E.A., Steeves, R.A., Lange, R.D., and Grace, J.T., Jr. (1968): Proc. Soc. Exp. Biol. Med., 128:844-849.

23. Odaka, T. (1970): Int. J. Cancer, 6:18-23.
24. Oliff, A.I., Hager, G.L., Chang, E.H., Scolnick, E.M., Chan, H.W., and Lowy, D.R. (1980): J. Virol., 33:475-486.
25. Quade, K. (1979): Virology, 98:461-465.
26. Racevskis, J., and Koch, G. (1977): J. Virol., 21:328-337.
27. Rasheed, S., Gardner, M.B., and Chan, E. (1976): J. Virol., 19:13-18.
28. Rowe, W.P., Pugh, W.E., and Hartley, J.W. (1970): Virology, 42:1136-1139.
29. Ruscetti, S.K., Linemeyer, D., Feild, J., Troxler, D., and Scolnick, E.M. (1979): J. Virol., 30:787-798.
30. Steeves, R.A., Mirand, E.A., Bulba, A., and Trudel, P.J. (1970): Int. J. Cancer, 5:346-356.
31. Teich, N.M., Weiss, R.A., Martin, G.R., and Lowy, D.R. (1977): Cell, 12:973-982.
32. Troxler, D.H., and Scolnick, E.M. (1978): Virology, 85:17-27.
33. Troxler, D.H., Parks, W.P., Vass, W.C., and Scolnick, E.M. (1977): Virology, 76:602-615.
34. Troxler, D.H., Yuan, E., Linemeyer, D., Ruscetti, S., and Scolnick, E.M. (1978): J. Exp. Med., 148:639-653.
35. Van Griensven, L.J.L.D., and Vogt, M. (1980): Virology, 101:376-388.
36. Witte, O.N., and Baltimore, D. (1978): J. Virol., 26:750-761.

Expression of Differentiated Functions in Cancer Cells, edited by R. F. Revoltella et al., Raven Press, New York © 1982.

Studies on the Biology and Genetics of Murine Erythroleukemia Viruses

W. Ostertag, I. B. Pragnell, A. Fusco, D. Hughes, M. Freshney,
*B. Klein,**C. Jasmin, †J. Bilello, †G. Warnecke,
and ‡K. Vehmeyer

*Beatson Institute for Cancer Research, Bearsden, Glasgow G61 1BD, Scotland; *Laboratoire d'Immunopharmacologie des Tumeurs, Centre Paul Lamarque, Hopital St.-Eloi, 34033 Montpellier, France, **ICIG, Department of Virology, 94800 Villejuif, France, †Institute of Physiological Chemistry, University of Hamburg, 2000 Hamburg 13, West Germany; ‡Department of Hematology, School of Medicine, University of Goettingen, 3400 Goettingen, West Germany*

Several retroviruses which cause acute leukemia, involving expansion of the erythroid cell lineage of adult mice, have been isolated and characterized (11, 22, 30, 33; Fusco, A., Pragnell, I. B. and Ostertag, W., unpublished). Some of these viruses induce mainly or exclusively the proliferative expansion of erythroid cells: the anemia inducing Friend virus (FV), FV-A, and the polycythemia inducing FV, FV-P (29, 41, G. Rossi et al., this volume). Rauscher virus (RV) induces increased proliferation (increase in relative cell density) of not only the splenic erythroid, but also the macrophage/granulocyte and the hematopoietic stem cell compartment (37). The myeloproliferative sarcoma virus (MPSV) induces similar, but more pronounced changes than Rauscher virus (16, 18, 29, 30). Moreover, MPSV, unlike any of the previously listed retroviruses, is also able to transform fibroblasts in vitro and elicits sarcomas upon intramuscular injection into young mice (A. Fusco, unpublished). AF1 virus, a previously unrecognized retrovirus, arose on passage of twice cloned helper virus of FV-P in, first, murine fibroblasts [virus: 643/22F (31)], and then in spleens of newborn mice (NIH Swiss, Balb/C, DBA/2 strains). AF1 causes splenomegaly and spleen focus formation in some adult mice if injected intravenously, and sarcomas, if injected intramuscularly. It also induces splenomegaly and sarcomas in newborn mice. This virus does not transform fibroblasts in vitro (A. Fusco, Pragnell, I. B. and Ostertag, W., unpublished). We decided to study the effect of these retroviruses with respect to host range, biology and molecular biology, in order to understand the effect of these viruses on erythroid proliferation.

Present address of W.Ostertag: Heinrich-Pette-Institute, University of Hamburg, 2000 Hamburg 20, West Germany.

401

STRUCTURE OF RETROVIRUS COMPLEXES CAUSING ERYTHROID
EXPANSION IN ADULT MICE

All of the above cited retroviruses appear to be virus complexes
of at least one, possibly two (FV-P of Friend cells, RV) defective
subunits, at least one, in one case (RV) possibly two replication
competent subunits (8, 9, 21, 31, 43). It has been generally assumed
that the replication competent helper virus is not involved in generating the biological specificity of these virus complexes (29, 41).
Recent experiments on cloned helper virus of the FV and RV complex have
however raised considerable doubts whether this generalisation is, in
fact, correct: helper virus of the FV complex, MuLV-F, and helper virus
of the RV complex, MuLV-R, may induce not only T cell leukemias, as
assumed previously, but also erythroid hyperplasia, chloroleukemia,
etc., although not very rapidly (29, 41, 42). It was thus necessary
to construct complexes of the above mentioned retroviruses by rescuing
the defective genome of the transforming virus from non-producer cells,
using different replication competent, but biologically "inert" cloned
MuLV helper viruses (e.g. amphotropic MuLV, MuLV-Gross or MuLV-Mol).
The defective (and putatively transforming) retrovirus subunit of the
FV (FV-A, FV-P), the RV and the MPSV complex was cloned in either
mouse or rat cells (2, 3, 7, 9, 30, 32, 35, 42). An SFFV-R$^+$, MuLV$^-$
murine transformed erythroid cell clone (RA1) is also available for
such pseudotype studies (23). Pseudotype studies on FV-A and FV-P
(9, 10, 13, 20) and on MPSV (30, and Fagg et al. in preparation)
indicate that biological specificity in adult mice as tested by these
studies is a property of the defective transforming virus. However,
since the supposedly innocuous helper viruses which can be used (MuLV-
Mol, MuLV-Gross, amphotropic MuLV) do not rescue SFFV (of FV-A, FV-P
or RV origin or MPSV as efficiently as the Friend helper virus (MuLV-F)
(10, 29, 30, 42), the interpretation of these studies has remained
doubtful. To overcome this difficulty and to be able to compare the
biological effects of the different defective transforming viruses in
adult mice, we decided to construct pseudotypes of MuLV-F with each
of the defective viruses (SFFV-F, SFFV-R, MPSV). This minimizes the
effect of differential rescue of defective virus and differential
spread of helper virus on injection of mice. Use of such pseudotypes
will however not overcome difficulties in interpretation of biological
results which may arise as a consequence of differential replication
of helper virus in possibly different target cells of the defective
transforming virus component. The latter deficiency can only be
overcome by studying the effect of the defective virus alone, e.g. by
integration of this virus into the germ line of mice (15), or by
constructing allophenic mice with nonproducer teratocarcinoma cells.
Both of these approaches are technically very involved and time con-
suming. Three kinds of nonproducer cells were used: for MPSV rescue,
the transformed rat NRK fibroblast cell clones MPV 6-6 #3 and p5-8 #1
(30), for SFFV-F rescue, the mouse fibroblast cell lines SC204 and
6S26 (3, 28), for SFFV-R rescue the mouse erythroleukemia cell clone
RA1 (6, 23). Virus can be rescued from these cell lines by exposure
to the twice cloned MuLV-F helper virus which is released by the SC1
cell line 643/22N. Rescued virus only shows two subunits, that of the
defective transforming virus, with 32S (SFFV-R, SFFV-F) or 33S (MPSV)
RNA, and that of the MuLV-F component (35S RNA). This is shown in
Figure 1a for the SFFV-R complex, in Figure 1b for the MPSV complex, and

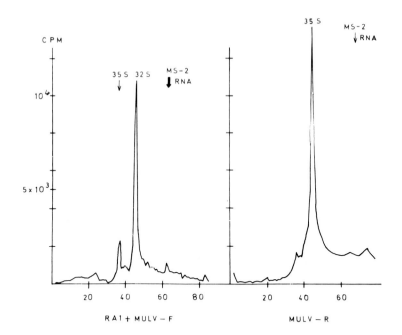

Figure 1a

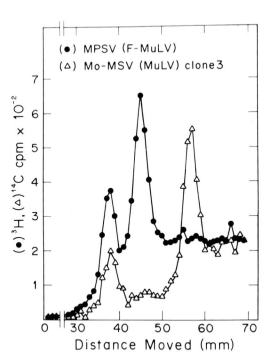

Figure 1b

Figure 1: Separation of subgenomic RNA of Rauscher virus of cell line RA1 [SFFV (MuLV-F)] (left panel of Figure 1a), of MuLF-F (right panel), and of myeloproliferative sarcoma virus [MPSV (MuLV-F)] (Figure 1b). The data of Figure 1a were obtained by Dr. J. Mol (23).

has been published for the SFFV-F complex (7, 24, 28).   Furthermore,
oligonucleotide fingerprint analysis showed that the two RNA components of each of these complexes were homogeneous and that the 35S
RNA species of the different complexes were identical.   The defective
32-33S subunits of the different complexes are distinctly different
(9, 23, 24 and unpublished data).

Unique properties of the defective transforming subunits were
further characterised by subtractive hybridisation using MuLV-F RNA
to remove sequences homologous to MuLV-F from cDNA made against the
total virus complex   (Table 1): SFFV-F of the FV-P complex thus has
specific sequences which hybridize largely also to RNA of xenotropic
virus (SFFV probe), hereas MPSV of the MPSV (MuLV-F) complex has
specific sequences (MPSV probe) which hybridize completely to Moloney
sarcoma virus RNA (31), and not to RNA of FV-P, or of xenotropic virus.
MPSV is thus a novel spleen focus inducing virus which does not share
specific sequences with SFFV-F or SFFV-R (31).   RV has previously been
shown by others to contain SFFV specific sequences (42).   RA1 nonproducer cells thus express high levels of SFFV-F related RNA
(unpublished).

TABLE 1.   Specific sequences of FV and of MPSV

Viral RNA	% specific cDNA hybridized		
	MPSV	MSV-Mol	SFFV-F
MuLV-F	6	0	3
MuLV-Mol	0	4	7
MPSV (5-8#1)	100	94	8
MSV-Mol	93	100	NT
MSV-Ki	0	NT	NT
MSV-Ha	1	NT	NT
Abelson	1	NT	NT
FV-P of F4-6	7	NT	100
FV-P of SC204	0	NT	103
NZB-X	1	NT	70
Balb/2-X	5	NT	66

BIOLOGICAL PROPERTIES OF RETROVIRUS COMPLEXES CAUSING
ERYTHROID EXPANSION IN ADULT MICE

Virus of the RV, FV-P, FV-A and MPSV complex was injected intravenously into 3-6 months old adult DBA/2J mice which have the $Fv-2^S$
allele.   Injection of these viruses causes splenomegaly within 7-21
days, as well as anemia (hematocrit 20-40% for FV-A, RV and MPSV) or
polycythemia (hematocrit 45-90% for FV-P).   Spleen and bone marrow
cells of these mice and of uninfected controls were seeded in methylcellulose medium containing either erythropoietin or burst promoting
activity from Wehi-3 cell supernatant), both or none (Table 2).

The erythropoietin was isolated from the urine of patients with
Fanconi anemia and purified extensively to remove residual BPA
activity (Fagg, B. and Ostertag, W., unpublished).   This erythropoietin does not promote development of early erythroid colonies

(10 day BFU-E) but is satisfactory for the development of late erythroid colonies (2 day CFU-E). Even high concentrations of this erythropoietin preparation do not promote optimal BFU-E formation in control spleen or bone marrow cells. Dialysed and concentrated supernatant of Wehi-3 cells, grown in serum free medium, contains BPA activity (25) and was necessary for the development of maximal numbers of BFU-E in bone marrow and spleen of control mice (Table 2). CFU-E development was linearly dependent on input of cells, whereas formation of BFU-E was linearly cell dosage dependent only at cell densities > 2-5 x 10^4 cells/ml (data not shown). Mice injected with virus of SFFV-P complex which was released by SC204, SFFV$^+$ MuLV$^-$, cells infected by MuLV were used for similar assays. Bone marrow and spleen cells of these mice, as expected, show much elevated levels of CFU-E with or without erythropoietin, thus confirming previous reports (29, 41). BFU-E cell density (number of BFU-E colonies per 10^6 bone marrow or spleen cells) in these mice is known to be largely unaffected (29, 41). Injection of FV-A also gave rise to an increase in the density of CFU-E in infected spleens but not as much in bone marrow (10, 29, 39, 41, Rossi et al., this volume). Spleen cells of MPSV infected mice show a large increase in CFU-E density. Most of the CFU-E developed only in the presence of low doses of erythropoietin (Table 2), but a small fraction (5-20% in different experiments) of these CFU-E did not require addition of erythropoietin. There were very few changes in CFU-E density of infected bone marrow cells. 10-12 day BFU-E of spleen and bone marrow of MPSV infected mice developed without requiring addition of Wehi-3 supernatant as a source of BPA (Table 2). MPSV induced CFU-E are linearly dependent on cell input, whereas BFU-E formation is linear only at a cell density of > 2-5 x 10^4 cells/plate.

TABLE 2. Erythroid colony forming cells in spleen and bone marrow of DBA/2 mice infected with FV-P, FV-A, RV and MPSV

Tissue	Virus used	Spleen Size	CFU-E		12 day BFU-E			
					No Epo		+ Epo	
			0	+Epo	No BPA	+BPA	No BPA	+BPA
			Colonies/10^5 cells					
Bone Marrow	None	1	2.2	136	0	0	0.1	20
	FV-P	18	2500	2300	0	N.T.	0	N.T.
	FV-A	9	1.0	480	N.T.	N.T.	N.T.	N.T.
	RV	7	13	590	0	1.5	8.9	23.9
	MPSV	11	9	302	0.25	0	27	23.5
Spleen	None	1	0.2	52	0	0	0	1.3
	FV-P	18	2200	2600	0	N.T.	0	N.T.
	FV-A	9	15	2100	N.T.	N.T.	N.T.	N.T.
	RV	7	16	4700	0	0	1.2	3.0
	MPSV	11	210	1920	0	0	4.5	3.8

RV [SFFV-R (MuLV-F)] infected mice were also tested for CFU-E and
BFU-E density in infected bone marrow or spleen and for their requirement for erythropoietin or BPA (Table 2).   The density of CFU-E in
spleen cells is largely increased, but only in the presence of
erythropoietin.   Development of BFU-E in spleen and bone marrow cells
was only optimal in presence of BPA.   However, at least 40-50% of the
BFU-E also develop without addition of BPA.   The effects of RV
infection thus are similar to those obtained on injection of mice with
MPSV and differ from those reported for mice infected with the FV
complex (FV-A or FV-P) (Table 2).   The results on RV could be the
effect of different heterogeneous genomic components (43): Van
Griensven and Vogt showed that RV of infected mouse spleen and of
infected tissue culture cell lines was heterogeneous and contained up
to four distinguishable subunits.   RV as used in these studies (43)
caused essentially the same biological effects (14, 37) as was shown
here for a RV complex with only two genomic subunits, SFFV-R (32S RNA),
and MuLV-F (35S RNA) (Figure 1).   The presence of one defective subunit is thus sufficient to account for the biological specificity of
RV and of MPSV.

Further similarities between the action of RV and of MPSV were
apparent: both RV (14, 31) and MPSV (16, 18) caused a marked expansion
not only of cells of the erythroid lineage, measured in colony forming
cells (cell density), but also of cells of the granulocyte/macrophage
series, and of pluripotent stem cells of spleen and peripheral blood.
These increases in number of colonies (cell density) were highest with
MPSV and were entirely absent on injection of mice with FV.   The
total number of CFU-C or CFU-S in the enlarged spleen of FV injected
was however also increased (12, 41).

The apparent lack of requirement for BPA of RV or MPSV infected
spleen and bone marrow BFU-E may reflect either BPA independence of
the infected target cell (BFU-E cell), or may be caused by the
release of BPA by MPSV or RV infected other hematopoietic cells,
(T cells or macrophages) or even nonhematopoietic cells.   More
detailed experiments involving infection of bone marrow or spleen
cells in vitro, as were done for FV (13) are necessary to allow
conclusions on the actual target cells of these viruses (Hankins,
Pragnell and Kost, in preparation).

HOST   RANGE   PROPERTIES   OF   RETROVIRUS   COMPLEXES   CAUSING
ERYTHROID   EXPANSION   IN   ADULT   MICE

Effects of the Fv-2 and Mpsv resistance loci

Several genes which are present in different allelic states in
different mouse strains appear to influence erythroleukemia induction
by competent retrovirus complexes (19, 26, 27, 29, 40, 41).   We have
centered our attention on genes which appear to influence availability
of differentiated target cells for infection or transformation with the
defective specific viral component of each virus complex, rather than
on genes, such as Fv-1, which have an influence on cellular resistance
to the replication competent helper virus.   All of the genes which
appear to influence transformation directly (supposedly mediated by the
specific defective transforming component) appear to be genes which
primarily have an influence on proliferation and differentiation of
hematopoietic cells.   Examples are the Fv-2 locus, the W and the Sl
loci.

TABLE 3. <u>Spleen focus formation and spleen weight, influence of the Fv-2 locus</u>

	FV-P		RV		MPSV	
	SFFU/ml	Spleen wt. <u>infected</u> control	SFFU/ml	Spleen wt. <u>infected</u> control	SFFU/ml	Spleen wt. <u>infected</u> control
C57BL $Fv-2^r$ $Mpsv^r$	0	1.05	0	1.5	0	1.0
C57BL $Fv-2^s$ $Mpsv^r$	1.5×10^5	10.6	1.2×10^4	5.1	3×10^3	4.9
DDD $Fv-2^r$ $Mpsv^s$	0	1.3	0	4.3	3.3×10^3	5.3
DDD $Fv-2^s$ $Mpsv^s$	1.7×10^5	11.4	1.0×10^4	3.9	5.8×10^3	4.7

The <u>Fv-2 locus</u> has a profound influence on cycling of BFU-E cells in the mouse (40). BFU-E cells which in $Fv-2^r/2^r$ mice appear to be largely in non-cycling are in cycling state in $Fv-2^s/2^s$ or $Fv-2^s/2^r$ mice. This difference in cycling may control the availability of the BFU-E target cells for SFFV or MPSV. While $Fv-2^r/2^r$ mice are resistant to leukemia induction by SFFV, $Fv-2^s$ mice are sensitive (Table 3). MPSV induces leukemia in C57 BL 6 $Fv-2^s$ but not in congenic C57 BL $Fv-2^r$ mice (27) (Table 3). MPSV, but not SFFV generated leukemia in DDD $Fv-2^r/2^r$ mice. This prompted us to suggest the presence of a second gene or genes in C57BL mice which confer resistance to MPSV. These Mpsv genes possibly may control the BPA sensitive "target cell" population of MPSV (see above). Differences in response to BPA of C57BL mice as compared to e.g. DBA/2 mice, which appear not to be regulated by the Fv-2 gene (Johnson, G., this volume) may be related to MPSV resistance. BPA is possibly a single hormone, reacting with receptors on hematopoietic stem cells, on early erythroid (BFU-E), and on early granulocyte/macrophage precursor cells (N. Iscove, this volume).

Any hypothesis which attempts to explain the action of MPSV (or RV) must account for the following:

(i) Their effects on three cell types, i.e. hematopoietic stem cells.
(ii) The relative lack of requirement for BPA of erythroid and mixed BFU-E colony formation.
(iii) The partial CSF independence of early myeloid cells.
(iv) The requirement for an MPSV resistance locus. The $Mpsv^r$ locus (loci) may in fact influence the control of cell proliferation of BPA sensitive target cells of MPSV.

In view of the similarity of biological effects of MPSV and RV
one might expect that RV, although similar to SFFV-F in genome composition, would be able to cause leukemia also in DDD Fv-$2^r/2^r$ mice
which appear to have the Mpsv sensitivity allele of the Mpsv locus
Unlike FV, RV induces splenomegaly as predicted, but not spleen focus
formation in these mice (Table 3).

TABLE 4.   Spleen focus formation and spleen weight, influence of
                      the W locus on leukemogenesis

Virus		W/W^v	$W^v/+$	$W/+$	$+/+$
RV	SFFU/ml	2.3×10^3	3.6×10^3	2.4×10^3	3.8×10^3
	spleen wt. infected control	5.5	5.1	5.3	5.7
MPSV	SFFU/ml	9.7×10^2	1.6×10^3	1.1×10^3	8×10^2
	spleen wt. infected control	2.5	3.8	2.5	1.9
FV (literature)	SFFU	0	$\pm$	+++	+++

Effects of the W and Sl loci
     The mutant alleles of the two gene loci, W^+ and Sl^+, W and Sl are
involved in the control of hematopoietic stem cell differentiation.
They cause macrocytic anemia and affect mainly the erythroid compartment (34). W/W^v, $W^v/+$ as well as Sl/Sl^d mice were resistant to FV
induced leukemogenesis (1, 38).   We have thus tested these mice for
spleen focus-formation and leukemogenesis by MPSV and RV (Table 4):
MPSV and RV, unlike FV, induced focus-formation and splenomegaly in
W/W^v and $W^v/+$ mice.   Moreover Sl/Sl^d mice were sensitive to MPSV
induced leukemogenesis.

TEMPERATURE SENSITIVE TRANSFORMATION DEFECTIVE MUTANTS OF MPSV

     MPSV is the only murine spleen focus-forming virus with the unique
ability to transform both fibroblasts and hematopoietic cells.   The
specific (fibroblast transforming) sequence of MPSV was indistinguishable from that of a conventional MSV-Mol (see above) by liquid
hybridisation.   The question can thus be raised whether the V_{mos}
sequence of MPSV is also the specific part of the MPSV genome
involved in transforming hematopoietic cells.   We approached this
problem by isolating mutants for the fibroblast transformation gene of
MPSV.   If the same transforming gene (functional unit) is responsible
for both transforming activities, these mutants should also be
defective for hematopoietic transformation.   A second approach to
solve the problem of how dual transformation can arise, would be to

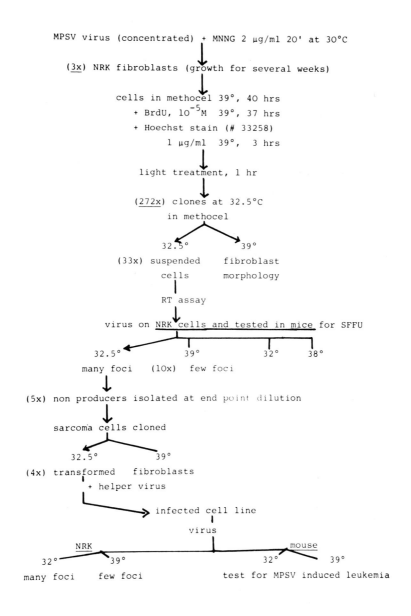

MPSV virus (concentrated) + MNNG 2 μg/ml 20' at 30°C

(3x) NRK fibroblasts (growth for several weeks)

cells in methocel 39°, 40 hrs
+ BrdU, 10^{-5}M 39°, 37 hrs
+ Hoechst stain (# 33258)
1 μg/ml 39°, 3 hrs

light treatment, 1 hr

(272x) clones at 32.5°C
in methocel

32.5° 39°

(33x) suspended   fibroblast
cells   morphology

RT assay

virus on NRK cells and tested in mice for SFFU

32.5°   39°   32°   38°

many foci (10x) few foci

(5x) non producers isolated at end point dilution

sarcoma cells cloned

32.5°   39°

(4x) transformed fibroblasts
+ helper virus

infected cell line

virus

NRK   mouse

32°   39°   32°   39°

many foci   few foci   test for MPSV induced leukemia

Figure 2: Selection scheme for ts mutants of MPSV.

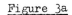

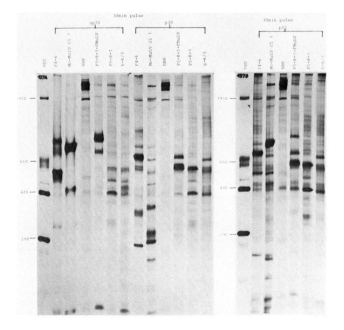

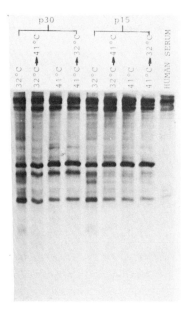

Figure 3: Immunoprecipitation of retrovirus related proteins of wild type (Figure 3a) and ts mutant (Figure 3b) MPSV nonproducer cells. MPSV nonproducer cells do not show gp70 related proteins. MPSV nonproducer p5-8#1 (Figure 3a) expresses a gag related polyprotein of ca. 60 K MW, MPV 6-6#3 (Figure 3a) nonproducer cells and ts 124 (Figure 3b) a gag related polyprotein of slightly higher molecular weight.

clone the MPSV genome in bacteria, and generate mutants directly (see below).

Ts mutants of murine sarcoma viruses, such as the Kirsten sarcoma virus (36), and the Moloney sarcoma virus (4, 17, 45, 46), have previously been isolated. They share the undesirable property that they are leaky (4, 17, 36, 45, 46) and that they revert to pseudo-wildtype phenotype at a very high rate (4, 17). The selection procedures which were previously used were thus not very satisfactory. We therefore decided to use an improved method to select for ts mutants using the basic procedure originally described by J. Wyke (45) to isolate ts mutants of Rous sarcoma virus.

The procedure which we used is outlined in Figure 2. MPSV was mutagenized with about half lethal dose of MNNG ($2\mu g/ml$). The mutagenised virus was used to infect NRK cells at permissive temperature ($32.5^\circ C$). The transformed NRK cells were grown at non-permissive temperature ($39.5^\circ C$) in methyl cellulose. Only those cells which are also of transformed phenotype at 39.5° should grow, those which are fibroblastic at this temperature should grow more slowly or not at all. BrdU was then added and is only incorporated by growing and not by nongrowing cells. The dye 33258 (Hochst) was added (5) and the cells were irradiated by visible light. The DNA of cells that had incorporated BrdU is broken by activation of BrdU. The Hochst dye increases the intensity of activation 10 x 100 fold. Virtually all cells that grown at 39.5° were thus killed and those cells that did not grow (do not incorporate BrdU) survived. Cloned surviving cell populations were tested for (1) ts morphology, (2) virus release at 32.5 and 39.5° C, (3) transforming capacity of virus released by these cells at 32.5 and $39.5^\circ C$. Cell clones were selected which showed ts morphology, released virus at a similar rate at permissive and nonpermissive temperature, but transformed NRK cells at least 100 fold better at permissive temperature than at non-permissive temperature. Virus from these cell clones was plated at end point dilution on NRK cells and foci were picked which contained MPSV, but not MuLV-F (nonproducer clones). Several nonproducer clones of independently derived MPSV ts mutants were thus established and were tested for morphology, and for growth in methylcellulose. All of the cell clones showed transformed morphology at permissive, but not at nonpermissive temperature. The nonproducer cells generated transformed, loose, colonies in methylcellulose at permissive, and not at nonpermissive temperature. The ts non-producer cell clones were also checked for viral protein synthesis at 32.5 and $39.5^\circ C$ (Figure 3b). The parental nonproducer MPSV cell clone, MPV 6-6 #3 has no env related glycoprotein as shown by immune precipitation (Figure 3), but synthesizes a virus related gag poly-protein, presumably coded for by MPSV, of 60-70 K (Figure 3a): this protein was precipitated with either anti p15 or p30, but not with anti p10 antisera. It is thus a gag polyprotein which is not processed and appears to be similar to proteins found in some MSV-Mol nonproducer cell lines (44). Nonproducer cells of the MPSV ts mutant 124/2 do not show differences in the rate of synthesis or degradation of this protein (Figure 3b) at permissive and non-permissive temperatures. This makes it unlikely that this particular MPSV ts mutant is in fact temperature sensitive for translation of the gag polyprotein. Ts 124 is thus more likely a ts mutant for the V_{mos} gene of MPSV.

TABLE 5.   MPSV ts mutants, recloned: fibroblast, spleen focus forming titres

	Fibroblast transformation			$37.5^\circ C$ DBA/2	Ratio $\dfrac{SFFU(*)}{FFU}$
	FFU/ml		FFU $\dfrac{32.5}{39.5}$	$\dfrac{SFFU}{ml}$	
	39.5°	32.5°			
+MPV 6-6#3	1.3×10^4	1.8×10^4	1.4	2.6×10^3	1.4×10^{-1}
ts 124/2/4	5.9×10^4	5.6×10^7	940	3.4×10^2	6.1×10^{-6}
ts 143/1/1	8×10^2	1.6×10^5	200	13	8.1×10^{-5}
ts 159/5/1	6.5×10^3	9.8×10^6	0		0

(*) SFFU at mouse body temperature (37.5°), FFU at 32.5°.

TABLE 6.   MPSV ts mutants: fibroblast and spleen focus forming titres

		Wild type MPV 6-6#3	ts 259
NRK cells (FFU)	32.5°	1.8×10^4	1.6×10^4
	39.5°	1.3×10^4	3.2×10^1
	ratio $\dfrac{32.5^\circ}{39.5^\circ}$	1.4	500
DBA/2J mice (SFFU)	32.5°	3.1×10^3	0
	37.5°	2.6×10^3	0
$\dfrac{SFFU}{FFU}$	37.5° and 32.5°	0.2	0

Ts nonproducer cells were infected with helper virus (MuLV-F) to rescue the ts mutant virus.   The virus complex was tested on NRK fibroblasts and showed 100-1000 fold decreased efficiency of fibroblast transformation at nonpermissive temperature (Table 5, 6):   the same ts virus isolates were also much less active in inducing leukemia at the nonpermissive body temperature $(38^\circ C)$ in DBA/2J mice (Table 5, 6).   Data on these three MPSV ts mutants thus suggest that the same functional unit of the MPSV genome, possibly the V_{mos} gene is

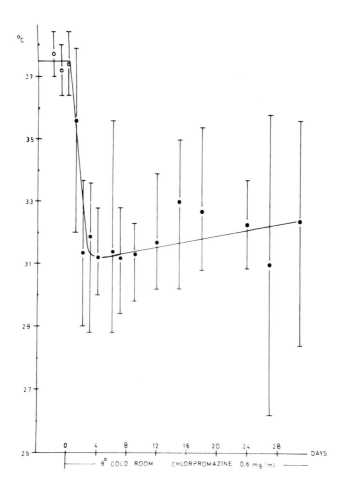

<u>Figure 4</u>: Lowering of body temperature of C57BL/6 mice by exposure to cold room temperature (9°C) and inclusion of chlorpromazine (0.6 mg/ml) to the drinking water of the animals. The results of two experiments (one using 10 mice, the other experiment using 5 mice initially) were pooled. The bars indicate the variability of body temperature. Similar experiments with essentially the same results were done with DBA/2J mice. Mortality of DBA/2J mice, however, during the course of the experiment is higher than with C57BL/6 mice.

in fact responsible for fibroblast and spleen focus–forming (leukemia inducing) properties.   In order to test leukemia induction in mice at permissive temperature it is necessary to be able to lower body temperature.   We therefore devised a protocol to obtain an average body temperature of mice of 32–33°C (Figure 4).   Using these conditions we were unable to obtain leukemia and focus formation at permissive temperature in mice on inoculation of these mice with ts virus (Table 6).

CLONING OF THE MPSV GENOME

We have recently constructed a library of recombinants between λ phage DNA and fragments of DNA from 6–6#3 MPSV nonproducer cells. A clone has been selected which carries an integrated MPSV provirus. DNA of this MPSV clone has been used to transfect and transform fibroblasts.   The potential for hematopoietic transformation of virus released from these transformed fibroblasts is at present being tested.

REFERENCES

1. Bennett, M., Steeves, R. A., Cudkowicz, G., Mirand, E. A. and Russell, L. B. (1968): Science 162: 564–565.
2. Bernstein, A., Mak, T. and Stephenson, J. (1977): Cell 12: 287–294.
3. Bilello, J., Colletta, G., Warnecke, G., Koch, G., Frisby, D., Pragnell, I. B. and Ostertag, W. (1980): Virology 107: 331–344.
4. Blair, D. G., Hull, M. A. and Finch, E. A. (1979): Virology 95: 303–316.
5. Conkie, D., Young, B. D. and Paul, J. (1980): Exp. Cell Res. 126: 439–444.
6. De Both, N. J., Vermey, M., van't Hull, E., Klootwyk–van Dyke, E., van Griensven, L. J. L. D., Mol, J. N. M. and Stoof, T. J. (1978): Nature 272: 626–628.
7. Dresler, S., Ruta, M., Murray, M. C. and Kabat, D. (1979): J. Virology 30: 564–575.
8. Dube, S. K., Kung, H. J., Bender, W., Davidson, N. and Ostertag, W. (1976): J. Virology 20: 264–272.
9. Evans, L., Nunn, M., Duesberg, P. H., Troxler, D. and Scolnick, E. M. (1980): Cold Spring Harbor Symp. Quant. Biol. 44: 823–835.
10. Fagg, B., Vehmeyer, K., Ostertag, W., Jasmin, C. and Klein, B. (1980): in "In vivo and in vitro erythropoiesis: the Friend system", ed. G. B. Rossi, Elsevier/North Holland: 163–172.
11. Friend, C. (1957): J. Exp. Med. 105: 307–318.
12. Golde, D. W., Faille, A., Sullivan, A. and Friend, C. (1976): Cancer Res. 36: 115–119.
13. Hankins, W. D. and Troxler, D. (1980): Cell 22: 693–699.
14. Hasthorpe, S. (1978): in "In vitro aspects of erythropoiesis", ed. M. J. Murphy, Springer Verlag, New York, Heidelberg, Berlin: 172–176.
15. Jaenisch, R. (1976): Proc. Natl. Acad. Sci. U.S.A. 73: 1260–1264.
16. Jasmin, C., Le Bousse, M. C., Klein, B., Smadja–Joffe, F., Mori, K. J., Fagg, B., Ostertag, W., Vehmeyer, K. and Pragnell, I. B. (1980): in "In vivo and in vitro erythropoiesis: the Friend system", ed. G. B. Rossi, Elsevier/North Holland: 183–192.

17. Klarlund, J. K. and Forchhammer, J. (1980): <u>Proc. Natl. Acad. Sci.</u> U.S.A. 77: 1501–1505.
18. Klein, B., Le Bousse, C., Fagg, B., Smadja–Joffe, F., Vehmeyer, K., Mori, C., Jasmin, C. and Ostertag, W. (1981): <u>J. Natl. Cancer Inst.</u>, in press.
19. Lilly, F. and Pincus, T. (1973): <u>Adv. Cancer Res.</u> 17: 231–277.
20. MacDonald, M. E., Mak, T. W. and Bernstein, A. (1980): <u>J. Exp.</u> Medicine 151: 1493–1503.
21. Maisel, J., Klement, U., Lai, M. M.–C., Ostertag, W. and Duesberg, P. (1973): <u>Proc. Natl. Acad. Sci. U.S.A.</u> 70: 3536–3540.
22. Mirand, E. A. (1967): <u>Proc. Soc. Exp. Biol. Med.</u> 125: 562–565.
23. Mol, J. N. M., Ostertag, W., Bilello, J. and Stoof, T. J. (1981), submitted.
24. Mol, J. N. M., Vonk, W. P., Pragnell, I. B. and Stoof, T. J. (1981): <u>J. Gen. Virology</u>, in press.
25. Moore, M. A. S. (1981): in "<u>Modern Trends in Human Leukemia</u>", ed. R. Neth, 4: in press.
26. Odaka, T. (1969): <u>J. Virology</u>, 3: 543–548.
27. Ostertag, W., Odaka, T., Smadja–Joffe, F. and Jasmin, C. (1981): <u>J. Virology</u> 37: 541–548.
28. Ostertag, W. and Pragnell, I. B. (1978): <u>Proc. Natl. Acad. Sci.</u> <u>U.S.A.</u> 75: 3278–3282.
29. Ostertag, W. and Pragnell, I. B. (1981): <u>Curr. Topics Microbiol.</u> <u>Immunology</u> 93, in press.
30. Ostertag, W., Vehmeyer, K., Fagg, B., Pragnell, I. B., Paetz, W., Le Bousse, M. C., Smadja–Joffe, F., Klein, B., Jasmin, C. and Eisen, H. (1980): <u>J. Virology</u> 33: 573–582.
31. Pragnell, I. B., Fusco, A., Arbuthnott, C., Smadja–Joffe, F., Klein, B., Jasmin, C. and Ostertag, W. (1981): <u>J. Virology</u> 38: in press.
32. Pragnell, I. B., McNab, A., Harrison, P. R. and Ostertag, W. (1978): <u>Nature</u> 272: 456–458.
33. Rauscher, F. J. (1962): <u>J. Natl. Cancer Inst.</u> 29: 515–543.
34. Russell, E. S. (1979): <u>Adv. Genetics</u> 20: 347–459.
35. Ruta, M. and Kabat, D. (1980): <u>J. Virology</u> 35: 844–853.
36. Scolnick, E. M., Stephenson, J. R. and Aaronson, S. A. (1972): <u>J. Virology</u> 10: 543–557.
37. Seidel, H. J. and Opitz, U. (1978): in "<u>In vitro aspects of</u> <u>erythropoiesis</u>", ed. M. J. Murphy, Jr.: 142–148.
38. Steeves, R. A., Bennett, M., Mirand, E. A. and Cudkowicz, G. (1968): <u>Nature</u> 218: 372–374.
39. Steinheider, G., Seidel, H. J. and Kreja, L. (1979): Experientia 35: 1173–1176.
40. Suzuki, S. and Axelrad, A. (1980): <u>Cell</u> 19: 225–236.
41. Tambourin, P. E. "Haematopoietic stem cells and murine viral leukemogenesis", in <u>Brit. Soc. Cell Biol. Symp.</u> (1979) 2: 254–316, Cambridge University Press, Cambridge.
42. Troxler, D. H., Ruscetti, S. K. and Scolnick, E. M. (1980): <u>Biochim. Biophys. Acta</u> 605: 305–324.
43. Van Griensven, L. J. L. D., and Vogt, M. (1980) <u>Virology</u> 101: 376–388.
44. Van Zaane, D. and Bloemers, H. P. J. (1978): <u>Biochim. Biophys.</u> <u>Acta</u>, 516: 249–268.

45. Wyke, J. A. (1975): <u>Biochim. Biophys. Acta</u>, 417: 91–121.
46. Yusa, Y. and Shimojo, H. (1977): <u>J. Gen. Virology</u> 36: 257–266.

ACKNOWLEDGEMENT

This work was supported by the MRC and by the Stiftung Volkswagenwerk.

Expression of Differentiated Functions in Cancer Cells, edited by R. F. Revoltella et al., Raven Press, New York © 1982.

The Relationship of Epidermal Growth Factor-Stimulated Protein Phosphorylation and the Protein Kinase Activity of the Rous Sarcoma Virus Transforming Gene Product

Eleanor Erikson, David J. Shealy, and R. L. Erikson

Department of Pathology, University of Colorado School of Medicine, Denver, Colorado 80262

The malignant changes caused by Rous sarcoma virus (RSV) are the consequence of the expression of a single viral gene termed src for sarcoma (28). The RSV src gene is apparently derived from a normal cellular gene, designated sarc or c-src (cell-src). The existence of c-src DNA and poly(A)-containing c-src RNA in normal uninfected vertebrate cells was demonstrated by molecular hybridization experiments with radioactive DNA specific for the RSV src gene (24-26, 29). The product of the RSV src gene is a phosphoprotein of M_r = 60,000, designated pp60^{src} (1, 2, 21). Because c-src nucleotide sequences are so closely related to src sequences, it was expected that a protein encoded by c-src would be closely related to pp60^{src}. Indeed, a phosphoprotein of M_r = 60,000 identified in normal uninfected cells appears to be the product of these sequences (3, 5, 7, 19). This protein, designated pp60^{c-src}, is present in normal cells at a level 50- to 100-fold less than pp60^{src} in transformed cells.

The src gene product, pp60^{src}, is closely associated with a protein kinase activity (ATP:protein phosphotransferase, EC 2.7.1.37) that has the unusual specificity of phosphorylating tyrosine residues in polypeptides (6, 9, 10, 11, 16). Moreover, a normal cell protein of M_r = 34,000 (34K) has been identified as a possible substrate of pp60^{src} kinase activity (11, 12, 23). This protein is specifically phosphorylated on tyrosine residue(s) in all RSV-transformed cells examined to date. In addition, this protein is phosphorylated in vitro by purified pp60^{src} at a site similar to that phosphorylated in the transformed cell. Although pp60^{c-src} prepared from normal avian cells is also capable of phosphorylating 34K in vitro (22), this reaction has not yet been demonstrated in normal uninfected avian or mammalian cells.

Cohen and associates have observed that epidermal growth factor (EGF) stimulates a tyrosine-specific protein kinase activity associated with plasma membranes (4, 27) and have speculated that this activity may be related to the activity of pp60^{c-src}. In order to determine more directly whether the EGF-stimulated protein kinase activity and pp60^{c-src} or pp60^{src} activity may be related, we studied the phosphorylation of 34K in both systems.

RESULTS

Because we had available antibody previously prepared against purified 34K (13), we used immunoprecipitation and analysis by polyacrylamide gel electrophoresis to study the effect of EGF stimulation on the phosphorylation of 34K. As shown in Figure 1, treatment with EGF resulted in approximately a 4-fold increase in phosphorous radiolabel in the 34K protein. Such an effect was not seen in normal chicken embryo fibroblasts under identical conditions. Phosphoamino acid analysis revealed that 34K prepared from unstimulated cells contained only phosphoserine whereas in 34K prepared from EGF-stimulated cells the majority of radiolabel was in phosphotyrosine, with some phosphoserine also present (about 4:1) (data not shown).

We have previously shown that the 34K protein purified from normal chicken embryo fibroblasts could serve as a substrate in vitro for the protein kinase activity associated with either the RSV transforming protein, pp60^{src}, or its homologue pp60^{c-src} prepared from normal avian cells (12, 22). To gain further insight into the phosphorylation of 34K under conditions of EGF stimulation we purified both the 34K protein and pp60^{c-src} from A431 cells. In vitro phosphorylation experiments revealed that A431 34K could serve as a substrate for pp60^{src} and for A431 pp60^{c-src}. The specific sites phosphorylated in vivo and in vitro were compared by two-dimensional analysis of tryptic phosphopeptides. Figure 2 shows that 34K radiolabeled in vivo under conditions of EGF-stimulation or in vitro contains two tryptic phosphopeptides. More importantly, mixing experiments reveal that the phosphopeptides comigrate under these conditions, indicating that most likely the same sites are phosphorylated.

DISCUSSION

In this communication we describe our initial effort to determine whether there is a common link between activity of the RSV-transforming protein pp60^{src} or its normal cell homologue pp60^{c-src} and the response of cells to growth factors such as EGF. Our results show that at least one normal cellular protein is phosphorylated in a remarkably similar way as the result of expression of all three activities. Thus, we can conclude from these studies that EGF stimulates a protein kinase activity in cells with high levels of EGF receptor that has a specificity similar to that of pp60^{src}/pp60^{c-src}. However, these data do not show that it is pp60^{c-src} that is responsible for the phosphorylation of the M_r = 34,000 protein because there may be other tyrosine-specific protein kinases that recognize the same sites in the protein as pp60^{c-src}. It is important to recognize this distinction because our previous studies have shown (13) that Fujinami sarcoma virus and PRCII sarcoma virus, which contain src genes distinct from the RSV src gene, also elevate the level of phosphorylation of the M_r = 34,000 protein in transformed cells and, moreover, examination of the phosphopeptides generated by tryptic digestion show that they are similar, if not identical, to those seen in response to RSV transformation. The transforming gene products of these viruses are antigenically distinct from pp60^{src} but may also be associated with protein kinase activities specific for tyrosine residues (14, 20). Thus, there may be several tyrosine-specific kinases with similar specificities. It is worth recalling this precedent for different protein kinases with similar specificities since cyclic adenosine monophosphate- and cyclic guanosine monophosphate-dependent protein kinases have similar substrate specificities, at least in vitro (15). In order to resolve these issues, we are in the process of searching for a protein kinase that may be directly involved with EGF responses.

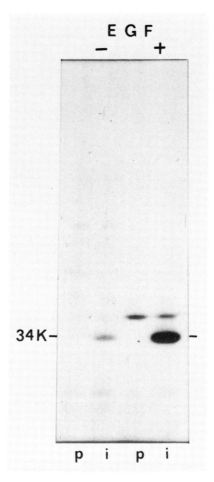

FIG. 1. Stimulation of phosphorylation of M_r = 34,000 protein in EGF-treated cells.

Cultures of human epidermoid carcinoma cells, A431, which had just reached confluency were labeled with 1 mCi/ml of [^{32}P]orthophosphate in phosphate-free medium containing 10% dialyzed fetal calf serum. After 30 min. EGF (Collaborative Research) was added to one culture to a final concentration of 400 ng/ml and 2.5 hr. later both cultures were harvested. The cells were lysed, clarified, and immunoprecipitated with preimmune or anti-34K serum as previously described (13). Protein A-containing Staphylococcus aureus, strain Cowan I was used to adsorb the immune complexes (17). Proteins were released from the bacterial adsorbent by treatment for 1 min. at 95° in buffer containing SDS and β-mercaptoethanol, and were resolved by electrophoresis through 10% SDS-polyacrylamide gels using the buffer systems described by Laemmli (18). Radiolabeled proteins were detected by autoradiography with the aid of Dupont Lightning Plus intensifying screens. p, preimmune serum; i, anti-34K serum.

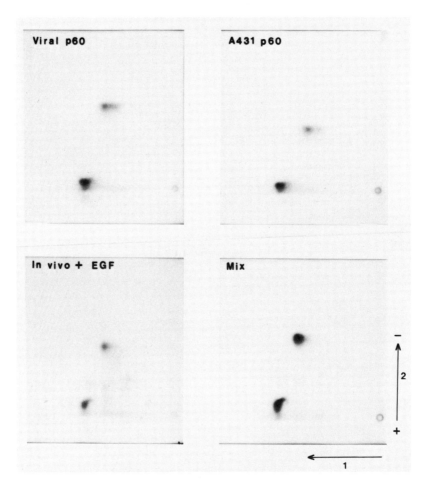

FIG. 2. Two-dimensional tryptic phosphopeptide analysis of the
M_r = 34,000 protein phosphorylated <u>in vitro</u> by RSV pp60^{src}, by A431
pp60^{c-src} and <u>in vivo</u> by EGF-stimulated protein kinase activity.
[^{32}P]-labeled 34K was prepared from EGF-stimulated A431 cells by immunoprecipitation and polyacrylamide gel electrophoresis as shown in
Figure 1. In addition, the 34K protein was purified from A431 cells
following the procedure described for chicken embryo fibroblasts (12).
No kinase activity was detectable in the native 34K preparation.
pp60^{src} was purified from RSV-transformed vole cells by immunoaffinity
chromatography (10, 11) and pp60^{c-src} was purified from A431 cells by
immunoaffinity chromatography on a column prepared with cross-reacting

immunoglobulin. The A431 34K protein was phosphorylated in vitro in the presence of $[\gamma\text{-}^{32}P]ATP$ by either pp60^{src} or A431 pp60^{c-src} as previously described (12). The products of the reaction were resolved by polyacrylamide gel electrophoresis. The radiolabeled 34K preparations were localized in the preparative gels by autoradiography, excised, eluted from the gels, precipitated, digested with trypsin, and fractionated by chromatography in the first dimension and by electrophoresis at pH 3.5 in the second dimension (8). Viral p60, 34K phosphorylated in vitro by RSV pp60^{src}; A431 p60, 34K phosphorylated in vitro by A431 pp60^{c-src}; In vivo + EGF, 34K prepared from radiolabeled EGF-stimulated A431 cells; Mix, equal counts of the second and third preparations were mixed and fractionated together.

REFERENCES

1. Brugge, J.S., and Erikson, R.L. (1977): Nature, 269:346-348.
2. Brugge, J., Erikson, E., Collett, M.S., and Erikson, R.L. (1978): J. Virol., 26:773-782.
3. Brugge, J.S., Collett, M.S., Siddiqui, A., Marczynska, B., Deinhardt, F., and Erikson, R.L. (1979): J. Virol., 29:1196-1203.
4. Cohen, S., Carpenter, G., and King, L., Jr. (1980): J. Biol. Chem., 255:4834-4842.
5. Collett, M.S., Brugge, J.S., and Erikson, R.L. (1978): Cell, 15:1363-1369.
6. Collett, M.S., and Erikson, R.L. (1978): Proc. Natl. Acad. Sci. USA, 75:2021-2024.
7. Collett, M.S., Erikson, E., Purchio, A.F., Brugge, J.S., and Erikson, R.L. (1979): Proc. Natl. Acad. Sci. USA, 76:3159-3163.
8. Collett, M.S., Erikson, E., and Erikson, R.L. (1979): J. Virol., 29:770-781.
9. Collett, M.S., Purchio, A.F., and Erikson, R.L. (1980): Nature, 285:167-169.
10. Erikson, R.L., Collett, M.S., Erikson, E., and Purchio, A.F. (1979): Proc. Natl. Acad. Sci. USA, 76:6260-6264.
11. Erikson, R.L., Collett, M.S., Erikson, E., Purchio, A.F., and Brugge, J.S. (1979): Cold Spring Harbor Symp. Quant. Biol., 44:907-917.
12. Erikson, E., and Erikson, R.L. (1980): Cell, 21:829-836.
13. Erikson, E., Cook, R., Miller, G.J., and Erikson, R.L. (1981): Mol. Cell. Biol., 1:43-50.
14. Feldman, R.A., Hanafusa, T., and Hanafusa, H. (1980): Cell, 22:757-765.
15. Hashimoto, E., Takeda, M., Nishizuka, Y., Kamana, K., and Iwai, K. (1976): J. Biol. Chem., 251: 6287-6293.
16. Hunter, T., and Sefton, B.M. (1980): Proc. Natl. Acad. Sci. USA, 77:1311-1315.
17. Kessler, S.W. (1975): J. Immunol., 115:1617-1624.
18. Laemmli, U.K. (1970): Nature, 227:680-685.
19. Oppermann, H., Levinson, A.D., Varmus, H.E., Levintow, L., and Bishop, J.M. (1979): Proc. Natl. Acad. Sci. USA, 76:1804-1808.
20. Neil, J.C., Ghysdael, J., and Vogt, P.K. (1981): Virology, 109: 223-228.
21. Purchio, A.F., Erikson, E., Brugge, J.S., and Erikson, R.L. (1978): Proc. Natl. Acad. Sci. USA, 75:1567-1571.

22. Purchio, A.F., Erikson, E., Collett, M.S., and Erikson, R.L. (1980): In: Cold Spring Harbor Conference on Cell Proliferation-Protein Phosphorylation, Vol. 8 (in press).
23. Radke, K., and Martin, G.S. (1979): Proc. Natl. Acad. Sci. USA, 76:5212-5216.
24. Spector, D.H., Smith, K., Padgett, T., McCombe, P., Roulland-Dussoix, D., Moscovici, C., Varmus, H.E., and Bishop, J.M. (1978): Cell, 13:371-379.
25. Spector, D.H., Baker, B., Varmus, H.E., and Bishop, J.M. (1978): Cell, 13:381-386.
26. Stehelin, D., Varmus, H.E., Bishop, J.M., and Vogt, P.K. (1976): Nature, 260:170-173.
27. Ushiro, H., and Cohen, S. (1980): J. Biol. Chem., 255:8363-8365.
28. Vogt, P.K. (1977): In: Comprehensive Virology, edited by H. Fraenkel-Conrat and R.R. Wagner, Vol. 9, pp. 341-455, Plenum Publishing Corp., New York.
29. Wang, S.Y., Hayward, W.S., and Hanafusa, H. (1977): J. Virol., 24:64-73.

Expression of Differentiated Functions in Cancer Cells, edited by R. F. Revoltella et al., Raven Press, New York © 1982.

Genetic Analysis of Pathogenic and Non-Pathogenic Avian Retroviruses

John M. Coffin, Kathleen F. Conklin, Philip N. Tsichlis, and *Harriet L. Robinson

*Department of Molecular Biology and Microbiology, Tufts University School of Medicine, Boston, Massachusetts 02111; *Worcester Foundation for Experimental Biology, Shrewsbury, Massachusetts 01545*

The avian tumor viruses can be classified into three groups depending on their pathogenicity and lifestyle (Table 1). The majority of isolates are the nontransforming viruses, such as the avian leukosis viruses (ALV), which are endemic in many flocks of chickens and are responsible for a variety of malignancies, most commonly B-cell lymphomas which have a long latent period (6 months or more). These viruses are transmitted horizontally, both from one individual to another and from mother to offspring via infection of the egg. The genome of these viruses consists only of information required for virus replication.

TABLE 1. Types of Avian Tumor Viruses

Type	Growth Rate	Pathogenicity	Transmission	Composition
Exogenous				
transforming	rapid	rapid	laboratory	gag-pol-env-src-U_3 or gag-onc-U_3
non-transforming	rapid	slow	horizontal	gag-pol-env-U_3
endogenous	slow	none	genetic	gag-pol-env-U_3

A rarer group of isolates includes the transforming viruses, which are related to (and probably derived from) the nontransforming viruses by acquisition of all or part of a cellular gene (generally called an onc gene) either in place of (as with most isolates) or in addition to (as with nondefective Rous sarcoma virus) the replicative information (for review, see 3, 7). These viruses induce rapid transformation in vitro and rapid disease in animals, with a latency of about 5-20 days, and their ability to induce disease is directly attributable to the product of the onc gene. There is little or no evidence for

horizontal transmission of transforming viruses and it is quite likely
that each isolate has arisen independently as a result of a recombination event between an ALV and a c-onc sequence in the animal from
which it was isolated. Recent evidence (10,18,19) has supported the
proposition (4,28) that the nontransforming viruses also cause disease
by modifying the activity of cellular onc genes. In particular,
integration of a provirus adjacent to a cellular onc gene (c-myc) is
a feature common to most ALV-induced lymphomas. The integration occurs
in such a way that the promoter within the 3' copy of the U3 region of
the proviral LTR could act directly to stimulate transcription of
c-myc (Figure 1).

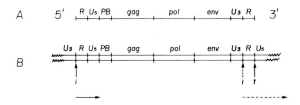

FIG. 1. The ALV genome and provirus. The top line shows the genome of
avian leukosis virus with the coding (gag, pol, and env) and non-coding
regions. The double line at the bottom shows the integrated provirus
with the long terminal repeat (LTR) of U3-R-U5. Probable sites of
initiation and termination of transcription are shown by i and t
respectively. Note that use of the initiation site in the 3' LTR would
lead to transcription into the cell genome.

The endogenous viruses of chickens are closely related to the
exogenous viruses (for review see 21), yet differ in important characteristics. First, their primary mode of transmission is genetic, as
stably integrated proviruses, with structural features identical to
those acquired by infection (12, 13, 25). These proviruses have been
classified by Astrin and coworkers (1, 2, 26) into a set of endogenous virus (ev) loci, depending on the phenotype they confer and
their site of residence (Table 2). The provirus associated with ev-1,
for example, is found in a very high proportion of white leghorn
chickens (26), yet is usually almost completely inactive transcriptionally (9) and confers no apparent virus-releated phenotype on cells

TABLE 2. Properties of Endogenous Proviruses

Locus	Frequency (% of chickens)	Expression (genomes/cell)	Defect
ev-1	99+	0.5-1	pol (no obvious deletion)
ev-2	5	0.1	none (inducible to RAV-0)
ev-3	16	100	gag-pol deletion
ev-6	14	100	LTR-gag deletion
ev-7	14	?	env?
ev-9	4	100	pol?
ev-10	3	?	none (inducible to C-ILV)

which contain it. The ev-2 provirus, by contrast, is also almost silent, yet it encodes complete infectious virus (RAV-0), and, under permissive conditions, ev-2-containing cells can be reinfected with the small amount of RAV-0 produced (8). Such reinfected cells acquire a new RAV-0 provirus which is expressed at levels more than 1000-fold greater than that of the inherited ev-2 (9). Clearly, there is some nonheritable block to transcription affecting the endogenous but not the genetically identical exogenous acquired provirus.

Even when expressed at high levels as a result of reinfection, RAV-0 replicates substantially more slowly than exogenous ALV (16, 23), and is completely nonpathogenic (17,22). These features are most likely related to one another and to the endogenous lifestyle, since it is easy to imagine that a pathogenic virus would be counterselected as an endogenous virus.

The studies described in this report were undertaken to learn more about the mechanisms of the control of virus replication and pathogenicity by using the endogenous viruses as a model system. We have found (i) that the endogenous viruses form a lineage distinct from exogenous viruses although they are very closely related to one another; (ii) that the low expression of inherited proviruses is associated with methylation of the proviral DNA; (iii) that the common provirus ev-1 lacks infectivity due to a mutation that leads to non-expression of pol; (iv) that the primary difference affecting growth rate between endogenous and exogenous ALV is in the U_3 region; and (v) that this difference is partly, but not entirely responsible for the difference in pathogenicity between these viruses.

RESULTS AND DISCUSSION

Relationship Between Endogenous and Exogenous Viruses

For a number of years, we have been obtaining T_1 oligonucleotide fingerprints of a variety of endogenous and exogenous avian tumor virus genomes and comparing their oligonucleotide maps (5, Coffin, et al., in preparation). This method of analysis is the most sensitive available (short of complete sequence analysis) for comparison of RNA's. A typical fingerprint displays about 30-40 unique oligonucleotides, containing about 600 nucleotides. A single base change is revealed as a loss or alteration in an oligonucleotide, so that two genomes differing by as little as 1% random divergence will yield fingerprints that

differ, on average, by 6 oligonucleotides. An example of this comparison is shown in Figure 2 for an exogenous virus and three different
endogenous viruses (i.e. products of different ev loci). It is
apparent that there are three classes of oligonucleotides: those
identical in all four viruses, those found only in endogenous viruses,
and those unique to a single isolate. Thus, endogenous and exogenous
viruses are closely related, yet form distant lineages, and the
products of different ev loci are closely related, distinguishable
one from the other. Figure 3 shows a collection of oligonucleotide
maps, based on that of RAV-0 (6). The oligonucleotide order and gene
assignment that we previously determined have recently been confirmed
by nucleotide sequencing (D. Schwartz, personal communication).
Oligonucleotides found in RAV-0 are shown as open regions; different
(or missing) oligonucleotides as shaded regions; and deleted or undetermined regions are shown as dotted lines. It is apparent that sequence differences between the groups of viruses are found in all parts
of the genome; however, they are greatest in the subgroup coding portion of env (6, 27) and in U3. The former difference is not surprising, since all endogenous viruses are of a subgroup (E) distinct from
that of all exogenous viruses (A-D) (21).

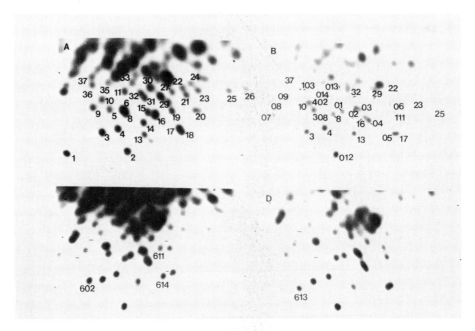

FIG. 2.   The genomes of an exogenous and 3 endogenous avian tumor
viruses. T_1 oligonucleotide fingerprints of labeled genome RNA of
(A) Pr-RSV-B; (B) RAV-0 (the product of ev-2); (C) C-ILV (ev-10); and
15B E virus (a recombinant between ev-1 and ev-7) were prepared as
described (5). The numbering of unique oligonucleotides follows
our usual convention, with identical oligonucleotides assigned the
same numbers. Only oligonucleotides not shared with RAV-0 are numbered
in C and D.

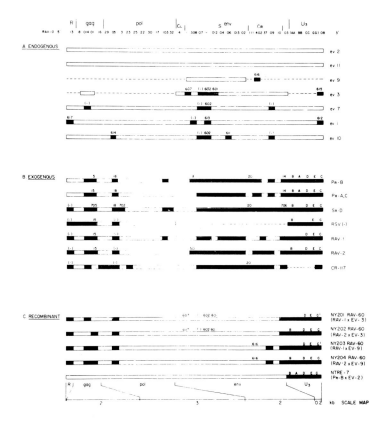

FIG. 3. <u>Oligonucleotide maps of avian tumor viruses</u>. The top line
shows the oligonucleotide map and gene assignment of the genome of
RAV-0 (6). The maps of other genomes are shown by comparison to
that of RAV-0, with open regions indicating the presence of identical
oligonucleotides and shaded regions the absence of RAV-0 specific
oligonucleotides. Deleted lines indicate deletions or undetermined
regions. The bottom line shows a scale map deduced from restriction
maps and the molecular weights of the gene products.

From the few oligonucleotide differences among the endogenous
viruses, we can infer the relationship scheme shown in Figure 4. We
conclude the following. (i) These viruses appear to be diverged
in three distinct lines from an ancestor most similar to RAV-0 (ev-2).
(ii) <u>Ev</u>-1, although by far the most widespread of the endogenous
proviruses in white leghorn chickens, is the most distantly related to
the others. (iii) The most distant relationship (between <u>ev</u>-10 and
<u>ev</u>-1) is 10 oligonucleotide differences, each probably the consequence
of a single base change. This would correspond to less than 2% random
sequence divergence. (iv) The pattern of defectiveness of various
loci (Table 2) has no particular relationship to their position in this
scheme, suggesting that the defects arose very late in the evolutionary history of each provirus.

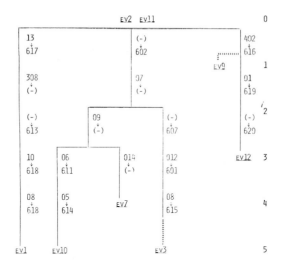

FIG. 4. <u>Relationships among ev proviruses</u>. The numbers adjacent to
the lines indicate the minimal sequence changes (by reference
to oligonucleotide numbers) necessary to change one virus genome to
another. The column at the right shows the number of such changes.
The dotted lines connecting <u>ev</u>-3 and <u>ev</u>-4 reflect the absence of
complete information for these proviruses.

Expression and Induction of the ev-1 Provirus

The <u>ev</u>-1 provirus is found in virtually all white leghorn chickens
(26) yet is expressed at a low level and confers no detectable phenotype. Those two characteristics are most likely unrelated, since the
<u>ev</u>-2 provirus is expressed at a still lower level (9), yet suscept-
ible <u>ev</u>-2 cells became sponanteously virus producing early in life.
An entry into the <u>ev</u>-1 problem was provided by the chance finding of
an embryo, number 1836 (<u>ev</u>-1, <u>ev</u>-6), whose fibroblasts spontaneously
produced a high level of non-infectious virions with a <u>gag</u> protein
composition resembling that of other endogenous viruses (Figure 5).
These virions also contained <u>env</u> proteins (most likely due to <u>ev</u>-6,
see below) but no <u>pol</u> products or reverse transcriptase activity,
accounting for the lack of infectivity. The production of virions
must have been due to <u>ev</u>-1, since <u>ev</u>-6 has a deletion including most
or all of <u>gag</u> (9, 13). Analysis of a number of sibling embryos
from the same cross, such as 1831 (<u>ev</u>-1) and 1837 (<u>ev</u>-1, 6) revealed
that only 1836 had this phenotype, suggesting that some nonheritable
alteration in this embryo was responsible for the spontaneous induction
of <u>ev</u>-1. Once such nonheritable modification hypothesized to affect
transcription is methylation of DNA at dC residues, specifically in
the dinucleotide dCdG (20). It was recently observed that treatment
of cells with the analog 5-azacytidine could lead to the rapid

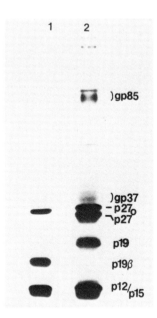

FIG. 5. Virions released from 1836 cells. Virions were sedimented
from supernatant medium of 35S-methionine labelled 1836 (lane 1) or
control ALV-infected cells (lane 2). The 1836 particles were immune-
precipitated with anti-gag antiserum and both preparations were analyzed by SDS-polyacrylamide gel electrophoresis and autoradiography.

demethylation of DNA and a variety of phenotypic changes (14). To
test the possibility that methylation might be involved in the
"repression" of the ev-1 provirus, 1831, 1836, and 1837 fibroblasts
were treated with 3µM 5-azacytidine for 24 hours, and the expression
of virus related proteins was monitored by immune precipitation of
35S-methionine labelled cell proteins with anti-gag antiserum
(Figure 6A). Untreated 1831 and 1837 cells (lanes 5 and 6) contained
no detectable gag related polypeptides, whereas 1837 cells contained
ΔPr76 and the usual pattern of processing products (lane 7). Five days
after azacytidine treatment, however, both 1831 and 1837 cells (lanes
8 and 9) synthesized an identical pattern of gag-related peptides
in amounts not distinguishably different from 1836, which was apparently unaffected by the treatment. That the expression of ev-1 induced
by 5-azacytidine was permanent is suggested by the continued expression
of ev-1 10 days after treatment (lanes 11 and 13) and even as late as
30 days after treatment (data not shown). That alterations in methylation are associated with this high level of expression is also
suggested by a direct analysis of the DNA of these cultures using
methyl-sensitive restriction enzymes (data not shown). Thus, methylation of dC residues seems to be intimately involved with the low
expression of ev-1, and, by extension, other endogenous proviruses as
well.

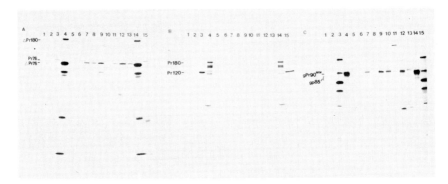

FIG. 6. Virus-related proteins of ev-1 containing cells. 1831, 1836, and 1837 cells were left untreated or were treated for 24 hours with 3μM 5-azacytidine. Five or ten days later, the cells were labelled for two hours with 35S-methionine and extracts were immuneprecipitated with (A) anti-gag, (B) anti-pol or (C) anti-env serum. 1831 cells are shown in lanes 5, 8, and 11; 1837 cells in lanes 6, 9, and 12; and 1836 in lanes 7, 10, and 13 of each set. Lanes 5-7, untreated, lanes 8-10, treated with 5-azacytidine, 5 days, lanes 11-13, treated, 10 days. The outside lanes show controls: lanes 1 and 2 uninfected cells; lanes 3, 4, 14, and 15, cells infected with marker viruses.

    The gels in Figure 6 also provide a clue as to the defectiveness of ev-1. In no case was any protein precipitated with anti-pol serum (Panel B), and no polypeptide larger than 76,000 was precipitated by anti-gag serum (Panel A), although in both cases the Pr180 gag-pol fusion protein was precipitated from control infected cells (lanes 4 and 14). Thus there seems to be a complete failure to synthesize any gag or pol-related protein larger than Pr76. This could be due either to a termination mutant immediately following gag, or (more interestingly) to a failure to process pol mRNA correctly. An additional defect in ev-1 was revealed by precipitation with anti-env serum using 1831 cells (Panel C, lanes 8 and 11) (the other cells contain ev-6 which encodes a high level of env protein). Although Pr90 env is synthesized and glycosylated, it is not processed to mature gp85 and gp37, nor is it incorporated into virions. Again, the basis for this defect is not known.
    The phenotype of ev-1 is of some virological importance, since most cells used for growth and analysis of avian tumor viruses contain this provirus, and we have found that recombinants with ev-1 which acquire a subgroup E host range can readily be obtained from stocks of exogenous virus grown on ev-1 containing cells. Indeed, we have recently found that a host range variant of RSV, which we had previously attributed to mutation (30), was in fact a recombinant with ev-1. Similarly, gag proteins with distinctive ev-1 size and peptide

markers are frequently found on recombinant viruses (24) and a recently described "mutant" has an identical env processing defect (15), and its genome contains underline{ev}-1 specific markers (K. Conklin, unpublished).

Role of the U3 Region in Growth and Oncogenicity

The region of greatest sequence divergence between the genomes of rapidly replicating exogenous avian tumor viruses and slowly replicating benign endogenous viruses is the U_3 region (6, 11). In previous experiments, we found that all recombinants between endogenous and exogenous viruses selected for subgroup E and rapid replication inherited the U_3 region of the exogenous parent (27, 28, 29), implying that the U_3 region difference was the only determinant encoding the difference in growth rate. We have recently confirmed this conclusion using the five recombinant viruses shown at the bottom of Figure 3. All of these viruses had identical growth rates in culture which were about 30-fold higher than that of RAV-O (data not shown). Note in particular that NTRE-7 is identical to RAV-O except for the exogenous U_3 region. Since the U_3 region contains the promoter for virus RNA synthesis (3,1), the difference is almost certainly due to a major (perhaps 10-30 fold) difference in promoter efficiency.

TABLE 3. Disease Induced by NTRE-7, RAV-60, and RAV-O

Tissue	Disease	Number of Cases		
		NTRE-7 (75)[a]	RAV-60 (87)[a]	RAV-O (58)[a]
mesenchyme	fibrosarcoma	2	1	0
	chondrosarcoma	1	0	0
	osteopetrosis	3	2	0
hematopoetic	anemia	0	2	0
	lymphoma	3	41	0
kidney	adenocarcinoma	1	0	0
	nephroblastoma	1	0	0
unknown	wasting	0	10	0

a. number of birds in each group

Based on these results, we suggested (28) that the most straightforward explanation for the nonpathogenicity of endogenous viruses was that the U_3 promoter was not efficient enough to give rise to oncogenic levels of downstream transcripts (see Figure 1). To test this point directly, the five recombinant viruses and RAV-O were inoculated into one-day old chicks. At three months, the chicks were tested for the level of viremia. Although there was a wide scatter in the results (due in part to variability in the immune response), the median level of circulating virus was that predicted from the cell culture results; i.e., the four RAV-O's and NTRE-7 were equal, and RAV-O was about 10-fold lower. Similar results were obtained by analysis of viral antigen in the bursa of Fabricius (the primary target organ). Thus, the U_3 region also encodes a relatively rapid replication rate in the whole animal. The birds were subsequently held until 1 year of age and

monitored for neoplasms associated with ALV infections. The results
are shown in Table 3. As previously reported (17), there was no disease at all associated with RAV-0 infection. However, all four
RAV-60's tested had a pathogenicity identical to that of RAV-1, a
control "standard" ALV; i.e. about 50% incidence of lymphoma with a
mean latency of about 30 weeks (22), and a small proportion of a
variety of other diseases with a latency of one year or more. To our
surprise, NTRE-7 had a very limited pathogenicity, amounting to some
13%, and there was no significantly higher incidence of any one
disease, in particular lymphoma or osteopetrosis. (Several isolates
of ALV induce osteopetrosis as their principal disease; preliminary
evidence suggests that this is also true of td Pr-RSV-B, the exogenous
parent of NTRE-7). Thus, although disease incidence induced by NTRE-7
was significantly higher that that of RAV-0, it was significantly lower
that that of the RAV-60's or ALV, and more closely resembled the "background" diseases seen with these viruses. These results imply that the
U_3 region (presumably by virtue of promoter efficiency) is important
to disease process, but that some other region of the genome also
plays a role, in such a way that results in "targeting" toward
particular cell types, to result in high incidence of lymphoma or
osteophetrosis, for example.

    At the moment, we have no definitive evidence for what the relevant
other region of the genome is or how it might affect such targeting.
Recent nucleotide sequence analysis confirms the structure shown in
Figure 3 for the genome of NTRE-7. The U_3 region is identical to that
of its parent, and there seems to be a crossover point within a
"spacer" noncoding region of about 290 nucleotides between the 3' end
of env and the beginning of U_3 (P. Tsichlis, unpublished). Comparison
with the RAV-60 genomes shown in Figure 3 suggests that the most
significant difference between these genomes and NTRE-7 is in the
position of this crossover, which in the RAV-60's is substantially
more 5', somewhere within env. It is conceivable that there is some
as yet unrecognized role of gp37 in this process. Alternatively,
the sequence 5' of U_3 is positioned in such a way that it could contain
elements specifically regulating promotion from the adjacent U_3 region,
but not the 5' U_3 region and thus control downstream promotion but
not replication.

    Unfortunately, these experiments have stretched the resolution of
fingerprinting techniques to its limit, and we are now resorting to
recombinant DNA technology to reassemble specific recombinant viruses
and to test these hypotheses.

REFERENCES

1. Astrin, S. (1978): Proc. Natl. Acad. Sci. U.S.A. 75: 5941-5945.
2. Astrin, S.M., Robinson, H.L., Crittenden, L.B., Buss, E.G., Wyban,
    J., and Hayward, W.S. (1980): Cold Spring Harbor Symp. Quant.
    Biol. 44: 1105-1109.
3. Bishop, J.M. (1981): Cell 1: 5-6.
4. Bishop, J.M., Courtneidge, S.A., Levinson, A.D., Oppermann, H.,
    Quintrell, N., Sheiness, D.K., Weiss, S.R., and Varmus, H.E.
    (1980): Cold Spring Harbor Symp. Quant. Biol. 44: 919-930.
5. Coffin, J.M. and Billeter, M.A. (1976): J. Mol. Biol. 100: 293-318

6. Coffin, J., Champion, M., and Chabot, F. (1978): J. Virol. 28: 972-991.
7. Coffin, J.M., Varmus, H.E., Bishop, J.M., Essex, M., Hardy, W.D., Martin, G.S., Rosenberg, N.E., Scolnick, E.M., Weinberg, R.A., and Vogt, P.K. (1981): J. Virol. (in press).
8. Cooper, G.M. and Temin, H.M. (1976): J. Virol. 17: 422-430.
9. Hayward, W.S., Braverman, S.B., and Astrin, S.M. (1979): Cold Spring Harbor Symp. Quant. Biol. 44: 1111-1121.
10. Hayward, W.S., Neel, B.G., and Astrin, S.M. (1981): Nature 290: 475-480.
11. Hishinuma, F., DeBona, P.J., Astrin, S., and Skalka, A.M. (1981): Cell 1: 155-164.
12. Hughes, S.H., Payvar, F., Spector, D., Shinke, R.T., Robinson, H.L., Payne, G., Bishop, J.M., and Varmus, H.E. (1979): Cell 18: 347-359.
13. Hughes, S.H., Toyoshima, K., Bishop, J.M., and Varmus, H.E. (1981): Virology 108: 189-207.
14. Jones, P.A. and Taylor, S.M. (1980): Cell 20: 85-93.
15. Linial, M., Fenno, J., Burnette, W.N., and Rohrschneider, L. (1980): J. Virol. 36: 280-290.
16. Linial, M. and Neiman, P.E. (1976): Virology 73: 508-520.
17. Motta, J., Crittenden, L., Purchase, H., Stone, H., Okazaki, W., and Witter, R. (1975): J. Natl. Cancer Inst. 55: 685-689.
18. Neel, B.G., Hayward, W.S., Robinson, H.L., Fung, J., and Astrin, S.M. (1981). Cell 23: 323-334.
19. Payne, G.S., Courtneidge, S.A., Crittenden, L.B., Fadly, A.M., Bishop, J.M., and Varmus, H.E. (1981): Cell 23: 311-322.
20. Razin, A. and Riggs, A.D. (1980): Science 210: 604-610.
21. Robinson, H. (1978): Curr. Topics Microbiol. and Immunol. 83: 1-36.
22. Robinson, H.L., Pearson, M.N., Tsichlis, P.N. and Coffin, J.M. (1980): In: Viruses in Naturally Occurring Cancer, edited by M. Essex, G. Todaro, and H. ZurHausen, pp. 543-552, Cold Spring Harbor Press, New York.
23. Robinson, H.L., Swanson, C.A., Hruska, J.F., and Crittenden, L.B. (1978): Virology 69: 63-74.
24. Shaikh, R., Linial, M., Coffin, J., and Eisenman, R. (1978): Virology 87: 326-328.
25. Skalka, A., DeBona, P., Hishinuma, F., and McClements W. (1980): Cold Spring Harbor Symp. Quant. Biol. 44:
26. Tereba, A. and Astrin, S.M. (1980): J. Virol 35: 888-894.
27. Tsichlis, P.N. and Coffin, J.M. (1980a): J. Virol. 33: 238-249.
28. Tsichlis, P.N. and Coffin, J.M. (1980b): Cold Spring Harbor Symp. Quant. Biol. 44: 1123-1132.
29. Tsichlis, P. and Coffin, J. (1979): Proc. Natl. Acad. Sci. USA 76: 3001-3005.
30. Tsichlis, P.N., Conklin, K.F., and Coffin, J.M.: (1980). Proc. Natl. Acad. Sci. U.S.A. 77: 536-540.
31. Yamamoto, T., deCrombrugghe, B., and Pastan, I. (1980): Cell 22: 787-798.

Expression of Differentiated Functions in Cancer Cells, edited by R. F. Revoltella et al., Raven Press, New York © 1982.

Continuous Lines of AMV-Transformed Nonproducer Cells: Growth and Oncogenic Potential in the Chick Embryo

Carlo Moscovici, Nancy Zeller, and M. G. Moscovici

Department of Pathology, College of Medicine, University of Florida, and Tumor Virology Laboratory, Research Service, Veterans Administration Medical Center, Gainesville, Florida 32602

Within the past few years, a large collection of data has accumulated with regard to the biology and molecular biology of avian defective leukemia viruses (6, 17, 18, 23, 34). This group of viruses has been shown to share some common features: i.e. they are all replication-defective; they are all able to transform cells of hemopoietic origin together with cells of connective tissue origin (the only exception is AMV, which does not transform fibroblast cells); and finally they all can induce leukemia in the chicken after short periods of latency. Hence, one could divide the numerous isolates of avian defective leukemia viruses studied so far into two large groups, affecting either the myeloid or the erythroid lineage of the chicken hemopoietic system. This arbitrary classification at present should be considered provisional, since some avian leukemia viruses may simultaneously interact and cause neoplasia in vivo with target cells of both myeloid and erythroid origin (C. Moscovici et al., in preparation).

Our studies have focused primarily on the avian defective viruses, particularly of avian myeloblastosis virus (AMV) that cause myeloid leukemia (23). Previous experiments have shown that after infection of hemopoietic cells with AMV, it was possible to obtain continuous lines of nonadherent transformed cells that could permanently release infectious virus (23, 26). These cells were also found to carry distinctive markers of myeloid differentiation (16).

Similar results were obtained with a long-term line of AMV-nonproducer cells (NPs), which has been recently described (26). This prompted us to study in detail the growth and differentiation of NPs and their biological characterization. The present study examines the fate of these cells when injected into the chicken embryo and the rescue of leukemogenic virus from injected NPs by superinfection of the helper in vivo. Results will be presented with regard to the differentiation and proliferation of transformed cells in an embryonic milieu, together with their role in the oncogenic response in the chicken.

MATERIALS AND METHODS

Cells

The NP AMV myeloblastic cell line originated from the infection of 17-day-old SPAFAS embryonic bone marrow cells with AMV-B at a low multiplicity of infection (m.o.i. of 0.01 to 0.001) (26). The infected cells were prepared in soft agar and developed into colonies, which were picked into linbro wells as described (32). Supernatant fluids from actively growing colonies were tested for the production of virus by reverse transcriptase and conventional biological assays. The NP cell

line GM 727 was obtained and has been maintained in culture for more
than 2½ years.

Two additional cell lines, 5YS and BM2, were originated from the
recovery of GM 727 cells from the yolk sac of an embryo and the bone
marrow of a bird after injection in ovum, respectively.

Myeloblasts derived from a leukemic bird that produced infectious
AMV-C cultured in vitro were also used.

Viruses

The nondefective helper viruses MAV-2 and RAV-7 were used in this
study. MAV-2 was cloned by plaque assay (24) and RAV-7 by the interference assay (35). AMV-B stocks originated from individual foci of
transformed yolk sac macrophages.

Cell Cultures

Bone marrow cultures were prepared from birds injected with NPs. The
tibias were freed of all muscle and membranes and rinsed three times
with Tris buffer. The cells were obtained by flushing media through the
bone marrow with a syringe. The cell clumps were broken up by pipetting
and were then seeded at a density of 75×10^6/100 mm dish. After 24 hr
the cells in suspension were transferred to another tissue culture dish.

The NP AMV myeloblasts were grown at a density of $6-10 \times 10^6$ cells/ml
in BT-88 (4) medium plus 160 µg/100 ml of folic acid.

Assays

The soft agar colony technique was used to isolate the NPs from bone
marrow and yolk sac cultures. The yolk sac cells were prepared as
described (25). The cells were mixed with soft agar medium (12) at a
density of 1×10^5/35-mm tissue culture dish. Bone marrow cells were
seeded at the same density in soft agar.

To test for the presence of virus in cell supernatants, we used
transforming assay (23), the plaque assay (24), and the reverse
transcriptase assay (8).

For cytotoxicity assays the NPs were washed twice in serum-free
medium and placed in the microtiter wells at a concentration of 1×10^6 cells in 0.1 ml. Next, 0.1 ml of the diluted test serum was added,
and the plates were incubated at 4°C for 30 min. Freshly isolated
chicken complement, 0.05 ml, was then added, and the plates were incubated at 37°C for 15 min. The cells were stained with trypan blue and
counted. Antiserum to chicken red blood cells and chicken red blood
cells were used as a positive control.

In Vivo Experiments

The NPs were washed once in Tris, and 0.1 ml samples of cell suspension at various concentrations were injected into 13-day-old (C/E SPAFAS
Inc., Norwich, Conn.) embryos via the chorioallantoic veins (5).

In the challenge experiments, 10^6 plaque-forming units of MAV-2
helper virus and 10^4 interfering units of RAV-7 helper virus,
respectively, in 0.1-ml aliquots were injected into the chorioallantoic
veins of the embryos by reopening the egg or into the wing web vein of
hatched birds. For the experiments with labeled NP, the cells were

washed three times in Tris buffer and 0.1 ml of the cell suspension was injected.

Weekly blood smears were made from all hatched chickens. Bone marrow, liver, and spleen samples from sacrificed birds were fixed and prepared for histological observation and stained with hematoxylin and eosin.

Detection of NP In Vivo with [125]IUDR Radioactive Labeling

In the preparation of [125]IUDR-labeled NPs, the cells were cultured for 72 hr with two changes of [125]IUDR medium. The labeling medium consisted of normal growth medium without tryptose phosphate broth and with 0.1 μCi/ml ^{125}I-iodo-2'-deoxyuridine ([125]IUDR) (specific activity 10^2-10^3 mCi/μg (New England Nuclear Corp., Boston, Mass.). Concentrations of [125]IUDR > 0.1 μCi/ml slowed the growth of the cells.

The percentage of labeled cells was determined by autoradiography (15). Briefly, a cytocentrifuge preparation of the cells was made and then dipped into a 1:2 dilution of NTB$_2$ emulsion (Kodak) and incubated for 7 to 14 days.

The technique used to detect the [125]IUDR-labeled NPs was described by Fidler (15) with the following modifications: Each embryo was injected with 3-10 x 10^6 [125]IUDR-labeled cells. A representative sample of the inoculum was counted and radioactively measured. The embryos were sacrificed 2 hr, 24 hr, and 4 days after injection of the labeled cells. The embryos and surrounding membranes and fluids were recovered. Solid organs and membranes were rinsed three times over a 3-day period with 70% ethanol to remove any nonspecific counts. Fidler (15) and Dethlefsen (9) have shown that radioactivity was associated with whole cell DNA in living cells.

As a control, the NPs were heat-killed at 70°C for 10 min. The cells were intact but not viable as determined with trypan blue staining and autoradiography. The killed labeled cells were injected at the same concentration as were the viable NPs, and the embryos were sacrificed after the same intervals of time. The organs, membranes, and fluids were measured for radioactivity.

Other controls included injecting free [125]IUDR, AMV-C-producer myeloblasts, normal bone marrow cells from a 1-week-old bird, and normal yolk sac macrophages from 13-day-old embryos. All the above control cells were labeled, injected, and radioactively monitored in the same manner as for the NPs.

All radioactive measurements were made with a well-type of scintillation counter having a sodium iodide crystal (Abbott Laboratories) with an efficiency of 54%.

Suicide Experiments

The suicide experiments were done as described (33). The [125]IUDR-labeled NPs were injected in ovum, and 48 hr later the eggs were injected again with either 0.1 mCi ^{3}H-thymidine (specific activity 72 Ci/mmol, in aqueous solution, New England Nuclear) or 0.005 μmol unlabeled thymidine in 0.1 ml; both were made isotonic. The embryos were killed 24 and 48 hr later. Half the yolk sac was measured for ^{125}I radioactivity to determine the number of NPs present, and the second half was seeded in soft agar so that the efficiency of the NP colony could be determined.

RESULTS

Origin and Maintenance of 727 NP Line

Three NP cell lines were developed as described in Materials and Methods. Of 14 single clones examined, only one, No. 727, developed into a cell line growing with a doubling time of 48-72 hr. The cells continued to grow in suspension at an ideal density of 6-10 x 10^6 cells/ml, preferably in 60-mm Falcon plastic dishes. Unless stated, most of this study was conducted with line 727.

Some of the properties of the 727 NP are listed in Table 1. The cells exhibit characteristics of myeloblasts. They are positive for Fc receptors, can phagocytize latex particles, are negative for complement receptors and immune phagocytosis, and produce colonies indistinguishable from AMV producer myeloblasts in soft agar. Some virus-specific products are made by these cells, and infectious virions were never detected by the reverse transcriptase assay or conventional biological assays. The NPs do however synthesize a virus that lacks genetic information for envelope glycoprotein and reverse transcriptase (13). This virus probably falls in the same category as the recently described defective leukemia virus OK10 (30). When superinfected with helper leukosis viruses, infectious AMV can be rescued from NP cells. In conclusion, the NPs have the same functional markers as do the producer myeloblasts described previously (16).

TABLE 1. Characteristics of AMV-induced nonproducer cell line 727

Fc receptor	Positive
Complement receptor	Negative
Nonspecific phagocytosis (latex particles)	Positive
Immune phagocytosis	Negative
GAG POL precursor protein (Pr 180)	Positive
GAG precursor protein (Pr 76)	Positive
GAG protein (P27)	$\pm$
ENV precursor protein (Pr 90)	Negative
AMV rescuability with helper virus	Positive
Type II colonies in semi-solid medium	Positive

Proliferation and Oncogenicity of NPs

From 5 to 35 x 10^6 NPs were injected into 13-day-old embryos (Table 2). Overt leukemia was not observed in any of the injected birds up to 1 year after injection.

We attempted to reisolate NPs from a few organs of birds injected with different amounts of NPs. Table 2 shows that indeed we were able to reisolate the NPs from bone marrows up to 4 weeks after injection of 35 x 10^6 NPs of line 727. Nonproducers were also reisolated from livers and spleens, respectively (data not shown). Interestingly, histopathologic examination of all the marrows in the group injected with line 727 at different cell concentrations showed that only one bird developed a myeloproliferative disorder, and this was at 4 months after injection.

TABLE 2. Retrieval of nonproducer myeloblasts (NP) from bone marrows of chickens injected as embryos

Time Elapsed[a] Post NP Injection	5-10 X 10^6 727 NP Injected/13-day-old embryo		35 X 10^6 727 NP Injected/13-day-old embryo		35 X 10^6 5YS NP Injected/13-day-old embryo	
	NP Recovered	Histopathology	NP Recovered	Histopathology	NP Recovered	Histopathology
24 hr	1 positive	1 normal				
5 days	1 positive	1 normal				
2 wk	7 positive 1 negative	8 normal	2 positive	2 normal	1 negative 1 positive	1 myeloprolif. 1 normal
3 wk	3 negative	3 normal	2 positive	2 normal	1 negative 1 negative	1 myeloprolif. 1 normal
4 wk	6 negative	6 normal	2 positive	2 normal	1 positive	1 myeloprolif.
5 wk	4 negative	4 normal	2 negative	2 normal	2 negative 1 negative	2 myeloprolif. 1 normal
6 wk	2 negative	2 normal	2 negative	2 normal	1 negative	1 myeloprolif.
3 mo	6 negative	6 normal				
4 mo	4 negative	1 myeloprolif. 3 normal			1 negative	1 negative
8 mo	3 negative	3 normal				
1 yr	8 negative	8 normal				
Total No. of birds examined	46		10		13	

Similar results were obtained when another NP line, namely 5YS, was
tested in vivo. Line 5YS originated from the reisolation of NPs from
the yolk sac culture of an embryo 5 days after the intravenous injection
of the 727 cell line. Table 2 shows that 5YS cells, when tested in vivo
in the same manner as for the 727 line, were being retrieved from bone
marrow cultures of chicken 4 weeks after embryonic injection. A marked
difference however was observed during histologic examination of the
bone marrows. They showed that a myeloproliferative disorder was present in 6 of 13 birds (46%), compared with 1 of 46 birds (2.1%) used
with the 727 group. The myeloproliferative disorder was still present
in birds killed after 5 and 6 weeks after injection (Table 2).
Reisolation of nonproducers at these late dates was unsuccessful in all
cases. It is difficult to determine whether this represents a limita-
tion of our cultural conditions, which rendered impossible the recovery
of even a few nonproducers, or whether the injected transformed cells
did go through a cycle of partial growth followed by a state of intermediate differentiation. Table 3 summarizes in a composite way the
results obtained with both 727 and 5YS cell lines.

It was surprising to find that no correlation existed between
myeloproliferative conditions and the absence of transformed cells in
the bone marrows. Additional experiments are in progress to determine
the real nature of these findings.

Finally, we tested the presence of cytotoxic antibodies against the
NPs in the serum of birds injected with NPs. Sera were tested from 1-
week to 1-year-old birds that as embryos had been injected with NPs. In
addition, sera were tested from birds with bone marrows either positive
or negative for NP recovery. Cytotoxic antibodies were not detected
against the NP in any of the samples, which suggested that the host was
not preventing leukemia via an immune response.

"Homing" of NPs in the Chick Embryo

To determine whether the NPs were destroyed, had survived, or had
proliferated in the embryonic environment, we labeled the cells with
[125]IUDR before injection. Autoradiography of the labeled cells indicated that 90% to 95% were indeed labeled following the protocol in
Materials and Methods. In the first set of experiments summarized in
Table 4, injection·of labeled NPs is compared with the injection of
heat-killed labeled NPs. The organs of the sacrificed embryos were processed as described, and the ethanol rinses were saved to represent the
nonspecific counts. The radioactivity persisting within the organs
after the ethanol rinses is indicative of [125]IUDR present in surviving
NPs (15). The label present in the ethanol rinses and the fluids of
the embryo is the result of release of [125]IUDR from dead cells. Most
of the radioactivity from the injection of heat-killed cells was nonspecific and was present in the embryonic fluids. By day 4, radioactivity
was increased in the body of the embryo, which may indicate reutiliza-
tion of broken down labeled DNA. In conclusion, the live injected NPs
survived and were found primarily in the yolk sac and also in the liver
of the embryo. More than 50% of the radioactivity was present in the
yolk sac as early as 2 hr after injection. The amount of radioactivity
in the yolk sac and liver was 10-fold greater than that seen with the
heat-killed NP controls. In addition, radioactivity was not detected in
some organs, which suggested that the NPs were specifically migrating or
"homing" to some chosen organs of the embryo.

TABLE 3. Summary of NP detection and histopathological findings in chickens injected with two NP lines

Line used	NP injected	Embryo age	No. embryos injected	No. birds examined	Time P.I.	NP recovered from bone marrow	Histopathology
727	5-10 X 10⁶	13 d	60a	46	1 d-1 yr	9	1 myeloprolif.
727	35 X 10⁶	13 d	10	10	2-6 wk	6	0
5YS	35 X 10⁶	13 d	17b	13	2 wk-4 mo	2	6 myeloprolif.

a,b14 and 4 embryos, respectively, died a few days after injection.

TABLE 4. Detection of [125]IUDR-labeled nonproducer (line 727) myeloblasts in ovum after injection of 13-day-old embryos with heat-killed or live cells

(% of total CPM)[a]

Organ[b]	2 h post-injection		24 h post-injection		4 d post-injection	
	Live	Heat-Killed[c]	Live	Heat-Killed	Live	Heat-Killed
CAF	1.5	33	2	18	34	33
Yolk	1	6	11	41	5	7
CAM	14	16	6	9	2	6
Yolk sac	53	5	63	6	17	2
Legs	1	1	1	2	5	6
Liver	7.5	0.5	8	0.5	4	1
Heart	0	0	0	0	0	0
Stomach	0	0	0	0	3	3
Head	1	3.5	2	6.5	11	8
Body	3	6	5	7.5	17	30
Nonspecific	18	9	2	9.5	2	4

[a]Percentages were based on total CPM injected into the embryos.
[b]Solid organs were rinsed 3 times over a 3 day period with 70% ethanol before counting.
[c]Cells were exposed to 70°C for 10 min before injection.
CAF = chorioallantoic fluid; CAM = chorioallantotic membrane.

TABLE 5. Detection of ^{125}IUDR-labeled nonproducer myeloblasts (NP) 24 h postinjection in ovum (% of total CPM)[a]

Organ[b]	Producer Myeloblasts	NP (Line 727)	NP (Line 5YS)	NP (Line BM2)	Controls Normal Bone Marrow	Normal Yolk Sac
CAF	1	2	3	1	7	22
Yolk	1	11	25	9	33	8
CAM	3	6	7	3	14	37
Yolk sac	78	63	24	44	14	11
Legs	1	1	3	3	4	1
Liver	8	8	17	14	6	8
Heart	0	0	0	0	0	0
Stomach	0	0	0	2	0	0
Head	1	2	4	3	5	3
Body	4	5	14	17	15	10
Nonspecific	3	2	3	4	2	31

[a]13-day-old embryos were used.
[b]Solid organs were rinsed 3 times over a 3-day period with 70% ethanol before counting.
CAF = chorioallantoic fluid, CAM = chorioallantoic membrane.

Table 5 shows the fate of the ^{125}IUDR-labeled cell types and NP lines. The data show that the AMV producer myeloblasts migrated in a manner similar to that of the NPs. Although there was some variability among the different NP lines, the majority of cells were still detected in the liver and yolk sac. Bone marrow cells from a 1-week-old chicken and from yolk sac cells of 13-day-old embryos were labeled with ^{125}IUDR and injected as normal cell controls. The normal cells did not "home" to the yolk sac. Most of the radioactivity was detected in the embryonic fluids or with the nonspecific counts, which indicated cell death.

The radioactivity studies demonstrated that the NPs survived in the embryo after injection. Table 6 shows evidence that the injected NPs proliferated in the yolk sacs of injected embryos. One can retrieve the NPs from the yolk sac by preparing a suspension of the yolk sac cells and seeding them in soft agar. The NPs from the yolk sac can still produce characteristic transformed colonies in soft agar. When the number of NP colonies per number of yolk sac cells seeded was compared with the known number of ^{125}IUDR-labeled NPs in the yolk sac, calculated by radioactively measuring the yolk sac, the colony efficiency of the NPs could be determined. If labeled NPs were proliferating after injection, the number of NPs, as measured by the radioactivity, should increase; therefore, the colony efficiency would increase as a function of time. In the control experiments (Table 6) the colony efficiency did increase with time after NP injection, which indicated cell proliferation. To confirm these findings, we performed suicide experiments with ^{3}H-thymidine because Suzuki and Axelrad (33) showed that when appropriate doses of ^{3}H-thymidine were used, the thymidine taken up by the dividing cells damaged the DNA and eventually killed the cells. In our experiments ^{3}H-thymidine was injected in ovum 24 hr after NP injection. The NP colony efficiency remained constant after the ^{3}H-thymidine injection, whereas injection of unlabeled thymidine did not affect the

TABLE 6. Colony efficiency of ^{125}IUDR-labeled nonproducer myeloblasts (NP) recovered from the yolk sacs of injected embryos[a]

Experiment[b]	2 h P.I. %	24 h P.I. %	48 h P.I.	72 h P.I. %	4 d P.I. %
Suicide exp. control	1.0	4.5	injected unlabeled thymidine	11	17
Suicide exp.			injected ^{3}H-thymidine	5	4.5

[a]Colony efficiency is determined by calculating the total number of NP present with ^{125}I measurements and comparing that number with the number of colonies that develop in soft agar: number of colonies of NP/number of yolk sac cells seeded $\div$ radioactive number of NP/total number of yolk sac cells = colony efficiency (%).
[b]Each experiment was done at least twice in triplicate.
P.I. = postinjection of NP.

increase in the colony efficiency that occurred in the control experiments. In conclusion, the NPs migrated within the embryo to specific organs, particularly the yolk sac, where they were able to proliferate.

Challenge of the NPs in Vivo

Another set of experiments was performed to determine how long the NPs would be viable in the embryo and still be able to release infectious AMV after superinfection of the NPs with helper virus.

The results are summarized in Table 7. The helper virus was indeed able to infect the injected NPs and induce the release of AMV, which caused acute leukemia. The helper virus could be injected either with the NPs or separately, for as long as 10 days later when the birds were 2 days old, and still induce overt leukemia. AMV was recovered from the plasma of the leukemic birds and from the supernatant fluids of the cultured leukemic cells. Helper virus injected into birds 2 weeks after hatching did not induce leukemia, due probably to the immunocompetence of the animals at that age.

Additional experiments were performed with embryos from chicken lines resistant to the pseudotype of the helper used for superinfection of the NPs. The results are shown at the bottom of Table 7. In the case of NP-injected C/C embryos challenged with RAV-7, leukemia surprisingly did not develop. However, when NP-injected C/BE embryos were challenged with MAV-2, one bird out of seven succumbed with leukemia. The leukemic cells and plasma from the leukemic bird contained infectious AMV.

TABLE 7. Induction of leukemia in vivo from nonproducer myeloblasts (NP) challenged with helper virus[a]

Exp.	No. Cells Injected/ Embryo	No. Embryos Injected	Virus Challenge Post NP Injection	No. Leukemic Birds
461	4×10^6	3[b]	Coinfection RAV-7	1/3
423	2×10^6	3	24 h RAV-7	3/3
440	5×10^6	17	48 h RAV-7	7/13
445	2.5×10^6	3	Post-hatching 2 d RAV-7	1/3
470	7.0×10^6	7	Post-hatching 2 wk RAV-7	0/7
432	5.0×10^6	8	4 mo RAV-7	0/8
525	10×10^6	10[c]	48 h RAV-7	0/10
532	10×10^6	7[d]	48 h MAV-2	1/7

[a]NPs were injected IV into 13-day-old embryos.
[b]Experiments 461-432 were of C/E phenotype.
[c]Experiment 525 was of C/C phenotype.
[d]Experiment 532 was of C/BE phenotype.

DISCUSSION

The purpose of this study was to determine whether virus-free transformed cells still carrying functional markers of the myeloid lineage were capable of expressing oncogenic potentials after injection into chick embryos. The study was conducted principally with one of the lines described earlier (26), which consisted of nonproducer myeloblasts originally obtained by infecting chicken bone marrow at a low m.o.i. of AMV and grown as a continuous line in suspension.

Several procedures were used to follow the living conditions of these cells upon reinjection into the host microenvironment provided by the chick embryo and the hatched chick.

Our data have essentially shown that NP cells, after injection into the host migrate to specific organs within 2 hr after intravenous injection of the embryos. More than 50% of NPs homed to the yolk sac and approximately 8% to the liver. Furthermore, the NPs could still be retrieved from the bone marrows, livers, and spleen of hatched birds 4 weeks after embryonic injection, but not later. At present it is a matter of speculation whether this represents a) a gradual extinction of the injected cells, b) differentiation of the transformed cells into normal components of myeloid lineage, or c) simple immunological recognition (unlikely) from the host. Further experiments will be necessary to opt for one of these possibilities. Nevertheless, two main findings emerge from this study. Both are correlated on one side with growth and a presumable control of transformed cells by the host microenvironment and on the other with viral leukemogenesis.

Hemopoietic microenvironments are involved, with many hormonal and biochemical factors controlling proliferation and differentiation of the hemopoietic stem cells (10, 28). Detrimental changes in this microenvironment can affect the growth and maturation of normal cells causing hemopoietic disorders like anemia and leukemia (7, 14, 27-29). It is not unreasonable to question whether the reverse could be true, i.e., that in our experiments a normal hemopoietic microenvironment could regulate and control an abnormal proliferation of transformed cells. Investigators have long suggested and recently proved that a normal embryonic environment can induce transformed cells to differentiate and develop normally (1, 20). A line of myeloid leukemic cells has been induced to differentiate in vivo in diffusion chambers placed in the peritoneal cavities of adult mice (19, 22). Furthermore, the exposure of several different rat tumors to embryonic indicators in the primitive streak of chick embryos causes the tumors to differentiate and lose their invasive properties (cited by Rubin, [31]).

We have demonstrated that the NPs survive well in the embryonic environment and in the bird during the first weeks after hatching, but a possibility remains that beyond this time the host mounts an immune response that is able to destroy the NPs. However, cytotoxic antibodies were never detected against the NPs in the sera of birds that had been injected with NPs in ovum. One would also expect that injection of NPs in ovum should create a tolerance in the hatched bird to the NP. Moreover, we recently found that NPs could be recovered from a 10-day-old bird that had been injected at hatching, which suggested that our SPAFAS kept in pens for years are more histocompatible than would be expected.

The 727 line of NPs practically lacked oncogenic potential even when 35×10^6 cells were injected in ovum (Tables 2, 3). In addition, all bone marrows examined histologically did not show any sign of disease. However, the 5YS NP line was able to induce myeloproliferative disorders in 6 of 12 birds injected with 35×10^6 cells. The 5YS line originated from the recovery of 727 NPs from the yolk sac of an embryo injected 5 days earlier. This line has the same properties as the 727 NPs in vitro. At present we cannot offer a plausible reason for these data except to propose that transformed cells with very low oncogenic potential, as in the case of line 727, may acquire by further passage in the host a major degree of malignancy. It remains to be explained, however, why the observed myeloproliferation disorder observed in several bone marrows remains controlled and does not develop, as one would expect, in an overt invasive leukemia. It is of interest that other reports on the in vivo behavior of neoplastic cells in mammals do also show the influence of the microenvironment on cell proliferation (2, 11, 21). Further experiments are in progress to assess the oncogenicity of 5YS and of BM2 lines. The latter will be of particular interest, since it is a cell line originated from line 727 but retrieved from bone marrow 2 weeks after chicks were hatched.

Control experiments were done with AMV and AMV-producing cells injected into genetically resistant embryos. Baluda (3) had already shown that injection of AMV-producing myeloblasts into susceptible embryos resulted in a leukemia caused by the virus produced by the cells and not by the cells per se. In our experiments C/BE chickens, which were also shown in vitro to restrict AMV-B transformation came down with leukemia caused by the superinfection of the NPs with MAV-2. The leukemic cells and the birds' serum had infectious AMV. One can argue that the amount of virus produced could overcome the genetic restriction and cause leukemia. However, injection of free AMV-B as a control indicates that this was not possible. This result suggests that the helper virus may actually increase the tumorigenicity of the NPs perhaps by increasing the growth rate or the production of AMV-specific products.

Recently, Duesberg et al. (13) have observed that NPs were found to release a defective particle (DVP) that contains avian tumor viral gag proteins but lacks envelope glycoprotein and a DNA polymerase. Whether some of the pathological results reported here may be related to the presence of DVP in our inocula is not yet certain. It should be kept in mind, however, that all established cell lines derived from the original 727, namely 5YS and BM2, all contained the defective virus particle. These studies may be useful in defining the growth control mechanism, or mechanisms, exerted by a normal host microenvironment on proliferating transformed cells.

ACKNOWLEDGMENTS

The authors would like to thank Dennis Chi and Gordon Thompson for their technical assistance. A particular thanks to Dr. Ronald Alexander for his expertise in interpreting the pathological findings.

This work was supported by National Cancer Institute Grant CA 10697, Postdoctoral Fellowship CA 09-126-04 (N.K.Z.), and by the Medical Research Service of the Veterans Administration.

REFERENCES

1. Andres, G. (1953): Experiments on the fate of dissociated embryonic cells (chick) disseminated by the vascular route. II. Teratomas. J. Exp. Zool. 122:507-536.

2. Aoshima, M., and Ishidate, M. (1976): Alteration of biological behavior of a rat leukemia by different routes of passage. J.N.C.I. 56:769-777.

3. Baluda, M. A. (1962): Properties of cells infected with avian myeloblastosis virus. Cold Spring Harbor Symp. Quant. Biol. 27: 415-425.

4. Baluda, M. A., and Goetz, I. E. (1961): Morphological conversion of cell cultures by avian myeloblastosis virus. Virology 15: 185-199.

5. Baluda, M. A., and Jamieson, P. P. (1961): In vivo infectivity studies with avian myeloblastosis virus. Virology 14:33-45.

6. Bishop, J. M. (1978): Retroviruses. Annu. Rev. Biochem. 37: 35-88.

7. Boggs, D. R. (1980): The hematopoietic microenvironment N. Engl. J. Med. 302:1359-1361.

8. Chen, J. H., Moscovici, M. G., and Moscovici, C. (1980): Isolation of complementary DNA unique to the genome of avian myeloblastosis virus (AMV). Virology 103:112-122.

9. Dethlefsen, L. A. (1969): Comparison of tumor radioactivity after the administration of either ^{125}I or ^{3}H labelled 5-iodo-2'-deoxyuridine. Cancer Res. 29:1717-1720.

10. Dexter, T. M. (1979): Haemopoiesis in long term bone marrow cultures. Acta Haematol. (Basel) 62:299-305.

11. Diamandopoulos, G. T. (1979): Microenvironmental influences on the in vivo behavior of neoplastic lymphocytes. Proc. Natl. Acad. Sci. (U.S.A.) 76:6456-6460.

12. Dodge, W. H., and Moscovici, C. (1973): Colony formation by chicken hematopoietic cells and virus-induced myeloblasts. J. Cell. Physiol. 81:371-386.

13. Duesberg, P. H., Bister, K., and Moscovici C. (1980): Genetic structure of avian myeloblastosis virus, released from transformed myeloblasts as a defective virus particle. Proc. Natl. Acad. Sci. (U.S.A.) 77:5120-5124.

14. Ershler, W. B., Ross J., Finlay, J. L., and Shahidi, N. T. (1980): Bone-marrow microenvironment defect in cogenital hypoplastic anemic. N. Engl. J. Med. 302(24):1321-1327.

15. Fidler, I. J. (1970): Metastasis: quantitative analysis of distribution and fate of tumor emboli labeled with ^{125}I-5-iodo-2'-deoxyuridine. J.N.C.I. 45:773-782.

16. Gazzolo, L., Moscovici, C., Moscovici, M. G., and Samarut, J. (1979): Response of hemopoietic cells to avian acute leukemia viruses: Effects on the differentition of the target cells. Cell 16:627-638.

17. Graf, T., and Beug, H. (1978): Avian leukemia viruses: Interaction with their target cells in vivo and in vitro. Biochem. Biophys. Acta 516:269-299.

18. Hanafusa, H. (1977): Cell transformation by RNA tumor viruses. In: Comprehensive Virology, edited by H. Fraenkel-Conrat and R. R.

Wagner, Vol. 10, pp. 408-483. Plenum, New York.

19. Honma, Y., Kasukabe, T., and Hozumi, M. (1978): Relationship between leukemogenicity and in vivo inducibility of normal differentiation in mouse myeloid leukemia cells. J.N.C.I. 61: 837-841.

20. Illmensee, K., and Mintz, B. (1976): Totipotency and normal differentiation of single teratocarcinoma cells cloned by injection into blastocysts. Proc. Natl. Acad. Sci. (U.S.A.) 73:549-553.

21. Ishidate, M., Aoshima, M., and Sakurai, Y. (1974): Population changes of a rat leukemia by different routes of transplantation. J.N.C.I. 53:773-781.

22. Lotem, J., and Sachs, L. (1978): In vivo induction of normal differentiation in myeloid leukemia cells. Proc. Natl. Acad. Sci. (U.S.A.) 75:3781-3785.

23. Moscovici, C. (1975): Leukemic transformation with avian myeloblastosis virus: Present status. Curr. Top. Microbiol. Immunol. 71:79-101.

24. Moscovici, C., Chi, D., Gazzolo, L., and Moscovici, M. G. (1976): A study of plaque formation with avian RNA tumor viruses. Virology 73:181-189.

25. Moscovici, C., Gazzolo, L., and Moscovici, M. G. (1975): Focus assay and defectiveness of AMV. Virology 68:173-181.

26. Moscovici, M. G., and Moscovici, C. (1980): AMV-induced transformation of hemopoietic cells: Growth patterns of producers and non-producers. In: In Vivo and In Vitro Erythropoiesis: The Friend System edited by G. B. Rossi pp. 503-514. Elsevier/North-Holland, Amsterdam.

27. Olofsson, T., and Olsson, I. (1980): Suppression of normal granulopoiesis in vitro by a leukemia-associated inhibitor (LAI) of acute and chronic leukemia. Blood 55:975-982.

28. Quesenberry, P. and Levitt, L. (1979a): Hemopoietic stem cells. I. N. Engl. J. Med. 301:755-760.

29. Quesenberry, P., and Levitt, L. (1979b): Hemopoietic stem cells. III. N. Engl. J. Med, 301:868-872.

30. Ramsay, G., and Hayman, M. J. (1980): Analysis of cells transformed by defective leukemia virus OK10: Production of non-infectious particles and synthesis of Pr76^{gag} and an additional 200,000 dalton protein. Virology 106:71-81.

31. Rubin H. (1980): Is somatic mutation the major mechanism of malignant transformation? J.N.C.I. 64:995-1000.

32. Silva, R. F., Dodge, W. H., and Moscovici, C. (1974): The role of humoral factors in the regression of leukemia in chickens as measured by in vitro colony formation. J. Cell. Physiol. 83:187-192.

33. Suzuki, S., and Axelrad, A. A. (1980): FV-2 locus controls the proportion of erythropoietic progenitor cells (BFU-E) synthesizing DNA in normal mice. Cell 19:215-236.

34. Vogt, P. K. (1977): Genetics of RNA tumor viruses. In: Comprehensive Virology edited by H. Fraenkel-Conrat and R. R. Wagner, Vol. 9, pp. 341-455. Plenum Press, New York.

35. Vogt, P. K., and Ishizaki, R. (1966): Patterns of viral interference in the avian leukosis and sarcoma complex. Virology 30:368-374.

Expression of Differentiated Functions in Cancer Cells, edited by R. F. Revoltella et al., Raven Press, New York © 1982.

Retroviruses and Differentiation

Jay A. Levy, Paul Volberding, *Hermann Oppermann, and **JoAnn Leong

*Department of Medicine, *Department of Microbiology and Cancer Research Institute, University of California, San Francisco, California 94143; **Department of Microbiology, Oregon State University, Corvallis, Oregon 97441*

SUMMARY

Retroviruses were originally detected in tumors of many animal species but their primary role in nature may be linked to normal developmental processes. Many of them are inherited in multiple copies in the genes of animals, and are associated with developing embryos and normal tissues and not malignancies. Results of research on a variety of animal model systems indicate that retroviruses can influence normal cell differentiation and may be important in regulating specific biologic functions. Infection by them can block melanin production by melanoma cells in vitro and prevent embryonal carcinoma cells from differentiating into nerve cells. Moreover, in the development of the embryo, the viral genome may be selectively expressed. The effect of the RSV src transforming protein, for instance, appears inhibited in embryo but not adult cells. In examining human systems, the placenta, a tissue with varied differentiated functions, offers an opportunity to examine the role of viruses in human development. Placentas from mouse and baboon have been a rich source of retroviruses and the syncytiotrophoblast layer of human placentas contains particles resembling these viruses. This layer also has virus-specific RNA-directed DNA polymerase and an inhibitor which blocks this enzyme's activity. Purification of the enzyme, its inhibitor and the ultimate cultivation of the placental viruses are objectives of our research. Conceivably these two biologic factors interact in regulating placental function. Final proof for the role of retroviruses in normal differentiation awaits further studies of their specific expression and function in well-defined stages of development.

INTRODUCTION

Retroviruses were initially discovered at the turn of the century in tumors of birds[1,2]. Subsequently they were found associated with malignancies of many different animals including mice, cats, hamsters, rats and cows [3,4]. With contemporary molecular techniques, integrated viral genomes have been detected and traced in animals through the evolutionary tree [5]. It has thus become apparent that these RNA viruses have been inherited in the animal species for millions of years and multiple copies of each virus are found integrated into the genome of animal cells [5,6].

451

These and other data strongly suggest that retroviruses were not conserved purely as oncogenic agents. They most likely have a role in other developmental processes (6). We have reported that inherited mouse type C viruses (MuLV) of the xenotropic (X-tropic) virus class can be found in embryos and normal adult tissues, associated with sperm, and in organs undergoing differentiation (6,7). Moreover, we have demonstrated that the inoculation of X-tropic MuLV into duck eggs prevents the normal development of the embryos (to be published, 6). In addition, we and others have noted that X-tropic MuLV do not produce malignant disease in heterologous hosts (6) but may be important in the immune response (6,8). These observations have led us to conclude that the principal role of retroviruses may be in early developmental processes (embryogenesis and differentiation) and not in maturation events associated with diseases such as autoimmunity and cancer (4). In examining this possibility we have studied several areas of research dealing with retroviruses and differentiation.

ASSOCIATION OF RETROVIRUSES WITH TISSUES AND CELLS UNDERGOING DIFFERENTIATION

The possible role of retroviruses in embryogenesis was investigated by examining developing eggs and embryos from many strains of mice for the presence of infectious type C viruses. We successfully isolated X-tropic MuLV from embryos of several strains of mice and have evidence that this virus is most likely first expressed in the blastula stage of mouse eggs (6), the time when differentiation begins. We also demonstrated that the X-tropic virus is recovered readily from mouse placentas and from embryonic pancreases, after the somite stage (6).

The interplay between retroviruses and differentiation was investigated using the C57 Black B16 mouse melanoma cell line. We observed that when these cells were treated with the viral inducer, iododeoxyuridine (IUDR), three types of endogenous MuLV were produced (9). The N and B tropic ecotropic MuLV which grow preferentially in NIH Swiss and BALB/c mouse cells respectively and an X-tropic virus which productively infects heterologous cells but not mouse cells (6). At the same time, the induction procedure caused a marked reduction in the amount of melanin produced and often led to the emergence of amelanotic cells. These amelanotic cells lost their tumorogenicity in mice but regained it once melanin production reoccurred, or "black" cells reappeared (10). We believe the induction of MuLV led to the expression of new antigens (e.g. viral) on the cell surface which resulted in an immunologic reaction by the host.

An important finding made in these studies was the loss of melanin concomitant with the production of retroviruses by the cell. In examining this observation further, we superinfected the mouse melanoma cells with ecotropic (mouse-tropic) MuLV and measured the extent of melanin production. It was substantially reduced (9). These results suggested that the mechanisms for melanin production and viral production were closely linked, perhaps via the amino acid, tyrosine. They also indicated that active MuLV production could compromise a normal differentiation function of mouse cells.

MOUSE EMBRYONAL CARCINOMA CELLS

Infection With Mouse Type C Viruses

In further studies aimed at defining the relationship of endogenous viral genes to differentiation, we have examined undifferentiated mouse embryonal carcinoma(EC)cells.These cells, originating from teratomas in mice, can differentiate in vitro into a variety of cell types including muscle, fat and nerve (11,12). Differentiation occurs if the cells are allowed to grow in stationary culture; it is prevented if they are transferred every 2-3 days (11,13). Some investigators have reported that undifferentiated mouse EC cells cannot be productively infected by MuLV (14,15). These retroviruses only replicated in the EC cells after differentiation had begun. These observations resembled those made by others, who had exposed mouse eggs to M-MuLV; productive infection did not take place (16).

We have demonstrated, using several undifferentiated EC cell lines, that the block to replication of infectious virus can be overcome by a high multiplicity of infection (MOI)(Table 1)(17). For instance, the PCC7S cell line derived from a teratoma in a 129-C57B1 recombinant mouse (18) became productively infected with the Moloney and AKR strains of ecotropic MuLV and the Moloney and Harvey strains of MSV when an MOI of 10 was employed. The cells, transferred every 2-3 days to prevent differentiation, released by the 5-6th passage as much as 1000 infectious particles per ml of supernatant fluid. The cells were also susceptible to productive infection by HIX, the Moloney and xenotropic virus envelope recombinant MuLV (19). They were resistant to X-tropic virus, even at an MOI of 100, as expected for this class of MuLV (6).

This observation with the PCC7S line was confirmed with other EC cell lines cultivated in the laboratory of Professor François Jacob, Paris, France (13,20). The EC lines could not be productively infected with MuLV at an MOI of 1, but released infectious virus when inoculated with the Moloney and HIX viruses at a multiplicity of 10 (Table 1). Two EC lines were particularly noteworthy: the PCC6 and the PCC4 line. The PCC6 line was established from an A/He mouse and cannot differentiate in vivo or in vitro (21). This line was productively infected with M-MSV and the HIX virus at a multiplicity of 10 but not with AKR-MuLV at an MOI of 1 (Table 1). The PCC4 line, derived from a 129 teratoma, differentiates only in vivo and not in vitro (13,20). It was consistently resistant to MuLV at MOIs of 1-10 as reported by others (14,22) but occasionally sensitive to MOIs of 16-100 (Table 2). Productive infection of PCC4 was observed with a high MOI of the Friend and Moloney strains of MuLV but not the Rauscher or AKR-MuLV. The efficiency of this infection was very low and indicated that there was a greater resistance to productive infection in this line than the other EC lines employed (Tables 1, 2). Furthermore, after 3-4 passages, the infected PCC4 lines,releasing up to 400 infectious particles/ml of supernatant fluid,ceased producing infectious virus. Low levels of MuLV were not present in the supernatant since cocultivation of the cells with mouse cells for several weeks did not uncover infectious virus. We have found, however, as recently reported by others (23), that non-virus producing infected PCC4 cells can be induced to re-release virus by treatment for 18h with IUDR (30μg/ml) and dexamethasone (10^{-6}M).

TABLE 1.   <u>Infection of mouse embryonal carcinoma cells with mouse type</u>
                              <u>C viruses</u>

Cell line	Mouse strain	AKR-MuLV	M-MuLV	M-MSV	HIX	X-MSV
PCC7S	129(C57B1)	+	+	+	+	–
PCC3/A/1(ND-1)	129	–	NT	+	+	NT
C17S1	C3H	–	NT	+	+	NT
PCC6	A/He	–	NT	+	+	NT
PCC4 AZA1	129	–	±	–	+	–

Cell lines and procedure are described in text. With all viruses,
except AKR-MuLV, an MOI of at least 10 was employed. AKR-MuLV was used
at an MOI of 10 with the PCC7S line and an MOI of 1 with the other EC
cell lines. A + sign indicates productive infection in which at least
100-1000 infectious particles/ml were consistently expressed. A – sign
indicates no detectable progeny virus. A ± sign indicates transient release of MuLV.

M-Moloney; MuLV-mouse type C virus; NT-not tested; HIX-Moloney and
xenotropic virus envelope recombinant MuLV; X-MSV-MuLV pseudotype of
Harvey mouse sarcoma virus.

A promising new approach at infecting the refractory undifferentiated EC cells with ecotropic MuLV has been the use of UV-irradiated
monolayer cells. SC-1 mouse cells, infected with M-MuLV, were UV-
irradiated so they would die in 12-24 hours. Uninfected PCC4 cells
were then added to these SC-1 cells shortly after the UV treatment. All
detectable SC-1 cells were lost after 24h, and PCC4 cells were subsequently passed every 2 days. By passage 7 when clearly no residual
SC-1 cells were left in the culture, titers of the Moloney virus released by the PCC4 cells were over 10^2 infectious particles/ml of
culture supernatant.

One surprising observation made with the PCC4 line was its apparent
sensitivity to the recombinant HIX virus. With an MOI as low as 0.6,
replicating virus was noted in the PCC4 cultures. Titers as high as
10^2 were observed by passage 4 and 5 and, with continual transfer of
the PCC4 cells, titers reached levels higher than 10^4 infectious
particles/ml of culture supernatant. By immunofluorescent testing (24),
most of the PCC4 cells infected by the HIX virus contained the MuLV
p30. The reason for the relative sensitivity of these EC cells to infection with HIX virus is not known, but it may have some relationship
to the X-tropic virus component.

These results with undifferentiated EC cells have demonstrated the
existence of an intracellular block to the replication of MuLV. However, this resistance can be abrogated by a high MOI. A similar observation has been made with the intracellular inhibitor associated with
the Fv-1 locus regulating sensitivity of mouse cells to N and B-tropic
ecotropic viruses (25,26). Since the inhibitor in EC cells restricts
all types of ecotropic MuLV, it is clearly different from that associated with the Fv-1 locus. Attempts by us to demonstrate a cytoplasmic
factor, using the extraction methods employed by Tennant <u>et al</u> (27) to
show the Fv-1 inhibitor, have been unsuccessful. Our results and
those of others would suggest that the block to MuLV infection by EC
cells can occur early and prevent efficient integration of MuLV.

TABLE 2.   Infection of PCC4 embryonal carcinoma cells with ecotropic
mouse type C viruses

Virus	MOI	Virus replication/No.attempts
F-MuLV	1-10	0/3
	16-30	1/2
	100	1/5
	1000	0/4
M-MuLV	1-10	0/3
	100	1/1
	1000	0/1
R-MuLV	10	0/2
	100	0/1
	1000	0/1
AKR-MuLV	1-16	0/2
	100	0/1
HIX	0.6-1	1/3
X-MSV	1000 -10,000	0/4

The PCC4 embryonal carcinoma cells were treated in suspension with
DEAE-dextran(25µg/ml), washed and resuspended in medium containing mouse
type C viruses (MuLV) at the multiplicity of infection (MOI) listed.
After 30-120 minutes at 37°C they were plated in 60mm petri dishes in
EMEM with 10% fetal calf serum. Cultures were passed every 2-3 days
and assayed for virus no earlier than 5 days after virus inoculation.
   F=Friend; R=Rauscher; See legend to Table 1 for other abbreviations.

A later block is also present which inhibits production of the presumably integrated virus. This latter mechanism for virus control
seems responsible as well for the cessation of MuLV production by some
EC cells which were initially releasing the virus.
   The relationship between differentiation and resistance to virus infection is not known but apparently one of the early steps in EC cell
differentiation may be a decrease in the factor(s) controlling virus
expression. Since PCC4 cells on occasion form epithelial-looking cell
types it is possible that successful infection and replication occurs
only when these cells appear in culture. One EC cell line has been
reported that releases MuLV only after differentiation has taken place
(28).
   Our results also suggest that EC cells may vary in the undifferentiated state. Although morphologic evidence for differentiation may not
be present, certain intracellular changes may have taken place in some
EC cells to make them more susceptible to infection by MuLV. In this
case, one could consider the PCC7S,C17S1, ND-1 and PCC6 more advanced
towards this differentiation property than the PCC4 cell line. Nevertheless, the unusual susceptibility of PCC4 to HIX virus must be given
further attention.

Effect of type C virus infection on differentiation of mouse embryonal carcinoma cells.

Besides this correlation of EC cell differentiation with enhanced
susceptibility to retrovirus infection, another important finding has
been the ability of productive infection to arrest the normal

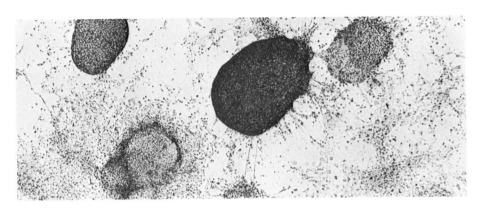

FIG.1.PCC7S embryonal carcinoma cells in the final stages of differentiation in culture. Aggregates of cells have formed and protrusions
resembling nerve axons have appeared. X34.

    differentiation pattern. The PCC7S line, when placed in stationary
culture, differentiates into cells resembling nerve (13,18). In the
first 5 days of culture the cells become confluent and then undergo
cell lysis for 24h in which 50-60% die. Subsequently, the residual
cells become epithelial-like and gradually form aggregates. By day
8-10, structures resembling nerve axons appear that link the aggregates
or descend down to the bottom of the culture dish (Figure 1). When the
undifferentiated PCC7S line was infected with Moloney MuLV or MSV, the
cells no longer aggregated to the same extent as uninfected cells and
nerve axons did not form (17). This effect was noted after 5-6 passages when most of the PCC7S cells, as determined by immunofluorescence
staining for MuLV p30, were infected by the virus. When these infected
PCC7S cells were examined for markers of differentiation, we found that
they could not be infected by SV40 virus nor did they contain tropo-
myosin and actin cables (experiments performed by F. Kelly and D.
Paulin, respectively). Thus, they maintained the characteristics of
undifferentiated embryo carcinoma cells (29,30).
    In studying these observations further, sublines of the infected
cells were begun by plating 5-10 cells in Terasaki wells. Ten established lines releasing M-MuLV were derived and all of these were unable to differentiate in culture. Infectious center testing of one
subline (200-C1A) indicated every cell was producing infectious MuLV
(17). To ascertain that we did not select for certain sublines unable
to differentiate, we established sublines from the parental PCC7S cells
by similar methods. Four of these were studied and all of them differentiated into nerves in 8-12 days. On subsequent infection with M-MuLV,
these lines also were blocked in differentiation.
    In following these latter cultures, we noted that the number of
cells releasing infectious virus was a necessary factor in the arrest
of differentiation. If less than 40% of the cells were producing infectious virus, a reduction in the differentiation pattern was not
detected. These observations have supported the concept that the cell
surface is an important factor regulating normal differentiation of
these cells (11). If a new antigen (retrovirus envelope) is placed on
the cell membrane, effective aggregation does not occur and the cells

remain essentially undifferentiated.

LACK OF TRANSFORMATION OF MOUSE EMBRYO CELLS BY ROUS SARCOMA VIRUS

In the preceding section we discussed the ability of undifferentiated mouse TC cells to prevent infection and replication of MuLV. In other studies we have noted a difference in the effect of certain viral products, in particular the avian Rous sarcoma virus (RSV) transforming protein src (31), on early passaged mouse embryo cells. We have reported that RSV can undergo phenotypic mixing with ecotropic and xenotropic MuLV (32). The resulting viruses, RSV(MuLV), differ from the parental RSV in their enhanced ability to transform mammalian cells and their capacity to replicate efficiently in these cells (32). The MuLV appears to serve as a helper for the infection and replication of RSV. Concomitant with these findings was the observation that the ecotropic MuLV pseudotype of the Bryan high-titered strain of RSV (BH-RSV) could produce foci of cell transformation in established mouse (3T3, SC-1) and rat cell lines but not in early passaged mouse embryo (ME) cells (Fig.2). The ME cells, however, could produce high titers of the ecotropic MuLV pseudotype of BH-RSV which transformed other mouse and rat cell lines. In fact, the highest titers of BH-RSV (MuLV) were produced by early passaged ME cells (32).

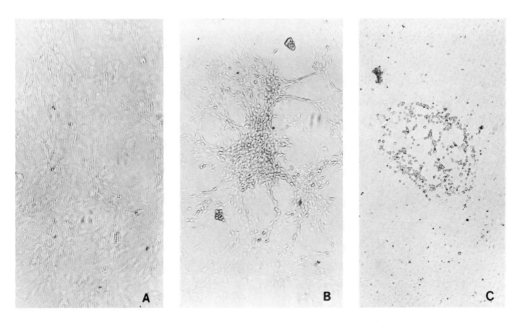

FIG. 2. Infection of mouse embryo, mouse 3T3 and rat (NRK) cells with the AKR-MuLV pseudotype of Bryan high-titered Rous sarcoma virus. Note the absence of focus formation in the mouse embryo cells. Replication of infectious focus-forming BH-RSV(MuLV) by the two mouse cell lines was comparable (see text). (A) NIH Swiss mouse embryo; (B) NIH Swiss mouse 3T3; (C) Rat (NRK) cells. X34.

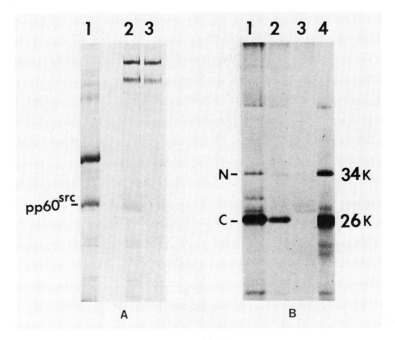

FIG. 3. A. Immunoprecipitation of pp60^{src} labeled in tissue culture
with ^{35}S methionine. Labeling and immunoprecipitation with tumor
bearing rabbit serum was performed exactly as described in Oppermann
et al (33). Lane 1: BH-RSV transformed BHK cell line; Lane 2: BH-RSV
(MuLV) infected mouse embryo cells; Lane 3: Mouse embryo cells.

     B. Partial proteolysis of pp60^{src} by staphylococcus protease
(V8). The pp60^{src} from a gel, as shown in Fig.3A was excised and
digested with V8 protease (33,34). V8 generates two primary fragments
of pp60^{src}, the amino-terminal fragment of MW 34,000 with little
methionine and the carboxy terminal fragment of MW 26,000 containing
the majority of methionine on pp60^{src}. Lane 1: BH-BHK; Lane 2: BH-RSV
(MuLV) infected mouse embryo cells; Lane 3: A corresponding section of
gel from uninfected mouse embryo cells; Lane 4: pp60^{src} of the
Schmidt-Ruppin strain for comparison.

     The reason for this block in expression of the RSV src gene product
by ME cells has been under study in our laboratory. Understanding the
mechanism for this control of BH-RSV src by embryo cells could help
explain the mode of action of this transforming protein and provide an
ultimate approach for arresting the effect of oncogenic proteins.
Initially, we examined acutely infected ME and mouse 3T3 cells for the
production of infectious virus. We found the amount of infectious BH-
RSV (MuLV) released from ME cells was equal to that produced by infected 3T3 cells. Titers ranged as high as $10^{5.3}$ FFU/ml as detected
in NRK (rat) cells. Moreover, infectious center testing of the ME and
mouse 3T3 cells indicated that,with the high MOI used, all the cells
were producing infectious BH-RSV (MuLV) as measured by focus formation
in NRK cells.

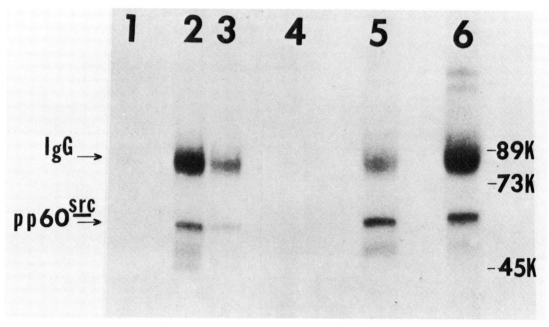

FIG. 4. Assay for pp60src protein kinase activity. Cytoplasmic extracts were prepared from cultures of about 10^6 cells. pp60src was
immunoprecipitated using tumor bearing rabbit serum. Protein kinase
activity in the isolated immune complex was assayed by addition of
γ - ^{32}P-ATP. The reaction resulted in phosphorylation of IgG and autophosphorylation of pp60src. Procedures were modified slightly from
those described (33). Because the samples were not heated, IgG heavy
and light chain were not split and migrated with an approximate MW of
85,000. Lane 1: Uninfected NIH 3T3 cells; Lane 2: NIH 3T3 cells infected with BH-RSV (MuLV); Lane 3: Another culture of NIH 3T3, separately
infected with BH RSV (MuLV); Lane 4: Mouse embryo cells; Lane 5: Mouse
embryo cells infected with BH-RSV (MuLV); Lane 6: BH-RSV transformed
BHK line (35).

We simultaneously examined the production of BH-RSV src protein in
these cells. As shown in Fig. 3A, we found that the RSV src protein was
present at a substantial level in the ME cells. A BH-RSV transformed
hamster cell line was used as a positive control (35). In uninfected
ME cells, no viral src protein was detected. We verified the identity
of this src protein in the infected ME cells by partial digestion with
staphylococcus protease (V8) using the methods of Cleveland et al (34).
The src proteins in BH-RSV transformed hamster cells and the ME cells
were not detectably different. Both had the carboxy-terminal fragment
of MW 26,000, characteristic for viral pp60src (Fig. 3B). Furthermore,
when the kinase activity of the src protein was evaluated no detectable
difference in the activity of this enzyme could be found in the mouse
embryo and 3T3 cells. The proteins from both mouse cells were auto-
phosphorylated and phosphorylated the rabbit IgG (Fig. 4). Thus,
the lack of morphologic change in the ME cells could not be explained
by a markedly reduced level of BH-RSV src protein or a lack of its

phosphorylating capacity. The mechanism for this effect may become
apparent when we analyze the location of the RSV src protein in ME cells
and the expression and phosphorylation of its target proteins.

It is noteworthy that the untransformed ME cells releasing the
MuLV pseudotype of BH-RSV were capable of morphologic transformation
when MSV was used. After superinfection of the cells with an amphotropic MuLV pseudotype of MSV, efficient focus formation occurred.

By these molecular studies, we have confirmed the biologic evidence
that ME cells can be infected by RSV (MuLV) and produce infectious
transforming viruses (32). Moreover, these recent results suggest that
mouse embryo cells,in contrast to adult cells, have a mechanism by which
they can prevent the morphologic transformation of the cells by the RSV
transforming protein. Confirmation of these results awaits further
studies with other strains of RSV. The relevance of these observations
to the ultimate control of cell transformation is an exciting area for
continued study.

RETROVIRUSES AND THE HUMAN PLACENTA

Presence of RNA-directed DNA Polymerase Activity in Human Placentas

Our interest in the role of retroviruses in normal development was
stimulated by the discovery of the mouse X-tropic virus, and its association with normal tissues (6). In attempts to find similar viruses in
human cells, we have focused on the human placenta which undergoes
differentiation during the process of embryogenesis. Retroviruses have
been detected in placentas of several animal species particularly pri-
mates (for review, see 36) and infectious mouse and baboon xenotropic
viruses have been readily recovered from this organ (6,37). Virus-like
particles have been consistently observed by electron microscopy (EM) in
human placentas (38,39) and antigens cross-reacting with known retrovirus antigens have been detected in this human tissue (40-42). The results of our studies on the human placenta over the past 5 years are
discussed below.

Initially we confirmed the EM findings of Kalter et al (38), and
found budding virus-like particles, similar to type D (and not type C)
viruses in the syncytiotrophoblast layer of 35% of human placentas (43).
Moreover, we detected the presence of virus-like RNA directed DNA polymerase (RDDP) activity in extracts of this placental layer from over 80%
of the more than 200 placentas examined (44). The enzyme was associated
with particles found at the sucrose density fractions of approximately
1.12, 1.15-1.17 and 1.24g/ml. After heating the fraction at 1.15-1.17
g/ml for 15 minutes at 37°C, the majority of RDDP was found at a density
of 1.24 g/ml - the known density for viral cores (44,45). These results
strongly suggested that RDDP activity was associated with virus particles. And, EM pictures of the 1.15-1.17 g/ml density fractions have
shown structures resembling retroviruses (44). We suspect the 1.12g/ml
density fraction contains aggregates of the placental virus detected in
the 1.15-1.17 g/ml density range. This placental enzyme has a Mg^{2+}
cation preference similar to that of known type D viruses and it uses
the $(rC_m)_n \cdot dG_{12-18}$ template very efficiently - a characteristic
generally reserved for virus-specific RDDP (45). The placental enzyme
is found in the cytoplasm since extracts of placental cells, free of
nuclei, contain RDDP activity.

TABLE 3. <u>Characteristics of the placental RNA-directed DNA polymerase</u>

1. Associated with particles found in sucrose density fractions of 1.12, 1.15-1.17 and 1.24g/ml.
2. Uses the $(rC)_n \cdot dG_{12-18}$ and the $(rCm)_n \cdot dG_{12-18}$ as template primers.
3. Intracytoplasmic
4. MW $\sim$70,000
5. Elutes off phosphocellulose column at $\sim$0.2M.
6. <u>Not neutralized by antisera to mammalian viral RDDP.</u>

In extensive studies aimed at defining the optimal conditions for demonstrating this placental RDDP activity we have observed that lysing the particle containing the enzyme depends on the relative levels of salt, protein, and NP40. Moreover, successful recovery of the enzyme requires the extraction of the placenta soon after delivery. For optimal results, we assay for activity in fresh placentas extracted in low salt and high protein using 0.5-2% NP40. Under these conditions, the enzyme is less sensitive to the detergent (Leong, J., Nelson, J.,Levy, J., in preparation).

We have also isolated the α, β, and γ polymerases from human placentas (Nelson, J., Libby, D., Leong, J., in preparation). The molecular weight of α(250,000) and β(30-40,000) and the template preference of these polymerases distinguish them from the RDDP enzyme we have detected. The placental virus-like enzyme differs as well from the γ polymerase which prefers manganese as a cation and has a molecular weight of 120 daltons (45). We have determined by glycerol gradients that the molecular weight of the placental RDDP is about 70,000 as is the MuLV enzyme (6). Moreover, the placental RDDP elutes off a DE52 column before any of the γ polymerase activity is detected, and comes off a phosphocellulose column at about 0.2M - characteristic of viral RDDP (45).

The placental virus-like enzyme, which is particle-associated, also differs from the human cell RDDP enzyme recently described by Gerard <u>et al</u> (46). This latter enzyme has a small molecular weight (30-40,000) and has not been found in any normal tissues, only human tumors. Finally, the placental RDDP has not been sensitive to neutralization by antisera directed against the enzymes from cat, mouse, baboon and simian retroviruses (44). In conclusion, the template and cation preference, the molecular weight, and the location of the placental RDDP, distinguish it from all the other known human cellular polymerases (see Table 3).

<u>Placental RDDP inhibitor</u>
We recently found that placentas which lacked the RDDP activity contained an inhibitor associated with the particles found in the sucrose density gradient fractions of 1.15-1.17g/ml (Table 4)(47). This inhibitor was not detected in any other sucrose density gradient fractions containing placental extracted material. The inhibitor acts selectively on the RDDP enzyme and not other ingredients of the assay system since its activity can be abrogated only by increasing the amount of the placental enzyme used (47). The highest inhibitor activity has been found in a placenta from a woman with a history of four spontaneous abortions.

TABLE 4.   Characteristics of the placental inhibitor of RDDP

1. Associated with particles found only in sucrose density fractions of 1.15-1.17g/ml.
2. Reversibly inhibits placental RDDP activity.
3. Intracytoplasmic.
4. Active against mammalian viral RDDP.
5. Not active against α, β, and γ polymerases.
6. Not a protease.
7. Not DNAase or RNAase.
8. Not an immunoglobulin.
9. Resistant at 85°C, unstable at 100°C.
10. Resistant to pH 2 and pH 12.
11. Resistant to trypsin and phospholipase C.
12. Resistant to ether extraction and ethanol/ether treatment.
13. Inactivated by chloroform/methanol.
14. Inhibits replication of type C viruses (preliminary data).

This inhibitor is very active against the RDDP from the placenta and from known mammalian type B, C and D retroviruses (47). It has no effect on the α and γ eukaryotic polymerases and only affects human placental β polymerase slightly. Thus, its specificity appears to be for viral RDDP.

By extracting the particulate fraction at 1.15-1.17g/ml with high salt and separating the soluble extract by centrifugation, we have recovered substantial amounts of the placental inhibitor. When we added this inhibitor preparation to cells chronically infected with mouse xenotropic virus a dimunition in the production of infectious virus was noted within 5 days. When it was added to cells prior to infection with the X-tropic MuLV, a 20% decrease in virus infectivity occurred. Incubating the inhibitor preparation directly with MuLV had no effect on the viral infectivity, and the inhibitor was not toxic to the cultured cells. These results are preliminary but suggest that the placental inhibitor may function in controlling retrovirus expression.

The nature of the inhibitor is not yet known. It has been partially purified by hydroxyapatite and DE52 cellulose chromatography. It is not a protease, DNAase or RNAase since it is unable to digest labeled proteins and nucleic acids (47). Moreover, immunodiffusion testing has indicated that it is not a human immunoglobulin. This observation was further confirmed with Biorad beads containing anti-human IgG, IgA and IgM antibodies. The RDDP inhibitor preparation is resistant to temperatures as high as 85°C but unstable to heating at 100°C for 10 min. Its activity is unaffected by conditions at pH 2 and pH 12 and by treatments with trypsin and phospholipase C (47). Moreover, inhibitor activity remained in the aqueous phase after ether extraction and in the organic phase after ethanol/ether treatment. Exposure to chloroform/ methanol, however, inactivated the placental RDDP inhibitor.

We believe the placental virus-like RDDP and its inhibitor interact to regulate viral information required for normal placental development. In this regard it resembles the known inhibitor for RNAase which fluctuates during cell growth (48).

Attempts to isolate the placental retroviruses

In attempts to isolate in pure culture the retroviruses observed in the syncytiotrophoblast layer of human placentas, we cultivated 56 cell lines established from 22 human placentas. They could be maintained in culture for up to 2 months in DME supplemented by 10% fetal calf serum,

1% non-essential amino acids, 2mM glutamine and 1% antibiotics (penicillin and streptomycin). The addition of hormones such as estrogen, insulin and dexamethasone to the medium did not enhance the growth of these placental cells. We also maintained 114 animal cell lines inoculated with minces of human placentas (Table 5). All these cell cultures were grown and passed weekly for 3 months in the media described above.

TABLE 5. <u>Cell lines established from human placentas.</u>

Trophoblast layer - maternal side	30
Trophoblast layer - fetal side	22
Amnion	4
Animal cell lines receiving minces of human placentas	154

Tissues from 22 placentas were used.

Virus production by the cells was assessed by the presence of RDDP activity in the culture supernatant using the $(rC)_n \cdot dG_{12-18}$ template primer (44). We obtained higher counts with an $(rA)_n \cdot dT_{12-18}$ template, but the $(rC)_n \cdot dG_{12-18}$ template primer helps select for virus-like RDDP activity (45). Cultures were considered positive when their supernatant contained RDDP activity at more than 4000 counts were minute (cpm) above background (300-1000 cpm). Moreover, only those cultures whose 30 min counts were at least twice that of the 15 minute count were considered positive.

The supernatants from the cell lines established directly from placentas never showed definite RDDP-like activity. Only three of the placental cell lines had any detectable enzyme-like activity in their culture fluid and this was noted only at an early passage. The animal cell lines inoculated with placental tissue minces also contained no RDDP activity in their culture fluid.

In further attempts at isolating the retrovirus detected in human placentas, we inoculated on tissue culture cells the sucrose density gradient fractions containing placental extracts having RDDP activity (44). In order to assay them on a large number of different animal cells, we placed cell lines with similar growth rates together in one culture. Up to 5 different animal cell types were used to establish eight <u>zoion</u> (<u>Gr.</u> animal) cell lines (Table 6).

TABLE 6. <u>Zoion Cell lines.</u>

Zoion 1	Zoion 2	Zoion 3	Zoion 4
Mallard duck embryo	Orangutan	Dog sarcoma	Racoon uterus
Bear lung	Gazelle lung	SC-1 mouse	Bovine embryonic kidney
Dolphin kidney	Armadillo trachea	Mink lung	Budgie embryo
Bat lung	Horse dermis		Moscovy duck embryo
	Quail embryo		Sea lion lung

Zoion 5	Zoion 6	Zoion 7	Zoion 8
Syrian hamster embryo	Mink lung	Sheep brain	Lion lymph node
Ringed neck pheasant embryo	Chinese hamster embryo	Bovine kidney	Lion kidney
Black-foot mongoose skin	D-17 dog osteosarcoma	Goat esophagus	Armadillo foreskin
		Bush Wallaby skin	Bearded seal connective tissue

TABLE 7. <u>Inoculations of placental extracts.</u>

Cell line	1.12g/ml	1.15g/ml	1.17g/ml
Human foreskin	8	8	1
Mink S+L–	7	8	1
SIRC (rabbit)	6	10	1
SC-1 (mouse)	3	6	
Mink lung	4	4	1
Rhesus monkey foreskin	3	3	1
D17 (dog sarcoma)	3	4	
Dog thymus	2	2	1
Cat S+L–	2	3	
Cat embryo	2	3	
Bat lung	3	3	
Horse dermis	3	2	
Goat esophagus	1	1	
Mongoose skin	1	1	
Z-1	6	6	1
Z-2	3	6	1
Z-3	2	4	1
Z-5			1
Z-6	3	2	1
Z-7	2	2	1
Total	64	78	12

Sucrose density fractions containing extracts from 12 placentas were inoculated onto the cell lines listed. The number of cultures receiving the material and subsequently cultivated is given. Z=zoion lines.

However, we found, in studies with Dr. Walter Nelson-Rees, Oakland, CA, that despite the initial similarity in growth, one cell line predomina-ted after 6-7 passages. Thus, we always begin with fresh mixtures of cells each time a placental extract is assayed. Since retroviruses can pass to non-permissive cells during cocultivation (6), we expect that if the placental virus grows in one of the cell lines that is later lost, it will get passed to the predominant cells in cultures. For these stu-dies, a total of 154 animal and zoion cell lines were inoculated with 3 different RDDP positive density fractions containing extracts from 12 placentas (Table 7).

These cell lines were maintained with weekly transfers for 6-8 months since the isolation of certain primate retroviruses required this period of time for their eventual recovery in substantial titer (49). The cul-ture fluids were assayed for RDDP activity every 3-4 passages. If a positive fluid was detected, the supernatant from the next passage of that cell culture was tested. During 5 years of study, supernatants from certain cells have been positive for RDDP activity on multiple occasions (Table 8). They came from 10 cultures out of the 154 hetero-logous cells inoculated with the sucrose density gradient fractions. These positive cultures received extracts from six of the twelve pla-centas studied. It is noteworthy that only certain cell lines inocula-ted with the fractions contained RDDP activity in their supernatants. Cell fluids from other cell lines, receiving the same extract, remained negative for the enzyme (Table 8).

TABLE 8. Cultures showing RNA-directed DNA polymerase (RDDP) activity after inoculation with placental extracts

Culture No.	Passages* in Culture	Range† in cpm	Cell line	Placenta No.	Sucrose density fraction inoculated (g/ml)	Cells+ negative for RDDP activity	RDDP activity° in cells receiving positive culture fluid
1977	42	1200-4400	SIRC	LE-1	1.13	Rhesus	+
1983	54	400-4000	SIRC	LE-1	1.16	monkey	
2226	90	700-5200	SIRC	5	1.13	Dog thymus,	−
2238	55	600-12,000	SIRC	5	1.17	mink lung, HuF	
2370	89	400-12,000	Mink lung	7	1.12	HuF, cat embryo, bat lung, horse dermis, dog, thymus, SIRC (rabbit), SC-1 mouse	−
2439	104	500-7000	D17	8	1.15	SIRC, bat, horse, HuF, cat, SC-1, mouse	−
2474	57	600-7300	Pig Kidney	9	1.12	Mink lung, HuF, bovine,	+
2490	49	600-5600	Dog Thymus	9	1.15	cat, bat, SC-1, SIRC, Z-2, Z-8	
2859	119	700-27,000	Cat E	12	1.15	HuF, dog, bat,	+
2860	102	700-19,000	Cat E	12	1.17	horse	

Extracts from 12 human placentas were inoculated onto animal cell lines (see text). Supernatants from the cultures listed showed RDDP activity on multiple occasions.

LE-1 - Placenta from a woman with lupus erythematosus. All other placentas were from women with no known disease.

*Cultures have been transferred weekly for the number of passages listed. RDDP assays were performed every 2-3 passages.

†Assays of RDDP were conducted using the $(rC)_n \cdot dG_{12-18}$ template primer. Specific activity of the ^3HdGTP was 5000 counts/pmol (44).

+These cell lines were inoculated with the same placental extract but did not have RDDP activity in their supernatant. Z=zoion; HuF= human foreskin cells.

°Fluid from the positive cultures was passed to fresh cells from the same cell line.

A + indicates RDDP activity periodically observed in these cultures.

The primary difficulty in evaluating the results of these virus isolation studies has been the fluctuation in RDDP activity observed with positive cultures (Fig. 5). Some cell culture supernatants for example, would have RDDP activity at passage 3 but lack this enzyme at passage 4. Then the enzyme would be redetected in fluids at passage 7 or 10 (Fig. 5). Similar observations with type C viruses grown in chronically infected cell cultures have been reported (50).

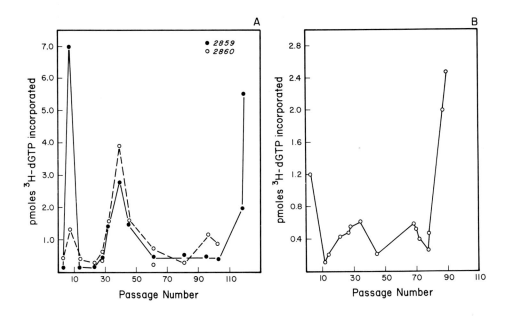

FIG. 5. RNA-dependent DNA polymerase (RDDP) activity in culture fluids
was measured at various subculture passage numbers. Approximately 10ml
of culture fluid was centrifuged at 10,000 x g for 10 min at 4°C. The
resulting supernatant was then centrifuged at 95,000 X g for 60 min at
4°C in a Beckman type 30 rotor. The resulting pellet was resuspended in
STE (0.01 M Tris-HCl, pH 7.8, 0.1 M NaCl, 0.001 M EGTA), 100 ul. A
30 ul aliquot was taken from each sample and assayed for RDDP activity
as described by Nelson, et al (44). Each point is the average of
duplicate samples and represents the number of pmoles (5,000 cpm/pmol)
of ^{3}H-dGTP incorporated into acid-precipitable DNA in a reaction using
$(rC)_n \cdot (dG)_{12-18}$. (A)cultures 2859 and 2860; (B)culture 2370.

We have maintained in prolonged culture those lines which have
periodically shown RDDP activity in their supernatant (Table 8). Recently, three of these seem to have RDDP in the culture fluid consistently
(Fig. 5). None of these cultures have contained mycoplasma nor viruses
such as the cat and mouse type C viruses. Thus, the RDDP activity
noted appears associated with an as yet uncharacterized particle released from the cells. We are presently focusing our attention on these
positive cultures with the hope of isolating a virus associated with the
RDDP activity.

Cell culture fluids from 61 cultures which have shown some RDDP activity have also been inoculated back on fresh parental cells and on
occasion to other animal cell lines. Out of 83 attempts, supernatants
from eight cultures have had periodic fluctuations in RDDP activity.
These cultures received fluids primarily from those cells showing frequent RDDP activity cited above (Table 8).

We have also attempted to demonstrate the presence of a retrovirus in
human placentas by other methods. We have cocultivated the placental
cells and heterologous cells releasing RDDP activity with non-virus

producing MSV transformed rat cells (51). On no occasion has a focus-
forming virus been detected. Moreover, immunofluorescent studies using
antisera from women with a history of lupus erythematosus and from normal women have not shown any clearcut evidence of antigens specific for
placental cells. Finally, cell lines releasing RDDP have been cocultivated with KC cells to determine if the fusion observed with Mason
Pfizer type D virus would take place (52). No fusing activity was
detected.

In summary, these results indicate that the syncytiotrophoblast
layer of human placentas contains virus-like particles detected by EM
and viral enzymes demonstrated by the RDDP assay. The isolation of a
virus in pure culture, however, has not yet been achieved. The most
promising results have been obtained with human placental extracts
in the sucrose density fractions at 1.12 and 1.15-1.17g/ml.

CONCLUSION

We have reviewed the results of several studies aimed at defining
a possible role of retroviruses in normal differentiation. Clearly,
viral infection of cells undergoing differentiation can bring about an
arrest in that process. Likewise, cells at certain stages of development may inhibit the expression of viruses and their viral proteins.
The relationship of our findings to human systems is not clear but we
have focused our attention on the human placenta which is a highly
differentiated organ and consistently shows the presence of virus-like
particles. Their similarity, morphologically, to animal retroviruses,
the presence of RDDP activity in the placenta, and the recent finding of
an inhibitor specific for this RDDP, suggests that these virus-like
particles may be necessary in placental function. The association of
retroviruses with processes of differentiation and their inheritance as
multiple copies in many animal species emphasizes their potential
importance in normal development.

ACKNOWLEDGEMENTS

The research by the authors was supported by USPHS grants, CA13086
and HD13740, a contract from the National Cancer Institute, a grant
(MV-18) from the American Cancer Society and a grant from the Lalor
Foundation. PV is a fellow of the Bank of America-Giannini Foundation.
The authors would like to thank Ms. Judy Joyner and Ms. Peggy Moody for
excellent technical assistance in the studies of human placentas.

REFERENCES

1. Ellerman,V.,Bang,O.(1908): Zentra Bakt Parasit Abt 2 Orig. 46:595-597.
2. Rous,P.(1911):Am.Med.Assoc.56:198-200.
3. Gross,L.(1978) Oncogenic Viruses. Pergamon Press.
4. Levy,J.A.(1977)Cancer Res.37: 2957-2968.
5. Todaro,G.J.(1975) Am. J. Pathol. 81:590-605.
6. Levy,J.A.(1978) In: Current Topics in Microbiology and Immunology, pp. 111-213. Heidelberg:Springer-Verlag, Vol. 79.
7. Levy,J.A.,Joyner,J. and Borenfreund, E.(1980):J.Gen.Virol. (51:439-443).
8. Moroni,C.,and Schumann,G.(1977):Nature 269:600-601.

9. Levy,J.A.,Rutledge.F.,Dimpfl,J.,and Silagi,S.(1979):J. Gen. Virol. 43:283-288.

10. Silagi,S., Beju,D., Wrathall,J., and Deharven, E.(1972) Proc. Natl. Acad. Sci. USA 69: 3443-3447.

11. Jacob, F. (1977): In: Immunological Reviews,Transplantation Reviews 33, edited by G. Moller pp.3-32. Munksgaard, Copenhagen, Denmark.

12. Martin,G.R. (1980):Science 209: 768-776.

13. Jacob,F.(1977): Proc. R. Soc. Lond. B. 201:249-270.

14. Peries,J., Alves-Cardoso,E., Canivet,M., Debons-Guillemin, M.C. and Lasneret,J. (1977) J. Natl. Cancer Inst. 59:463-465.

15. Teich,N.M., Weiss,R.A., Martin,G.R. and Lowy,D.R. (1977) Cell 12: 973-982.

16. Jaenisch,R.,Fan,H., and Croker,B.(1975) Proc. Natl. Acad. Sci. USA 72: 4008-4012.

17. Levy,J.A. (1980)(Abstract)Proc. Am. Assoc. Cancer Research: 311.

18. Fellous,M.,Gunther,G., Demler,R., Wiels, J., Berger,R., Guenet,J.L., Jakob,H., and Jacob, F. (1978): J. Exp. Med. 148: 58-69.

19. Fischinger,P.J., Nomura,S., and Bolognesi,D.P. (1975): Proc. Natl. Acad. Sci. USA 72:5150-5155.

20. Nicolas,J.F., Avner,P., Gaillard,J. Guenet,J.L., Jakob,H. and Jacob, F.(1976): Cancer Res. 36:4224-4231.

21. Debons-Guillemin,M.C., Canivet,M., Salle,M., Emanoil-Ravicovitch,R., and Peries,J. (1978): C.R. Acad. Sc. Paris,   286 :1547-1549.

22. Gautsch,J.W. (1980): Nature 285:110-112.

23. Speers,W.C., Gautsch,J.W. and Dixon,F.J. (1980): Virology 105: 241-244.

24. Avery,R.J.,and Levy,J.A. (1978): J. Gen. Virol. 39:429-449.

25. Lilly,F., and Pincus,T. (1973): Adv. Cancer Res. 17:231-277.

26. Duran-Troise,G., Bassin,R.H., Rein,A., and Gerwin,B.I. (1977): Cell 10:479-488.

27. Tennant,R.W., Schluter,B., Yang,W.K., and Brown,A. (1974): Proc. Natl. Acad. Sci. USA 71:4241-4245.

28. Huebner,K., Tsuchida,N., Green,C., and Croce,C. (1979): J. Exp. Med. 150:392-405.

29. Kelly,F., Guenet,J.L., and Condamine,H. (1979): Cell 16:919-927.

30. Paulin,D., Perreau,J., Jakob,H., Jacob,F., and Yaniv,M. (1979): Proc. Natl. Acad. Sci. USA 76: 1891-1895.

31. Brugge,J.S.,and Erikson,R.L. (1977): Nature(Lond.) 269:346-348.

32. Levy,J.A. (1977): Virology 77:811-825.

33. Oppermann,H., Levinson,A.D., and Varmus,H.E. (1981): Virology 108: 47-70.

34. Cleveland,D., Fischer,S.G., Kirschner,M.W., and Laemmli,U.K.(1978): J. Biol. Chem. 252:1102-1106.

35. Sarma,P.S., Vass,W., and Huebner,R.J. (1966): Proc. Natl. Acad. Sci. USA 55:1435-1442.

36. Panem,S. (1979): In: Current Topics in Pathology, edited by E. Grund-mann and W.H. Kirsten, pp.175-189. Springer-Verlag, Berlin Heidelberg.

37. Benveniste,R.E., Lieber,M.M., Livingston,D.M., Sherr,C.J., Todaro, G.J., and Kalter,S.S. (1974): Nature(Lond). 248:17-20.

38. Kalter,S.S., Helmke,R.J., Heberling,R.L., Panigel,M., Fowler,A.K., Strickland,J.E. and Hellman,A. (1973): J. Natl. Cancer Inst. 50: 1081-1088.

39. Vernon,M.L., McMahon,M.J., and Hackett,J.J. (1974): J. Natl. Cancer Inst. 52:987-989.

40. Strand,M., and August,J.T. (1974): J. Virol. 14;1584-1596.
41. Sawyer,M.H., Nachlas,N.E.,Jr. and Panem,S. (1978): Nature 275: 62-64.
42. Klavins,J.V., Shapiro,S.H., Wessely,Z., and Berkman,J.I. (1980); Annals of Clinical and Laboratory Science 10;137-142.
43. Dirksen,E.R., and Levy,J.A. (1977); J. Natl. Cancer Inst. 59: 1187-1192.
44. Nelson,J., Leong,J. and Levy,J.A. (1978); Proc. Natl. Acad. Sci.USA 75: 6263-6267.
45. Sarngadharan,M.G., Robert-Garoff,M., and Gallo,R.C. (1978): BBA 516: 419-487.
46. Gerard,G.F., Loewenstein,P.M., and Green,M. (1980): J.B. Chem. 255; 1015-1022.
47. Nelson,J.A , Levy,J.A., and Leong,J.C. (1981); Proc. Natl. Acad. Sci. USA 78;1670-1674.
48. Roth,J.S. (1967): Methods Cancer Res. 3;151-243.
49. Sherwin,S.A., and Todaro,G.J. (1979): Proc. Natl. Acad. Sci. USA 76; 5011-5055.
50. Panem,S., Prochownik,E.V., Knish, W., and Kirsten, W. (1977): J. Gen. Virol. 35:487-495.
51. Levy,J.A., Kazan, P., Varnier, O. and Kleiman,H. (1975): J. Virol. 16:844-853.
52. Rand,K.H., Long,C.W., Wei,T.T.,and Gilden,R.V. (1974): J. Natl. Cancer Institute 53:449-452.

Expression of Differentiated Functions in Cancer Cells, edited by R. F. Revoltella et al., Raven Press, New York © 1982.

On the Relationship Between the Transforming onc Genes of Avian Rous Sarcoma and MC29 Viruses and Homologous Loci of the Chicken Cell

P. Duesberg, T. Robins, W.-H. Lee, K. Bister, *C. Garon, and *T. Papas

*Department of Molecular Biology, University of California, Berkeley, California 94720; *Tumor Virus Genetics Laboratory, National Cancer Institute, Bethesda, Maryland 20205*

ABSTRACT

The relationship between two classes of retroviral onc genes and cellular structural homologs termed proto-onc genes was studied. The type I Rous sarcoma virus (RSV) src gene, which is unrelated to essential virion genes, and the specific part (mcv) of the type II MC29 virus onc gene, which is a hybrid that also includes part (Δ) of the structural gag gene of retroviruses (Δgag-mcv), were found to have complete sructural homologs in cloned chicken DNA based on fingerprinting RNA-DNA hybrids. Both cellular loci are not linked to any other virion sequences. Since Δgag is not present in the proto mcv-locus, the onc gene of MC29 does not have a complete homolog in the cell. Presumed host markers of certain viral src genes, said to be experimentally transduced from the cell, were not detected in the proto src-locus. The cellular mcv-locus was found to be interrupted by one sequence of non-homology relative to the viral counterpart; the src-locus is known to be interrupted by six. We deduce that there is a close qualitative sequence-homology between viral onc genes and cellular proto-onc genes. However, due to the different arrangements of onc-related sequence in viruses and cells and to scattered single nucleotide differences in their primary structures, functional homology between onc genes and proto-onc loci cannot be deduced. Considering the genetic structures of RSV and MC29 and those of the corresponding cellular DNA loci it follows that the generation of viruses like RSV and MC29 by transduction of cellular sequences into the genome of a retrovirus must have involved rare, illegitimate recombinations and specific deletions.

INTRODUCTION

The hallmark of the transforming onc genes of acutely transforming retroviruses such as Rous sarcoma virus (RSV) and avian myelocytomatosis (MC29) virus, is a onc-specific, coding RNA sequence that is unrelated to virion genes which are essential for virus replication (7, 12, 15). Over a dozen different onc-specific sequences have been identified in various oncogenic viruses (15). Based on analyses of the genetic structures and the products we have recently distinguished two types of onc genes (6, 7). The coding sequence of type I consists entirely of specific sequences. The original example is the src gene of RSV (13, 26)

471

which encodes a 60 kd protein (8). The onc gene of avian myeloblastosis virus is another example in the avian tumour virus group (16). The coding sequence of type II onc genes is a hybrid consisting of a specific sequence and of elements of essential virion genes typically including a partial (Δ)gag gene. The original example is the onc gene of MC29 in which both Δgag and a specific sequence, termed mcv, function as one genetic unit, that encodes a 110 kd gag-related, probable transforming protein (33, 3). The hybrid onc genes of Fujinami sarcoma virus (29) and avian erythroblastosis virus (4) are other examples in the avian tumour virus group.

Retroviruses with onc-genes are acutely and inevitably oncogenic in susceptible animals (15). However such viruses are rarely found in natural cancers indicating that they do not play a significant role in natural carcinogenesis (18). Several retroviruses with onc genes like Harvey (21), Kirsten (25), and Moloney (34) sarcoma viruses and the murine Abelson (1) acute leukemia and the MC29 virus-related OK10 acute leukemia virus (35) have been isolated from animals that developed tumours after inoculation with lymphatic leukemia viruses that do not contain onc genes. The rare, spontaneous or lymphatic leukemia virus-induced occurrence of retroviruses with onc genes and the complete lack of evidence for an epidemic, horizontal spread of retroviruses with acute onc genes have raised several critical questions about the origin of these viruses. (i) Are viral oncogenes stored in covert form in normal cells? (ii) How do viruses with related onc genes (like MC29 and OK10 or Harvey and Kirsten virus) appear in seemingly independent spontaneous cancers? (iii) Are lymphatic leukemia viruses involved in the emergence of viral oncogenes? These questions were first addressed by the oncogene hypothesis of Huebner and Todaro (23). The oncogene hypothesis postulates that viral onc genes are present in normal cells and may cause cancer if induced by carcinogens or other oncogenic agents. Subsequently, it was hypothesized that genetic elements with a potential of becoming viral onc genes can be transduced by retroviruses and can evolve into viral onc genes (44, 45).

An experimental test of the oncogene hypothesis became possible with the identification of onc gene-specific sequences initially in RSV (13, 26), then in Kirsten and Harvey sarcoma viruses (31, 38, 39, 47) and later in many other avian and mammalian retroviruses (7, 15). The first direct evidence of sequence homology between cellular DNA and onc-specific sequences was obtained in the cases of Kirsten and Harvey sarcoma viruses (38, 39, 47) and later also with those of Moloney sarcoma (17), Rous sarcoma (42), MC29 (41, 43) and other viruses. These results lend indirect support to the oncogene and transduction hypotheses. However these experiments did not determine whether viral onc genes (referred to as the quantitative model) or structural relatives of viral onc genes with possibly different functions (referred to as the qualitative model) were detected in normal cells.

In the case that viral onc genes have direct counterparts in normal cells, as postulated by the quantitative model, cellular transformation by viruses with onc genes is thought to be due to enhanced gene dosage (2). In accord with the quantitative model it was proposed that viruses without viral onc genes cause cancer by integrating proviral DNA adjacent to, and consequently promoting the expression of, cellular genes related to viral onc genes (22). Specifically, it was concluded the "downstream promotion" of a cellular MC29-related proto-mcv sequence is the cause for lymphomas in chicken infected by lymphatic leukemia viruses (22). In the murine system the quantitative model derives support from experiments which showed transformation of 3T3 fibroblasts with cellular sequences homologous to the specific-sequence of Moloney sarcoma virus(MSV) after ligation with terminal sequences of MSV (36) or with cellular sequences homologous to the transforming region of Harvey MSV again after ligation with viral terminal sequences (10). However with regard to the relevance of these experiments for the quantitative model one would have to know whether viral and related cellular sequences encode functionally similar transforming proteins. In addition it would be critical to know whether only viral or also cellular promoters could induce onc-related sequences to transform cells in order to exclude the possibility that besides promoter functions other functions are encoded in the viral terminal sequences. [It would also be interesting to know whether viral promoters could also transform cells by inducing cellular sequences unrelated to viral onc genes.] The quantitative model appears to be most directly supported in the avian system by the claim that partial src deletions of RSV which lack over 75% of src (19, 20, 49, 50) including one src-terminus (20, 27, 52) can reproducibly transduce src from the cells of infected chicken to regenerate RSVs which have been termed recovered (r)RSVs (19). Proof for the transductional origin of the src genes of rRSVs has been based on presumably host-derived oligonucleotide and peptide src markers (20, 49, 50, 52).

In an effort to distinguish between the quantitative and the qualitative model we have compared here a prototype of each of the two classes of viral onc genes to DNA of their cellular homologs: the src-gene of a Rous strain that was reportedly transduced from the cell (49, 50) and the hybrid Δgag-mcv gene of MC29.

RESULTS

a. The complexities of the cellular src-related locus and viral src are about the same, but the cellular locus is not linked to viral sequences outside src.

We have recently identified about 20 RNase T_1-resistant oligonucleotides in the src genes of 10 strains of Rous sarcoma virus including two reportedly transduced form the cell (30). The purpose of this study was to determine the degree of variability among src genes of different viral strains and to identify markers of transduction in src genes thought to be transduced from the cell (49, 50, 52). The study concluded that src genes of all RSV strains tested are completely allelic, differeing only in scattered single base variations (30). Fig. 1C shows the fingerprint of the about 20 src oligonucleotide of rRSV 14-2 which was isolated by Vigne et al. (37, 49, 50). This fingerprint was obtained form rRSV 14-2 (^{32}P) RNA hybridized by a src-specific cDNA. src-specific cDNA was prepared by annealing rRSV 14-2 cDNA with unlabelled RNA of an isogenic src-deletion mutant which lacked the 1.6 kb src gene and about 200 additional nucleotides mapping adjacent to the 5' end of src [see Fig 1 nucleotide positions -200 to about 1600 of src (9)] (30). After hybridization the reaction mixture was incubated with RNases A, T_1 and T_2 to degrade unhybridized RNA. Subsequently the RNase-resistant hybrid was isolated and the RNA melted and fingerprinted (Fig. 1C, ref. 30). The oligonucleotides x and y derive from the 200 non-src nucleotides mapping adjacent to the 5' end of src in rRSV 14-2 RNA (Fig. 1C).

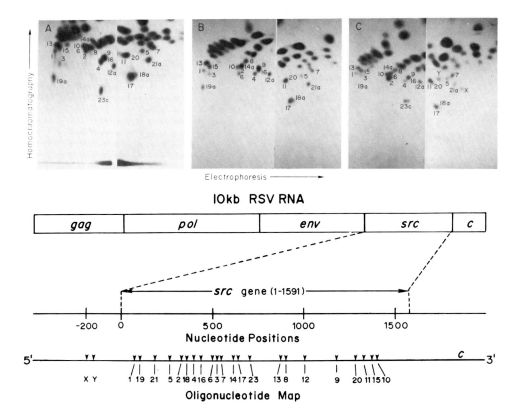

FIG. 1. *Src*-specific oligonucleotides of a RSV strain termed rRSV 14-2, hybridized by DNA of the cellular *src*-related locus. (A) rRSV 14-2 (^{32}P) RNA (0.25 μg or 1 x 10^6 cpm) was hybridized for 8 hr at 40°C in 10 μl 70% formamide, 0.3 $\underline{M}$ NaCl, 0.03 $\underline{M}$ Na citrate, and 10 m$\underline{M}$ Na-phosphate at pH 7 with about 20μg of *src*-related DNA of the chicken cell cloned in a lambda phage CS3 that had been degraded for 12 min at 95°-100° in 0.3 $\underline{N}$ NaOH. The reaction mixture was then incubated in 200μl 0.3 $\underline{M}$ NaCl 0.03 $\underline{M}$ Na-citrate pH. 7.0 for 30 min at 40°C with RNase T$_1$ at 50 units/ ml and the hybrid was prepared and fingerprinted as described (30). To enhance resolution of oligonucleotides electrophoresis was on cellulose acetate strips at pH 2.5 over a distance of 30 cm. The strip was then cut and each half was chromatographed on a 15 x 30 cm commercial DEAE cellulose thin layer plate (30). The splice marks in the middle of A to C represent the junctures of the two half-fingerprints. The diagrams show the genetic map of the 10 kb RSV RNA genome and the location of *src*-oligonucleotides and non-*src* oliginocleotides x and y on the known oligonucleotide map (30) and partial nucleotide sequence (9) of RSV. The letters associated with oligonucleotide numbers identify the rRSV 14-2 specific alleles of variable *src* oligonucleotides (30). (B) A rRSV 14-2 (^{32}P) RNA λCS3 DNA hybrid was prepared as for (A).

The reaction mixture was then incubated in 200 μl 0.3 M NaCl, 0.03 M Na-citrate pH 7.0 with RNases A (5 units/ml), T_1 (50 units/ml) and T_2 (10) units/ml) at 40°C for 30 min and the hybrid isolated by gel exclusion chromatography. After phenol extraction the hybrid was melted and the RNA digested with RNase T_1 and fingerprinted as for (A). (C) rRSV 14-2 (^{32}P)RNA (0.25 μg or 1 x 10^6 cpm) was hybridized for 2 hr as for (A) with src-specific cDNA, prepared by hybridizing 0.5 μg rRSV 14-2 cDNA with 5 to 10 μg RNA of an isogenic src-deletion mutant termed td Schmidt-Ruppin RSV-D21 (30). The reaction mixture was then processed as for (B).

The composition of <u>src</u> oligonucleotides and oligonucleotides x (4U, 3C, G, C, 2AU, A_2C) and y (2U, C AC, AU, A_2G) has been described elsewhere (30). The genetic structure of RSV [5'<u>gag-pol-env-src-c</u> 3' (7, 15)] and the location of the above oligonucleotides within the known oligonucleotide map (30) and nucleotide sequence of RSV (9) have been determined and are diagrammed in Fig. 1.

To determine whether the <u>src</u>-related locus of the chicken (40, 42) contains all sequences represented by the <u>src</u> oligonucleotides of rRSV 14-2, rRSV 14-2 (^{32}P) RNA was hybridized to DNA of the <u>src</u>-related locus of the chicken cloned in lambda phage. The particular clone was a gift of G. Cooper and has been termed λCS3 (40). After digestion of the reaction mixture with RNase T_1, the hybrid was isolated and the RNA was digested with RNase T_1 and fingerprinted. As is shown in Fig. 1A the resulting fingerprint contained all <u>src</u>-oligonucleotides shown in Fig. 1C. However it lacked all known, non-<u>src</u> virion oligonucleotides of rRSV (37) even olignucleotides x and y from the adjacent non-coding 5' region as well as all known oligonucleotides of the adjacent 3' <u>c</u>-region (30) (cf. Fig. 1). Therefore, we can conclude that (i) the complexities of the viral <u>src</u> and the cellular <u>src</u>-related locus are about the same and (ii) that the cellular <u>src</u>-related locus is not linked to any viral sequences outside <u>src</u> including probable non-coding sequences mapping directly adjacent to <u>src</u>. This extends the results of others (24,40) that <u>src</u>-related loci of the chicken are not linked to other coding or non-coding sequences of endogenous retroviruses.

b. <u>The cloned cellular src-related locus does not contain a putative tranductional src oligonucleotide marker of rRSV 14-2.</u>

Previous analyses conducted by us (30, 37) and others (20, 49, 50, 52) have indicated that the <u>src</u> genes of rRSVs contain parental and non-parental <u>src</u> oligonucleotides. As we have shown recently probably all of these non-parental oligonucleotides represent point mutations of allelic parental counterparts (30). Since all rRSVs from one laboratory (49, 50) and some of those from another (20, 52) contained one non-parental oligonucleotide, i.e., the 23c allele of oligonucleotide 23, that was also not found in other RSV strains (30) it has been argued that this oligonucleotide is a marker of cell-derived <u>src</u> sequences (49, 50, 52). [Other RSV strains contain different alleles of oligonucleotide 23, e.g., oligonucleotide 23a or 23b (30)].

To test this possibility directly we have asked whether the 23c allele can be detected in the λCS3 clone which, as shown above in

Fig. 1A, contains a homolog of oligonucleotide 23. n order to determine whether the cellular locus contained the rRSV-specific 23c allele, a rRSV 14-2 RNA -λCS3 DNA hybrid, which had been incubated with RNases A, T_1 and T_2 to degrade mismatched sequences, was fingerprinted. As can be seen in Fig. 1B the hybrid lacked src oligonucleotide 23c. By contrast a RNase A, T_1 and T_2 -resistant hybrid formed with homologous src-specific cDNA contained oligonucleotide 23c (Fig. 1C).

We conclude that the 23c allele of src oligonucleotide 23 is not present in the chicken src locus of λCS3. Hence it appears unlikely that this src marker was directly transduced from this cellualar src-related locus. It is possible that src-related loci of chicken may differ in scattered base changes. However if one concedes that cellular src-related loci vary in single bases one can no longer use single base changes as markers of src transduction, since src genes, like other viral genes, are also subject to spontaneous point mutations (30).

   c. Structural relationship between a normal chicken DNA locus and the onc gene of MC29

   In order to compare sequence-relationship between a representative hybrid onc gene and a cellular counterpart, we have anlayzed here the homology between MC29 RNA and the mcv-related chicken locus (41) cloned in lambda phage. A lambda phage containing the mcv-related locus termed λ proto-mcv3 was selected by screening a chicken library with molecular-ly cloned proviral MC29 DNA as a hybridization probe (Robins, T., Bister, K., Garon, C., Papas, T. and Duesberg, P., unpublished). We have used the same library of chicken DNA that had been used to select the above src-related locus (11).

   The chicken DNA of our λ proto-mcv3 recombinant phage measured about 17 kb. To locate the MC29-related sequence in the recombinant phage a heteroduplex was prepared with proviral MC29 DNA prepared from a recom-binant lambda phage (28). The cloned fragment of MC29 DNA extended from the 5' end of the viral genome to a restriction endocuclease Eco RI site at about 2.5 kb from its 3' end. It also included about 4.5 kb of quail cell DNA mapping adjacent to the 5' end of MC29 DNA (28). The genetic structure of MC29 has been determined previously to read 5' Δgag-mcv-Δenv-c 3' (5, 14, 33) and is schematically represented in Fig. 3. It can be seen in Fig. 2 that the MC29-related sequence of the chicken was located in two discontinuous regions of 0.9 and 0.7 kb respectively and was interrupted relative to viral DNA by a 1 kb region of non-homology (see arrow in Fig. 3). Based on the heteroduplex and the known structure of the cloned fragment of MC29 DNA (28) the cellular 0.9 kb region was identified as co-linear with the 5' half and the 0.7 kb re-gion as co-linear with the 3' half of most or all of the mcv sequence.

   In order to determine whether the cellular MC29-related DNA contains the complete onc gene of MC29 or only part of it, the RNA of a RNase T_1-resistant hybrid formed between MC29 RNA and λ proto-mcv3 DNA was fingerprinted. As shown in Fig. 3A this hybrid contained all eight MC29-specific oligonucleotides defined previously, i.e. nos. 1, 3, 6, 7b, 8b, 15, 26, and 120 but no other MC29-oligonucleotides. Treatment of the hybrid with RNases T_1, A and T_2 prior to fingerprint analysis virtually eliminated oligonucleotides nos. 3 and 7b (Fig. 3B). Under the the same conditions of digestion none of the eight MC29-specific oligonucleotides are eliminated from a MC29-specific cDNA hybrid (33) or from a MC29 RNA hybrid formed with an endonuclease BamHI-resistant

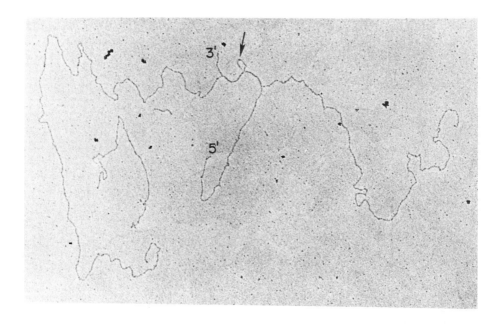

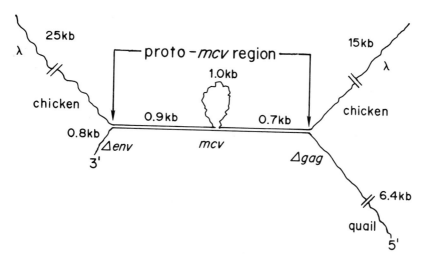

FIG. 2. *Electronmicrograph of a heteroduplex formed between a fragment of molecularly cloned MC29 DNA and the cellular MC29-related locus of the chicken cloned in lambda phage.* Procedures for heteroduplex formation and analysis have been described (28). The MC29 DNA used was a restriction endonuclease Eco R1-resistant DNA fragment that extends from the 5' end and includes about 4.5 kb quail cell DNA adjacent to the 5' end of the viral DNA (28). DNA of the λ proto-mcv3 clone includes the MC29-related locus flanked by about 6 to 7 kb chicken DNA at either side and then by the two arms of the lambda phage vector (Robins, et al., unpublished). The arrow marks the 1 kb sequence of nonhomology that interrupts the MC29-related sequence of λ proto-<u>mcv3</u>. The diagram reports length measurements of the respective DNA regions of the heteroduplex in kilobases.

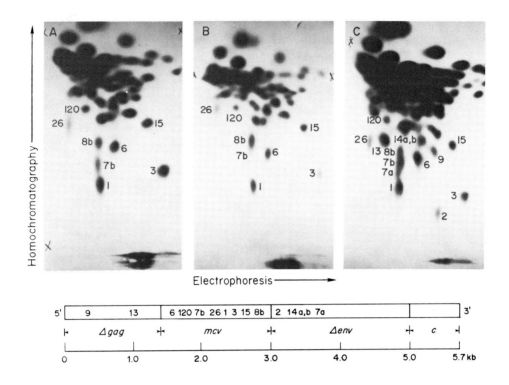

FIG. 3. *The MC29 oligonucleotides hybridized by DNA of the cellular MC29-related locus and by cloned viral DNA.* (A) MC29 (ring neck pheasant [RPV]) (^{32}P)RNA (0.25 μg or 1 x 10^6 cpm) was hybridized with 25 g μg of alkali-degraded λ proto-MCV3 DNA as described for Fig. 1. After treatment of the reaction mixtrue with RNase T$_1$ as described for Fig. 1 the RNA of the hybrid was fingerprinted as described (6, 14, 33). The MC29-specific (mcv) oligonucleotides are fingerprinted and numbered as in previous publications which also describe their compositions in terms of RNase A-resistant fragments (5, 14, 33). The genetic structure of the MC29 genome (5' Δgag-mcv-Δenv-c 3') is schematically represented at the bottom of the figure. The order of all oligonucleotides identified here on the known viral oligonucleotide map (5, 14, 33) is recorded in the diagram. (B) The mcv-oligonucleotides from a hybrid formed as in (A) but isolated after treating the reaction mixture with RNases A, T$_1$ and T$_2$ as detailed in Fig. 1. (C) The mcv-oligonucleotides and some gag and env-related oligonucleotides from a RNase A, T$_1$ and T$_2$-resistant hybrid formed with a restriction endonculease BamHI-resistant fragment of molecularly cloned MC29 DNA. The hybrid was prepared as for (B). The MC29 DNA fragment included most of the Δgag, all of mcv and about 0.3 kb of Δenv of the MC29 genome (28). Some Δgag and Δenv-related oligonucleotides are at higher molar concentrations than the mcv-oligonucleotides, because both MC29 and RPV helper virus contribute gag and env-oligonucleotides.

fragment of MC29 DNA which was cloned in pBR322 (Fig. 3C). This fragment includes the 3' part of Δgag, all of mcv and the 5' end of Δenv (28). It can be seen in Fig. 3C that all mcv oligonucleotides were recovered at near equimolar ratios. The molar recovery of some gag and env-relted oligonucleotides was higher since the hybrid was formed with excess DNA and hence also includes gag and env-oligonucleotides of the helper virus. The gag-oligonucleotide 20a has not been identified previously in MC29, but has been analyzed in CMII under the label 17b (5) and in OK10 under the label 20a (6). The map location of all MC29-oligonucleotides described here on the MC29 RNA genome is diagramemed in Fig. 3; these include the eight mcv oligonucleotides in addition to the gag oligonucleotides nos. 20a and 13 and the env oligonucleotides nos. 14a, 7a and 2.

Based on homology with MC29-specific oligonucleotides and on the size of heteroduplexed sequences, we conclude that the complexities of the primary sequence of the cellular MC29-related locus and of the viral mcv are about the same. However, no oligonucleotides of virion sequences outside mcv, in particular no gag-ralated oligonucleotides were detected in the MC29 RNA-λ proto-mcv3 DNA hybrids analyzed here (Fig. 3), although the mcv-related sequence of λ proto-mcv3 is flanked by 7 kb of chicken DNA on either side (Fig. 2). This conclusion is consistent with unpublished evidence of Sheiness et al. (quoted in ref. 41) that a 10 kb restriction enzyme-resistant fragment of proto-mcv DNA lacks sequences related to essential virion genes. It would appear that the cellular locus analyzed here does not contain an entire, structural homolog of the Δgag-mcv gene which is thought to be the onc gene of MC29 (5, 14, 33).

DISCUSSION

Are cellular src-related sequences experimentally transducible?

Clearly, transduction of onc genes with coding sequences unrelated to essential virion genes such as src would be direct evidence for a functional homology between viral src genes and cellular src-related sequences and hence support for the quantitative model. Since src transduction has been said to occur experimentally, we have analyzed here a reportedly transduced src gene for host markers. We have found that the only presumably transductional src oligonucleotide marker of the reportedly transduced src gene studied by us (30, 37) and others (49, 50) is not found in the cellular src-related locus cloned in λCS3.

Even if we assume that src-transduction cannot be proven by biochemical src markers, because viral and cellular src-related sequences are too similar, the transduction frequencies reported in the above system cannot be reconciled with the evidence that the src-related locus is not linked to any other viral sequences (Fig 1, ref. 24, 40). It has been reported that, in this system, src deletions that lack either the 5' end (20, 52) or the 3' end (27, 49) as well as deletions that retain both ends (20, 52) nevertheless transduce src at the same high rate of over 50% within two months (19, 50). This appears surprising since illegitimate recombination with proto-src would be required for src transduction by deletions lacking one end of src while the more efficient and plausible homologous recombination would suffice to regerate src from deletions with two residual src termini and proto-src. Reproducible transduction involving illegitimate recombination appears also unlikely

in view of the followng examples: Since both replication-defective
RSV(-) (15, 51) and Moloney sarcoma virus (15, 31, 36) share sequences
adjacent to their 3' boundary of their respective src or onc-specific
sequence with their respective helper viruses, they should each be able
to form non-defective sarcoma viruses by one homologous recombination
with helper virus near the 3' end of src and one illegitimate recombination at the 5' end of src.   Yet there is no evidence for the formation
of nondefective RSV (46) or Moloney sarcoma virus (32, 46) despite
extensive passage of these viruses in animals and cell culture.   This
type of recombination should in fact be more frequent than that reported
between partial src deletions lacking one src-terminus and proto-src
because there is abundant direct evidence for recombination between
related retroviruses (14, 15, 48) but no direct experimental evidence
for recombination between a retrovirus and a cell.   Furthermore, in viral recombination no introns need to be removed from viral src.

Hence it cannot be excluded that cross-reactivation among non-
overlapping src-deletions possibly present in the stocks of src-deletion
mutants used to generate recovered RSVs, rather than transduction, was
the origin of the src genes of recovered RSVs (30, 37).   This is
suggested because long-term persistence of stable heterozygotes had been
described previously in retroviruses subjected to extensive biological
cloning even under selective conditions, non-permissible for the host
range of one of two viral components (32, 48) and because the partial
src-deletions used to generate rRSVs were not molecularly cloned (19,
27, 50).

On the origin of oncogenic viruses

Although our evidence casts doubt on the idea that the specific src
sequence of recovered RSVs originated recently by experimetal transduction from the cell, the close relationship between src and the cellular
src-related sequeces argues that such an event occurred at one time in
evolution of RSV.   Likewise does the similarity between mcv and proto-
mcv argue for a cellular origin of viral mcv.

However, in view of our previous results that onc-specific sequences
are located within viral RNA genomes at very specific sites (5, 7, 12,
15), transduction of these sequences must be a complex process for the
following three reasons:

(i) Since the src and mcv-related cellular loci lack any detectable linkage to other virion sequences, transduction must involve double
illegitimate recombination.

(ii) Moreover the six introns (relative to src) of the proto-src
locus (40) ond the one intron (relative to mcv) of proto-mcv (Fig. 2)
would have to be deleted in order to make these sequences co-linear with
the known viral onc genes.   [This is also true for the cellular homologs
of other viral onc genes (7)]. It is conceivable that this is accomplished by a splicing mechanism during or after transcription.   However
since the src-related mRNA of normal cells measures about 3.5 kb but viral src mRNA only about 2 kb (53) and since the MC29-related mRNA of
normal cells measures about 2.8 kb (41) but the mcv-sequence of MC29
only about 1.6 kb, it cannot be assumed that cellular splicing removes
the intervening sequences of non-homology upon transcription, until this
is directly demonstrated.   It is acknowledged that normal cells contain
a protein that is similar to the viral src gene product (2).   However,
it remains to be demonstrated that this protein is indeed translated

from the cellular 3.5 kb RNA and that the protein is potentially oncogenic.

(iii) Finally in the case of type II onc genes, such as the Δgag-mcv gene of MC29, specific deletions of virion genes of the transducing retrovirus would have to occur in order to form the Δgag hybrid onc genes (cf. Fig. 3).

All of these events must occur during the course of an infection of a single animal by a retrovirus in order for a transmissible recombinant virus to emerge. Alternatively the formation of an oncogenic virus could proceed in many steps leading to stable, vertically transmissible proto-types of oncogenic viruses such as the 30S defective retroviruslike RNAs found in certain normal cells (15). In this case not all of the above events would have to occur during the infection of a single animal. Instead an oncogenic virus could be generated by a relatively minor genetic change from an endogenous pre-existing precursor (15).

Qualitative or quantitative model?

Due to a total lack of direct evidence at this time for the function of cellular src-and mcv-related DNA, it is difficult to assess whether onc-specific sequences and their cellular structural homologs are also functionally related as postulated by the quantitative model (2) or different as postulated by the qualitative model.

We have detected minor differences between the primary structures of viral and cellular sequence counterparts: For example the src oligonucleotide marker, 23c, had an allelic but no identical counterpart in the cellular src -related locus of the chicken cloned in λCS3. Likewise did mcv-oligonucleotides nos. 3 and 7b of MC29 have allelic but no identical counterparts in λ proto-mcv3. Since the permissible range of sequence variation that does not affect onc gene function is not known, we cannot deduce whether these qualitative differences could explain the apparent functional difference between viral and cellular sequences.

Further it is uncertain at this time whether the sequences that interrupt the src and mcv-related sequences of the cell are indeed noncoding introns. It is possible that these sequences together with oncrelated sequences encode products that are qualitatively different from viral transforming proteins.

However a clear qualitative difference was detected between the Δgagmcv gene of MC29 and the cellular homolog of MC29 which lacks Δgag altogether. Hence proto-mcv cannot represent a structural counterpart of the onc gene of MC29, although the role of Δgag in transforming function of the viral Δgag-mcv protein remains to be determined. This view is nevertheless compatible with the hypothesis of Hayward et al. (22) that expression of the cellular proto-mcv locus without Δgag is the cause of lymphatic leukemia. Clearly a lymphatic leukemia is qualitatively different from the acute leukemias, carcinomas and sarcomas caused by MC29 (15).

In conclusion our evidence supports the qualitative model in the case of type II onc genes of MC29, since only a part of the hybrid onc gene is found in uninfected cells, but does not at this time distinguish between the two models in the case of type I onc genes, like src. To distinguish further between the two models it would be necessary to determine whether the gene products of cellular, structural homologs of viral onc-sequences are also functional homologs of viral onc genes; and whether experimental transduction of cellular onc-related sequences by molecularly cloned retroviruses without functional <u>onc</u> genes generates oncogenic viruses.

ACKNOWLEDGEMENTS

We are grateful to Mike Botchan and his staff for assistance with DNA cloning and Mike Kriegler for review of the manuscript. This work was supported by NIH Research Grant CA 11426 from the National Cancer Institute.

REFERENCES

1. Abelson, H. T. and Rabstein L. S. (1970):Cancer Res. <u>30</u>, 2213-2222.
2. Bishop, J. M. (1981):<u>Cell</u> 23:5-6.
3. Bister, K., Hayman, M. J., and Vogt, R. K. (1977):<u>Virology</u> 82:431-448.
4. Bister, K. and Dueserg, P. H. (1979):<u>Proc. Natl. Acad. Sci</u> 76: 5023-5027.
5. Bister, K. and Duesberg, P. H. (1980):<u>Cold Spring Harbor Symp</u>. <u>Quant</u>. <u>Biol</u>. 44:801-822.
6. Bister, K., Ramsay, G., Hayman, M. J., and Duesberg, P. H. (1980):<u>Proc</u>. <u>Natl</u>. <u>Acad</u>. <u>Sci</u>. 77:7142-7146.
7. Bister, K., Duesberg, P. H. (1982) in "Advances in Viral Oncology" ed. G. Klein, Raven Press, New York, in press.
8. Brugge, J., and Erikson, R. J. (1977):<u>Nature</u> 269:346-348.
9. Czernilofsky, A. P., Levinson, A. D., Varmus, H. E., and Bishop, J. M. (1980):Nature <u>287</u>:198-203.
10. DeFeo, D., Gonda, M. A., Young, H. A., Chang, E. J., Lowy, D. R.,Scolnick, E. M., and Ellis, R. W. (1981):<u>Proc</u>. <u>Natl</u>. <u>Acad</u>. <u>Sci</u>. 78:3328-3332.
11. Dodgson, J. G., Strommer, and Engel, J. A. (1979):<u>Cell</u> 17:879-887.
12. Duesberg, P. H., and Bister, K. (1981): In: <u>Cancer</u>: <u>Achievements</u>, <u>Challenges and Prospects for the 1980's</u>: edited by J. Burchenal and H. Oettgen. Grune and Stratton, New York, pp. 111-136.
13. Duesberg, P. H. and Vogt, P. K. (1970): <u>Proc</u>. <u>Natl</u>. <u>Acad</u>. <u>Sci</u>. 67:1673-1680.
14. Duesberg, P. H., Bister, K., and Moscovici, C. (1979):Virology 99:121-134.
15. Duesberg, P. H. (1980):<u>Cold Spring Harbor Symp. Quant. Biol</u>. 44:13-27.
16. Duesberg, P. H., Bister, K., and Moscovici, C. (1980):<u>Proc. Natl. Acad</u>. <u>Sci</u>. 77:5120-5124.
17. Frankel, A. D., and Fischinger, P. J. (1976):<u>Proc. Natl. Acad. Sci</u>. 73:3705-3709.
18. Gross, L. (1970):Oncogenic Viruses. Pergamon Press, New York.
19. Hanafusa, H., Halpern, C. C., Buchhagen, D. C., and Kawai, S. (1977): <u>J</u>. <u>exp</u>. <u>Med</u>. 146:1735-1747.
20. Hanafusa, H., Wang, L.-H., Hanafusa, T., Anderson, S. M., Karess, R. E., and Hayward, W. S. (1980):In: <u>Animal Virus Genetics</u>, edited by B. Fields, R.Jaenisch and C. F. Fox, pp. 483-497. ICN-UCLA Symposia on Molecular and Cellular Biology. Academic Press, New York. pp 483-497.
21. Harvey, J. J. (1964) Nature 284:1104-1105.

22. Hayward, W. S., Neel, G. B., and Astrin, S. M. (1981):<u>Nature</u> 290:475-480.
23. Huebner, R. J., and Todaro, G. J. (1969):<u>Proc. Natl. Acad. Sci.</u> 64:1087-1092-1094.
24. Hughes, S. J., Stubblefield, F., Payvar, F., Engel, J. D., Dodgson, J. G., Spector, D., Cordell, B., Schimke, R. T., and Varmus, H. (1979): <u>Proc. Natl. Acad. Sci.</u> 76:1348-1352.
25. Kirsten, W. M., and Mayer, L. A. (1967) <u>J. Nat. Cancer Inst.</u> 39:311-335. 26. Lai, M. M.-C., Duesberg, P. H., Horst, J., and Vogt, P. K. (1973): <u>Proc. Natl. Acad. Sci.</u> 70:2266-2270.
27. Lai, M. M.-C., Hu, S. S. F., and Vogt, P. K. (1977):<u>Proc. Natl. Acad. Sci.</u> 74:4781-4785.
28. Lautenberger, J. A., Schulz, R. A., Garon, C. F., Tsichlis, P. H., and Papas, T. S. (1981):<u>Proc. Natl. Acad. Sci.</u> 78:1518-1522.
29. Lee, W.-H., Bister, K., Pawson, A., Robins, T., Moscovici, C., and Duesberg, P. H. (1980):<u>Proc. Natl. Acad. Sci.</u> 77:2018-2022.
30. Lee, W.-H., Nunn, M. and Duesberg, P. H. (1981):<u>J. Virol.</u>: 39: 758-776. 31. Maisel, J., Klement, V., Lai, M. M.-C., Ostertag, W., and Duesberg, P. H. (1973):<u>Proc. Natl. Acad. Sci.</u> 70: 3536-3540
32. Maisel, J., Dina, D., and Duesberg, P. H. (1977):<u>Virology</u> 76: 295-312.
33. Mellon, P., Pawson, A., Bister, K., Martin, G. S., and Duesberg, P. H. (1978):<u>Proc. Natl. Acad. Sci.</u> 75:5874-5878.
34. Moloney, J. B. (1966) Nat. Cancer Inst. Monograph 22:139-142. 35. Oker-Blom, N., Westermark, H., and Rosengard, S. (1970) in "Progress in antimicrobial and anticancer chemotherapy" Vol 2, p 103-106. University Press, Baltimore. 36. Oskarsson, M. McClements, W. C., Blair, D. G., Maizel, J. V., and VandeWoude, G. F. (1980): <u>Science</u> 207: 1222-1224.
37. Robins, T., and Duesberg, P. H. (1979):<u>Virology</u> 93:427-434.
38. Scolnick, E. M., Rands, E., Williams, D., and Parks, W. P. (1973):<u>J. Virol.</u> 12:458-463.
39. Scolnick, E. M., and Parks, W. P. (1974):<u>J. Virol.</u> 13:1211-1219.
40. Shalloway, D., Zelenetz, A. D., and Cooper, G. M. (1981):<u>Cell</u> 24: 531-541.
41. Sheiness, D., Hughes, S. M., Varmus, H. E., Stubblefield, E., and Bishop, J. M. (1980):<u>Virology</u> 105:415-424.
42. Stehelin, D., Varmus, H. E., Bishop, J. M., and Vogt, P. K. (1976): <u>Nature</u> 260:170-173.
43. Stehelin, D., Saule, S., Roussel, M., Sergeant, A., Lagrou, C., Rommens, C., and Raes, M. B. (1980):<u>Cold Spring Harbor Symp. Quant. Biol.</u> 44:1214-1223.
44. Temin, H. M. (1971):<u>J. Nat. Canc. Inst.</u> 46:3-7.
45. Temin, H. M. (1980):<u>Cold Spring Harbor Symp. Quant. Biol.</u> 44:1-7.
46. Tooze, J. (1973):<u>The Molecular Biology of Tumor Viruses</u>. Cold Spring Harbor Press, New York.
47. Tsuchida, N., Gilden, R. V., and Hatanaka M. (1974) <u>Proc. Natl. Acad. Sci.</u> 71:4503-4507.
48. Tsichlis, P. H., Conklin,K. F., and Coffin J. M., (1980):<u>Proc. Natl. Acad. Sci.</u> 77:536-540.
49. Vigne, R., Neil, J. C., Breitman, M. L., and Vogt, P. K. (1980): <u>Virology</u> 105:71-85.

50. Vigne, R., Breitman, M., Moscovici, C., and Vogt, P. K. (1979): Virology 93:413-426.
51. Wang, L.-H., Duesberg, P. H., Kawai, S., and Hanafusa, H. (1976): Proc. Natl. Acad. Sci. 73:447-451.
52. Wang, L.-H., Halpern, C. C., Nadel, M., and Hanafusa, H. (1978): Proc. Natl. Acad. Sci. 75:5812-5816.
53. Wang, S. Y., Hayward, W. S., and Hanafusa, H. (1977):J. Virol. 24: 64-73.

Expression of Differentiated Functions in Cancer Cells, edited by R. F. Revoltella et al., Raven Press, New York © 1982.

Expression of MHC Products in Human Cell Lines Treated with Interferons

M. R. Capobianchi, **F. Ameglio, *†A. Dolei, and **R. Tosi

*Istituto di Virologia, University of Rome, Rome; **Laboratorio di Biologia Cellulare, C.N.R., Rome; †Cattedra di Patologia Generale, University of Camerino, Italy*

Interferons (IFN), besides being antiviral agents, exert a number of biological activities on cell functions (1), including inhibition of cell division, modulation of differentiation, enhancement of phagocytosis, altered expression of cell surface antigens and regulatory properties on the immune response(2). As for the latters, plasmamembrane structures, particularly the antigens controlled by the major histocompatibility complex (MHC), play a critical role . It has already been reported that IFN enhances the expression of MHC antigens, both in human and mouse systems (2).

We focused our attention on the influence of human IFN on the expression of MHC products in a wide spectrum of human cell lines, i.e. E_1SM (normal) and MG_{63} (osteosarcoma) fibroblasts; Namalva B lymphoblastoid cells; M_{10} and M_{14} (melanoma) and Hep2 epithelioid cells. Methods and experimental design were performed as in (3). Treatment with IFN did not cause any toxic effect or cell death in our hands; protein synthesis was almost unaffected and an antiviral state was always established (not shown).

HLA-A,B,C, Ia antigens as well as β_2-microglobulin (β_2-m) were quantitatively determined by radioimmunoassays (RIA) as in (3-4). This method allowed us to quantitate both cell-associated and shed products. All cell lines tested expressed cell-associated HLA-A,B,C and β_2-m, whereas Ia antigens were expressed only by Namalva, M_{10} and M_{14} cells. As for the shedding, all cell lines released β_2-m. HLA-A,B,C was released by Hep2, M_{10} and M_{14}. Ia antigens were released only by M_{10} and M_{14} cells. The degree of antigens expression varied enormously, according to the cell line tested. To be noted the lack of quantitative correlation between HLA-A,B,C and β_2-m expression, for both cell-associated and shed products (see legend to Fig. 1).

As shown in Fig.1, treatment with β IFN caused a dose-dependent enhancement of the expression of cell-associated HLA-A,B,C, β_2-m and Ia in cells that already expressed detectable amounts of them. IFN, however, did not switch-on the expression of silent

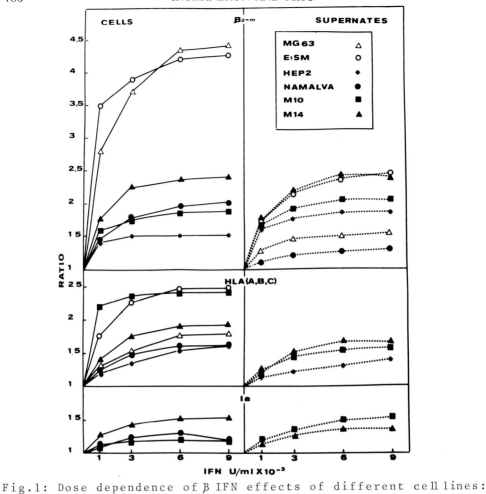

Fig.1: Dose dependence of β IFN effects of different cell lines: Cultures were seeded with/without different doses of partially purified IFN for 24h, then cell lysates (solid lines) and dyalized supernates (dotted lines) were tested by RIA for β_2-m, Ia and HLA-A,B,C. Data are expressed as ratio of values of antigen concentrations ($IU_{50}/10^6$ cells) of treated/ untreated cultures. Basal levels of cell-associated (C) and shed (S) antigens in each cell lines are the following:

M_{10} : Ia: C 402, S 12; HLA-A,B,C: C 14, S 10; β_2-m: C 84 , S 44
M_{14} : Ia: C 39, S 10; HLA-A,B,C: C 12, S 10; β_2-m: C 85 , S 115
Hep2:Ia-negative;   HLA-A,B,C:C 78, S 1400; β_2-m: C133, S 269
Namalva:Ia:C 19, S neg.; HLA-A,B,C: C 13,S neg.; β_2-m:C11,S 35
E_1SM: Ia neg.; HLA-A,B,C: C 20, S neg.; β_2-m: C 39, S 217
MG_{63}: Ia neg.; HLA-A,B,C: C 32, S neg.; β_2-M: C 40, S 166

MHC genes. The enhancing effect of β IFN was also seen on shed products from those cells which already released detectable amounts of antigens.The effect of α IFN on cell-associated HLA and β_2-m was previously reported (2), whereas the enhanced expression of these antigens after treatment with β IFN is a new finding. On the other hand, Ia expression was reported to be unaffected by α IFN (2). In view of that, we extended the studies to the expression of single gene products of the Ia system, i.e. DC1 and DRw2, in Namalva cells, that do not shed Ia molecules from the plasmamembrane. In addition, we compared the effects of α and β IFNs, in order to see whether different types of IFN exert different effects on the Ia system. As shown in Table 1, there were no major differences between the effects of α and β IFNs on the expression of the Ia antigens, as an enhancement was seen both for Ia <u>in toto</u> and for single gene products expression. However, it must be pointed out that in another cell line, i.e. M_{14} (3), the expression of total Ia was not mainly affected by α IFN being instead enhanced after treatment with β IFN, dose-dependently.

These findings indicate that different IFN types can have different effects on plasmamembrane proteins. Ia antigens are present only on some cell types in the body, and thus can be considered as "differentiation antigens". Moreover, they are probably the product of immune response (Ir) genes. The presence of multiple Ia loci products, the possibility of different functions and tissue distribution, and, lastly, the possibility of differential sensitivity to IFNs, should be taken into account when considering the mechanism by which IFN may modulate the immune responses.

Work supported in part by a grant fron C.N.R., Progetto Finalizzato Virus, Contratto n. 81.00308.84.

Table 1: Expression of Ia products in Namalva cells treated for 48 h with 2000 U/ml of α or β IFNs. Data, obtained by RIA, are expressed as $IU_{50}/10^6$ cells.

	Ia	DC1	DRw2
Control	13.2	5.6	17.5
+α IFN	18.1	6.8	25.4
+β IFN	15.5	7.6	20.7

REFERENCES
1) Stewart W.E. (1979). <u>The Interferon System</u>, Springer Verlag New York.
2) Sonnenfeld G. (1980). <u>Lymphokine Reports</u>, 1:113.
3) Tosi R., Tanigaki N., Centis D., Rossi P.L., Alfano G., Ferrara G.B. and Pressman D. (1980). <u>Transplantation</u>, 29:302
4) Dolei A., Ameglio F., Capobianchi M.R. and Tosi R., submitted.

Expression of Differentiated Functions in Cancer Cells, edited by R. P. Revoltella and M. Pontieri, Raven Press, New York © 1982.

Establishment of Functional T Cell Lymphoma Lines from Antigen-Specific T Cells Infected *In Vitro* with Radiation Leukemia Virus

P. Ricciardi-Castagnoli, E. Barbanti, F. Robbiati, *G. Doria, and *L. Adorini

*CNR Center of Cytopharmacology, Department of Pharmacology, University of Milano, 20129 Milano; *CNEN-Euratom Immunogenetics Group, Laboratory of Radiopathology, CSN Casaccia, 00060 Roma, Italy*

The immune response is the resultant of a complex network of cellular interactions among thymus-derived lymphocytes (T cells), bursa-derived lymphocytes (B cells) and accessory cells. These cellular interactions, largely mediated by soluble factors, represent a most sophisticated system of defferentiated functions. However, lack of availability of cloned, antigen-specific, functional T cell lines has delayed, until recently, a detailed analysis of the differentiation process in T cell lineage.

Murine T cell lymphomas have been induced in several ways including infection with oncogenic viruses (7), exposure to ionizing radiations (5) or injection of carcinogens (4). However, the T cell lymphomas so far established according to these procedures have unknown antigenic specificities and therefore they are not suitable for a functional analysis of T cell differentiation (10). Recently, antigen-specific, functional T cell clones have been obtained by somatic cell hybridization (15), by cell culture in interleukin-2-containing media (13), and by Radiation Leukemia Virus (RadLV)-induced transformation of antigen-specific T cells (3).

RadLV, originally isolated by Lieberman and Kaplan (8) from radiation-induced thymic lymphomas, has a restricted tropism for T cells (9). T cells can be infected not only by virus injection but also by a short in vitro exposure to RadLV. However, in vitro infected cells became transformed only after injection into histocompatible hosts and they give rise, in 3-4 months, to donor-type thymomas. Using this method T cell lymphoma lines with helper ac-

489

tivity have been obtained, by Kaplan and co-workers (3), from
spleen cells of mice injected with 2,4 dinitrophenylated keyhole
limpet hemocyanin (DNP-KLH). These cell lines were capable of replacing carrier-primed helper T cells in a secondary anti-DNP antibody response <u>in vivo</u>.

ESTABLISHMENT OF HEN EGG-WHITE LYSOZYME-SPECIFIC SUPPRESSOR T CELL LINES

In this report we describe the establishment of hen egg-white
(HEL)-specific suppressor T cell lines obtained by RadLV-induced
transformation of HEL-specific suppressor T cells. This antigen
has been chosen because it is a very well characterized protein
and a large panel of related lysozymes and defined peptides are a-
vailable. Moreover, the antigenic and idiotypic regulation of the
anti-lysozyme response has been extensively studied and the basic
features of the cellular interactions involved are well documented
(14). In mice of H-2^b haplotype, genetically non responder to HEL,
intraperitoneal HEL-CFA priming induces suppressor T cells which
are antigen-specific, I-J positive and bear idiotypic determinants
(1, 6). These suppressor T cells have been used to establish HEL-
specific T cell lines, according to the protocol outlined in fig.1.

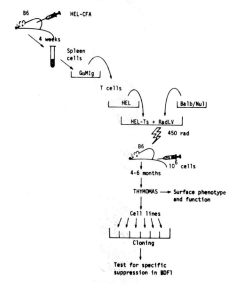

Figure 1. Experimental protocol to establish HEL-specific T
cell lymphoma lines.

Suppressor T cells from HEL-primed C57BL/6 (H-2^b) mice, selected by sequential passage over anti-immunoglobulin and antigen-
coated plates, have been infected <u>in vitro</u> with RadLV obtained from

culture supernatant of the BALB/Nu$_1$ cell line, chronically infected by the replicating virus (1). The infected T cells were then
injected into sublethally irradiated syngeneic hosts. Thymomas developed in 30% of the injected mice and they were analyzed for T
cell markers by immunofluorescence. Among the 6 thymomas tested
one showed the expected surface markers for suppressor T cells
(Thy 1.2$^+$, Ly 2$^+$, I-J$^+$, sIg$^-$) and cell-free extracts obtained from
this lymphoma demonstrated HEL-specific suppressive activity in a
T cell-dependent lymph node proliferative assay (12). Cell lines
from this thymoma were then established in vitro for further studies.

Functional analysis of HEL-specific suppressor T cell line products

The suppressive activity of T cell lymphoma products obtained
by RadLV-induced transformation of spleen cells from HEL-primed B6
mice has been routinely assessed on cells from HEL-primed BDF1 mice,
semisyngeneic to B6 and responder to HEL. A representative experiment demonstrating HEL-specific suppression of the T cell dependent
proliferative response is shown in fig. 2. HEL-specific proliferative response of HEL-primed lymph node cells from BDF1 mice is suppressed by the addition of culture supernatant from HEL-specific T

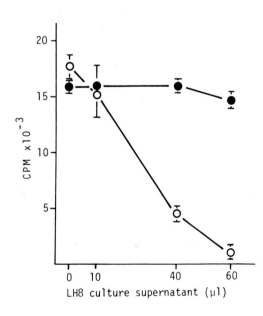

Figure 2. HEL-specific suppressive activity of culture
supernatant from LH8 cell line.
Four x10^5 lymph node cells from
BDF1 mice immunized a week previously with 10 μg HEL-CFA were
cultured with 100 μg/ml HEL
(O——O) or with 50 μg/ml PPD
(●——●). Culture supernatant
was obtained from 24-hour cultures of LH8 cells (2x10^5/ml)
and added at the beginning of
the culture. Thymidine incorporation was measured 5 days later. Results are expressed as
arithmetic mean and standard
error of counts per minute (CPM).

cell lines whereas the response to PPD, an antigen unrelated to
HEL but present in the CFA used for immunization, is not affected.
Culture supernatants from HEL-specific T cell lymphoma lines are
also able to suppress the in vitro anti HEL plaque-forming cells
(PFC) response of lymph node cells from HEL-CFA primed BDF1 mice
stimulated in culture with HEL conjugated to sheep erythrocytes

(HEL-SRBC) (2). In this case lymphoma cell extracts were purified
by adsorption to and elution from HEL immunoadsorbents and only the
eluted material exerted suppressive activity. Culture supernatants
added to lymph node cells stimulated in vitro with SRBC did not sup
press the anti-SRBC PCF response. Culture supernatants from HEL-
specific T cell lines injected at the same time of HEL priming are
also able to specifically suppress the anti-HEL PFC response (L.A-
dorini et al., manuscript in preparation). The suppressive activity
of T cell products from HEL-specific lymphoma lines demonstrates
an exquisite fine specificity because the response to ring-necked
pheasant egg-white lysozyme, a molecule closely related to HEL, is
not suppressed. Suppression of HEL-specific antibody response induced by injection of T cell products is genetically restricted and
the suppressive factor appears to act at the helper T cell level.

Biochemical analysis of HEL-specific cell line products

To isolate HEL-specific molecules lymphoma cells were biosynthetically labelled with ³H-leucine. Culture supernatants were then
collected, concentrated by ultrafiltration and reacted with antigens
linked to Sepharose 4B immunoadsorbents. After extensive washing
the bound material was analyzed by fluorography after resolution
on polyacrylamide slab gels containing 10% sodium dodecyl sulfate
(SDS-PAGE).

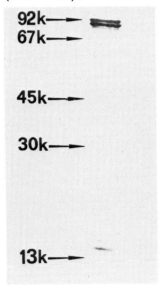

Figure 3. SDS-PAGE analysis of HEL-
binding molecules. SDS-PAGE analysis
was performed on culture supernatant
obtained from HEL-specific T cell lymphoma lines biosynthetically labelled
with ³H-leucine, and conjugated to HEL-
Sepharose 4B. After solubilization
under reducing conditions the sample
was loaded onto a 10% SDS-polyacrylamide slab gel and processed for fluorography. Molecular weight markers were,
from top to bottom: phosphorilase B
(92.500 d), bovine serum albumine
(69.000 d), chicken ovalbumine (46.000
d), carbonic anhydrase (30.000 d) and
cytochrome c (12.300 d).

As demonstrated in fig. 3, HEL-specific T cell lymphoma products
are resolved in two major sharp bands with an approximate molecular
weight of 85.000-90.000 d. Experiments in collaboration with M.

Cecka and M. Feldmann, University College, London, have demonstrated that cell extracts from ^{35}S-methionine labelled HEL-specific T cell lymphoma line can be sequentially adsorbed and eluted from anti-V_H and HEL immunoadsorbents. When resolved by SDS-PAGE the eluted material shows two close and sharp peaks of radioactivity with an approximate molecular weight of 85.000 d. These peaks were not observed when the radiolabelled proteins were eluted from anti-V_K or KLH immunoadsorbents.

Therefore, T cell products from HEL-specific T cell lymphoma lines contain antigen-binding site and the framework structure of Ig heavy chain variable region (V_H), both on the same molecule.

CONCLUSIONS

Differentiated T cells preselected for a given antigenic specificity and immunological function can be immortalized by RadLV-induced transformation and their antigen-specific products can be obtained in large amounts. Structural, genetic and functional studies of these molecules should give, in the near future, clear-cut answers about the nature of the T cell receptor and the generation of diversity in functional T cells. RadLV-induced transformation does not interfere with the expression of T cells specificity and function and both suppressor and helper T cells can be transformed. Therefore, these antigen-specific T cell lymphomas, easily cloned and functionally stable, represent a very promising material for the study of differentiation events in the T cell lineage.

AKNOWLEDGMENTS

This work has been supported by C.R.N. Progetto Finalizzato "Controllo della Crescita Neoplastica" and by CNEN-Euratom Association Contract.

REFERENCES

1. Adorini, L., Miller, A., and Sercarz, E.E. (1979):J. Immunol., 122: 871-877.
2. Adorini, L., Doria, G., and Ricciardi-Castagnoli, P. (1981): Lymphokines, In press.
3. Finn, O.J., Boniver, J., and Kaplan, H.S. (1979): Proc. Natl. Acad. Sci. USA, 76: 4033-4037.
4. Haran-Ghera, N. (1967): Proc. Soc. Exp. Biol., 124: 697-702.
5. Haran-Ghera, N. (1967): Brit. J. Cancer, 21: 739-745.
6. Harvey, M.A., Adorini, L., Miller, A., and Sercarz, E.E. (1979)

Nature, 281: 594-596.

7. Kaplan, H.S. (1967): Cancer Res., 27: 1325-1339.

8. Lieberman, M., and Kaplan, H.S. (1959): Science, 130: 387-388.

9. Lieberman, M., and Kaplan, H.S. (1976): Blood cells, 2: 291-299.

10. Lieberman, M., Decleve, A., Finn, O., Ricciardi-Castagnoli, P., Boniver, J., and Kaplan, H.S. (1979): Int. J. Cancer, 24: 168-177.

11. Ricciardi-Castagnoli, P., Lieberman, M., Finn, O., and Kaplan, H.S. (1978): J. Exp. Med., 148: 1292-1310.

12. Ricciardi-Castagnoli, P., Doria, G., and Adorini, L. (1981): Proc. Natl. Acad. Sci. USA, in press.

13. Schreier, M.H., Iscove, N.N., Tees, R., Aarden, L., and von Boehmer, H. (1980): Immunological Rev., 51: 315-336.

14. Sercarz, E.E., and Metzger, D.W. (1980): Springer Semin. Immunopathol., 3: 145-170.

15. Taniguchi, M., Takei, I., and Tada, T., (1980): Nature, 283: 227-228.

Expression of Differentiated Functions in Cancer Cells, edited by R. F. Revoltella et al., Raven Press, New York © 1982.

Reversible Suppression of the Differentiation Program in RSV-Transformed Quail Myogenic Cells

*F. Tatò, S. Alemà, **G. Cossu, and **M. Pacifici

*Gruppo di Microbiologia e Patologia Generale, **Istituto di Istologia, Università di Roma, and Istituto di Biologia Cellulare, CNR, Rome, Italy*

Transformation with Rous sarcoma virus (RSV) blocks the expression of the differentiation program of cells belonging to several different lineages (6,7). This block is dependent upon the presence and functional expression of the viral src gene, as demonstrated by use of temperature-conditional transformation mutants (7). For example, when primary cultures of skeletal myogenic cells are infected by ts-RSV and maintained at the permissive temperature (35°), the cultures become enriched with morphologically converted, replicating mononucleated cells. At the restrictive temperature (41°), the great majority of myogenic cells withdraw from the cell cycle, fuse into multinucleated, cross-striated myotubes and synthetize muscle-specific proteins (4,8).

However, a closer examination reveals the presence of oligo- or multi-nucleated myotubes also at permissive temperature (see Holtzer et al., this volume). The differentiation observed at 35° could be ascribed either to the presence of untransformed (uninfected or transformation-defective infected) cells or to a reduced transforming ability of ts mutants. A first argument against these two possibilities stems from the observation that the extent of this phenomenon could be influenced by culture conditions. A formal demonstration that RSV-infected, fully transformed cells can overcome the pp60 src-induced block of differentiation, was obtained by isolation of clonal strains of quail myogenic cells, transformed by the parental wt-strain of RSV.

Isolation of clonal strains of wt-RSV-transformed quail myogenic cells

Quail embryo presumptive myoblasts were infected with the wt-Prague strain of RSV of subgroups A and C (PR-A and PR-C). The cells were then cloned in soft agar according to standard·procedures. Of the many clones obtained, fifteen of them from each of the two groups of transformed cells; were picked up and further expanded. The majority were eventually found to be myogenic in nature and no substantial differences were observed among different clones. Therefore,only the features of a representative clone are reported here. In clone QM(PR-A)11,confirming earlier results obtained with uncloned cells,a small proportion of

495

differentiated cells could be detected by immunofluorescent staining with antibodies raised against skeletal muscle myosin.

Spontaneous differentiation of RSV-transformed muscle cells is modulated by culture conditions

We have developed a growth promoting medium (GM) and a differentiation promoting medium (DM), which respectively suppress or amplify the spontaneous differentiation of transformed presumptive myoblasts.

In GM, the great majority of transformed cells display a round-shaped morphology and less than 1 per cent of total nuclei is in what can be recognized as small multinucleated myotubes (Fig.1a). In DM, on the contrary, a sizeable fraction (up to 30 per cent) of total cell number form clearly distinguishable myotubes (Fig.1b). These myotubes,however, exhibit peculiar characteristics : they often have a flattened,irregular shape and nuclei are confined to a centrally located area of the sarco-plasm. Immunofluorescent studies show that myosin is not organized into the muscle-specific sarcomeric, striated myofibrils and is rather diffuse or preferentially located in the perinuclear region of the myotube. Cultures grown in DM express significant levels of other muscle-specific products, such as AChR, AChE,and the MM isozyme of CPK.

It is possible to further manipulate this system by using DMSO or HMBA, typical inducers of erythroid differentiation (5). These compounds prevent in a reversible manner terminal differentiation of RSV-transformed muscle cells promoted by DM. This inhibitory effect is not observed in uninfected muscle cells and is similar to that exerted by the same compounds on rat myogenic cell lines (1).

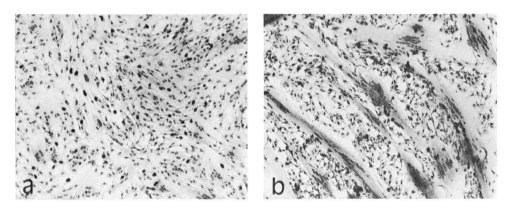

Fig.1. Micrographs of QM(PR-A) clone 11 grown for three days either in GM (a) or in DM (b), stained with Wright's solution. (x80)

CONCLUSIONS

It is widely accepted that transformation and differentiation represent antithetic states for a given cell type. For instance, in RSV-infected myogenic cells, the action of pp60 src , the viral transforming gene product (3), prevents the progression into the ultimate compartment of the skeletal muscle lineage (7). Using ts-transformation mutants, it has been demonstrated that, after shift to 41°, the reversion from the transformed state is accompanied by the resumption of the normal pathway of differentiation (4,8). Our results complement these observations and show that wt-RSV transformed muscle cells are in a metastable state from which they can escape and spontaneously differentiate. This property is susceptible to modulation by the appropriate changes in the micro-environment or by adding specific compounds. These findings provide formal evidence that reversion of RSV-transformed cells, assessed by the expression of specific genes associated to the normal phenotype, can be evoked by epigenetic mechanisms (2).

It remains to be seen whether the spontaneous differentiation of RSV-transformed cells represents the full expression of the myogenic repertoire and what is the fate of pp60 src inside these cells.

This research was partially supported a grant from the C.N.R. under the P.F.Virus-subprogetto Virus Oncogeni.

REFERENCES

1. Blau, H.M. and Epstein, C.J.(1979): Cell, 17:95-108.
2. Braun, A.C. (1981): Quart. Rev. Biol., 56: 33-60.
3. Collet, M.S. and Erikson, R. (1978): Proc. Nat. Acad. Sci. USA, 75: 2021-2024.
4. Fiszman, M.Y. (1978): Cell Diff., 7: 89-101.
5. Friend, C. (1979): In: The Harvey Lectures, Series 72, pp. 253-282. Academic Press, New York-London.
6. Giotta, G.J., Heitzmann, J. and Cohn, M. (1980): Brain Res., 202: 445-458.
7. Holtzer, H., Biehl, J., Pacifici, M., Boettiger, D., Payette, R. and West, C. (1980): In: Results and Problems in Cell Differentiation, Vol. 11, edited by R.G. McKinnell, M.A. DiBerardino, M. Blumenfeld and R.D. Gerard, pp. 166-174, Springer-Verlag, Heidelberg .
8. Moss, P.S., Honeycutt, N., Pawson, J. and Martin, G.S. (1979): Exp. Cell Res., 123: 95-106.

Expression of Differentiated Functions in Cancer Cells, edited by R. F. Revoltella et al., Raven Press, New York © 1982.

Biological and Biochemical Studies of Revertant Clones from Avian Sarcoma Virus Transformed Rat Cells

Ugo Rovigatti

Istituto Fisiologia Generale, Universita Degli Studi Di Roma, 00100 Rome, Italy

In order to study the expression of a transforming gene (src) and its control over the transformed phenotype, I have analysed several revertant rat cell clones obtained from a clone, A^+12, originally transformed by Avian Sarcoma Virus (ASV). I have previously reported[1] that the revertant clones but not the normal parental cells (Rat-1) can be retransformed in the presence of the following agents: 1) dexamethasone (Dex) at a concentration of 10^{-6} M; 2) 12-0-tetradecanoyl phorbol-13-acetate (TPA) at a concentration of 160 nM and, 3) superinfection with a non-transforming but replication competent Murine Leukemia Virus (MuLV). Dex effects appear to be reversible, but a small percentage of the cells retransformed in the presence of TPA and all the foci obtained after MuLV superinfection maintain a stably transformed pheontype. I have further investigated these effects by biological and biochemical experiments.

Cells from the original transformed clone (A^+12), the original revertant (A^+12IIR),[2] several subclones of A^+12IIR, and the retransformed clones have been plated in liquid or semisolid medium or on top of a normal cell monolayer in the presence or absence of the different inducers. No direct effect of the inducers on the Efficiency of Plating (EOP) of the different clones in the various conditions has been evidenced.

The possible involvement of the original transforming virus (ASV) and gene (src) was investigated following a different approach. Revertant clones were isolated from 3R, a cell clone originally transformed by a mutant of ASV temeprature sensitive for the expression and maintenance of transformation (LA 339, non-permissive temperature: 39.5°C). Different foci of retransformed cells were then induced in these revertants at the permissive temperature (35°C) by adding Dex or TPA or by superinfecting the cells with MuLV. Table 1 shows the effects of a 48 hr shift to the non-permissive temperature on these retransformed foci phenotype. It is evident that the phenotype is ts in the revertant clones obtained from 3R, while the foci induced in A^+12IIR are non conditional.

A preliminary analysis of the integrated viral sequences is presented. The parental transformed (A^+12) and revertant (A^+12IIR) clones show a similar pattern of ASV integrated sequences after digestion with Sac I and Eco RI and hybridization with an ASV specific probe (kindly

---

Present address: Institute for Cancer Research, 7701 Burholme Ave., Philadelphia, Pennsylvania 19111.

499

TABLE 1.   Revertant clones of ts ASV cells tested at 35°C and 39.5°C for the presence of ts foci

Phenotype of original transformed clone	Revertant clone	Transformed foci marked at 35°C		Transformed foci after shift to 39.5°C for 48th	Phenotype of cells sub-cultured from transformed foci	
					ts	wt
ts	3R CR10 (from 3R)	Dex	26	0	12	0
		TPA	37	0	10	0
		MoMuLV	69	0	7	0
wt	A^+12IIR	Dex	36	36	0	15
		TPA	29	29	0	7
		MoMuLV	61	60	0	26

provided by Dr. H. Hanafusa). On the other hand, all the and retransformed clones appear to have substained considerable rearrangements and losses of integrated viral sequences. Further studies are in progress in order to elucidate the origin and mechanism of the proviral rearrangements and possible involvement in the retransformation process.

1. Rovigatti, U.G., Weiss, R.A. and Wyke, J.A. (1980): Cold Spring Harbor Meeting on RNA Tumor Viruses, p. 107.

2. Wyke, J.A. and Qusole, K. (1980): Virology, 106:217-233.

Expression of Differentiated Functions in Cancer Cells, edited by R. F. Revoltella et al., Raven Press, New York © 1982.

Differentiation in Retroviruses Transformed Cells: Establishment of a New System of Epithelial Origin

G. Vecchio, A. Pinto, G. Colletta, P. P. Di Fiore, A. Fusco, M. Ferrentino, M. Grieco, and *N. Tsuchida

*Centro di Endocrinologia ed Oncologia Sperimentale del C.N.R., Istituto di Patologia Generale, II Facoltà di Medicina e Chirurgia, Università di Napoli, 80131 Napoli, Italy; *The Wistar Institute, Philadelphia, Pennsylvania 19104*

Transformation of differentiated cells by retroviruses provides new oppurtunities to study the relationships between the establishment of the cancerous state and the expression of cellular differentiated functions.

Recently several systems have become available which exploit the oncogenic potential of retroviruses for cells expressing well defined markers of differentiation. Most systems so far reported are concerned with cells of mesenchimal origin such as blood cell lineages precursors transformed in vitro by leukemogenic viruses (3, 10, 14, 15, 17) or differentiated cells belonging to one of the several pathways of the mesodermal differentiation, such as cells of chondrocytic or myoblastic derivation transformed in vitro by sarcomagenic viruses (7, 11, 13).

We have recently demonstrated that the transforming potential of at least one of the mammalian sarcoma viruses, the Kirsten murine sarcoma virus (Ki MSV) , is widened to include also cells of non mesenchimal origin such as epithelial cells from the rat thyroid gland (8).

In the present paper we will present an outline of the results obtained by transforming in vitro undifferentiated as well as differentiated cell lines.

MATERIALS AND METHODS

T-79, FRT-L and FRT cells have been obtained from Fisher rat thyroid glands as described by Ambesi-Impiombato et al. (2) and by Ambesi-Im piombato and Coon (1) and cultivated as described in Table 1.

TABLE 1.   Growth properties and differentiated functions of epithelial
           thyroid cells used for transformation

Cell line	Growth[a] medium	Doubling time	Iodide uptake	TG[b] secretion	TSH binding
FRT	+ 5% c.s.[c]	24 h	−	−	+
T-79	+ 0.5% c.s. + 6H[d]	4 days	+	+	+
FRT-L	+ 5% c.s. + 6H	36-48 h	+	+	+

[a] Growth medium was prepared according to Coon and Weiss (5)
[b] Thyroglobulin
[c] Calf serum
[d] 6H are: insulin, hydrocortisol, transferrin, thyrotropin,
        somatostatin, and the trypeptide glycil-hystidil-lysine.

   The NRK 58967 clone and C 127 cells were grown in Dulbecco's modified
Eagle's medium containing 10% foetal calf serum.
   The Ki MSV (Ki MLV) and Ki MSV (Mo MLV) were obtained from supernatant fluids of the NRK 58967 clone and C 127 cells respectively (16).
   The infection with viruses, the tumor induction with transformed
cells, the measurements of thyroglobulin secretion and iodide uptake
have been described elsewhere (8).
   The reverse transcriptase assay and the soft agar colony assay were
also performed according to published procedures (4, 12).
   Labeling of intracellular proteins with ^{35}S-Methionine and immunoprecipitation of labeled proteins with a p 21 anti-serum were performed
according to the methods described by Shih et al. (16).

                              RESULTS

   T-79 and FRT-L cells are well differentiated epithelial thyroid cells;
they show typical signs of thyroidal differentiated functions such as
iodide uptake, thyroglobulin synthesis and secretion and membrane binding of the specific thyroid stimulating hormone (TSH) (2). They
are also dependent for optimal growth on a mixture of six factors (TSH,
insulin, hydrocortisol, transferrin, somatostatin and the trypeptide
glycil-hystidil-lysine).
   FRT cells are undifferentiated since they do not trap iodide from the

medium, nor synthetize thyroglobulin. They are also not dependent for growth in vitro on the mixture of six growth factors (1), however they show TSH membrane binding and morphologically resemble epithelial cells in culture (see Table 1).

We have infected all these epithelial cells with the Ki MSV (KiMLV) strain of the Kirsten sarcoma virus and the FRT-L cells also with the Ki MSV (Mo MLV) strain of Ki MSV at various multiplicities of infection. Moreover, we infected both FRT and FRT-L cells with the leukemogenic helpers (either Ki MLV or Mo MLV) alone, in order to clarify whether these viruses posses any ability to derange the normal cellular differentiation pathway.

Evidences that infection and cellular transformation of the cell lines had taken place is presented in Table 2.

All cell lines infected with Ki MSV (Ki MLV) and Ki MSV (Mo MLV) began to release, into the culture medium, reverse transcriptase containing particles and virus capable of transforming fibroblasts in culture (FFU). The strongest evidence of transformation is represented by the ability of the infected cells to grow in a semi-solid medium (as measured by the soft agar colony assay) and by the ability to induce tumors when injected subcutaneously into syngeneic animals (all the tumors induced show the typical features of carcinomas).

Moreover, some of the transformed cell lines have also been tested for the presence of the p 21 protein, which is believed to represent the src gene product of the Ki MSV (16). Two cell lines, the FRT-L KiKi and the FRT-L KiMol, have been found to synthetize considerable amounts of this protein (see Table 2).

Cells infected by Ki MLV alone behave, as expected , in a quite different manner in that they do not show any of the transformation markers and their supernatant fluid, though positive for the reverse transcriptase assay, is not capable of transforming fibroblasts in culture.

In Table 2 are also reported the results obtained with two tumor lines (FRT Tumor and T-79 Tumor) obtained by cultivating in vitro trypsinized explants from two tumors induced into syngeneic animals by FRT cells transformed by Ki MSV (Ki MLV) (FRT KiKi) (8) and by T-79 cells transformed by Ki MSV (Ki MLV)(T-79 KiKi) (9).

These two lines behave like the parental lines as far as the transformation markers are concerned, but are unable to release virus into the culture medium as demonstrated either by the reverse transcriptase assay or by production of foci of transformation in fibroblasts.

Since T-79 and FRT-L are well differentiated cells, we have also investigated the effects of transformation on the expression of the differentiated phenotype after infection with both Ki MSV (Ki MLV) and Ki MSV (Mo MLV). The results of such studies are summarized in Table 2.

Virus transformation causes in these systems a complete loss of all the differentiation markers, such as thyroglobulin secretion, iodide

TABLE 2. Transformation of epithelial differentiated and undifferentiated rat thyroid cells by various strains of the Kirsten sarcoma virus

Cell line	Type of virus used	Culture medium (Coon's modified Ham F-12)	Virus production		Transformation markers		P 21 Src	Differentiation markers		
			RT[a]	FFU[b]	growth in soft agar	carcinoma[c] induction		TG[d] secretion	iodide uptake	sensitivity to "6H"
FRT-KiKi	KiMSV(KiMLV)	+5% c.s.	+	+	+	+	N.T.	−	−	−
FRT-Tumor	FRT-KiKi (From an FRT-KiKi induced tumor)	+5% c.s.	−	−	+	+	?	−	−	−
FRT-Fibro KiKi	KiMSV(KiMLV)	+5%c.s.	+	+	+	+	N.T.	−	−	−
T-79KiKi	KiMSV(KiMLV)	+0.5% c.s.	+	+	+	+	N.T.	−	−	−
T-79Tumor	KiKi induced (From a T-79 tumor)	+0.5% c.s.	−	−	+	+	?	−	−	−
FRT-LKiKi	KiMSV(KiMLV)	+5% c.s.	+	+	+	+	++	−	−	−
FRT-LKiMLV	KiMLV	+0.5 c.s. + 6H	+	−	−	−	N.T.	+	+	+
FRT-LKiMol	KiMSV(MoMLV)	+5% c.s.	+	+	+	+	+++	−	−	−

[a] Reverse transcriptase assay (pMol ^{3}H dTTP incorporated / 10^6 cells)
[b] Focus forming units
[c] Assayed by transplanting 2×10^6 cells into syngeneic rats
[d] Thyroglobulin

uptake and the dependence on the six factors for an optimal growth
in vitro.

In Fig. 1A is presented, as an example, a growth curve of FRT-L
transformed by Ki MSV (Mo MLV) showing a clear loss of growth dependence on the six factors. Similar results were obtained with the two
tumor lines. On the contrary FRT-L do not seem to have been altered
from the differentiated point of view, after the infection with Ki MLV
alone. These cells (FRT-L Ki MLV) in fact, as shown in Table 2, still
secrete thyroglobulin and trap iodide from the culture medium.
Moreover as presented in Fig 1B, they retain a total growth dependence
on the six factors, like the normal FRT-L cells do.

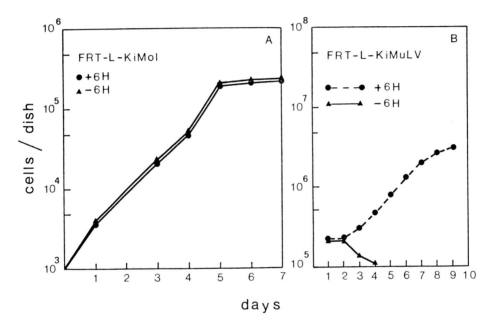

FIG. 1., Growth curves of FRT-L KiMol and FRT-L KiMLV in the presence
and in the absence of the six growth factors (see Materials
and Methods).

This result clearly rules out the possibility that the leukemic
genome plays a role in the differentiation block induced by transformation with KiMSV (Ki MLV).

DISCUSSION

This paper describes the establishment of a new system of cell transformation in vitro by retroviruses, i.e. epithelial thyroid cells
transformed by the Kirsten murine sarcoma virus. Some of the results
obtained with this newly developed system have already been described

(8, 9). In our opinion the system described here lends itsels to interesting type of analysis. The system consists of epithelial cells of endodermal origin transformed by a sarcoma virus. This shows the ability of Ki MSV to transform in vitro also cells which are not of mesenchimal origin. This observation is important in view of the fact that epithelial cancer accounts for the great majority of tumoral growths in humans.

The system described allows to study the relationships between neoplastic transformation and the expression of a normal differentiated phenotype. Several efforts have been performed recently, aimed to develop new in vitro models characterized by having the greatest resemblance to physiological conditions. The cell lines used in the present report are higly differentiated and continue to express in vitro the typical differentiated features of thyroid tissue. The markers of differen tiation are easily detectable and are of high significancy in that iodide uptake and thyroglobulin secretion both play a critical role in the physiological activity of the thyroid gland in vivo . The results so far obtained have demonstrated clearly that:

1. The Ki MSV transformation interferes with the pattern of differentiation by blocking the expression of at least two of the differentiated functions of the thyroid cells in culture;

2. The Ki MSV transformation of undifferentiated FRT cells does not modify the differentiation patterns of these cells which remain undifferentiated after transformation;

3. The helper viruses, such as Ki MLV alone, are unable to modify the pattern of differentiation of the differentiated cells, then confirming that the block in differentiation is a specific feature of the Ki MSV genome.

Further studies are in progress in our laboratory to investigate the relationships between the expression of the p 21 src gene product and the expression of differentiated phenotype by taking advantages of molecularly cloned fragments of the Ki MSV genome (18), molecularly cloned rat thyroglobulin gene (6) and newly developed system of transformation of FRT-L cells by a temperature sensitive mutant of the Ki MSV.

REFERENCES

1. Ambesi-Impiombato,F.S. and Coon,M.G. (1979), Int. Rev. Cytol. Suppl., 10:163-171.
2. Ambesi-Impiombato,F.S.,Parks,L.A.M. and Coon,M.G. (1980), Proc. Natl.Acad. Sci. U.S.A., 77:3455-3459.
3. Beug,H.,Von Kirchbaum,A.,Doderlein,G.,Coscience,J.F. and Graf,T., (1979), Cell, 18:375-390.
4. Colletta,G.,Di Fiore,P.P.,Ferrentino,M.,Pietropaolo,C.,Turco,M.C. and Vecchio,G., (1980), Cancer Res., 40:3369-3373.

5. Coon,M.G. and Weiss,M.C., (1969), Proc. Natl. Acad. Sci. U.S.A., 62:852-859.

6. Di Lauro,R.,Obici,S.,Verde,P.,Tramontano,D.,Avvedimento,E.V., (1981) presented at the annual European Thyroid Association meeting, Lucca Italy, September 1981.

7. Easton,T. and Reich,E., (1972), J. Biol. Chem., 247:6420-6431.

8. Fusco,A.,Pinto,A.,Ambesi-Impiombato,F.S.,Vecchio,G. and Tsuchida,N., (1981), Int. J. Cancer, in press.

9. Fusco,A.,Pinto,A.,Tramontano,D.,Tajana,G.,Vecchio,G., and Tsuchida,N., submitted.

10. Gazzolo,L.,Moscovici,C.,Moscovici,M.G. and Samarut,J., (1979), Cell, 16:627-638.

11. Holtzer,H.,Bichel,J.,Yeoh,G.,Meganathan,R. and Kaji, A., (1975), Proc. Natl. Acad. Sci. U.S.A., 72:4051-4055.

12. Mac Pherson,I. and Montaignier,L., (1964), Virology , 23:291-294.

13. Pacifici,M.,Boettiger,D.,Roby,K. and Holtzer,H., (1977), Cell 11:891-899.

14. Raschke,W.C.,Ralph,P.,Watson,J.,Sklar,M. and Coon,H., (1975), J. Natl. Cancer Inst., 54:1249-1253.

15. Rosemberg,M.,Baltimore,D. and Scher,E.D., (1975), Proc. Natl. Acad. Sci. U.S.A., 72:1932-1936.

16. Shih,T.J.,Weeks,O.M.,Young,H.A. and Scolnick,E.M., (1980), J. of Virology, 31:546-556.

17. Sklar,M.D.,White,W.J. and Rowe,W.P., (1974), Proc. Natl. Acad. Sci. U.S.A., 71:4077-4081.

18. Tsuchida,N. and Uesugi,S., (1981), J. of Virology, in press.

ACKNOWLEDGMENTS

This work was supported by C.N.R. contract N°80.00650.84 of the Progetto finalizzato virus and in part by the Progetto finalizzato controllo della crescita neoplastica.

Expression of Differentiated Functions in Cancer Cells, edited by R. F. Revoltella et al., Raven Press, New York © 1982.

Common Mode of Action of Different Inducers of FL Cell Differentiation

L. Harel, C. Blat, *F. Lacour, **T. Huyn, and **C. Friend

*Institut de Recherches Scientifiques sur le Cancer, Laboratoire de Dynamique Cellulaire, B. P. N. 8, 94082 Villejuif, France; *Institut Gustave Roussy, C.N.R.S., Laboratoire d'Immunologie, 94800 Villejuif, France; **Mollie B. Roth Laboratory, Centre for Experimental Cell Biology, Mount Sinai School of Medicine, City University of New York, New York, New York 10029*

We have shown that the aminonucleoside of puromycin (AMS), an analogue of adenoside, is a potent inducer of Friend erythroleukemic (FL) cell differentiation, and that the induction of differentiation by AMS is inhibited by the addition of inosine or adenosine to the medium (1).

The mechanism of action of the various compounds that stimulate FL cells to express a program of differentiation remains unclear (2). It was reported that, in other cell lines, AMS inhibits ribosomal RNA synthesis (3,4) and decreases the RNA content of heteroploid cells (5), with this effect being prevented by addition of inosine to the medium. To gain further understanding of the mechanism of FL cell differentiation, it was of interest to study the mode of action of AMS and inosine on these cells.

By labelling the cells with ^{3}H uridine or ^{32}P, we verified that AMS, at the concentration (20 nMoles/ml) which induces 80 to 90% differentiation, inhibits RNA synthesis in these cells as it does in other cell lines (6).

When ^{14}C inosine was added to the medium, most of the radioactivity was incorporated, as expected, in ATP, GTP and RNA of the cells. The synthesis of these molecules was decreased in AMS treated cells compared to the controls. However, RNA synthesis from labelled added inosine was not as inhibited as RNA synthesis in AMS treated cells in the absence of inosine (6).

We next investigated the effect of the addition of inosine to the medium (at the concentration of 7.5 nMole/ml which prevents AMS induced differentiation) on the content of proteins, ATP, GTP and RNA of the cultures at different times after seeding the cells.

The rate of cell growth and the synthesis and accumulation of pro-

tein in cells treated with AMS or AMS + inosine were decreased as
compared with those in control cells. However, the inhibitions of protein synthesis and cell growth were similar, so the protein content per
cell was not appreciably changed in AMS and AMS + ionosine treated
cells compared to the untreated controls.

In the presence of AMS, the ATP/protein ratio and the GTP/protein
ratio were slightly modified, while the synthesis and accumulation
of RNA was more inhibited than the synthesis and accumulation of proteins. Thus, the RNA/protein ratio (Table 1) was decreased as early
as 24 hours after the beginning of treatment with AMS. Addition of inosine to AMS was able to overcome much of the inhibitory effect of AMS
on RNA accumulation and increase the RNA/protein ratio, which approached the level of untreated controls. These results point out a correlation between the decrease in RNA/protein ratio and the differentiation of FL cells.

We do not know the mode of action of the different inducers of FL
cell differentiation. However, it was reported (7, 8) that Me_2SO decreases the RNA and protein synthesis in these cells.

It was therefore, of interest to verify whether Me_2SO and sodium
butyrate, another potent inducer of differentiation also changed, the
RNA/protein ratio in FL cells during the precommitment time. Table
2 shows the results. With each of the three inducers, the RNA/protein
ratio was decreased compared to the untreated control and the cells
continued to multiply with a RNA content (and probably a ribosome
content) of about 60% of the untreated control cells.

TABLE 1. μ RNA/mg Protein in Cells at Different Times

Treatment of the cells	24 h.	48 h.	72 h.
No treatment	167	143	134
+ AMS	128	100	88
% difference	-23	-30	-34
+ AMS+Inosine	134	123	130
% difference	-14	-13	- 3

The cells were grown in the absence or presence of AMS (5 μg/ml)
or of AMS (5 μg/ml) with inosine (20 μg/ml). At the times indicated,
the content of protein and RNA were determined. The results are the
means between two experiments and four determinations.

TABLE 2. u RNA/mg protein in cells at different times

Treatment of the cells	24 h.	48 h.	72 h.
No treatment	141	135 ± 1	109 ± 1
+ Me$_2$SO	79 ± 3	85 ± 5	70 ± 5
% difference	- 44	- 37	- 36
+ Butyrate	75 ± 3	80 ± 5	63 ± 2
% difference	- 47	- 41	-42
+ AMS	94 ± 6	78 ± 8	60 ± 2
% difference	- 24	- 42	- 44

At different times after seeding the cells in the absence of the inducer or in the presence of AMS (20 uM), Me$_2$SO (2%) or butyrate
(2 mM), the RNA/protein ratio of the cells was determined. The
percentage of benzidine-positive cells scored at 96 hr in the cultures treated with AMS, Me$_2$SO, or sodium butyrate was 80%, 77% and
70%, respectively, as compared to 4% in the control cultures.

In conclusion, our results suggest that an inhibition of RNA synthesis which is not coordinated with a parallel inhibition of protein synthesis is the event required for FL cell differentiation. This hypothesis is
also supported by the report that actinomycin D, a well-known inhibitor of ribosomal RNA synthesis, is also an inducer of FL cell differentiation (9).

A non-coordinated inhibition of RNA and protein synthesis has also
been observed during myoblast differentiation (10), which the 45 S
precursor rRNA being inhibited, although the rate of synthesis of ribosomal proteins remains the same.

REFERENCES

1. Lacour, F., Harel, L., Friend, C., Huyn, T.N. and Holland, J. (1980)
   Proc. Nat. Acad. Sci. U.S.A.; 77, 2740-2742
2. Friend, C. (1980) :In: Differentiation and Neoplasia, edited by McKinnell, R.G., DiBernardino, M.A., Glumenfeld, M. and Bergan, R.D.,
   pp. 202-210
3. Farnham, A.E., and Dubin, D.T. (1965):J. Mol. Biol. , 14:55-62
4. Studzinski, G.P., and Ellem K.A.O. (1966):J. Cell. Biol., 29:411-421
5. Studzinski, G.P., and Ellem , K.A.O. (1968):Cancer Research:28, 1773
   -1782

6. Harel, L., Blat, C., Lacour, F. and Friend, C. (1981):Proc.Nat.Acad. Sci.U.S.A., 78:3882-3886

7. Sherton, C.C., and Kabat, D. (1976):Dev. Biol., 48:118-131

8. Harel, L., Lacour, F., Friend, C., Dubin, P., and Semmel, M. (1979): J.Cell.Physiol. , 101:25-32

9. Terada, M., Epner, E., Nudel, U., Salomon, J., Fibach, R., Rifkind, R.A., and Marks, P.A. (1978):Proc.Nat.Acad.Sci.U.S.A. , 75:2795-2799

10. Krauter, K.S., Soeiro, R., Nadal-Ginard, B. (1980):J.Mol.Biol., 142: 145-159

Subject Index